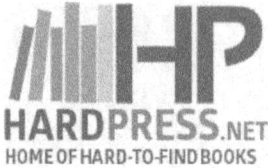

HARDPRESS.NET
HOME OF HARD-TO-FIND BOOKS

Health at Home, or Hall's Family Doctor :
Showing How to Invigorate and Preserve Health,
Prolong Life, Cure Diseases, Understand the
Physical Conditions of Maternity, and the Proper
Management of Infants ...
by William Whitty Hall

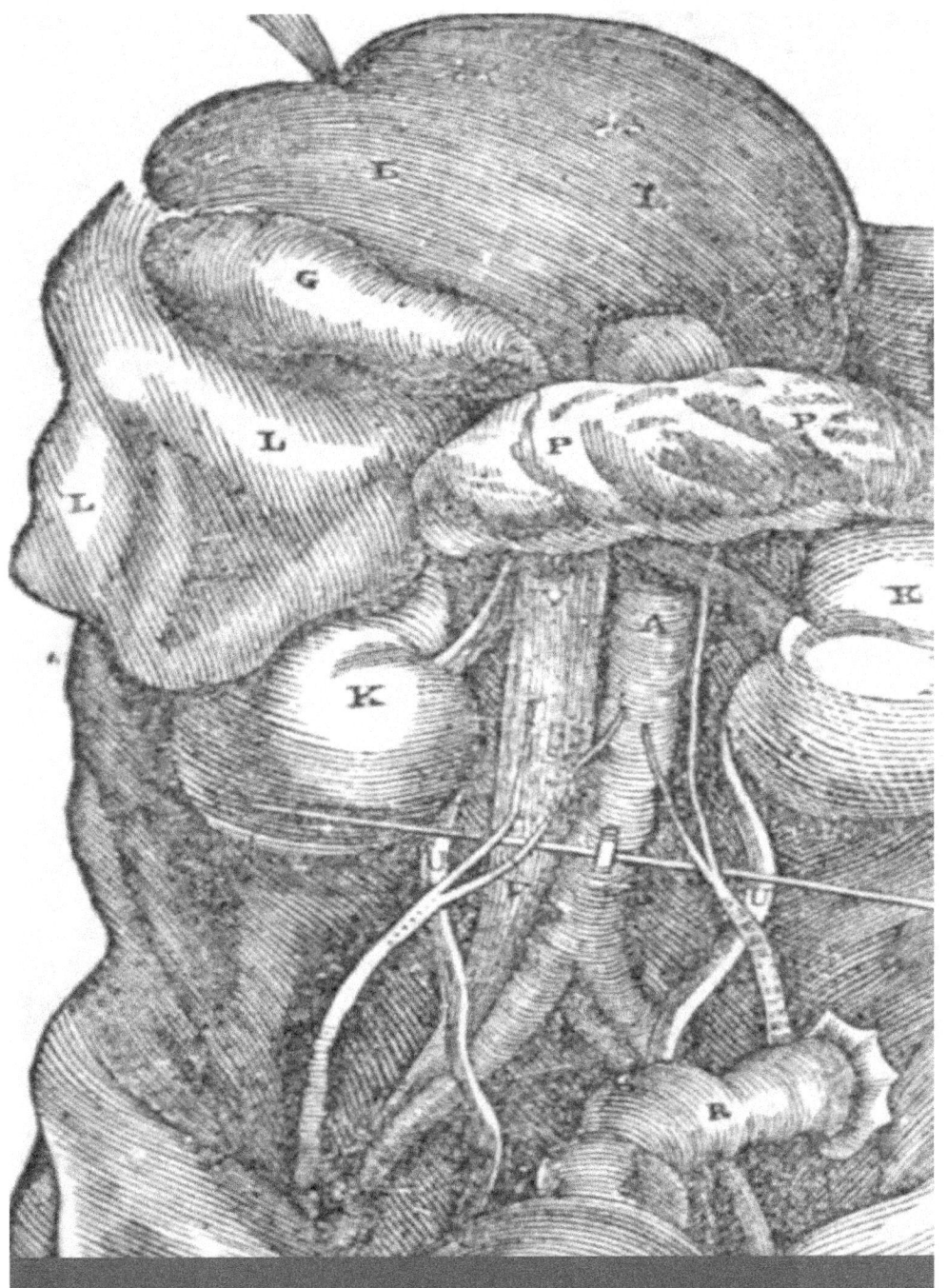

Health at home, or Hall's family doctor : showing how to ...

W W Hall

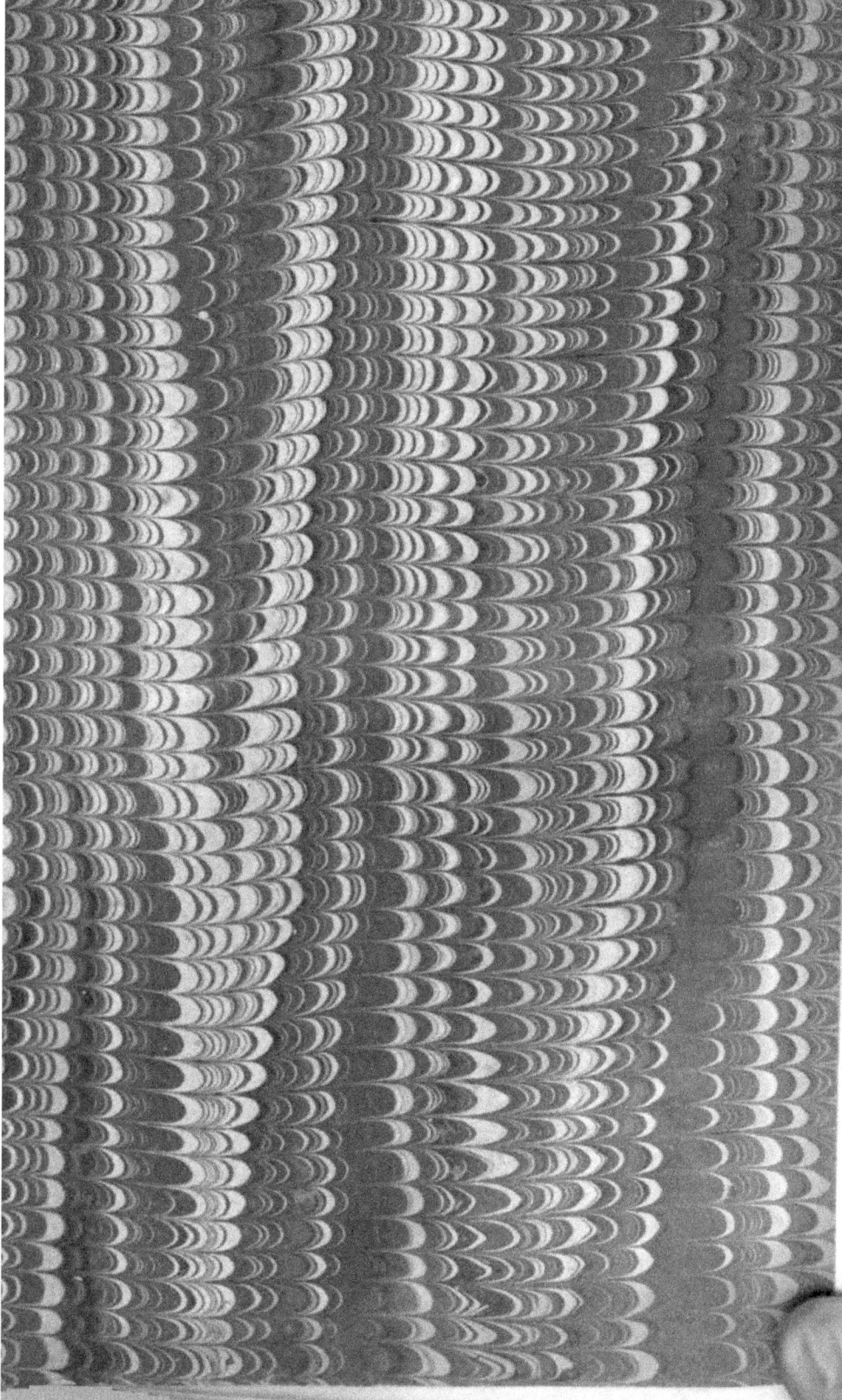

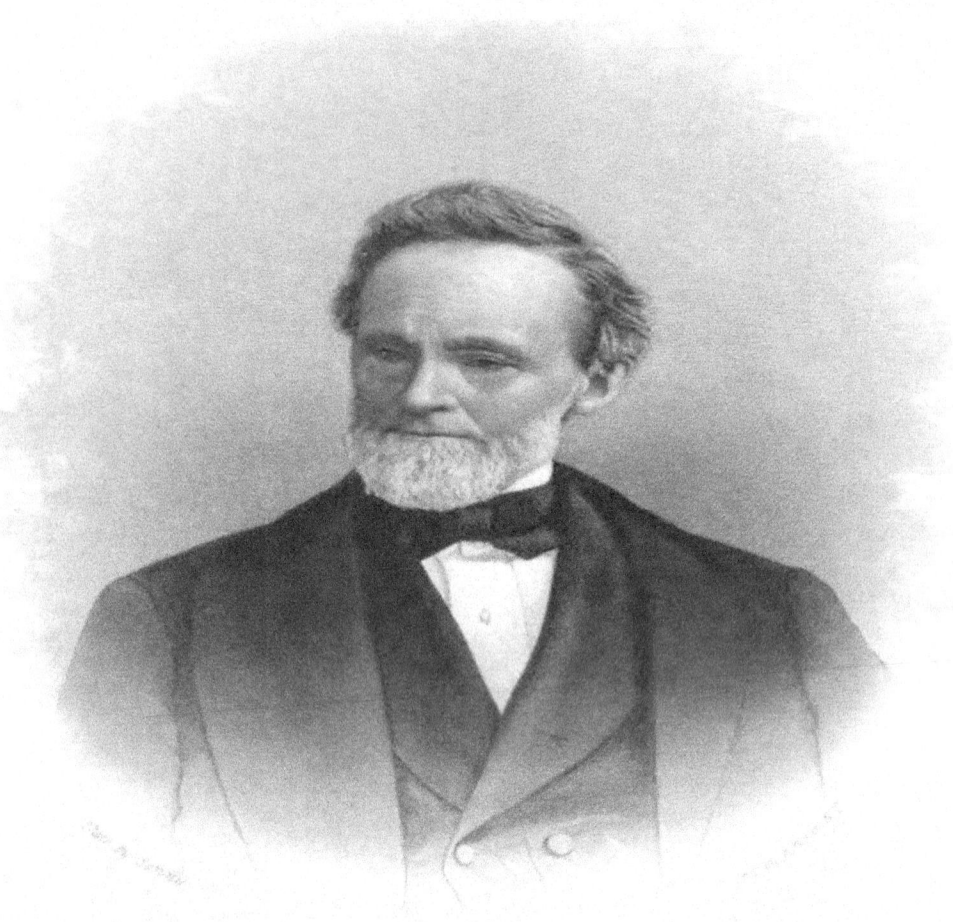

Very Truly Yours
W. W. Hall

EDITOR OF HALL'S JOURNAL OF HEALTH

HEALTH AT HOME,

OR

HALL'S

FAMILY DOCTOR:

SHOWING HOW TO INVIGORATE AND PRESERVE HEALTH, PROLONG LIFE, CURE
DISEASES, UNDERSTAND THE PHYSICAL CONDITIONS OF MATERNITY, AND
THE PROPER MANAGEMENT OF INFANTS, AND DISCUSSING THE
ENTIRE PHYSICAL WELL-BEING OF MAN, WITH A VERY
LARGE COLLECTION OF THE LATEST AND MOST
VALUABLE MEDICAL PRESCRIPTIONS.

BY

W. W. HALL, A.M., M.D.,

EDITOR OF HALL'S "JOURNAL OF HEALTH," AUTHOR OF "HEALTH BY GOOD LIVING," "SLEEP," "BRONCHITIS
AND KINDRED DISEASES," ETC., ETC.

JAS. BETTS & COMPANY,

HARTFORD, CONN., CINCINNATI, OHIO, AND CHICAGO, ILLS.
1873.

PREFACE.

THE bite of an insect, a midnight sickness, an accidental poisoning, have many times proved fatal while the messenger was sent for a physician; when on the kitchen-hearth, in the ice-box, the store-room, the dairy, the hen's nest, the big road, and the spring branch there were remedies more available for cure than the surgeon's knife or the physician's skill; more powerful for good than any drug ever taken from the shelf of the apothecary; but no one knew it, and the patient died. A main object of this book is to give such information as will enable the most unlettered reader to avail himself promptly of those means for saving health and life, which Nature and Providence have thrown broadcast around him in wonderful profusion.

Entered according to Act of Congress, in the year 1872, by
W. W. HALL, M.D.,
In the office of the Librarian of Congress, at Washington.

CONTENTS.

INTRODUCTION.

THE sting of a wasp or bee or yellow-jacket has often proved fatal within five minutes, when the prompt application of hartshorn to the wound, and a few drops swallowed with water, would have antagonized the poison and saved the life; but in a dozen houses in the country there might not be found a drop; look under the head of " bites and stings," and it will be seen that a bit of soap or a handful of wood-ashes stirred in a glass of water makes a hartshorn substitute in half a minute; or if there be not a wood fire in a mile, a handful of moist earth grabbed from the first mud puddle or pond or brooklet's edge contains hartshorn and other curative elements, which, if applied in the shape of a poultice, gives instant relief to the sufferer.

Towards midnight, after the first sleep, the hateful croup usually fixes its dreadful fangs on the unconscious child. What avails it in the country, miles away from a physician or a drug store, that this, that, or the other remedy is " good for " the disease, when neither physician nor remedy could be had for hours; and all this while the mother is in agony, and the infant sufferer clutches its throat for breath! But turn to the proper heading in the book, and it will be seen that no medicine known is so potent for cure as a boiling tea-kettle and a bit of flannel; or as a lump of ice or snow, with a handful of salt, applied to the throat in a silken pad or bag.

The terrible cramp colic, so often fatal before the dawn, can be relieved within an hour with a milk emetic, and flannels wrung in boiling water, applied to the stomach.

Has a child or other member of the household swallowed a rank poison? Turn to the article, and it will be seen in an instant that the number of poisons and their antidotes are legion; yet all are comprised in two divisions,—those which cause no pain whatever, and those which occasion fearful sufferings in the throat; that in both cases there are two things to be done: to dilute the poison, and get it all out of the stomach the earliest moment possible ; the painful kind is to be met with drinking warm milk or tepid or even cold water, until the stomach can hold no more, then a feather or finger in the throat will cause instant and copious vomiting ; if there is no pain, then a more speedy method is to stir a tablespoonful each of salt and mustard in half a glass of water ; the instant it reaches the stomach it begins to return, bringing everything else with it ; and in either case, lest some of the poison might be left, go to the hen's nest, take a fresh egg or two or more, and swallow the whites ; or if there is not a cow or a hen in fifty miles, do without them ; use warm water for the milk, and a tablespoonful of flour stirred in half a glass of water, and drink down rapidly ; it is a good substitute for the albumen of the egg.

It is in such ways an effort is made to instruct the people how to avail themselves of Nature's remedies for the cure of disease, when neither medicines nor physicians are possible of securement ; as in the accidents and burnings and maimings in connection with railroad travelling and disasters at sea.

The truth is, with some little understanding of the nature of disease, and some little genius for shifts and devices, half the ordinary ailments of humanity, in cases where at all curable by any human instrumentalities, can be successfully treated on a rock in the sea, on an iceberg at the poles, if there is fire, fresh air, and water.

To be sure, it is easier to get rid of our ailments by taking a sugar-coated pill, or some rank poison diluted and concealed in a glass of whiskey toddy ; and there is many a man, who, rather than be bothered with a bath or a sweat, or a wet pack, would greatly prefer swallowing the bolus of an Allopath, although it were as big as a pigeon's egg, or toy with the pin-head pellets of Homœopathy ; hence the book is so arranged as to give a man his choice of remedies and modes of cure. But the aim in all cases is to set before the reader certain cardinal points.

First, the nature of the disease. Second, the remedy proposed. Third, how that remedy accomplishes the object, that the patient may know whether the means used are doing what is wanted, by the manifestations they are making, and if not, and in order to lose not a moment unnecessarily, he may turn his attention to some other remedy acting in a like manner, or he may adopt some expedient presented to his own mind, which might produce the desired effect ; indeed, it is in this way that some of the most valuable methods of cure ever devised have in a sense been accidentally fallen upon by the necessities of some extraordinary emergency, wherein the most proper thing to be employed was not at hand. In these ways it is hoped the book will be more serviceable to the public at large than any of its predecessors.

There is a single idea in the article on " Congestion " which will at once clear from the mind at least one-half of the

MYSTERY OF MEDICINE,

and show how it is possible for one remedy to cure a hundred diseases. A house may be set on fire in many different ways ; the effect of the fire is one, destruction ; the remedy is one, water. Congestion may be brought about in a hundred different ways, in a hundred different parts of the body, giving rise to a hundred different diseases or symptoms ; but the cause is one, congestion. The one thing to be done is the removal of that congestion ; whatever does that will cure, if applied in time, whether it be by general hygienic measures, or by pure air, cleanliness, exercise, and rest, or by hydropathic means, or the surer and more direct allopathic instrumentalities, as, for example, by the use of the " Liver Pill," which all are instructed how to make, and which is destined to save multituds.

The uninformed reader will be surprised to learn the curative virtues of some of the most familiar things in any common household ; and surely it is the duty of all, especially of those who live in out-of-the-way places, to acquaint themselves with at least some of these, for in many instances it would be to the saving of human life.

Take, for example, the varied uses of a good article of hog's lard. Two or three folds of woollen flannel dipped in hot hog's lard will most promptly remove the pain or swelling from the bite of hornet, wasp, or bee. 2. Warm, fresh, unsalted hog's lard is one of the very best things to dislodge any live insect from the ear. 3. A quarter of a pint of warmed lard drank every fifteen minutes before breakfast, will sometimes dislodge a tape-worm, head and all. 4. Hog's lard rubbed well into a swollen limb, with the hand, patiently, often removes the swelling and any deep-seated pains attending them.   5. Half a pint of hog's lard, taken on three successive mornings, has relieved cases of the most obstinate and unmanageable constipation, even when croton oil and injections had failed.   6. If the skin, in scarlatina, is daily well rubbed with hog's lard or bacon rind for ten days, it will allay the heat of the skin, remove the soreness of the throat, lessen the risk of dropsy, and prevent the spreading of the disease, by confining to the body those small solid particles, which, otherwise escaping from the skin, would be breathed into the lungs of others and swallowed into their stomachs, and thus infect the blood.   7. The intolerable itching which attends erysipelas is mitigated and entirely controlled by persistent inunctions with hog's lard.   8. Persons who work in woollen factories, where the material has to receive hog's lard on it before it can be worked up, are remarkably exempt from consumptive disease, while those who live in cotton factories are specially liable to it.   9. Inunctions daily and abundantly of the parts of the skin infected with itch will cure almost any ordinary case.   10. The night sweats of consumption are often modified and sometimes removed by rubbing hog's lard into the skin every night, if sleeping in the same woollen nightshirt, which becomes impregnated with the oil.   11. There is no remedy which affords more instantaneous relief from the effect of swallowing acrid poisons than drinking hog's lard, which not only soothes the scalding heat in the throat, but dilutes the poison in the stomach, and by continuing to drink it until the stomach is full, a feather in the throat will bring it all up, poison and all.   12. And how could you make doughnuts without hog's lard ? Here, then, are a dozen most valuable remedial agencies found in the varied applications of hog's lard.   Surely it is well to know these things, and any book must be valuable, a main object of which is to utilize things which are most commonly at hand, with a view to alleviate pain, restore health, and save life.

A young man in a farmer's family accidentally dropped an open penknife, which struck the arm of a little girl playing on the floor.   The blood flowed alarmingly fast ; the father mounted a horse, and rode at full speed for the nearest physician, who lived five miles away, to find that he had started an hour before to go ten miles in an opposite direction, to visit a patient who was in a dangerous condition, and was not expected to return until next morning.   A message was left, and in the most dreadful apprehension and suspense the father turned his face homeward. Meanwhile the little child had bled to death ; the mother was thrown into convulsions, and expired. On learning the facts as he entered the house at nightfall, the father went through into the garden, threw himself into a well, and was drowned.

If a common handkerchief had been tied loosely about the arm, above the wounded artery, a stick run through between the handkerchief and the skin, and twisted round tightly, the bleeding would have been stopped in sixty seconds, and the child saved ; but nobody in the house knew this.

It is to provide families and individuals with such knowledge as will enable them to act efficiently under the emergencies of sickness or accident, that this book is written, and also for the wiser few who, from a sense of duty and intelligent principle, make it a point to inform themselves of the best means of preserving health ; and to that other class, less fortunate, but larger by infinity, who by ignorance or carelessness have lost that health.

To the former, this book will be an encouragement and a counsellor. To the latter, a safe guide. But both are earnestly advised, as a means of comprehending the whole scope of this volume, to read and re-read, with a patient and wise care, the articles

ON CONGESTION, AND PRINCIPLES OF MEDICAL PRACTICE,

which may give the mind such a clear idea of the essential nature of disease, of its oneness, of the value of medicine when judiciously administered, and of the simplicity of its operation, that its practice will ever after be considered, not a guess-work, not a feeling in the dark, not an incomprehensible agency, but a power, acting on fixed principles in nature with encouraging frequency, with a gratifying efficiency, and a gladsome result.

It is intended, as far as practicable, to give the one or two distinctive symptoms of each disease, to enable the reader to clearly ascertain what it is, leaving out the many symptoms which, although of more or less importance, are yet common to a variety of ailments ; hence their enumeration would but hinder the mind in coming to a satisfactory decision as to the real nature of the sickness, instead of helping to that result ; while the time lost in coming to a conclusion, and the hesitancy involved in employing remedies, with a feeling of uncertainty about their applicability, may occasion a loss of time and opportunity which in some cases would be fatal to the patient.

The general plan of the book is to enable the person who consults it to decide just what is the matter, what is the nature of the disease, what are the most appropriate remedies at hand, how they are intended to act, and in what way they are expected to yield desirable results.

The reader is first instructed as to the best means of relieving and curing his ailments without medicine; if prompt and favorable results do not follow, then to employ such as the

OLD-SCHOOL ALLOPATHIC PHYSICIANS

have found to be most available in the course of centuries in the hands of eminent educated men; at the same time, in several cases of common diseases, the remedies employed by those who favor the water-cure treatment are named, for there can be no doubt that the judicious employment of cold and warm water in the treatment of disease is very efficacious. The principles of

HYDROPATHISTS

in reference to cleanliness, dress, air, exercise, sunshine, the use of fruits, of coarse bread made of the material of the whole grain, whether of wheat, corn, rye, or oats, merit the approbation of intelligent men; but the Old School practitioners have always taught these things. There is virtue also in

HOMŒOPATHY.

Hence reference is made in some cases to their practice, for Allopathic physicians in all ages have made it an invariable rule to use any means and any remedies which, after a fair experiment, have been found to be uniformly successful; but, to be adopted, they must stand the test of repeated trials in every variety of circumstances and for a series of years; on the other hand, they are slow to discard a valuable remedy, and, in spite of an occasional failure, continue to use it with confidence.

THE GREAT REMEDY.

In nearly all forms of sickness, except cholera, diarrhœa, and dysentery, relief is obtained, and the foundation for a permanent cure is laid, by securing a full and free evacuation of the bowels, which may be done in half an hour by the administration of an enema of milk-warm water, or within two hours by giving a table-spoonful or two of Epsom salts or castor-oil. A more deep-search-ing, efficient, and certain relief is obtained by the purgative pills. But if the patient is not pressed for time, desires to avoid medicine, and prefers to get well with the least shock to the system, and with the greatest promise of permanency, it is unquestionably safe to adopt the following course :—

First, Give the whole skin a thorough washing with white soap and warm water.

Second, Secure a well-ventilated room, into the windows of which the sun shines most of the day.

Third, Eat nothing whatever from noon until next morning, drinking meanwhile as much cold water or hot tea as may be agreeable.

Fourth, Eat thrice a day, at not less than five hours interval,— nothing whatever between,—as much as is wanted of fresh butter, cold, coarse bread, berries, fruits, melons, tomatoes, and boiled rice ; not over three articles at the same meal, and no fluids within half an hour.

Fruits, berries, and melons are most efficient remedies when in their natural state, fresh, ripe, and perfect ; if preserved, those in glass vessels are safest.

If the principles of treatment just named were promptly carried out in the common forms of sickness, half the ailings of humanity would be cured, if curable by any means ; but the masses procras-tinate, and seem to prefer to eat, and physic, and die ; for such of those who, for want of means, or from distance, cannot promptly obtain the aid of an educated medical practitioner, this book has been written.

PRELIMINARIES.

No regular systematic order is pursued in the treatment of the various subjects discussed in these pages, for this is often tedious to the reader; besides, if two diseases, nearly allied, such as two different kinds of fever, are brought side by side, the unprofessional student would, in reading the two, be likely to become confused, and find himself unable to decide satisfactorily what the ailment under investigation was.

Nor has reference been made to differences of opinion among educated physicians as to special points of theory and practice, for these differences are often mere shades not more diverse than

"Tweedle dum and tweedle dee."

Then again, such discussions take up time and space unnecessarily, will inevitably unsettle the mind of the common reader, and after all, in very many cases of such diversity, there exists no difference whatever in the principles of treatment; most generally it is in the vigor of its application—in giving a little more or less of the same medicine.

One advantage of this line of procedure is, that in studying the nature of a particular disease, the mind has a single object in view, hence can the more readily give its undivided attention to a thorough investigation, and will thus be better able to arrive at a proper comprehension of its real character, its true nature, and its actual requirements. There is another incalculable advantage in this promiscuous discussion of subjects: many things can be treated which would come under no particular heading, and yet are of the very first importance in the promotion of the comfort, convenience, health, and well-being of families remote from cities and large towns, and also from reliable sources of information. For example, in the article on Accidents reference is made to the sufferings, torture, and terrible deaths by burning, from the explosion of kerosene lamps; occasion is there taken to explain how any person of very common intelligence might ascertain with absolute certainty whether the specimen of kerosene in the house could explode by any possibility. Look, again, at the article on

SHAVING,

which could not readily be brought under the heading of any disease or subject pertaining to health, and yet the information imparted is of prime importance to every man who shaves, for it not only tells how to manage the razor and strap and brush in a way to afford a comfortable shave, but how, in the easiest manner possible, to guard most effectually against the possibility of becoming a victim to that loathsome affection, the

BARBER'S ITCH.

The manner in which the explanation of medical terms may be used to elevate the style of conversation in reference to health and disease, is worthy of special attention. The reader has only to look to the index for the common name or for the scientific name of any medicine or plant or disease; one refers to the other, and thus a most grateful sense of satisfaction results. For example, very few might know what "mountain tea" was, proclaimed to be a certain cure for cancer, yet under the name of "tea-berry," or of "wintergreen," or of "pipsissewa," it becomes most familiar, and a farmer could, in half an hour's walk, get enough to load a wagon, thus saving him the trouble and expense of writing to the city, or to some more learned person than himself, to know what "mountain tea" was, how much it would cost, and how it could be sent; meanwhile days and weeks and months might elapse, and life itself might pass away.

In reading any page, if a phrase or term is not known, or if more definite or extended information is desired, look to the general index for that term, and on referring to the page a full explanation of it will be given, and so of the medicines advised.

It will be observed that comparatively few medicines are brought to notice, and these are of the most familiar and common kind, easily obtained at an ordinary village drug store. They are thus common because the most of them have been used for ages, and have been found serviceable and reliable by successive generations of distinguished medical men; for example, calomel, blue mass, rhubarb, opium, salts, castor-oil, ipecac, tartar-emetic, aloes, quinine, hartshorn, and a few others are representative medicines of their class; they are the great standbys; with them, comparatively speaking, everything can be done; without them, nothing; not that there are not remedies which, to some extent, and even quite efficiently, might accomplish all they do under favorable circumstances, but it never can be told whether they will or not. Some of them will do what is desired, if fresh and well prepared (this is specially true of all extracts and vegetable remedies); but if not well and carefully prepared, or if old, they are worthless, and that cannot be known until they have been given and their effects vainly looked for. Meanwhile time is lost, even life itself. No intelligent man wants to be trifled with in this way. All the medicines above named will keep many years without any deterioration whatever—are as good at the end of twenty years as on the day they were purchased; hence supplies can be obtained to any extent desired, or carried any distance, and their virtues can be relied on; besides, they occupy but little space, and the whole cost for the use of an ordinary family for half a lifetime need not exceed half a dozen dollars, and above all with the inestimable advantage of certainty of effect.

These medicines, either alone or in combination, if judiciously administered, will accomplish everything that is really necessary and safe, that all other medicines together can: they will purge, they will tonify; they will deplete, and they will build up; they will cool, and they will warm; they will soothe, and they will sweat; they will break down a fever, and disperse a chill; and there is scarcely a pain possible to the human frame which they will not alleviate or wholly remove.

Not that there are not many other valuable medicines which may accomplish similar things; but it is with those named as with a set of tools,—a good workman can make anything, from a box to a bureau, with an axe, a saw, a hammer, and a chisel; he could do it with a whole chest of tools with more elegance, but they are not indispensable. Besides, many medicines have virtues attributed to them which they cannot fairly claim; in truth, there is a fashion in medicine as there is in tailoring,—a running round in the course of years to the same cuts and styles. Some medicines are discarded for an age; then an enthusiastic youth brings them into notice, and they "have a run." The mountain-tea of to-day, for which thousands have been inquiring with so much eagerness, for the cure of cancer, was greatly praised for its virtues seventy years ago, by one of the eminent names in medicine ; but it failed to answer the expectations of subsequent experiments, and for half a century it was of no special importance. Perhaps the only advantage of a great variety of medicines is that some are more readily taken by fastidious patients than others.

Then again, in employing the great mass of remedies on the shelves of the apothecary, they being generally mild in their action and slow in their effects, they have to be taken frequently, several times a day, and for a long time, before decided effects for good manifest themselves; and then it is easy to slide into the most pernicious practice of taking something every day, and this is the actual result in many thousands of families; not a day, by any chance passes, in which some one or more of them is not taking medicine of some kind or another ; brought about in large part by the extensive advertisements of patent medicines, which are asserted, with such positiveness, to cure the worst cases of the ailments to which they apply ; and yet, these families fail to see, with the every-day fact staring them in the face, that the more medicine they take, the more they have to take, and yet, withal, they do not get well.

Another aid to this large consumption of medicine and its frequent use is found in the practice of Homœopathy.   There is no pain or symptom or irregular feeling possible to humanity, no condition of body, no state of mind which is not natural or healthful, for which a remedy is not presented.   Whether the symptoms be fixed or evanescent, whether severe or scarcely perceptible, the globules are resorted to, with the inevitable effect of nurturing the habit of taking something for everything.   If, for example, a man is angry, furious, he must take chamomile.   If there is fright with his anger, aconite is better.   If an anger which makes the cold chills run over him, arsenic is more appropriate.   If he gets mad and keeps mad, that is, becomes sulky, then bryonia is the champion.   But suppose it is an anger which cherishes itself with a silent grief, and the person goes away to some lonely spot and broods over the case by the hour, then ignatia will make him all right.   If, on the other hand, it is a petulant anger where everything done to appease only makes the matter worse, then he must have nux vomica, a virulent poison ; but if he is so fearfully incensed as to threaten insanity, veratrum album is the sure deliverer from the threatened mad-house

JEALOUSY.

If a man is jealous, vehemently so, he must take hyoscyamus; but if to such an extent that he may become insane, then the most appropriate globule is lachesis.

UNFORTUNATE LOVE.

If a young man is in such an uncomfortable position that he cannot get his sweetheart to love him, or the old folks won't let her marry him, and he is about to jump into the river, he should take aur. If he is jealous, and is only happy when he is talking about it to somebody, hyoscyamus will help him. If he is pining away into his grave, then ignatia mara is the cure-all. But if he goes farther, and is about to give up all life, he must speedily resort to repeated doses of lach. If he is rapidly becoming a skeleton, nothing but skin and bone, with night sweats, then he must take acid phos. But if he is really a worthy youth, of high character and unexceptionable morals, goes to church, teaches Sunday-school, and always attends prayer meetings, then he must, without any delay, if the young lady will not love so much worth, take staph. Any one must see that the very best thing for a young man to "take," under such unfortunate circumstances, would be a good switching; if a young lady, an out-and-out spanking. And so the book goes on, to the length of three columns, prescribing for every mental affection, such as anxiety, grief, home-sickness, forebodings, rage, and the like; still there is philosophy in this, since states of the mind often induce bodily disease, and there may be cases where medication is advisable; but if a person takes medicine for every trifling ailment of body or mind, and this medicine has to be taken several times a day, followed up day after day for many days occasionally, the inevitable result is, that a day never passes in which a family does not have to resort to the medicine chest, and the house is turned into a hospital; the conviction that disease is present becomes fixed in the mind, and half of life's joys are eaten out; clouds rest where there should be sunshine, and gloom where gladness.

If medicines have to be taken for mental conditions, they should be such as act promptly, decidedly, and with great efficiency.

Three or four tablespoons of castor oil, as much salts stirred in a glass of warm water, or the loss of a pint of blood from the arm, would, in a single hour or less, revolutionize the whole circulation, and make the entire mental atmosphere as clear as a bell. Still, a far better method than these would be to diminish the amount eaten and drank at least one-half, and spend the time between after breakfast and sundown in vigorous walking or horseback exercise; and still better, in steady, continuous, productive labor. These things, either of them, would inevitably not only wake up a better circulation, but would wear out of the system those humors and poisonous particles which were the cause of these mental and bodily conditions, so antagonistic to health and the enjoyment of life.

There are many cases of mental disturbance which could be happily rectified, not by pellets and potions, not by idle exercise, or by laborious and more productive employment, but by a higher and a really ennobling pastime—simply going out and doing somebody a good deed, or a kind act; a visit to the degraded, to the poor, to the sick, to those in great misfortune, and with a will to alleviate sorrow, to heal and to cheer, combined with the feeling of thankfulness which should arise from this opportunity of comparing the conditions of the helper and the helped, would have the tendency to change for the better the whole mental state of the chief actors in works like these; at other times a short visit to a cheery neighbor—one brimful of frolic and fun—would scarcely fail of highly beneficial results.

But after all, the short sharp rule for those who suffer from mental disturbances; for the nervous, for the highly imaginative class—and it is a large, a very large one—who are prone to magnify the slightest mishaps, trials, and inconveniences to mountainous proportions, is to

BE BUSY,

to be fully employed, to have every hour filled up,—so busy, in fact, as not only to have no idle time, but to be a little pushed; these are the happiest people, these are the healthiest, these are the fortunate and honored ones, who keep the world moving; a prescription this, which, in a vast variety of cases, in a great majority of cases, will be more efficient than any medicine of the apothecary, whether pellet, pill, or potion.

2

PRINCIPLES OF MEDICAL PRACTICE.

All diseased conditions arise from one great cause, an unequal circulation of the blood in the whole body, or in some part of it, at times not larger than the head of a pin : the severest torture of toothache and neuralgia is the result of the deranged condition of the circulation at some one point along the nerve of that part.

On the other hand, good health is the result of a natural, equable distribution of the blood to every portion of the human system.

The highest effect of medical practice in the dispersion of disease and the recovery of health is directed towards equalizing the circulation ; lessening it if too rapid, as in inflammation ; hastening it if too slow, as in shivering or chills, and other forms of suffering. For example, if a part is burning with fever, it is because too much arterial blood is sent to that part, and with too great rapidity ; hence we cut it off by gently bathing it with cold water, which invites the blood to a slower motion, and the man is well, for the fever has disappeared.

If the feet are cold it is because the blood is ceasing to circulate, is losing its life and heat ; we put them in warm water, this heats the blood, invites a more vigorous flow, and soon all is well again.

If you can bring warmth to a cool part, or cool a portion of the system which is in a fevered condition, you cure all the diseases which arise from too much cold or too much warmth.

Another condition of disease is where a very large amount of arterial or red blood is carried to a limited portion of the body, to the eye for example, or to the brain. We call this inflammation of the brain, and the man soon dies, unless relief is obtained ; unless the eye is relieved the sight is soon lost. The most instantaneous method of relief in such cases is to place the patient in a chair, or set him up in bed, open a vein in the arm, and let the blood run until he is about to faint, and the man is safe for the hour, and proper treatment afterwards establishes the safety, because the whole amount of blood in the body is diminished that much ; the blood to each particular part is diminished that much ; and by this diminution in the diseased part— diseased because there was too much blood there—there is a return to the natural condition of healthful circulation ; if actual

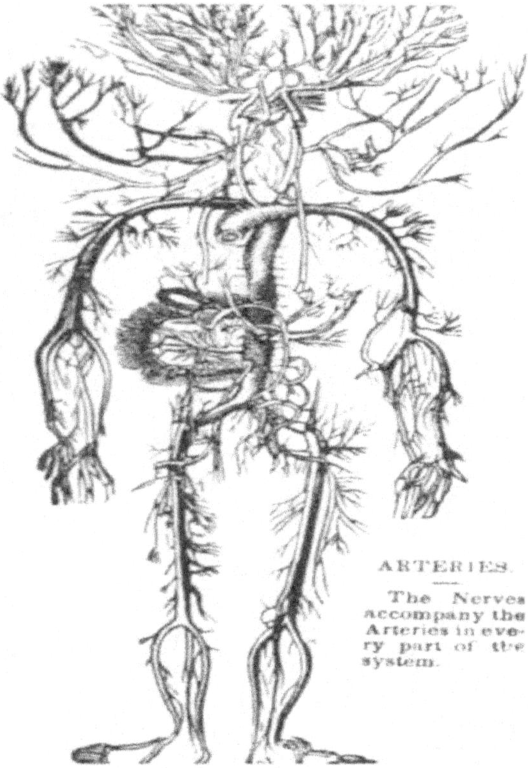

ARTERIES.

The Nerves accompany the Arteries in every part of the system.

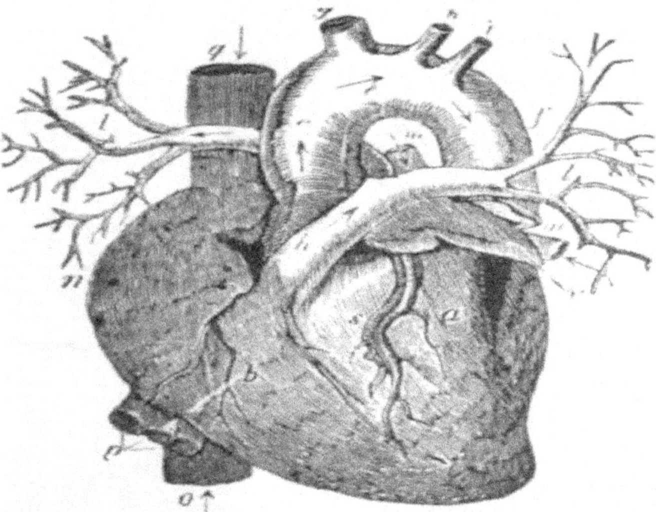

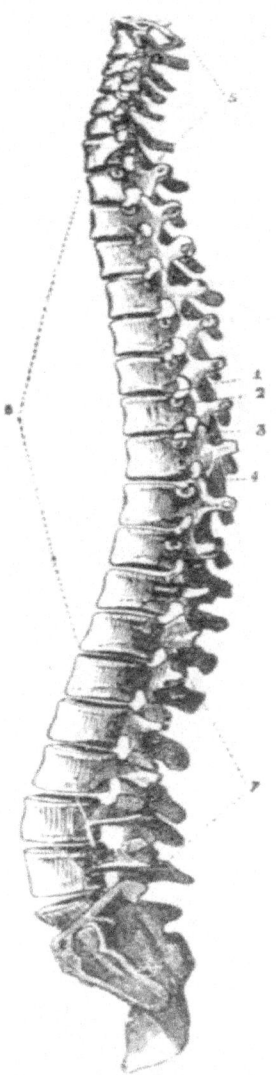

THE HEART AND ITS CIRCULATION.

BACK BONE, OR SPINAL COLUMN.

faintness is induced the whole flow of blood to the diseased part is arrested, giving that part perfect relief and perfect rest for the time being. But suppose there is a diseased condition resulting to a part because there is too much blood in the veins instead of the arteries; then there is no redness, as in the arteries, because the blood of the veins is dark-colored; then the part is dark-colored, as in the result of a blow; or there is no blood, as in the paleness of cold; and instead of the sharp pain of rapidly moving arterial blood there is the dull hurting of slow moving venous blood, so slow sometimes as almost to stop.

But whether the pain is sharp or dull, it is the result of too much blood being there; and in proportion as a remedy lessens the amount of blood by taking it away from the spot, out and out, as with leeches, or by inviting the excess of blood a short distance away to some point which, being in health, can better bear that excess, in such proportion do we give relief. A mustard plaster, for example, placed over the spot of an internal hurting, draws the blood to the surface, and relief is almost instantaneous.

But relieving pain and scattering disease and restoring health by the immediate extraction of blood from the part, although efficacious and instantaneous, is liable to abuse and to other objections; hence we come to the use of internal remedies, which are called drugs or medicines, accomplishing the same object, but in a more roundabout way, not so speedily but more enduring, and with less harm in several directions.

As the point to be arrived at is to lessen the amount of blood in the diseased part, the only thing necessary to be done is to lessen the amount of fluids in the whole system, and this is to lessen the amount of blood, for all these fluids are made out of the blood; and to that extent the whole amount of blood is lessened as effectually as if by the lancet.

A boil, just ready to burst, gives intense suffering; lance it, and allow a few drops of the yellow matter to flow out, and relief is instantaneous; give a cathartic medicine in almost any bodily pain or suffering, as two or three tablespoons of castor-oil, or two or three tablespoons of Epsom salts dissolved in a glass of water, and in a few hours several pounds of fluid are discharged from the body, affording in very many cases a most welcome relief.

Sometimes a more speedy deliverance is effected by the use of

an enema, which see, or " Rectal Bath," for this unloads the
system of a large amount of solid matter, sooner than salts or
oil.

There is a gentler, safer, and more permanent relief from bodily
suffering, as a result of too much blood being in any particular
part, but is not so expeditious; it is by giving medicines which
are said to " act on the liver," stimulate it, make it work (see
Liver and Biliousness); this is because a large part of the blood
of the body passes through the liver, and while it is in, its
quantity is largely diminished by being used to make bile, which
is passed directly into the bowels and out of the body, hence a
great deal more blood enters the liver than leaves it in the
shape of blood; thus any medicine, any remedy which makes the
liver work more actively, in thus making bile, diminishes the
quantity of blood in the body, and gives great relief.

But suppose the liver becomes so full of blood, its blood-chan-
nels clogged up, preventing any blood from passing along, then
this large escape of fluid from the system is arrested, the evil of
overfulness increases every moment, and every moment aggravating pain and intensifying the diseased condition.

The reader has now a complete idea of the principles of the
practice of medicine in the treatment of disease and pain and
suffering. It is narrowed down to the simple points of regulating
the quality and quantity of the blood: if it is too thick, it will
not run out; it clogs the machinery, it dams up the stream,
arrests the flow, and that is death. If there is too much blood,
there is distention of the blood-vessels: they carry too much blood
to a part, and disease and pain attack that part, to disorganize and
destroy it effectually, unless relief is obtained.

But there is another way of lessening the amount of blood in
the body, far better than any one, or all, mentioned above. Bleeding is depressive and in other ways objectionable. The use of
mustard plasters and setons and blisters is inconvenient and
painful. To give violent cathartics, or even more moderate purgatives, is troublesome, nauseous, and otherwise disagreeable. In
most cases better headway can be obtained and more human lives
saved if an attempt is made in all cases to diminish the amount
of blood, and equalize the circulation by

DIET AND EXERCISE.

All the blood is made out of what we eat; every mouthful of food taken makes that much more blood, and is used in no other way than to make blood. If, then, there is too much blood in the whole body, or in any part of it, causing disease or suffering, we begin at the very foundation by refusing to make any more blood; by refusing to eat an atom; and as each grown person eats and drinks several pounds a day, it is readily seen that abstinence from food stops at once the supply of blood. This is the medical treatment which blind instinct prompts the brute creation to adopt. A sick animal will not eat, or, if at all, most sparingly; hence the little disease observed in the animal creation, dying, as it does, by violence or age.

If the supply of blood is stopped in a case of disease by abstinence from food, the whole amount in the body is necessarily diminished, every second of a man's existence, by the ordinary laws of the system; because the glands of the body are in operation more or less actively every second of our being. Their office is to diminish the amount of blood passing through them, as above explained as to the liver; among the glands are the kidneys; they pass off a pound or more every day; the liver another; the whole skin may be considered a gland, and it passes off from the body in twenty-four hours, in the shape of visible and invisible perspiration, another pound or two of matter; then there are other places of discharge, the ears run wax, the eyes run water, the nose runs quite an amount in twenty-four hours; hence a man not eating or drinking anything for a whole day would necessarily weigh a pound or two or more less, all in the shape of fluids, and these fluids being abstracted from the blood, the volume of blood is thus diminished several pounds by natural operations which we cannot prevent; nature instinctively comes to our aid by actually helping us to a desirable result by taking away our appetite, and in some cases making even the sight and smell of food nauseating.

THUS IS DIETING MADE EASY,

Nature paving the way for the cure. But man may come in turn to aid nature in her attempts at cure by the exercise of his better reason; he can hasten the diminution of the quantity of blood in the system, as a means of relieving himself of suffering and disease, by

MUSCULAR EXERCISE.

All bodily motion necessarily involves a loss of fluid and solid substances; of fluids in insensible and visible perspiration, amounting to a pound or more in twenty-four hours; and of solid particles which are worn off by the friction of the muscles and other components of the system, as all friction implies waste and loss; a hard steel razor loses some of its substance, weighs less every time it is drawn along the strap; otherwise it would not be sharpened by the operation. If a knife is sharpened upon the edge of a table or bench, it will be very soon seen that the wood is wearing away; all rubbing together wears off, detaches particles; and when it is remembered that in the human body there are several hundred muscles, and bands, and bones, moving on and across one another; that the whole thirty or forty feet of the intestines are in incessant motion- one against another; that the heart is always throbbing; that pulses in every part of the body are beating forever, it must be apparent that there is unceasing waste of solid particles, which no sooner are they detached than they are hurried along bodily towards the rectum, or the great receptacle of the solids of the body; or they are dissolved into the minutest particles and are conveyed by the fluids of the system into the bladder, and then passed outwards in the urine, as seen in the sediment deposited on the bottom of the chambers, as a solid substance; these losses occur day and night, by the incessant motion of parts over which we have no control; these are called involuntary motions, and wear off and out of the body a pound or more of its substance in a day, although we may remain in bed all the time; but when, in addition to these, the voluntary actions of the muscles are put in operation, the hands and arms and feet and legs, with the various bends of the body, not less than two, three, or even half a dozen pounds may be passed out of the body in twenty-four hours, thus diminishing very largely the amount and bulk of the blood, lessening pain and inflammation, and returning the body to its healthful condition. Small wonder is it then that exercise, work, steady, unhurried labor, has such a decided, even powerful effect towards removing every variety of disease from the body, bringing back to it health and strength, and vigor and activity.   Thus there are several distinct methods of curing disease, all efficient in their way, and more or less in repute by turns in the progress of the ages.

First. By direct bleeding, using the lancet or leeches.

Second. By the use of blisters, mustard plasters, irritants, or other modes of diverting the blood from the diseased part.

Third. By the use of medicines which act on the bowels, or liver, or skin, as by the employment of castor-oil or salts for the bowels, calomel for the liver, and "sweats" for the skin, all these diminishing the amount of blood in the body.

Fourth. By ceasing to eat for a season, as food makes blood, and ceasing to eat cuts off the supplies, while the necessary operation of the system uses up rapidly what is on hand. Hence, if we eat or drink nothing for two or three days, the weight of the body is diminished several pounds.

Fifth. By active exercise we work off and out of the body the waste, worn off, useless, and poisonous particles in the system to the extent of several pounds every day.

CONGESTION.

The doctrine of congestion of the blood is the key which unlocks the entire system of medical practice, and makes of it a harmonious whole, a system which is beautiful in its simplicity, its efficiency, and truthfulness.   Its literal meaning is a pressing together and wedging in, and in this connection applies to the circulation of the blood, which comes out from the heart all bright and sparkling with warmth and life and vigor, entering the largest arteries, which divide and subdivide, getting continually smaller in their branches until they are almost invisible, everywhere depositing those atoms of nutriment with which it was freighted when it left the heart; and, having thus gone to the remotest portions of the body, unloading itself of all its nutriment, each infinitesimal ending artery inosculates, joins on to a corresponding vein quite as small, with this difference, the great aorta as it comes from the heart divides off into lessening branches continually, until they are immensely numerous and small, the volume of blood diminishing all the time, by the amount of nutrient particles it parts with, all full of life; the blood-vessels on the other hand, called the veins, get larger and fewer, and more full of blood at every inch of their progress; this blood, not carrying with it the life of the body, but its death, for it is really the washings out of the system, containing its mere refuse, useless, impure, and dead particles, so loaded is it with these, that it is not sparkling and bright with its cheery and warming red, as in the arteries, but it is dark, lifeless, and dead, finally conveyed in one single channel, one large vein which empties itself directly into the heart, to remain there but a moment, for it is hurried on to the lungs, where meeting with the pure air drawn into them, it parts with its impurities, hands them over to the air just taken into the lungs, which absorbs them and carries them out in each expiration, and rising upwards as it passes the lips and nostrils, it makes its way to the regions above the head, above the houses, above the trees, above the clouds, there to be renovated and made full of life again; again to descend to the earth and enter the nostrils to repeat its purifications and to impart its life, just as all the water of the earth and seas rises to the heavens after use here, and is returned to the earth again in its purity, in the shape of the refreshing showers and of

THE BEAUTIFUL SNOW.

The arteries and veins which convey the blood have thin coats, their sides are elastic, distensible, and of a material barely compact enough to convey the blood onwards; but are capable of distention to an extent that they may become so thin as to be pervious to the more watery particles of blood, for blood is a combination of blood and water. Not only may the thinner water pass through the sides of these distended blood-vessels, if the blood is unnaturally jammed in, but if that jamming is increased, the blood itself, thick as it is, will ooze through; and if the jamming continues the congestion increases, the sides give way, and there is

RUPTURE OF A BLOOD-VESSEL,

Which we know, if in the lungs, endangers life; if in the head, it is apoplexy and death. In some great emotions of the mind men perspire freely; it is not the warm, healthful perspiration of ordinary exercise, but of a deathly clamminess; this phenomenon was exhibited in the Redeemer's passion, when "he sweat, as it were, great drops of blood." This is the result of a general congestion. This is what is going on in the hour of death when great drops of water stand beaded on the forehead; it is seen again in the

COLLAPSE OF CHOLERA,

when the whole body seems drenched in a cold perspiration. These statements all show that under the influences of

CONGESTION

the more fluid particles of the blood come out of the blood-vessels when that congestion is moderate; in an increased degree, blood itself coming out.

These same operations of oozing out go on in every part of the system, in every gland of the body, in all its interior operations and conditions, giving name to diseases in many cases, according to the degree of the congestion. And it will be of exceeding interest, if the intelligent reader is at leisure, to follow it out to its legitimate issues in reference to several parts of the body.

Suppose there is a large accumulation of blood in the lungs, we call it pneumonia, but it is more commonly known by the more appropriate designation of

CONGESTION OF THE LUNGS.

There is too much blood in their blood-vessels, they are too full, they are so much distended, indeed, that blood itself does actually make its way out of the blood-vessels into the lungs themselves, not in a stream but in the form of minute particles, oozing through the distended sides, a kind of sweating, and mixing with the saliva it has the appearance of iron-rust, it is rusty-colored; this is a distinctive symptom of

INFLAMMATION OF THE LUNGS.

If the veins of the lungs are congested to a high degree, their sides ooze out large drops of blood, and we have the expectoration of

DARK CLOTS OF BLOOD.

But when this congestion goes on to a still greater extent the sides burst, blood flows into the lungs in a stream, creates a great tickling of the bottom of the neck, at the little hollow, and we have

HÆMORRHAGE OF THE LUNGS.

In a moderate degree of congestion of the brain there is an oozing out of the thinner parts of the blood, and it is called

WATER ON THE BRAIN.

If the congestion is more decided, a drop of blood escapes and that is death by

APOPLEXY.

If there is a moderate congestion along the bowels, there are thin, watery passages ; we give it the name of

DIARRHŒA.

If that congestion becomes more aggravated, blood escapes from the distended vessels, and we have

DYSENTERY.

If the eye is moderately inflamed it "waters ;" if the congestion becomes more decided a redder fluid appears, and we say of the eye that it is

"BLOOD-SHOT."

These examples show that ordinary diseases are readily accounted for by the doctrine of congestion, which is nothing more nor less than an over amount of blood in the veins or arteries of the part, and that the severity of attacks of sickness is directly in proportion to the degree of the congestion in the small blood-vessels of the parts, either in the veins or arteries, and so it is with all classes of fevers, and that long catalogue of complaints connected with the varied degrees of congestion of the liver, the spleen, and in short the whole glandular system.

But this same law of congestion holds good in reference to diseases of the throat and lungs. All throat complaints arise from a congested condition of the blood-vessels, as will be seen in any case by opening the mouth, when it will be found that the whole back part of the throat is either of a fiery red, showing that the arteries are over-full of blood, or of a dark or dusky hue, indicating that the veins are congested.

When there is a high condition of congestion in the throat of a child who has taken a severe cold, the more fluid parts of the blood ooze out at the sides of the distended blood-vessels, and as it oozes out, each particle comes in a drop; this unites with another drop and spreads, then unites with others until there is a thin coating all over the inside of the windpipe, almost as evenly spread over as if laid on with a brush ; but no sooner is this done than it hardens, as the gum on the bark of a tree begins to harden as soon as it is exposed to the air, and the process of oozing or exudation goes on, constantly toughening and thickening, until the whole cavity of the windpipe is filled up with it, thus stopping the breath, and the child dies. Sometimes before entire closure, means are successfully used in detaching that tough leathery substance, and it comes away in patches, or in some instances has been ejected in the shape of the windpipe, or a hollow reed, and the child is saved.

When the lungs become steadily and slowly congested in connection with a cold or cough the thinner part of the blood oozes out in drops ; these harden, and that is

TUBERCLE ;

And being allowed to go on, it becomes consumption, the ordinary consumption of the lungs, called Thysis by physicians, but spelled

PHTHISIS,

and is equivalent to the disease which is expressed by the common people in the country by saying the

LUNGS ARE AFFECTED.

It would deeply interest a few, but would weary the many, to go into a minute detail of all the diseases of the human body, which could be easily explained by the doctrine of congestion; but that point, in the light of the statements made, being taken for granted, it is of great value to trace out the deduction which may be legitimately drawn from the doctrine, and it is wide-sweeping.

If the great majority of all our more familiar diseases arise from congestion of the blood-vessels, either the arteries or veins, and if this congestion simply means that there is too much blood there, relief and ultimate cure consists in diminishing the amount of blood, drawing it away or off from those parts, and this is the doctrine of

DERIVATION,

In the practice of medicine, which means, strictly, drawing the flow from one part to another—from a part that has too much, and is weak or painful from that cause, to a part that is healthy and thriving, and therefore can bear an excess, at least for a while. A very severe pain on the inner walls of the belly will be relieved by putting a mustard plaster on the outside, because it draws the blood from the inside, which is diseased and suffering, to the outside, which is not diseased at all. This is curing an ailment by Derivation.

But, as said in another article, the blood can be lessened in four or five ways, by the

Lancet,
Leeches,
Dieting,
Medicines,
Working.

But from one cause or another, nine persons out of ten, even of the educated and cultivated classes, will, for various reasons, prefer to take some medicine which will accomplish the object, as that can be done with the least expense of time, and money, and trouble.

There are three kinds of medicines advised in these pages to be taken for the purpose of diminishing the volume, the amount, the weight of the blood in the human body—

Laxatives,
Cathartics,
Purgatives.

Laxatives loosen the bowels; they act quickly, and bring away a large amount of water—several quarts in a few hours—sometimes thus lessening the amount of blood very rapidly: among these are salts, castor-oil, jalap, and others.

Cathartics are those which act on the bowels less rapidly, bringing away more of solid substances; such as rhubarb, aloes, gamboge, and others.

PURGATIVES

are meant in these pages to be those medicines which are slower in their action than laxatives and cathartics, but are less weakening and take deeper hold, hence do more good, they being said to act on the liver; among this class of medicines are first and best, and surest always, calomel, next blue mass, podophyllin or May apple, taraxacum or dandelion, extract of black walnut, and others.

The reason that medicines which act on the liver do a more decided good is, that a large part of the blood of the body passes through the liver, and if it is congested even partially, the passage-way is stopped and the blood remains in the interior portion of the body, laxatives and cathartics affecting that which is nearer the surface, and thereby accomplishing only a partial or temporary good. If we can compound a medicine which will not only reach the stomach and upper bowels and lower bowels, but the liver too, then there will be the certain effect of clearing out the whole system and of meeting all the requirements of the case.

If, then, most of our ordinary diseases arise from congestion, if there are medicines which can remove that congestion, then it follows that to a very great extent:

The cause of disease is one and the same.

The thing to be done is one and the same.

The remedy to do that thing is one and the same; that is,

The cause is one—congestion.

The cure is one—to remove that congestion.

The remedy is one—purgation.

That purgation is surest, safest, and best which is accomplished by a combination of medicines, each of which has a distinct locality of action ; then the whole together acts on the liver, the stomach, the upper, the lower bowels, and on the alimentary canal. (See Purgative Pills, including the whole philosophy of their action and the rules for their administration.)

The uniform, universal action of these pills is to carry out of the body, within twelve hours, several pounds of solid and fluid matter, and to that extent diminish the supply of blood to the whole body in general, and to the ailing part in particular.

The broad fact is now laid down for the especial consideration of the reader, that nine-tenths of all ordinary diseases are promptly benefited or eventually cured by the judicious administration of the purgative pills.

PATENT MEDICINES.

It is a very common thing to see a medicine advertised in the papers as good for some particular disease, and in reading the circulars sent out with them it will be found that these medicines are good for a variety of diseases which seem to general readers to be wholly different, and yet to the experienced physician they are known to be essentially the same, as, for example, when diarrhœa and dysentery and bilious fever prevail in a neighborhood at the same time, the cause is one—miasma, making the blood thick, causing the three varieties of disease, according to the concentratedness of the cause, the time of exposure to its influence, and the degree of resistance possessed by different constitutions ; but the cause being one, the effects being different only in degree, the remedy is one and the same ; the same medicine will cure them all, the purgative pills, because they act on the bowels, bringing away a large amount of liquid and solid substances.

If you apply to six physicians for the cure of the same set of symptoms, for example, foul tongue, poor appetite, and chilliness, all will pronounce it the same disease,

BILIOUSNESS,

Yet each one will give directions of a varying character, but on close examination they will be found to be seeking to obtain one object—an evacuation of the bowels.

Professor Austin Flint, of New York City, has written one of the most comprehensive and learned volumes on the Allopathic Practice of Medicine; showing him to be one of the highest order of medical scholars : in three cases out of four, whatever may be the diversity of his remedies, some one of them will act in the direction of opening the bowels.

If then, on being called to any ordinary disease, whether it has occurred within a day or a week, or has been hanging about the system for years, the very first inquiry to be made is, have the bowels acted within twenty-four hours? if not, make them act, and with a day's "strict diet," which see, keeping the patient quiet, warm, clean, in a pure air, it will be a rare thing to find no improvement; it will be a very common occurrence that a report for the better in all respects will be certainly made. This action of the bowels diminishes the quantity of blood, which, with the dieting and the warmth, will amount to a couple of pounds, if not more. One of the next most frequent occurrences is, the feet are cold or the whole body is chilly,—that is, there is too little circulation in the feet or skin, the warm arterial blood has collected in excess somewhere else in the body; oftenest in the head; warm the feet in hot water, warm the skin by drinking a quart of hot tea, and tucking up in bed, these operations draw the blood to the feet and to the skin, the circulation is equalized, and as soon as that is established the man is well,—for establishing the circulation, making it equable in all parts, is removing the congestion from the ailing part.

One of the most successful practitioners of medicine on Red River, Louisiana, many years ago, was a colored man who had once been the body servant of a surgeon in the army. Swamp fevers and kindred diseases abounded; his main remedy, one used in almost every case, was warm water applied to the body in such a way as to draw blood where it was wanting, and to drive it away from parts where it abounded; this was equalizing the circulation. Very few have reached adult life who have not observed that when they became ailing, dull, depressed, irritable, with an ugly feeling all over, a free action of the bowels was putting a sun in the sky; it changed the whole physical and mental condition. Hence, one of the very earliest impressions to be made on the minds of the young, even as early as five or six years of age, should be in reference to the condition of the bowels, the absolute importance of going to the privy every day, drawing their attention to the fact in connection with their various ailments. That purgation is safest, surest, and best which affects the stomach, liver, and bowels in their whole extent.

To that end the purgative pill is employed, made of calomel, rhubarb, aloes, gamboge, and tartar emetic. See p. 806.

The Calomel is to act on the liver.

The Rhubarb is to act on the upper intestines.

The Aloes is to act on the lower intestine and rectum.

The Gamboge is to intensify and make more certain the action of all of them, so that there may not be often occasion to take anything after the pills, in order to work them off.

The Tartar Emetic is to relax the whole system, and thus make it more amenable to the action of the medicine.

As the above-named remedies will be used so often, and in so many connections, it will answer a good purpose if the reader will make himself thoroughly acquainted with their nature, their qualities, and their various uses.

CALOMEL

is worth all the other medicines known to man. It is called mercury, more familiarly known as quicksilver, which with common table salt is made by the chemist into that white, tasteless, smooth-feeling powder which we call Calomel, from two Greek words, Kalos and Melas, meaning a good black, from its resemblance to Æthiops mineral in some of its qualities, so that in taking calomel we take really what is made out of quicksilver and salt. It will doubtless be satisfactory to the reader to have this plain definition of a medicine which is so often used in all civilized lands.

Its chief value is in the certainty of its action on the secretions, mainly on the liver, in a manner more or less direct. If the liver

Inasmuch, then, as calomel is the surest and best and most efficient medicine in the world to clear out the channels of the liver, so that the blood may not be detained in it, but may pass through to other parts of the system, to perform its various offices, and to make that bile whose presence in the body in that shape answers indispensable purposes, it is clear that calomel is an appropriate medicine to be given in every disease which is incompatible with a free and equable circulation of the blood throughout the body, that is, a medicine which will have more or less good effect, in one or more directions, in every disease known to man, because by its action on the liver directly, in compelling it to make bile, and on the bowels indirectly, as this bile has to pass out of the body, from the liver into the bowels, making them operate, purging them, its nature and its effects on the system ought to be understood by every intelligent person.

Calomel could be made into five-grain pills with a very small amount of gum-arabic water, and their efficiency will be retained for a quarter of a century.

In the course of years it was found that calomel might act on the liver, but could not get into the bowels from obstruction, they being costive, then as a result constipation would keep the calomel in the system, and salivation or mercurial fever would result; hence it was thought advisable to combine with calomel some medicine which would as certainly act on the bowels as calomel would act on the liver. Rhubarb was known to be a good medicine to move the bowels proper, but occasionally all its effects would be spent before it reached the lower and large bowel, the rectum, which was sometimes so impeded with fæces that nothing would pass; it was then decided to combine aloes, a bitter medicine which seemed to act on the rectum, or gamboge or colocynth, the object being to make it as certain as possible that not only the liver but the upper and lower bowels, and the largest of all, the rectum, should be acted on, and thus make it sure of its effects without the necessity, as a general rule, of having to take anything else to carry off the calomel, but that it should carry itself off.

It occurred to the writer that if another medicine were added, which would relax the system and at the same time would cause water to flow from the stomach and upper bowels, and thus help to dilute and soften the hard mass of substance which is always present in costiveness, then a less amount of the other medicines would be needed; any nauseating medicines would do, but that is best which keeps the longest, which is surest in its action, and at the same time is least bulky. Tartar emetic combines in perfection all these requisitions. A pill made of five grains of calomel and one-fifth of a grain of tartar emetic will have more beneficial effects than a pill of ten grains of calomel, because of its relaxing power. The following combination of medicines has been devised by the writer to make a

CATHARTIC PILL

which could be safely and beneficially taken in every form of disease in which it was desirable to act on the liver or to move the bowels, each pill containing

> Two grains of calomel,
> Two grains of rhubarb,
> One grain of colocynth,
> One-fifteenth of a grain of tartar emetic.

It is better to mix up enough to make sixty-four pills, because in mixing with water so as to make the whole of a doughy consistence, the mass can be rolled out in a long shape, and can be divided into halves until the last divisions make two pills each. This is a good way to have each pill contain its proper amount of ingredients and of a proper size; the long roll, divided in the centre, would give sixteen pills to each; divide these two equally, then each division would give eight pills, the next four, the next two, or sixty-four in all.

For ordinary purposes take two or three pills at a time, and they should act on the bowels within ten hours; if not at the end of ten hours, take a tablespoon of castor-oil every hour until there is an action. Each person should notice for himself how many are necessary to act on his bowels within ten hours, and then take that number.

If two pills act in five or six hours, then only one should be taken, as it is better that the calomel should remain in the system ten or twelve hours before it is hurried out; it does more good the longer it remains without causing an action of the bowels, provided it is not longer than twelve hours. All medicines taken to act on the bowels should be given at bed-time, the person not having eaten anything for at least five hours, for the stomach being empty, the medicine will act more directly, promptly, and thoroughly on the system than if it has to act through a mass of food or liquids, besides being less likely to cause disturbance of the bowels and vomiting. Life has been lost a thousand times by an indiscretion in eating, after taking emetic or purgative medicines: these leave the whole intestinal canal in a debilitated condition, as well as the digestive functions; hence while medicine is acting on the bowels, and for twenty-four hours after it has been taken, the food should be light and small in quantity; the almost universal rule should be, eat thrice a day, at not shorter intervals than five hours, so as to have all the food in the stomach digested and carried out of it before more is taken in; these three meals should generally be made of any kind of soup, with bread crust or toasted bread broken into it, or a bowl of tea with cold bread and butter; then gradually increase the amount of solid food. The above diet is specially applicable after taking a dose of purgative pills, or a liver pill.

LIVER PILL.

Each one contains four grains of calomel, one grain of ipecac., and one-tenth of a grain of tartar emetic, carefully mixed with water; this will keep good for a lifetime. To make them in quantities, take sixty-four grains of pulvis ipecacuanhæ; six grains of tartar emetic, and two hundred and fifty-six grains of calomel, mix them together in their dry state most thoroughly, then add as much water as will make the mass of a doughy consistence, roll it out in a long roll, and divide it into sixty-four pills.

These pills ought not to be taken oftener than once a week, unless advised by a physician, simply because there is some risk of salivation, and because, further, in endeavoring to get well by taking any medicine, it is better to take as little as possible, and as seldom as possible, so as not to wear out its virtues, and so as to have something to fall back upon in more serious sickness; for most medicines begin to lose their effect in time: the system becomes accustomed to them, and more has to be taken, and at shorter intervals; finally no reasonable amount seems to have any effect. Very much as it is with liquor; at first a teaspoonful of brandy will make the head light, will exhilarate; but if habitually used, the time will come when half a glass of brandy will be required to do what the first teaspoonful did.

It is best to take the liver pill at bedtime, not having eaten anything or drunk anything within four or five hours; for if the stomach is full of food, the pill is dissolved at once, and the tartar emetic may cause vomiting; if the stomach is empty, the ingredients dissolve slowly and take hold more efficiently; the person soon goes to sleep, and escapes the nauseating effects altogether. It usually operates next morning and once or twice more during the day, sometimes weakening considerably, at others little, but always passing off in a few hours. When the patient begins to feel hungry, that if he had a bowl of nice hot soup he would relish it and it would do him good, and it certainly will if some stale toast or crust bread is broken into the soup; for it seems to have come to light recently that there is very little nourishment in meat soup, especially without something more solid, as bread or mashed potatoes; but the warmth of the soup is a positive advantage, since warmth in disease has great curative powers. Soup may be alternated with hot teas or broma or cocoa, with cold bread and butter.

On the day after a pill has acted, the diet may approach the regular habits of the patient.

If a pill does not operate within twelve hours, take about one tablespoon of castor-oil, which repeat every hour until it does operate.

A pill acts more efficiently, touches the liver more effectively, if it is ten or twelve hours before it causes an action of the bowels than if it operated earlier.

This pill begins to have its effect on the system in about two hours, as do the purgative pills; one effect is to stimulate, to cause more or less of an excitement, a kind of warmth or fever. Thus when either of them is given with a view to stop the chill of

FEVER AND AGUE

which is expected to come on in about that time, such a result pretty certainly takes place.

If, on the other hand, a liver pill is taken to arrest diarrhœa safely and healthfully, in about two hours the severest looseness of bowels will be very often found to cease; in fact, two or three liver pills at a dose will seldom fail to arrest the most fearful discharges of

ASIATIC CHOLERA.

The first effect of these pills, although given to cure costiveness and constipation, is to arrest the looseness, and then in a few hours more to cause passages with bile in them; the frequent, colorless passages are present from the fact that there is no bile in them; an unnatural action is going on in the system, by which the bile is locked up in the liver; the pills act on the liver, they unlock it, the bile flows out, and all goes on well. Sometimes the pill nauseates uncomfortably, but bear with it, as it will do the more good.

If there is a griping or a rumbling in the bowels at the end of four or more hours after it has been taken, you may know that it is having an effect, and that in due time it will give a good operation.

This griping in the bowels is not the result of any ingredient in the pill, for then it would always follow taking a pill, whereas it frequently does not take place. This griping is the result of acrid bile and other substances which are floating along downwards and out of the body, from having been unloosed, dislodged by the pill, and shows how needful it was to have taken the pill. Sometimes the bile is so acrid as to be described by patients as burning like fire at the exit from the body.

Many persons can take one of these pills at bedtime, and go to work next day as if nothing had happened, making no change in anything except in the eating during the day on which it was acting. The general rule should be, if its action debilitates much it is better to remain in the house and lie down awhile.

Let it be remembered that any weakening effect of the pill is but transient, passes off before the close of the day; and many times it has happened that persons who have taken a pill at night, not having felt hungry for a long time, are surprised at the feeling of being able to eat almost anything before the close of next day.

Bilious persons have taken these pills habitually for many years, whenever they

GET OUT OF SORTS,

without any special diminution of their good effects, and have urgently counselled that the mode of preparing them might not be permitted to pass away with the life of their maker. Some advantages which they possess, are :—

First.—They are small in size, hence are swallowed more easily.

Second.—They will keep good for a lifetime.

Third.—Can be easily and safely transmitted by mail.

Fourth.—If broken, their pieces will do as much good as if whole.

Fifth.—If a pill cannot be swallowed, it may be beaten into a powder, put on a spoon-handle, turned deftly, and placed on the back part of the tongue, and washed down with .cold water, and do as much good as any other way; or the powder may be placed between layers of boiled rice, or soft bread, or jelly, and swallowed.

Sixth.—It has no taste.

Seventh.—The calomel is so heavy that when it once gets into the stomach it falls to the bottom, and scarcely any amount of straining will throw it up. Once down, it stays down.

Eighth.—It does not require frequent repetition; as a general rule, a pill a week is all that is needed. If a person has to be taking medicine two, three, or four times a day and night, to be repeated and kept up for weeks and months, such person will soon come to feel himself a permanent invalid; besides, those who are all the time taking medicine are all the time sick, and will be always sick.

Ninth.—This pill rarely requires to be followed by other medicine; it works itself off in almost all cases. This is accomplished by the relaxing properties of both the tartar emetic and the ipecac.; hence these are important ingredients.

Tenth.—As much cold water may be drunk after the pill has been taken and during its action as the patient may desire; only if liquid is swallowed within an hour of taking the pill, nausea and vomiting may be the result.

As the pill causes two or more actions during the day, it is not important to have an action of the bowels on the day after its operation; for usually, if the bowels were regular before, they return to their regularity in two or three days; if they do not, it is better to take some castor-oil night and morning, not enough to purge, but merely enough to cause one full free action every twenty-four hours. Sometimes a single teaspoonful at a dose, morning and evening, will answer the purpose. Some persons require more, and some less. Each one must observe for himself how much he requires, and be governed accordingly. The one great point to be aimed at is one full, free action of the bowels during every twenty-four hours; take as much oil as will accomplish that in divided doses. A larger amount might be taken, a tablespoonful or more at a time; but the objection to that course is, large doses act quickly, harshly sometimes, debilitate, and leave the bowels costive for a day or two. Teaspoonful doses are not liable to these objections. There is no more danger in getting wet after taking one of these pills than there would be in getting wet after one had not been taken.

The uses to which this pill is applicable are very numerous; the symptoms which they are calculated to meet, if taken as above suggested, and the different ailments of the body which they will alleviate, dislodge, or remove cannot be mentioned in any single page of this volume. There is scarcely an ache or pain or distress in any part of the body which it is not pretty certain to alleviate or modify, if not to cure out and out.

Its tendency is, and always will be as long as there is life enough in a man to take an impression from it, to purify the blood, to make it thinner and more capable of flowing healthfully and actively through the veins and arteries; in short, it corrects bad blood; and as all pain is neuralgic (see Neuralgia), it tends to ease all pain. It acts on the liver, hence it is applicable to all diseases which arise from a disordered liver. If the bowels are costive the pill will remove it; if the bowels are loose the pill will arrest it, or make it a healthy looseness; if there is heaviness or dulness or oppression in the head, the pill will disperse it before it has had time to act on the bowels.

It is applicable when the appetite is poor, fitful, changeable, or when there is none at all. If there is

BAD TASTE IN THE MORNING

in the mouth, a judicious use of the pill, of exercise, and diet will remove the bad taste. If in the morning, on rising,

THE TONGUE IS COATED,

the coating will be removed with a little perseverance. If the

EYES ARE YELLOW,

it will clear them; if the skin is pumpkin-like it will restore it to its natural hue. If the

URINE IS SCANT

or high-colored this pill will increase its quantity, and will render it clear, copious, and healthful.   In all cases of

HEADACHE

arising from a torpid liver, usually accompanied with

COLD FEET,

cold hands, and chilliness, no remedy is more effectual than this, if these things are of recent occurrence; but for cold feet and hands and chilliness, which have been so long present as to have become habitual, other means must be added, but the pills will give an aid to these other means which no other medicine possibly can. In all fevers this pill cannot be taken amiss, now and then, because an over-quantity of blood in the liver, or engorged bile, is inseparable from all feverish conditions of the system.

Notwithstanding the efficiency of this pill, it ought not to be taken as long as a person can conveniently avoid it by using hygienic measures.   It is better in almost all cases of sickness, except those which are urgent, to try first what good can be done by

Abstinence from food,
Quiet and repose,
Good genial warmth,
Personal cleanliness,
Out-door activities.

These five things persevered in judiciously will moderate any form of human ailment, and will cure half of them, if not more; but when these have had a fair trial for a day or two, do not take a pill, but call in a physician if you are able, or if convenient; if not, then take a pill on the conditions before described; it can be always done with safety, and will seldom fail of a good result. Now and then we come across a person who has some peculiarity of constitution, called by physicians

IDIOSYNCRASY,

which will not tolerate a particular medicine; but this is rare and can be only told by an opportunity of making an experiment; in such cases, other medicines should be used whose effects are as nearly similar as possible.

ONENESS OF DISEASE,

AND the oneness of medicine as a remedy, is well worth the attention of the unprofessional reader, and parents especially. If a man of average intellect is advised to " take something " for his ailment, and it does him good, cures him, anybody's pills, or any old woman's tea, he is enthusiastic in its praise. This enthusiasm increases with every experience he has of its unmistakable efficacy. It will not be long before he finds himself thinking that if it has done him good in one disease, it may do him good in another, although apparently a very different malady. Lo and behold, it cures that too, and in a short time you find the man advising his favorite as a cure for everybody and everything. He treasures up in his own mind every case of success, and at length begins to think of setting up a patent medicine shop. Many have done it, and have made fortunes. Outsiders wonder why physicians did not find this out long ago, and every such person begins to feel, if he does not say, " I believe I know about as much as any of the doctors."

One half dozen medicines, skilfully employed, will cure more diseases than all the million others that are in the world. Nature will cure half of all the ailments of humanity, if you will only let her alone. The tincture of Thyme (time !) will cure half the remainder. But when people get sick they will not " take time ; " they tell the doctor they cannot afford it, they must take medicine, and get well right away. A day's loss to a workingman, or a struggling widow, means nothing to eat on the morrow. If you are really sick, go to a good doctor, hand him a fee, get his advice, and follow it. Do not get an opinion out of him, and then slip off without pay. The

" LIVER PILL "

has been in use fifty years, and it will cure fifty different diseases, aches, and pains. Its composition is made known.

If a well-made machine has a thousand wheels, more or less connected in their movements, and you stop one, you stop all. The human body contains a great many glands, manufactories, and wheels. Stop the great one, the heart, and you stop all. "Slow" one, and you "slow" all. Put upon one organ a thousand horse-power extra, and make it run a mile a minute, such as a tremendous dose of brandy, and the other organs will run like lightning.

The liver is one of the great controlling organs of the body. Regulate its working healthfully, and the other parts of the machine dependent on it will run healthily too. And in some way or other, almost every part of the human body has a more or less direct connection with the liver, sympathizing with its action. Hence, any medicine acting on the liver so as to restore it to a healthy working, necessarily restores all the other parts which depend on it.

The pill in question does affect the liver, and is called a "Liver Pill," because it acts on the liver infallibly.

THE LIVER PILL

may be given to advantage in all forms of disease which are associated with constipated bowels, with fevers, headache, cold feet, foul tongue, variable appetite, nausea, or pain.

One should be taken at a time, and if it does not operate within twelve hours, then take a tablespoon of castor-oil, or as much salts in a glass of warm water, every two hours, until there is a discharge from the bowels; or an injection may be given instead of the oil or salts, although it will not be as efficient in its action.

The pill should be made to act as above, because it contains a small amount of calomel, which may now and then cause salivation if it is allowed to remain too long in the system. But this pill contains ingredients which usually have the effect to act on the stomach and bowels, irrespective of the calomel, thus making it unnecessary to take anything after them to work it off.

It is not advised to take one oftener than once in five or six days, as, if taken at too short intervals, it might salivate. It is intended to act on the liver, to thin the blood, to lessen its quantity, to improve its quality, to make it good and life-giving.

FEVERS

of all descriptions will be benefited and cured by the judicious administration of this pill, from time to time, until the patient begins to feel as if bread and butter and roasted meat would taste very good. No other medicine is really needed; meanwhile , the system should be allowed to rest. If every trifling symptom is prescribed for, it will be found in a short time that some kind of medicine is to be taken almost every hour of the day and night, until outraged nature begins to reject everything, and scarcely tolerates a glass of the purest water.

The system will sooner rectify itself if left alone to the recuperative powers of nature, the pill being given merely to aid her a little in clearing the liver of the obstructions in it, so that the blood may pass on readily to other parts of the body. Each person should note how many are required to cause one operation within twelve hours, for some are more sensitive to the action of medicine than others, and sometimes a motion may be more urgently needed than at others. In such cases it would be better to take an additional pill, in order to be more certain of its effect, and that this effect should be more full and free.

LOOSE BOWELS.

One of these pills will cure any ordinary case of loose bowels, if the patient will go to bed at once, wrap up warm, and eat nothing for a day or two but boiled rice, with a small amount of boiled milk, using no other liquid whatever. But in taking this pill for diarrhœa, which is the physician's name for loose bowels, if it does not stop the passages within two hours, it is proof that a large enough dose had not been taken. Hence, at the end of two hours, if the bowels are still running off, give another, and pay more attention to giving the body rest, and keeping it warm.

This pill will keep good, in a dry place, for twenty years. It contains no dangerous ingredients ; and if all other medicines are abstained from, and cleanliness and pure air and warmth and quiet are secured, with a moderate diet, there is scarcely a disease of any ordinary character which will not be benefited by it, for the simple reason that it will always do more or less towards purifying the blood, lessening its quantity, and giving it a more healthful circulation. With this a person may travel the world over without the need of any other remedy to supplement his medicine-chest; because, in the large majority of ordinary attacks of sickness, quiet, warmth, rest, pure air, and abstinence from all food for twelve or twenty-four hours, will inaugurate an immediate improvement, which would result in cure, if the means stated were persevered in. At the end of fifteen or twenty hours after taking a pill, the patient should eat something, if there is a decided feeling of hunger; if not, wait for it, even if it is for three or four days, taking care not to eat at shorter intervals than five hours, eating moderately of only two kinds of food, bread being one.

But, although this is incomparably the best course to pursue, there are circumstances which make it necessary to have more immediate relief. Thus, at the first attack of sickness, if the bowels have not acted freely within twenty-four hours, take an emetic; if this is not convenient, then take one of the pills, and await its action.

If within three or four hours after taking the pill there is an action of the bowels, it is *not* from the pill; hence, if at the end of twelve hours there is not an action of the bowels, bring about such action with an enema, although they were moved within four hours after the pill was taken.

It is important to know if the pill is working favorably, which is ascertained by the color and consistence of the discharges from the bowels. If the discharges are large in amount, and somewhat thicker, or more consistent than mortar, if they are very offensive, if they are light, bright yellow, the pills have done good, but more if they are green, and more still if they are dark or black. Sometimes they are described as being

"BLACK AS TAR,"

these being indications of the different degrees of torpidity, or congestion of the liver. Hence, whatever medicines persons take, the discharges from the bowels afterwards should be scrutinized, to be able to decide on the beneficial effects of the medicine, if no physician is in attendance, and for his satisfaction, if you have one.

Sometimes nature herself throws off very yellow, green, or black discharges, thus showing that she has vigor enough to relieve herself of the diseased conditions of the system ; and although these passages may be free and frequent, if they are of greater consistence than water it is a

HEALTHFUL DIARRHŒA,

and nothing ought to be taken to arrest it ; but this is often ignorantly done, to serious and sometimes fatal injury, under the impression that it is a diseased condition, hurtful to the system, when in reality it is an effort of nature to cure herself. In the case, however, of green flocculent passages from infants, means should be taken to correct them. The pill usually acts in about ten or twelve hours, and then again once or twice during the day. In proportion as the discharges are thin, light-colored, and weakening, the pill has failed of its proper effect. Then more attention should be paid to warmth, rest, abstinence from food, unless hungry ; then take boiled rice with boiled milk in small quantities ; have a stout woollen flannel bound very tightly about the abdomen, some fourteen inches broad, and long enough to have a double layer in front. If the passages still continue, keep quiet and wait. Nothing more will be needed.

The value of this pill will be more intelligently appreciated by a simple enumeration of the diseased conditions to which it is applicable, the most of these symptoms being more or less directly associated with a torpid condition of the liver, although it is rare that more than two or three are present in any one case at a time.

Appetite Variable,	Diarrhœa,
Bad Taste,	Discouragement,
Belching,	Dizziness,
Bitter Taste,	Drowsiness,
Brownish Spots,	Dry Cough,
Chilliness,	Dry Throat,
Choking Sensation,	Dulness,
Cold Feet,	Dyspepsia,
Colic,	Flashes of Heat,
Constipation,	Flatulence,
Despondency,	Fulness of Stomach,

General Distress,

Gloominess,

Headache,

Heaviness at Stomach,

Internal Heat,

Low Spirits,

Nervousness,

Numbness,

Pain in Back,

Pain in Breast,

Pain in Bowels,

Pain in Shoulders,

Pain in Sides,

Palpitation,

Piles,

Raising Blood,

Rush of Blood,

Sallow Skin,

Sore Bowels,

Sore Throat,

Urine Unnatural,

Unsocial,

Yellow Skin,

Yellow Eyes.

It would be interesting and instructive to point out how these various symptoms may and do arise from a disordered condition of the liver, but want of space forbids.

In addition to all these ailments, which are directly reached by the Liver Pill, there is scarcely a pain or an ache in the whole human body which will not be more or less modified by one full, free, thorough operation.

In addition, it will cure almost any curable case of

FEVER AND AGUE;

Will break up the chills in a single day, sometimes, although of many months' duration, by simply taking one of them two hours before the expected chill. If two of them are taken one day and the chill is not broken, is not prevented from occurring, take three the next time. The philosophy of this action is that the pill at once begins to excite an activity in the circulation, which compels a more lively flow of the blood, throws it out from the centres of the body to the circumference, and thus prevents that stagnation, that congestion of the blood, which is the immediate cause of the chill. Then if the chill is prevented, there is no reaction to cause a fever and its consequences of debilitating perspiration. To make the matter sure, take another dose two hours before the next expected chill, and the work is done, but with much greater certainty if, when the pill begins to act on the bowels, about three grains of quinine are taken in water every two hours, until the time for the chill of the next day has passed, omitting the quinine after ten o'clock at night until daylight next morning, so as to allow the patient to sleep, the diet meanwhile being on the general principles of three meals a day, at not less than five hours' interval, of bread and butter and meat at breakfast and dinner, and at supper bread and butter only, with a cup of hot tea.

Here, then, is a pill of such constituents as will make it act on the stomach, liver, and bowels, and doing so, modifies all the symptoms which arise from their deranged condition.

It sometimes happens that a constipated condition of the bowels will give rise to forty or fifty different symptoms in as many different persons at least, not more than two or three of any of them found in the same persons; and an ignorant mind noticing the results in this connection, could be very readily led to attribute to this pill

A MIRACULOUS POWER.

But it is easy to see that any other means which would have the effect to clear out the system of its accumulations would give the same good results.

A due consideration of the subjects mentioned will serve to show reflecting persons that there is a oneness in disease, and in its remedy, which vastly simplifies the practice of medicine, and which removes from it much of the mystery which hangs around it in the minds of a large class of the community. And a proper reflection on the whole matter leads to the legitimate result, that the practice of medicine, in the hands of educated men of experience and skill, is more of a science than most persons think it is.

PRELIMINARY OBSERVATIONS.

Educated physicians at home and abroad agree that books on Family Medicines have done more harm than good. As far as this is so, the injury done has arisen more from certain omissions than from actual faults in the books themselves. It is intended to supply these omissions in this volume.

4

THE FIRST

main defect has been the failure to mention in plain terms some of the general principles of the practice of medicine—the failure to designate the different diseases so clearly that they might be recognized by persons of ordinary comprehension, it being necessary to know what was the matter with a man before it could be decided what to do for him. This book can be consulted most advantageously if the reader will spend some of his leisure time in the study of this preliminary chapter, and not leave it to be read when the mind is disturbed by the actual presence of disease in himself or some member of his family.

GOOD NURSING

will cure a large number of diseases without any medicine whatever, and when drugs are required, adds very greatly to their efficiency. All ordinary diseases demand

Rest,
Warmth,
Pure Air,
Nourishment;

And that is the best nurse who secures these to the patient the soonest and in the largest proportions.

All diseases come under one of two classifications—Acute or Chronic.

CHRONIC DISEASES

are named from the Greek word *chronos*, which means time, duration; hence chronic diseases are those which last for a long time—for months and years—such as bronchitis, consumption, dyspepsia, rheumatism, and others.

ACUTE DISEASES

Are those which are sharp, short, severe, run their course in a few days, such as cholera, colic, croup, diphtheria, diarrhœa, dysentery, fever, and others like them.

It is for the treatment of acute diseases, those which involve severe suffering and require immediate attention, that books of family medicine are mainly written; and in this connection it is a positive humanity to prepare such a book, because there are multitudes of cases where it is impossible to procure the services of a physician in a reasonable time. Even in large cities, at certain hours of the day, a messenger will be gone several hours before he can succeed in finding a doctor unengaged or at his office. In the country the inconvenience is increased manifold; the doctor's office is one, two, or ten miles or more away; on the arrival of a messenger he is often found to have gone five, ten, or a dozen miles off in another direction, leaving it altogether uncertain when he will return; he may have gone on a consultation visit or on a case of confinement; and to allow a person to endure the agonies of cramp, colic, of facial neuralgia, of internal bleedings, of suffocating croup, or the terrible asthma, for weary hours and days without any intelligent efforts to help, alleviate, arrest, or cure, is dreadful to think of. It is to meet this imperative want of millions of families—to meet it safely in all cases, in many, efficiently, it is hoped—that this book is written; and it has been a sweet and ever-sustaining thought all through its preparation, that when the writer's already extended pilgrimage is ended, many a critical malady may be arrested, many a dangerous disease averted, many an agonizing pain subdued and soothed and eradicated from the persons of those who have trusted themselves to his teachings, even if they be but followed until

THE DOCTOR COMES.

One of the general principles to be carried out in the treatment of almost all diseases is to

UNBURDEN THE SYSTEM.

In every sickness to which the human body is liable, there is something within it which ought not to be there, and to get it out is to cure. Disease is a burden, to lessen which, to remove, is to alleviate, to cure.

ILLUSTRATION.

If a man has eaten more than he ought to have done, the stomach is overburdened, he begins to feel dull, heavy, sleepy; next comes a feeling of oppression, shortness of breath, faintness, sickness, paleness of face, the perspiration breaks out on the forehead, and he feels as if he was almost ready to die. Get the food out of his stomach, relieve it of its load by an emetic of large draughts of warm water, and in an hour, it may be, he feels as well as he ever was.

CONSTIPATION

is the failure of a daily action of the bowels for thirty-six hours or more; then the system is burdened by carrying one or more pounds of food over what is natural and habitual; if this state of things is allowed to continue, the machinery of life clogs up, it fails to work well, and sickness is inevitable because the whole body is overburdened; remove that burden, let something be done to open the bowels, to cause to pass out of the body the accumulations of several days, and health returns. In a very extensive sense

DISEASE IS A UNIT.

In a sense quite as extensive, the cure of all curable diseases is a unit also; one cause, one remedy; the body is burdened by something within it which is unnatural to it, which ought not to be there: it is burdened, remove that burden, and the cure follows. The cause is one, the manifestations are multitudinous, the disease is various, according to the part of the body, according to the locality of the organ which feels the burden most.

A cold in the Head is an Influenza.
"　　　　　　Nose is a Catarrh.
"　　　　　　Throat is Laryngitis.
"　　　　　　Windpipe is Croup.
"　　　　　　Branches of Windpipe is Bronchitis.
"　　　　　　Lungs is a " Bad Cold."

It is sufficiently near the general truth to say, that in all diseases the blood is changed, it is in an unnatural condition, it contains particles which do not belong to it in its healthy state, it is burdened by having to carry along the veins and arteries foreign matter, it requires more power to freight it along, the pulse must beat faster or stronger, for it is the pulse which is the moving force and carries this life of the body to its furthest extremities, and if it has to work faster or harder it gets tired sooner, our strength is prematurely exhausted, and we are weak, and weakness is an element of all diseases.

If, then, you can remove the foreign particles from the blood, you remove the burden, and the man is well again.

It requires a certain amount of force to carry the blood through the body in its natural, healthy state; but if the blood has foreign particles in it, making it bad blood, that is, thicker and heavier than is natural, the force of fever is used by nature to carry it onwards, hence fever is nature's cure; artificial stimulants are the physician's cure, or purgation, which diminishes the quantity of blood to be moved and makes its motion easier.

NURSING THE SICK.

GOOD nursing, a judicious attention to the sick and all the surroundings of a sick-bed, would cure many cases of disease without the use of any medicine whatever; in other cases, where medicine cannot be borne, in consequence of the great debility of the patient, or the exhaustion of the system, it has been successful in restoring health and life for many years. And if families would heed the suggestions which follow, with reasonable fidelity, the attention of a physician could often be dispensed with, to say nothing of the comfort afforded to the sick and suffering, with all their discouragements and despondencies.

1. The sick-room should be up-stairs, if possible. There are certain pernicious emanations from the earth, besides the raw dampness and heaviness which vitiate the air, and otherwise render it pernicious to the invalid. If there is no second story, the higher the bed from the floor the better. Pallets on the floor, cradles, lounges, cots, and trundle-beds should be exchanged for high bedsteads.

2. By all means place the sick in the room in the building which faces the sun for the greater part of the day, although it may not have as many windows as others, and although it may be smaller, for the sunshine keeps it light and cheerful; it keeps it warm, a healthful warmth; it keeps it dry, and besides imparts

a life to the atmosphere breathed, which of itself is a very important element in bringing back vitality to an exhausted frame.   A
merchant in New York City noticed in the progress of years, that
his chief clerks sickened soon after they came to him, and one or
two of them died.   The thought occurred to him one day, that it
might be because the apartment where the books were kept was
so surrounded by buildings that the sun did not shine into any of
the windows for a single moment during the day.   Being a man
of culture, energy, and of a generous nature, he decided instantly
to have his books kept in the sunniest room in the building, with
the result of the immediate and continued improvement and
eventual recovery of permanent good health on the part of the
person then in his employ.   If, then, the want of sunshine is a
cause of actual and even fatal disease to young and hearty persons, as all the young men were when they first came to the merchant, much worse, incalculably worse results would follow, if
those who were already sick occupied rooms where no cheering,
warming sunshine ever came.

3. The bed should be so situated as to be easily approached
from both sides; and, if convenient, have the head towards the
north, to enable the patient to face the sunshine, to look on the
out-doors, which has of itself a cheering effect, lessens the monotony of the sick-chamber, and tends to divert the mind from the
condition of the body, thus allowing time to pass more pleasantly.
It may be fancy, or it may be fact, that certain electrical currents
are passing between the poles, and their course being longitudinal
to the body, and for other considerations, may have decidedly
advantageous results to the sick.   Such an opinion has been given
by different men, whose positions and abilities entitled them to
the respect and confidence of educated people.   The idea, however, may have readily arisen from the circumstance that if the
sick-bed has its head to the north, it gives the patient the easy
opportunity of seeing the glad sunshine all the time.

4. A good ventilation, a constant supply and resupply of pure,
cooling, out-door air, is of inestimable advantage to the sick. The
fact may be well repeated that an English physician was called
to attend a poor family of several members of different ages.
One by one had been taken sick, until every member was an invalid in the depth of winter.   The usual medicines seemed to fail
of their ordinary good effects; one or two of the family died

Soon after that, in one of his visits, the physician's attention was drawn to the fact that a window-pane had been broken, and the family expressed great apprehension of taking cold, as their means were limited, and it had been very necessary to be economical with their fuel. To make less do, every crevice of door and window had been carefully stuffed to keep out the cold, with the result of preventing ventilation, and occasioned the rebreathing of vitiated air all the time. The physician had repeatedly drawn their attention to the importance of opening a door or window every day for a short time, even several times a day; but he had noticed that his suggestions had remained uniformly unheeded, the bugbear of expense and taking cold being ever present to the inmates. Under the circumstances he considered the breaking of the glass a piece of great good fortune, and put obstacles in the way of repair in such a way as to defer it as long as possible. The result was immediate and most striking. Within a day or two the invalids began to improve, and all of them eventually recovered.

5. If a fire is kept on the hearth in cold weather; and in warm, a large lamp or candle is kept burning day and night, and the inner door always kept open, there is a continual draught passing along the floor towards the fire-place, which carries before it and up the chimney the most deleterious gases in the room, for the heaviest and most poisonous of these are always near the floor.

If the door cannot be left open all the time, it may be done a few minutes at a time, every hour or two. In other cases, the window might be elevated. If this cannot be done without causing a draught of air upon the patient, provide a board two or three inches broad, and just as long as the window-sash; lay it on the sill lengthways, edge up, under the sash. This causes an opening at the joining of the upper and under sash, through which a draught of air is driven upward toward the ceiling, where it is warmed, and gives way downward to other cool air coming in constantly, thus giving an out-door air warmed to supply the patient all the time. If needed, additional bed-clothing can be supplied, thus securing two most important conditions for the invalid: First, a pure out-door air to breathe; second, comfortable bodily warmth.

6. There should be no standing liquid of any description in a sick-room, not even the purest cold water; because, like a pane of glass of a very cold morning, the cold water causes the tainted

atmosphere of the sick-room to settle on its surface, and condense into oily drops, which under a microscope exhibit various impurities, even yellow matter, to drink which would be disgusting. If not drank, the same particles are made gaseous by the warm air of the room, are evaporated, mingled with the air, and breathed into the lungs, to be incorporated directly with the blood.

7. Everything perishable by evaporation should be removed from the room, as food and fruits of every description, because their smell, their exhalations, contaminate the air; every atom helps to make it less pure.

8. All medicines, bottles, and vials, or anything else which reminds of medicine, should be kept out of sight, except at the moment of administering them.

9. There should be no clothing hanging about in the room, and as little drapery about the bed and windows as possible, for these hold dust and absorb odors, and keep them in the room. For the same reason it is usually better to have no carpet on the floor, except a strip alongside of the bed, for carpets retain dust and dampness; and if any liquid is spilled on them it is not dried for days, and odors accumulate. Still, if the patient is quite ill, or greatly debilitated, or has been ill for a time, a carpet is indispensable, as it deadens the sound of feet and moving of chairs, which would otherwise interfere with the quiet and sleep of the patient. In all diseases sleep is better than medicine, and promotes cure more than anything else.

10. The qualifications of the nurse are so varied and so important, that great care should be taken and no expense spared to secure a good one. Women are generally better than men; although, if the patient is pretty helpless, and requires to be moved in and out of bed much, strength is a requisite.

The nurse should be either specially attached to the invalid, or should be a friendly acquaintance, with whom the patient has had pleasant associations, for these things secure a more devoted attention than hired services. At the same time intelligent capability and experience are to be preferred in a stranger to pure affection only.

The nurse should be firm, and quietly decided; of a kindly, gentle nature, and sympathetic; not hasty nor touchy, but calm and deliberate; at the same time spry, active, prompt. And not least, by any means, but of the very first importance, there should be a cheerful confidence and composure in the expression of the face all the time.

There are many things which the nurse should not do, and others which should be studiously avoided. And to do these properly a good judgment is indispensable. She should not wear a silk dress, or any other fabric which gives a rustling noise; for repose and quiet are essential in sickness, and whatever disturbs a doze or wakes from sleep, or rouses up just as sleep is coming on, is a great misfortune.

All short, sharp, sudden movements should be watched against, as they tend to alarm the patient. All suddenness should be avoided, all impatient or alarmed exclamations, everything which has the slightest tendency to discompose the invalid.

Mere visitors should not be allowed to remain in the sick-room more than five minutes, just long enough to allow a friendly greeting, and the expression of a hope that soon all will be well again, with the communication of such intelligence as might make a pleasant impression on the mind. Avoid questioning very sick persons as to the state of their health. They seldom know exactly how they are; are rarely good judges of their condition. They may feel as if they did not know whether they were any better or worse, and the very effort to come to a truthful decision in their own minds is at times quite exhausting, especially if the questions are repeated by the nurse or every visitor. A good nurse will know how the patient is without inquiry a great deal better than the patient, than convalescents especially; for as persons are getting well, particularly from serious or long illness, they are very desponding, and often think they are going to die, when it is clear to the physician and nurse that the crisis is just over, and that recovery is quite certain.

Nor should the nurse ask the patient if anything is wanted, or what he will have. Nine times out of ten the sick don't know what they want, and instinctively avoid the effort of deciding what they want. Besides, they are very apt to want what it would be very unwise to give. Then it is mere trifling to ask the question.

A competent nurse can anticipate a patient's needs, leaving wants out of the question; can tell better than the patient what is required, and what is best to be done.

Whatever is said to a patient should be as hopeful and assuring as is compatible with truthfulness ; and it is only necessary to suggest that every expression should be avoided which is calculated to excite apprehension or even disquietude, such as " You have changed a great deal," " I would not have known you," " You are very sick," " I am afraid you will not get well," and yet these things have been said to the sick.

Never whisper in a sick-room, or speak in a low tone. Let everything uttered be in a clear voice, distinctly enunciated, so that the patient may hear it. This self-evident propriety is too. often disregarded by even rational people. Never look sideways at a patient, or seem to be scanning him. On the other hand, never stare. The moment you are out of conversation, leave the room. It is not uncommon to see a person sit with his eyes fixed on the patient for one, two, or more minutes, not knowing what to say, compelling the sick one to keep up the conversation ; or, if they do talk, the remarks are of the most commonplace kind.

Never wake a patient, even to give medicine or to dress a wound, for sleeping is a healing process, giving strength and life. In almost all sickness a tendency to sleep is a favorable sign.

Let the patient alone. This is said in reference to many who wait on the sick who are incessantly doing something, either fixing up the room, adjusting the bed-clothes, or making some change, all of which tend to break up the quiet so necessary to an invalid. On the other hand, if the patient is in his right mind, and seems disposed to talk, or is inclined to ask questions, then it is advantageous to engage in conversation, but do not allow it to fall into a line of despondency. The good nurse will know how to lead the way to subjects which are interesting and cheering.

It is better to have two nurses in serious cases, so as to alternate several times in the twenty-four hours, for a sleepy or an overtaxed nurse can easily kill a patient whose life is hanging by a thread.

Avoid as much as possible bringing in a new nurse, especially a stranger. It discomposes the patient. The introduction into the house of a new servant is disquieting to healthy people.

It is better to have a woman to nurse a man. There is a gentleness, a sympathy in woman. There is a magnetism in her touch, in the softness of her voice; a carrying away the mind to mother and sister, which is peculiarly grateful to a sick man. Besides, a woman has that instinctiveness of perception of what is needed, of what would add to the patient's comfort in a thousand little ways, which is of infinite advantage.

On the other hand, a man nurse is best for a woman, who feels all the time as if she wanted strength under her, firmness. It is best for a sick woman to feel all the time she "must." She will bend to a man's will; she would to a woman's, never. She imperatively needs confidence, reliance, some one to look to. This gives courage and hopefulness, very necessary elements as helps in recovery from disease.

The patient should have all the clothing of the body changed once a day; and, if possible, the bed should be made night and morning. And several times during the day and night the bedclothes should be raised up from the body and let fall again, so as to drive out the confined air; or they should be thrown back towards the feet, to allow a full airing, while both bedclothes and body clothing should be kept most scrupulously clean. If at any time a drop of blood or other soiling should take place, the garment should be changed.

Prevent all surprises to a patient, especially disagreeable ones. To this end allow no one not of the household to enter a sickroom without first acquainting the sufferer, and getting permission; ascertaining also that it is a hearty assent.

The nurse owes several duties to the medical attendant,—

First. Be able to give a clear, plain, and connected history of the case since his last visit. Mention all striking occurrences; if instructions have not been strictly followed; if the medicines have not been taken as directed, or if taken, rejected before they could operate; notice the color, quantity, and consistence of all the bodily discharges, and if possible, especially in critical cases, preserve them, outside the doors of the house, for his inspection. There are times and conditions when life depends on these things.

Second. Notice whether the patient sleeps much or little; if there is any tendency to being out of his mind, to mutterings, or moanings, or sighs.

Nursing is an art, a science, an acquisition. Many a time a disease is conquered, but the patient fails to get well for want of proper attention, from injudiciousness in eating, to avoid which a good nurse will always make it a point to ascertain clearly and distinctly from the physician what the patient is to eat, how often, and how much, until he returns.

As a very general rule, sick persons should not eat oftener than at intervals of five hours, unless so weak that but very little if anything can be taken at a time. Then it may be better to eat oftener, at less intervals; but these are rare exceptions, and it is better to let the physician mark them out. One rule is always applicable: take but a few mouthfuls of any strange or unusual food or drink. Require the patient to-eat slowly, and cut up all food very fine. Meats especially should be in pieces not larger than a pea, for then they are more easily dissolved in the juices of the stomach, as small bits of ice are sooner melted in a glass of water than large ones.

RECAPITULATION.

1. Be quiet.
2. Be decided.
3. Be composed.
4. Be firm.
5. Be sympathetic.
6. Consult your patient's wants, but do it as seldom as possible, to save him from the mental labor of comparing and weighing reasons, and deciding for himself.
7. Never seem to compel your patient to do anything, but lead him to do what is right; this is the triumph of good management.
8. Be clear in all your communications, and distinct in every word or syllable you say, without being loud or severe. The very effort at listening is sometimes exhaustive of the little strength the invalid has.
9. Never peep, nor poke, nor pother.
10. No trickeries nor deceptions in the sick-chamber.
11. Be always on the alert.
12. Sameness is terrible to one who has been long an invalid; hence, make some change in the room every day; not many, one or two at a time. Either change the position of some one or two things already in the room, or introduce a picture or painting, or even a bunch of flowers; these often enliven a room very much;

at one time on the mantel, at another on the table, or in the window. Flowers of bright colors are best, if placed in among green sprigs, avoiding those of a strong or coarse odor. If a picture, let it be lively; let it be of the spring time, of childhood, or pastures green, with the lambkins or the little chickens; something which will remind of youth and innocence. These may appear to be small matters to the well and hearty, but to the poor invalid, who has been at death's door for weary weeks and months, and is just rising up to light and life again, they have an incalculable value, and for their sake and good, especial attention should be given to the suggestions.

The effervescing, the overflowing, the irrepressible good-humor of Franklin made a way for him wherever he went; in Christian America, in the halls of Congress, in infidel France, in the age of her disgraceful and inhuman and bloody revolution, Franklin was alike successful in carrying out his political purposes. What a life lights up in every eye, how instinctively a private company or a public crowd make way for a man who is known to be full of fun, to be a jovial soul. But good nature has its foundation in good health, in an industrious, temperate life, with a loving heart at the bottom of it all. And how much more will it help to buoy up the spirits of the invalid, and antagonize the depressions which so retard the recovery of the sick!

SICKNESS

and pain and suffering are the result of an unequal circulation of blood in the body, too little at one point, too much at another; equalizing that circulation, so that each part of the system shall have its natural and healthful share, is appropriately called

THE PRACTICE OF MEDICINE,

And the persons who bring about this result are termed Physicians, from the Greek word *Phusis*, which means Nature, as the physician brings about the natural order of things in the body.

In the early ages, when a man was sick he would place himself at the entrance of the town, or at the gate of the city, in the hope that some one passing might be able to tell him what would effect a cure, from his having had the malady himself. It was then very natural for the man who was thus cured to speak of it to others who might be afflicted in the same or in any similar way, and for the sake of going to headquarters the question would be put, What was his name, where does he live, "what did he do to thee? How opened he thine eyes?"

This man being visited at his house, taking up his time to restore a stranger to health, and succeeding, would be entitled to more than the mere thanks of one who had been so much benefited, and in gratitude the convalescent would compensate him to a certain extent in the form of a present. This is the method to this day in Heidelberg and other parts of Germany; the physicians there make no charge for their services, but leave it to the patient to give what he pleases.

It is very easy to see that after a man has been called upon at first for one disease, then for a similar affection, he would naturally extend his knowledge and his skill from the mere force of observation and experience, and in the course of years would become skilful and of repute.

In the progress of civilization the sick could not visit the physician, but he, being well, could visit the sick; and as this would take time, it very naturally came about that he should be paid for his services, and, as in all other callings, fix his own price, as physicians now do. But in these later years, when all things—time and skill, among others—have high values, and as in civilization it is the tendency of the poor to become poorer, and the rich richer, only the rich and the well-to-do can pay for personal medical services; the masses cannot indulge in the luxury of having a physician drive to their doors in his carriage, for the use of him, his vehicle, his horses, and his coachman has to be paid for; hence these poor people must suffer in patience until time, the great restorer and destroyer, brings about the result of health or death.

It would seem, then, a humanity for a physician to write his experiences, and those of others, in the course of ages and centuries, for the benefit of those who are too sick to come to him, and too poor to have him come to them. In this way, the cost of a single medical visit in a great city would supply a family with a volume, giving information by which the name and nature of ordinary ailments could be known, telling what things would benefit and cure such ailments, and how best to use them to that end. Such is the object, aim, and end in the preparation of this volume, as also to meet other requirements of emergencies in sickness and accident when there is no time to wait—when something must be done on the spot, or the man is dead; an artery has been divided, and the red blood spurts out in jets so rapidly that if not arrested on the instant, as in the case mentioned in the preface, a life becomes extinct in a few moments, but could be saved had it been known that a common handkerchief tied loosely around the arm above the wound,—that is, between the wound and the heart,—a short stick run through it and twisted down until the blood ceases to flow, would give time for the surgeon to arrive and stanch the wound. A member of the family takes by mistake a large amount of laudanum or a swallow or two of oxalic acid dissolved in water, or corrosive sublimate in liquid form, both used for domestic purposes; something must be done within ten minutes or death ensues. It is a positive humanity to have in the house a book giving plain information which will save life, by turning to the proper chapter, where it will be seen that there are two kinds of poisons, those which are called "corrosive," and those which are constitutional, requiring less haste; it is there seen that all corrosive poisons give a sensation of scalding in the throat on the instant; constitutional poisons, such as morphia, opium, paregoric, laudanum, and the like may be swallowed without any hurting or pain, and their effects come on slowly, usually giving abundant time to obtain a physician. In the case of the virulent or corrosive poison something must be swallowed on the instant which will not only soothe the throat in its passage to the stomach, but will rapidly mix with the swallowed poison in the stomach, and dilute it so largely that it will be prevented from burning the coats of the stomach, as it did the throat; here nothing could be more appropriately done than to swallow half a pint of sweet oil, an article which almost every family has in the house. That is the best kind of oil to be taken, because it is the mildest; if that cannot be obtained, then butter, as soon as it can be made thin enough by melting to admit of swallowing, or linseed oil, in fact any greasy or oily thing, hog's lard, goose grease, and the like. The principle is, swallow instantly some kind of mild, oily substance which will antagonize the poison in the manner named.

If, on the other hand, laudanum or morphia or any other narcotic has been swallowed in dangerous quantities, the first best remedy is to mix a tablespoonful of salt and a tablespoon of ground mustard; stir them rapidly in a glass of warm or cool water and drink it down; on the instant of its reaching the stomach it will so irritate it as to cause vomiting and the whole contents will be thrown up, poison and all; the principle being to get it out of the stomach before it can have any injurious effect; then, for fear every particle of the poison might not have been ejected, swallow the whites of two or three eggs; if the hurry is great, swallow yolk, whites, and all; but it is the white of the egg which has a chemical effect on the poison, making it innocuous; if eggs are not at hand, drink a cup of strong coffee, which also antagonizes all poisons in small quantities of the nature of opium, morphine, and the like.

So it is with reference to every variety of accident which is liable to befall any member of any family, a book in the house which can be turned to with confidence, which gives safe directions and with perfect plainness, is of an incomparable value in · the household of the crowded city as well as at the secluded hut or farm-house in the country; for persons who have lived long in a great city have come to the knowledge of cases where a physician could not be had within an hour or two or three, or at midnight in storms of wind or rain or hail; or about eleven o'clock in the forenoon, when city practitioners are on their rounds of visiting for the day, many of them not to return for three or four hours. In the country, it is still more disastrous to need medical aid at midnight, or on an emergency in the day-time; the doctor's shop two, three, or ten miles away, and no other physician within as many miles in any direction; for reaching his house in time to learn that he has gone in an opposite direction to superintend a confinement, and there is no knowing when he will return; and as every household is liable to have such and similar cases to occur at any time, it is scarcely less than a criminal negligence to have no

" FAMILY DOCTOR "

in the house in the shape of a plain and reliable health-advising book, such as this volume aims to be. It is true that such books are almost universally condemned by educated physicians, as doing more harm than good, which is possible; but that results from a defect in the book, and not the principle on which it is sought to be distributed all over the country. Medical books for family use hitherto have failed to meet the family wants in several most important respects. They failed to designate the ailment with sufficient clearness to enable the ordinary reader to decide certainly whether the symptoms observed were those of a malady in hand ; it was necessary to know what the disease was, before they could obtain the information needed as a means of cure.

They failed to tell the nature of the disease, what conditions were induced by it, and how the remedies removed those conditions.

They failed to tell how the remedies employed were expected to operate; hence, in many cases, where the medicine was old and had lost its power, while the patient was waiting to get better from its use, not knowing how it should act, invaluable time was lost. In ordinary family medicine-books, in describing any particular disease, a dozen or more symptoms are mentioned as attending that disease ; but perhaps on the very next page, another disease would be described with nearly all the symptoms of the other ; hence the person seeing these two descriptions would be unable, without long study and painful uncertainty, to decide in his own mind what was the disease in hand.

It is well known among medical lecturers that in speaking of different diseases to the young gentlemen attending the first year's course, they frequently imagine that they have each disease as it is lectured upon.

In these pages these objections are sought to be obviated ; for example, take one case which will exemplify all—very few know the difference between diarrhœa and dysentery. The same causes can produce both diseases. There are quite a number of symptoms common to both, such as fever, thirst, quick pulse, frequent passages, no appetite, pain, restlessness, dry skin, a feeling of despondency, of utter giving up, as if the bed was the most comfortable place possible, and no desire to leave it—all these things may be said of both ailments, yet no hint is given by which it could be told with positive certainty which was the disease present. The principles proposed in this volume relieve the reader from such a vexing uncertainty; for, instead of mentioning a dozen different symptoms, the one or two things are named without which one of these diseases could not possibly be present:

5

thus, dysentery means a discharge of blood from the bowels; bleeding piles is also a discharge from the bowels; but the thing which makes it dysentery, and it being present, and always present, rendering it absolutely impossible for it to be anything else than

DYSENTERY,

is the fact that these bloody discharges are always attended with an intolerable tormina and tenesmus, as the doctors express it—a distressing bearing down and straining; there is an urgent feeling of desire to go to stool; but on attempting to do something, to evacuate, nothing comes; or, if anything comes, it is a little blood, not at all satisfying of the desire to discharge. Dysentery, then, is a discharge of blood from the bowels, with a distressing sensation, and unless it is blood it cannot be dysentery. In some cases, in most cases, afterwards, in treating of the subject, it may be necessary to mention other than the distinctive symptoms of the disease; but it is our plan to first give, as far as possible, the very few symptoms which belong to the disease, and no other.

The point aimed at when a case of sickness is presented, is to direct the reader's mind to the prominent, to the most striking symptom, the one which most impressively strikes the attention; for example—

CROUP,

the peculiar cough which, when once heard by a mother, can never be forgotten or mistaken, is a cough belonging to no other known disease, a kind of barking, wheezing cough, bringing nothing with it; and to make it more certain, if indeed anything else were required to show that it was croup, there is the distressing breathing, short and heavily.

The reader is made acquainted with the essential nature of the disease, that it is a closing up of the windpipe by the gradual formation of a tough lining getting thicker and thicker until the windpipe is clogged up, and breathing and life cease together. It is explained that the object of the remedies used is to detach this substance, to loosen it, so that it may come away in whole or in part; if then, within a few moments, the whole formation comes away in a body or in detached pieces, then the mother knows in an instant that the remedy has taken effect, that what was intended to be done has been done, and that a cure is certain. But suppose this explanation of the nature of the disease and of what the medicine was intended to accomplish had not been made, the medicine would have been blindly given, and not knowing what it was expected to do, the anxious, trembling, and despairing parent waits in agony, and while she waits, if the medicine had lost its virtue, the child dies.

For these reasons it is hoped that this family medicine book will supply a want which has never been met by any of its predecessors at home or abroad, not only in these particulars but in many others, which the intelligent reader will find out as he turns over the pages.

It is earnestly desired to impress on the mind

TWO ESSENTIAL THINGS.

1st. Call a doctor wherever you can, and thus relieve yourself from a very painful feeling of responsibility and a most distressing sense of groping in the dark ; and

2d. Read at leisure, when not disturbed with a case of sickness in the family, the first chapters of the book under the heading of Sickness,

Principles of Medical Practice, and

Congestion.

These will give you a clear and comprehensive idea of the whole theory of the nature of disease and the philosophy of the practice of medicine. You will then have such an intelligent view of the scope of the book, that the perusal of any chapter and the management of any case yourself, when a physician cannot be had, will be a source of the very deepest interest, and will enable you to observe disease with an understanding and with an intelligence which will be deeply gratifying.

It was said in the beginning that disease consisted in the irregular circulation of the blood, and that its cure was accomplished by equalizing this circulation, causing the blood to be sent to every part of the body in its natural and healthful quantity. The physician does not send it there ; he has only to remove obstructions, to remove an overloading, that is, to clear out channels which are filled up (see article on "Congestion"), and Nature takes the remainder of the work in hand. In all diseases there is excess of blood somewhere; take away that excess and the circulation assumes its natural conditions, as a spring rebounds to its proper place the moment the pressure is removed.

The practice of medicine, then, consists in equalizing the circulation in such a manner that no part of the body shall have more than its natural healthful share of blood. There are half a dozen ways of causing the blood to be distributed in proper proportions to the different parts of the body, but the office which medicine is to perform in bringing about this result will be exemplified in these pages in connection with the treatment of the various diseases to which the human body is exposed; it is designed here to show what is first to be done in all ordinary cases of sickness, what is most applicable and most efficient, and how to make the application which seldom or never comes amiss.

Warmth, quiet, and purgation are the very first things to be brought about in an attack of sickness. These, better than all others, withdraw excess of blood from the parts suffering, and send it to such as most require its life-giving influences. Warmth, by inducing more or less of perspiration, lessens the quantity of blood in the body, besides rendering it more liquid, for cold congeals it.

Purgation, as explained under its proper heading, also diminishes, to a large extent, the quantity of the blood, and removes a vast amount of the solid wastes and worn-out and effete matters, which, if allowed to remain, would only poison the blood, and thus render it unfit for the purposes of life.

Warmth is best secured by being put to bed, the clothing tucked closely in at the sides, drinking meanwhile large draughts of any pleasant tea, or even simple hot water. If the feet are cold, place close up to them hot bottles or bricks wrapped in woollen, which will maintain the heat longest; if this is not sufficient, bottles of hot water may be placed at the arm pits, and cushions of warm salt, or ashes—which are lighter—over the pit of the stomach; if these are managed in such a way as to induce free perspiration, and this is kept up half an hour, or long enough to give considerable relief, then it is important to cool off very gradually, requiring half an hour to do it; first laying one covering half back, then three-quarters, as far down as the knees, giving the legs and feet extra covering; then it may be well to place one arm out from under cover, then another, and so on until the patient is comfortably cooled, and yet feels comfortably warm. But these good effects would be greatly increased if, before putting the patient to bed, an enema was administered (which see); or, if the bowels have not acted within twenty-four hours, take a dose of castor-oil (which see); or, better still, a purgative or liver pill, as a means of more radical relief and a permanent cure. There is scarcely a fever that can be named, not a single malady of the throat, lungs, or bowels, not a pain or ache in the whole body, which would not be more or less alleviated by the treatment named, if anything could alleviate.

If parents could be persuaded, could be made to feel that it was their duty to render themselves adepts in administering the few remedial means just alluded to, and do it promptly, it would forestall more than half the sufferings from ordinary ailments; if adopted the moment a person is known to have taken cold, it would avert and cut short off nine-tenths of all the colds to which humanity is liable, and thus prevent an incalculable amount of sickness, suffering, and premature death.

While medicines are a great blessing when judiciously administered, the time comes to every one, sooner or later, when they utterly fail of their legitimate effects, for

MAN IS BORN TO DIE.

There are other cases where the patient is in the condition of one of old, who "suffered many things of many physicians," and was nothing better, but rather grew worse! Sometimes such a result arises from the fact that the appropriate medicine has not been administered.

When the medicine seems to do no good, then cease taking it, and aim to recover from the sickness by attending to the

GENERAL HEALTH.

And it is especially requested that the chapter on that subject should be read repeatedly, thoughtfully, and with great care; in fact, it is of vital importance for the following reason :—

Medicine sometimes brings the patient forward to a certain point of health, there it seems to lose all further effect; then the only means left of completing the cure are those which keep up the general health to the highest possible point; for in doing this the blood is to that extent purified, made health-giving, vitalizing, and as it is sent to the most distant parts of the body, as well as to those parts which are inaccessible to the physician, these parts are vitalized, and health is gradually restored.   Very many cases of

INCIPIENT CONSUMPTION

Could be arrested if means were adopted to keep up the general health in the manner described in the article under that heading.

One of the most prevalent of all female diseases, for which innumerable washes and lotions have been devised from time immemorial, has never yet been remedied permanently and radically by any of them, or by any medicine, except in proportion as these have had an influence in keeping up the general health.   Many persons find themselves in a condition expressively described in the sentence : "The least thing in the world gives me a cold."   There may be no specific disease in the system at the time, no special organ is particularly out of order to which medicine might be directed, there is only a general want of vigor to resist the ordinary causes of bad colds.   The best means of breaking up this remarkable susceptibility to colds is to improve the general health, that is, give greater purity to the blood ; that purity gives it a vigor of circulation which wakes up all the activities of the constitution, and very generally produces effects such as described.

ILLUSTRATION.

During this writing a young lady of twenty, in Boston, was taken with bleeding at the lungs, in small quantities, repeated during several days, a hard heavy cough, difficult breathing on lying down, and excessive debility, with no appetite.   Several of her schoolmates had recently been taken in the same way and died; these symptoms pointed to the lungs as the diseased part ; they were so full of blood that the vessels were barely able to contain it, in fact some little was oozing out all the time ; the face was pale, the tongue very much coated, showing that the blood was tending internally about the lungs and liver and heart.   Both lungs and liver needed prompt relief ; the want of it too long would endanger life, in fact had been fatal to several others.   As soon as attention was brought to the case,

All eating from the instant was prohibited.

To be kept warm in bed.   To take a liver pill.

That pill acted, of itself, very largely within twelve hours; within twenty hours after the pill was swallowed the patient was hungry! The face regained its natural color,

THE BLEEDING CEASED,

the tongue was clearing off, the cough disappeared altogether; in two days the patient got about again, and no further medical attention was needed, because of the prompt action of the friends without that loss of time, hoping it would pass off of itself when the debility was all the while increasing, and the heart and lungs becoming more and more oppressed; in this case the calomel cleared out the gorged, congested channels of the liver, diminished largely the bulk of the blood, as explained in the article on "Congestion," and the patient saved from the prescription of the physician several hundred miles away; a case very grave, and to the point as illustrating the doctrine of

CONGESTION,

of too much blood at a part, as the cause of disease; and the philosophy of the treatment, in diminishing the quantity of the blood in the whole body, and proportionally of the part affected, as a means of cure, by means of medicines which act upon the liver and the bowels also.

It is of little consequence where pain and disease are, in what part of the body, in ordinary ailments; the course to be pursued is the same—diminish the amount of blood in the body, and that diminution will make itself felt in any ailing part.

BATHS AND BATHING.

THE room in which a bath is taken should be at seventy-five degrees F., or, in the absence of a thermometer, it should not be so cool as to cause an unpleasant sensation of coldness when the body emerges from the water.

For ordinary purposes of cleanliness the bath should be of warm water with soap, rubbed well in with the hand or sponge, reaching every part of the body possible, rinsing off afterwards so that there shall be no soap left on the skin; in wiping dry with a towel, friction should not be spared, laying the towel flat on the hand, keeping the mouth closed, then rub with a will nearly as hard as the hand can press, then for a minute or two more rub in the same way all over with the hands; this tends to soothe and soften the skin and impart a pleasant warmth to the surface.   In taking this warm cleansing bath the water should indicate ninety-five degrees F.; seventy-five, for a cold bath; eighty-five, tepid; a hundred and five, hot.   In taking a tepid or   .

COLD BATH,

the head should be wet with cold water, or forehead and face well washed with cold water, before getting into the bath tub.   If the feet are cold, they should be soaked in hot water, half leg deep, until completely warm, before getting into the bath.   These baths should be taken rapidly, the hands kept gently rubbing the limbs and body all the time, so as to keep up the circulation and thus prevent a feeling of chilliness, and, for the same reason, as soon as the body is out of the water it should be promptly and actively rubbed with a towel until perfectly dry, for if a feeling of chill runs over it, in the water or out of it, a great deal more harm has been done than good, by the whole process; in addition, dress quickly, and if not perfectly comfortable as to warmth, take a brisk walk immediately, or chop or saw wood, or do some other thing which will restore the circulation; if at night, or the weather is unsuitable, either go to a good fire, or into the kitchen, or to bed and wrap up, or dance vigorously until a sensation of comfortable warmth has been brought about, for persons have taken a chill in the bath which has resulted in death.   The precaution should always be taken, in all forms of bathing, to stand on a piece of woollen carpet or mat in emerging from a bath, because it is essentially important that the feet should be warm; for coming in contact with the cold floor or oil-cloth a chill may be sent through the whole body.   A gentleman in the advanced stages of consumption attributed his disease to standing on a piece of zinc on the bath-room floor, after taking his bath and while rubbing himself dry.

TIME FOR BATHING.

Persons in vigorous health, near the sea or river or lake, may safely walk half a mile before breakfast, jump in over head, swim around for five or ten minutes; dress quickly, walk rapidly home and take breakfast, and be all the better for it in summer-time. But for all ordinary purposes, a bath should be taken about ten or eleven o'clock in the forenoon; having taken breakfast three hours earlier, for the human system is more vigorous at that time of day than at any other hour of the twenty-four, as it is at its lowest ebb about five o'clock in the morning, hence it is that more persons die at that hour than at any other of the twenty-four, under ordinary circumstances.

A bath can do no good, but will always do harm, if the person is

TIRED.

Nor should any kind of bath be taken sooner than three hours after a regular meal, nor later than an hour or two before eating. Many persons have been found dead in the bath-room from taking a bath soon after a hearty dinner, even a warm bath.

BATH FOR FEVER.

If a person goes into a cold bath to cool off a fever, a hurtful and dangerous shock and chill may take place; it is safer and better, far more comfortable, and more efficient in cooling off the body, to have the water at eighty-five, bathe for a while, then gradually reduce it, but by no means to the extent of causing an uncomfortable feeling of coldness. It is safer to bathe in warm water to cool off a fever of the whole body, throwing the water upon it, running off, and thus allowing the evaporation to carry off the surplus heat.

In all forms of bathing, hot, cold, or tepid, a damp towel or wetted cap should be worn on the head, or if the hair is short, it should be wetted several times. The most effective way of doing which is to douse the whole head and ears under water, the object being to prevent an excess of blood from going to the head; fatal apoplexy has resulted in many cases from failing to take this precaution, of keeping the whole head wet or cold in all forms of bathing. The articles used for wiping off the body after a bath should be soft.

If a person takes a bath in a frail or feeble condition of the system, the whole body should be invested in a sheet the moment of emerging from the water and rubbed dry with it; this prevents chilliness; then the whole surface of the body should be rubbed with the hands, all over the body as far as can be reached in every direction, mouth closed, bearing on with the hands as hard as convenient; this aids in promoting the circulation, in expanding the lungs, and softening and warming the skin; if the person is feeble, then this hand-rubbing should be performed by an attendant; in either case it should be done with rapidity and energy, and completed within three minutes if there is any tendency to chilliness, for if a single chill runs over the body, or along the back, during or soon after the bathing, more harm has been done than good, hence any feeling of chilliness should be guarded against with great care; after dressing rapidly, the invalid should go to the fire or into the sunshine, while those who are able should take a brisk and extended walk, or engage in some form of vigorous exercise involving muscular activities in the open air, to invigorate the circulation and bring it to a healthful glow to the very extremities of the system; sometimes in feeble persons it is best to go to bed, wrap up warm, and perhaps go to sleep, for to them rest from the tiredness or fatigue of the bath is of more importance than exercise, the warmth of the bed being a greater aid towards keeping up the circulation than motion of the limbs. But in all cases of bathing, if after a couple of hours there is a sense of weakness or fatigue or tiredness, an indisposition to move around, then the bath has been an injury.

A HALF-BATH

is taken by sitting in a vessel of water, six inches deep, feet extended, wetting the head and forehead first with cold water; then rubbing the limbs with the hands and throwing the water on the body and back, all being done in two or three minutes by the patient or an attendant, according to the strength. If it is required to be done quickly, one person should rub the legs, another the back, and the bather the front part of the body; this gives him some exercise and tends to prevent chilliness, all hands rubbing briskly but lightly, throwing up the water on the body.

PLUNGE-BATH.

Go to the river or lake or sea-shore, undress quickly, wet the head and forehead well, jump in head over heels, swim around a few minutes, wipe dry, dress quickly, and walk away rapidly. This is for a healthy person, in warm weather. In cold weather there should be a tub or box of water four or five feet deep, broad enough to allow the bather to place the hands on the sides and jump in or out; allow the water to come to the chin, and conduct the whole operation to prevent chilliness. If the person is feeble this bath should be taken in bed, and should be performed by attendants; only a limb or small part of the body to be uncovered at a time, an arm or a limb extending over the side of the bed, using a soft towel dipped in tepid water, rubbing dry quickly with a soft cloth and then using the hands with quick friction. Judiciously done this is a great comfort to one having a burning fever in the hands and feet; if the body is hot it is very agreeable to treat the back in this way, but in all these forms have a care not to weary the patient much, for weariness predisposes to chilliness, which would be unfortunate, and in the reaction would increase the heat and fever. This mode of bathing, for purposes of mitigating fever, may be performed several times a day.

TOWEL BATH.

With all the clothing off, standing on a woollen mat, having wetted the head and forehead, dip a cloth in the water, press it out so as not to dribble, lay it flat on the palm of the hand, and with mouth closed and chest protuberant, rub the whole body well. This for a healthy person answers the purpose of a bath and cleanliness, can be done in one's own room every morning in a few minutes, and without soiling the nicest carpet; it may be done to advantage every morning in summer and in winter, answers the purpose of a regular bath very well; it should be followed by a minute's rapid hand-rubbing, dressing quickly; the whole operation, at least in winter, not to exceed three minutes.

THE DRIPPING SHEET.

Dip a sheet in water of the required temperature, and taking it by the two corners, extending it, place it on the bather, very much as a shawl is placed by another on a lady's shoulders. This sheet should reach to the floor, and should envelope the whole person, rubbing with both hands over the sheet. After rubbing a minute over the back of body and limbs, put the sheet in the water again and place it on the front of the body, and proceed as before.

DOUCHE-BATH.

The water should be as high as eighty degrees; two, three, or half a dozen pails of water should be thrown on a person in quick succession, he turning around all the time, so that all parts of the body may receive the water; if the floor is slanting, or the person stands on slats laid across the floor, then the water runs off.

THE PACK-BATH

is a remedy on which hydropathists place great reliance, and when properly managed is of very great efficiency in a variety of diseases, but liable to abuse, as other valuable remedies are. It is better taken on a lounge or cot, having ready for use several blankets or comfortables, to spread upon it, with a pillow. Over these spread a wet sheet—not dripping—reaching to below the knees, making the upper part to extend high enough up to be wrapped around the head, lie on the back, the arms at the sides, draw the sheet quickly from the further side under the chin, and tuck it under on the side next the operator, and all along down the body to the feet. Next treat the near side of the sheet in the same way, then the blanket and the comfortables, being careful to wrap these round the feet well, to keep them warm; if they seem inclined to be cold, place hot bottles or bricks or blankets to them, outside the blanket which folds them.

If, before taking the pack, there is any particular pain or ailment in any portion of the body, any extra amount of blood, venous or arterial, such as over the lungs, heart, and stomach, wring a flannel of several thicknesses in water and lay it over the part before wrapping the wet sheet.

If it was previously found that the person was much inclined to chilliness in getting on the wet sheet, lay a strip of flannel, six or eight inches broad, several folds, wrung out of hot water, on the wet sheet, so as to lie against the backbone inside the sheet; lay a cool towel on the forehead, and allow the patient quiet and sleep if desired, the attendant being present; remain in the sheet until comfortably warm, which usually happens in half an hour; sometimes an hour elapses in persons of feeble circulation. Feeble persons should have a dry sheet thrown around them the instant of emerging from the pack; others may take a rapid general bath.

THE SITZ-BATH.

Take a common-sized tub with enough water to enable the patient to sit in it without its overflowing; remove all the clothing, except shoes and stockings, and as soon as seated in the bath have the whole body enveloped with a comfortable or blanket; if the feet are cold, they should be placed in a vessel of warm water, having the head wrapped in a wet cloth, remaining in the bath near half an hour.

FOOT-BATH.

It is better to have a wooden pail, not very broad, so that it need not require a great deal of hot water when a hot foot-bath is taken, for when such a one is necessary, it is important to add hot water from time to time, that it may be at least as hot when the feet are taken out as when put in.

In taking a hot foot-bath, the vessel should be deep enough to allow the water to come up near the knees.

A TOE-BATH

is advantageous sometimes after a hot bath, to cause a reaction. In such cases there should be cold water enough to cover the toes when the feet are in, both in at once, and to remain in not longer than half a minute; such a bath adds greatly to the efficiency of a hot bath. As soon as the feet are taken out of the water, rub them dry, and hold them to a blazing fire, if convenient, having them rubbed with the hands until perfectly dry and warm in every part.

FOMENTATIONS

are valuable remedial means, often removing distressing pains and dangerous congestions. Let the patient lie on a doubled blanket, have a flannel of half a dozen thicknesses wrung out of very hot water placed on the feet, draw the dry blanket over the body to keep it warm, tuck it in on both sides, and then spread over the other bed-clothing; as soon as the wet blanket begins to feel cool, say in ten minutes, then apply another hot one, hot enough to feel comfortable, being careful to have a cold, wet cloth on the head, and to have the feet wrapped up warm; when satisfactory relief has been obtained, remove everything, wash quickly in cool water, say of eighty-five degrees, and dry; the object being by the warm applications to open the pores of the skin and allow free exhalations, so as to relieve the parts; then by the cold water to close the pores of the skin, and thus drive back the blood, to prevent that new accumulation which would but renew the trouble which it was the object to remove.

TO TAKE A SWEAT

Get in a sitz-bath, with the feet in a hot bath, all as warm as can be well borne, cover the whole body, and add hot water from time to time as the other cools; keep the head well wet with cold water all the time; after the perspiration has continued long enough, take quickly a half-bath or dripping sheet, at not lower than eighty degrees, for an instant only and go to bed at once.

The favorite hydropathic method of curing a bad cold, recently taken by a healthy person, is to take a profuse sweat, go instantly to a pack of eighty degrees, followed by a dripping sheet, go to bed, and for two or three days eating sparingly of coarse breads, fruits, and vegetables.

STOMACH BATH

may be of hot water or cold; if it is wished to cause vomiting, drink water of the most sickening temperature to the patient, from ninety to a hundred degrees, a teacupful every five minutes until the stomach relieves itself fully; when desirable to keep up the vomiting, continue the water; if the person is sick at stomach to begin with, vomiting usually takes place by the time a pint or two of water has been swallowed. The stomach is sometimes " washed out" with cold water when it is feverish or when there is great thirst; this may be a means of causing an action of the bowels; or on rising in the morning, free action of the bowels is induced by after breakfast, if several glasses of cold water are drunk.

RECTAL BATHS,

or injections, clysters, or enemas (the last is the name preferred by physicians) means throwing up into the rectum, or lower bowel, fluid substances, mainly for the purpose of obviating constipation, either by dissolving the hardened fæces, or by causing such a distention of the parts as to excite the natural desire for their expulsion. Pure water is usually employed, cool or warm or tepid ; they all act in the same way—distend the bowel. It is usually best to have the temperature most agreeable to the patient ; sometimes a little salt is added to the water in the belief that it has some stimulating effect on the parts, above that of cold water. Half a pint or pint may be thrown up, enough to produce the intended effect of a contraction of the bowels, which is an operation like that of emptying a bladder of fluid by pressing it with the hand, only that the bowel causes the expulsion by the power it has of contracting upon itself.

This is a method of relieving the system when there is urgency, or when all medicines fail, as is sometimes the case. Under such circumstances an enema is permissible, but to employ it frequently as a means of avoiding constipation, or of removing costiveness, is objectionable, because the oftener it is done the more nature seems to require the aid, oftener and oftener, until such a habit has been established that the bowels are evacuated only when an injection is taken, and a lifetime habit is established of taking an injection every day, which involves an immense amount of trouble and inconvenience and discomfort, and yet there are not a few who have arrived at this most unnatural condition of things, from not knowing the tendency of injections persisted in.

When persons cannot swallow, both food and medicines have been thrown up the rectum as a substitute for taking them into the stomach, but with not any very encouraging results.

VAGINAL BATHS,

or injections, are used as a means of cleansing the parts and of giving them tone. In cases of leucorrhœa great good has been done by the use of water, as cleansing, but much injury by impregnating it with astringents, such as alum, the infusion of white-oak bark, buchu, and similar substances, for they are not curative, they only palliate, give temporary relief, thus losing valuable time which ought to be employed in the cure, in the eradication of the malady; for the longer it remains in the system the more it debilitates, and the more difficult it is of removal.

LOCAL BATHS.

Sometimes it is of advantage to throw a stream of water against a particular part of the body to remove swelling, or painful inflammations or congestions; very painful sprains and strains have been greatly benefited by this means; sometimes a stream of water along the spine is of very great service. In cities and private houses where water is supplied by means of pipes, the following expedient will afford the means of such local baths, vaginal or otherwise: Have an india-rubber tube of any convenient length, large enough at the end to be drawn over the mouth of the faucet through which the water is to come; to the other end have an ivory mouth attached, with a fixture which by a turn will let on or shut off the water; with such an apparatus water can be directed in a stream to any portion of the body, and can be made to subserve many valuable purposes.

Where there are no water-pipes, have a barrel of water in the room above, with a hole in the floor, or raise the barrel several feet in the same room, or have it outside on an elevated platform, attach to it a tube like the tube above named, only longer; the quantity and force of the water used can be regulated by the stop-cock or screw at the ivory end.

WET BANDAGES

can be made to subserve a variety of good uses; if properly managed great medicinal effects can be accomplished by them. The best material for the purpose is soft Irish linen of a heavy material, although common muslin will answer a good purpose.

ABDOMINAL BANDAGES

when applicable, should be from six to fourteen inches broad, and long enough to go around the body once and a half, so as to have two thicknesses in front; wet one so as not to dribble, and when applied, put another bandage over that of muslin or wool, to be broader than the wet one, so as to overlap the edges of the wet one and keep in the steam. These bandages should be wetted every three or four hours, often enough to prevent them from getting dry; the object of keeping a wet cloth next the skin is to warm it, keep it warm, open its pores, and thus give exit to matters in the form of vapor or steam which are causing the disturbance. To derive the fullest advantage from the application of wet cloths, the dry ones should be so adjusted as to keep touching the skin all the time, for if they do not, not only does the steam escape, but cold air gets in and chills the part, thus aggravating the trouble. Many persons fail to get the full, or sometimes any advantage from these

LOCAL STEAM BATHS,

from want of attention in this particular item, especially when applied to the throat for the ordinary soreness of a common cold or from hoarseness. If no special benefit is derived from a throat bandage after a few applications, it is better to discontinue them. It is only in acute cases, such as last a day or two in connection with a common cold, that throat bandages are advised.

WET JACKETS

are used to advantage in fevers; they can be made in effect with a broad bandage to cover the chest or abdomen, or both, or a real jacket with holes for the arms; in either case there should be three or four thicknesses in front; they need not be dampened at the back, especially if there should be a disposition to chilliness.

WET CAPS.

These may be made very useful in headaches, and are always safe to be worn in going into a bath of any kind. Take a piece of linen long enough to reach around the head above the ears, and about four inches broad when doubled; sew the ends together, and gather up the upper edges so as to cover the head. Wet with cold water, let it come over the forehead, and re-apply the water before it gets a little dry; the point is to keep it wet all the time, as by the evaporation it keeps the head cool, relieves fever and inflammation, and sometimes gives relief in severe headaches.

COMPRESSES

are wet cloths applied to limited surfaces, and should be of several thicknesses, dipped in hot, tepid, or cold water, pressed out so as not to dribble, laid flat on the part, then a dry cloth of two or three folds laid over them in such a way that it shall extend an inch or more beyond the wet edges, to keep in the steam, the warm, moist air, which by the evaporating influences and effects caries off the ill-humors and fever which occasion the trouble.

Sometimes a piece of oiled silk is preferable to the dry cloth, as it is less bulky, and answers the object desired more perfectly.

THE EYE-BATH.

There are various circumstances wherein bathing the eyes in warm or cold water, or both alternately, does great good; the best plan, if they are feverish and hot, or are bleary, is to have a basin of quite warm water, and flap it up against the closed eye with the hand in such a way that the hand or fingers shall not strike opposite the eye-ball; let the palm of the hand be bent outwards, thus carrying more water against the eye, and let the ends of the fingers strike against the bridge of the nose or side of it; this warm water at every dash carries away heat by the evaporation, and is very grateful to the eye; then, if agreeable, open the eyes in the water as long as you can hold the breath, this may be repeated once or twice; then use cold water in the same way, first the flapping a few times only, then open them or not in the cold water, as may be agreeable or beneficial, but the cold water should be used rapidly, the object being to close the pores and prevent the excess of blood coming to the eye which caused the fever, by diminishing the calibre of the blood-vessels, for the smaller that calibre, the less blood can come, and cold does contract them.

Such a bathing is very grateful just before going to bed, when the eyes have been much used in reading or fine sewing, especially if they feel hot, or if there is a fulness or other uncomfortable feeling about them.

When persons wake up in the morning with eyelids glued together, it will be found a great comfort to have a basin of warm water brought, put the face in it, and open the eyes in it, and then go on as before; thus the hard matter will be softened, and removed by the finger-ends instead of the finger-nails, which is too common, and is always very hurtful to the eyes and eyelids—always irritating them, and setting up more or less of an inflammation. If warm water is not at hand, take some saliva on the finger-ends, and rub it first along the closed seam of the eyelids, and when softened a little, press down the lower lid, and rub the saliva in the upper face of it, and then so with the upper; in this way the matter will be dissolved, and can be removed with the balls of the fingers; the saliva being one of the mildest, blandest, and most penetrating fluids in nature, it is admirably adapted to the uses just named; but let it be repeated, any hard matter caked or matted at the edge of the eyelids or end of the eyelashes, should not be removed by the finger-nail. It is a common prejudice, that the finger-nails are poisonous in reference to their application to sores; it is because of their irritating and inflaming effect, in dragging particles away that are attached instead of allowing them to remain until they drop off; the result of the latter course would always be, that the sores would get well sooner, and with less liability to leave a scar.

SHOWER-BATHS

should fall on the head covered with a stout cap, or folded towel placed on the top of the head. It is better that the water should come in double streams. If necessary to be poured from a pail, or the spout of a pitcher, it should not be over a foot or two above the head. These baths should be taken rapidly, the dry rubbing to follow without delay, then dress, and go to a warm apartment, or take a brisk walk or other active muscularities, to rouse the circulation.

WHEN TO AVOID BATHING.

When followed invariably by headache, chilliness, or other discomfort.

When a decided glow does not follow the operation, although there may be no actual chilliness.

Avoid cold baths when the skin is moist, for the pores of the skin are open, and the sudden closing of them may cause chilliness or internal local congestions, more or less dangerous.

Not within an hour of eating a regular meal, or at least two hours after.

Not when tired or debilitated, as, for example, after a long walk or ride, or at the close of an over-busy day.

Not when very hungry.

OUT-DOOR BATHING

is only beneficial under the same laws as in-door bathing, that is, when there is no feeling of chilliness when the body emerges from the water; even if the feeling of coldness is merely sufficient to call the mind to the fact, with the least unpleasantness, such a bath is positively injurious.

SEA-BATHING

is advantageous, or at least agreeable, to persons in health, but then they do not need it.

In warm weather invalids may sometimes derive benefit from it when they can be taken into the water in a vehicle without fatigue, the air and water still and warm, remaining but a short time, the wiping dry, and the dressing and undressing, to be attended to by others.

The sea-bathings at public watering-places for persons not in good health are attended with more harm than good. To begin with, lives are lost by drowning every year. Sometimes persons receive wrenches from the dashing of the waves unexpectedly, from which they do not recover for days and weeks, sometimes not for life. Every person, sick or well, must look upon the trouble of dressing and undressing for a bath at a public sea-shore resort with unmixed repugnance. The exposure to the direct rays of a hot summer sun is anything but agreeable, and is sometimes positively dangerous; there may be a breeze, yet the hot sun's rays beat directly on the head for all that; then wading out of the water into the deep, hot, dirty sand, getting it between your toes and leaving your feet dirtier than before, is wholly disagreeable; if you wade out in your shoes, the inside of them is never clean, more or less sand will get in, and then the slushing and sloshing of the dirty water within the shoe is anything but agreeable. There is a gumminess about sea-water which has the effect to varnish over the skin, even though the sea-water is wiped off dry. There is no way to dress clean after a sea-bath unless the body is rinsed off in clean fresh water. Altogether, sea-bathing at public resorts is troublesome, dangerous, and an unmistakable indecency; and there are no facilities at any sea-side resort for sea-bathing to be taken to advantage by invalids.

It is not denied that persons are benefited at times by going to the sea-shore; but the fewest number of invalids are there, in reference to whom it can be said with any certainty that any benefit derived was the result of sea-bathing; the simple change of air, of scene, of cookery, of associations and habits, having advantages which in many cases are wrongfully attributed to sea-bathing.

TEMPERATURE OF BATHS.

To remember easily, it is sufficient to say that—
A cold bath is fifty degrees, or under.
A tepid bath about seventy-five.
A warm bath about a hundred.
A hot bath about a hundred and ten.
A vapor bath about a hundred and fifteen.
A cold bath is tonic.
A tepid bath is cleansing and calming.
A hot bath relaxes the muscles and excites the circulation.

NOTES FOR OUT-DOOR BATHERS.

The best kind of bath in the world, and the healthiest, is a plunge-bath in the river or lake or ocean, before breakfast; such a bath is for vigorous persons who don't need it. The young, the old, the invalid, the sedentary, should observe the following precautions:
Bathe about midway between meals.
The best time is in the forenoon.
Wash the forehead plentifully in cold water, or the whole head and face, before bathing.
Let the bathing be done rapidly, within ten minutes.
If after a walk, and there is any perspiration whatever, undress leisurely, out of any draft of air, but get into the water before there is the very slightest indication of chilliness.
If there is for an instant a feeling of chilliness, while in the

water, or when you emerge from it, the weather is too cold for you, and you should leave for the house instead.

Under all circumstances, as soon as you leave the water wipe dry, dress, and walk towards home without one moment's unnecessary delay.

APOPLEXY

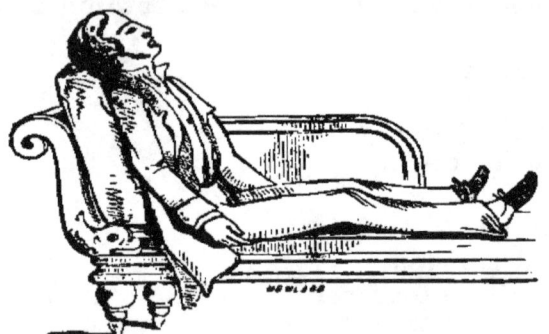

Is a sudden prostration of sense, motion, and consciousness, in consequence of an excessive amount of blood being sent to the brain through the arteries, shown by flushed face and eyes, violent beating of the arteries, and swollen veins at the sides of the neck. The pulse is full and slow, the face is turgid, or of a dusky hue, the breathing is measured, and often of a snoring character. There are two kinds of apoplexy: one called "congestive," where the blood-vessels are very full; the blood is, as it were, impeded in them, but still remains within them. In "hemorrhagic apoplexy" the blood is forced along the arteries to such an extent that in some weak spot the vessel gives way and the blood presses out into the brain in a clot. Sometimes violent coughing or vomiting produces the same effect, the uniform result being death, but not always or necessarily; for the clot is sometimes absorbed, and on the examination of the brain, years after, when the person has died of some totally different disease, the proof of a previous clot is obvious.

Apoplexy seldom occurs in young persons; is much more rare in women than in men; there is an increasing liability to it with increasing years; after thirty, more and more begin to die with it, until at fifty it becomes alarmingly frequent, in proportion as communities are more desperate in their effort for wealth and position and distinction, as in large cities, especially in New York, where the struggle for money sweeps all other considerations aside, and everything is made to yield to its accumulation. A man's thoughts are active and keen in proportion to the supply of good arterial blood to the brain, at the same time deep thought attracts blood there in unusual quantities, and stimulants of all kinds increase the flow of the blood to the brain, hence they are said to "excite" us. Heavy feeding does the same thing by causing more blood to be made, hence the blood-vessels of the brain must convey more and require a greater force and capacity and strength to carry the increased quantity. Hence gluttonous persons and wine-bibbers, gourmands and liquor-drinkers are peculiarly liable to apoplexy; so are public speakers, because the brain is all alive to the subject, and this very activity invites the blood there in increasing quantities, and everything which does that invites apoplexy, such as a heavy strain—all see how the blood gathers in the face under such a strain—or in running or wrestling, or in any of the active games; violent bursts of anger do the same thing, or great emotions, of whatever sort. Hence the wisdom of all, especially after fifty, is in seeking repose, avoiding all strains and liftings and rapid motions, all laborious efforts, physical or mental; exercise of the body should be slow, continuous, and steady; avoid all running up-stairs, all running to catch a public vehicle; cultivate also a quiet mind, a calmness and sobriety of deportment; by so doing, and maintaining the "general health" (which see), persons liable to apoplexy, or of an apoplectic make and age, stoutness of build, shortness of neck, with large features, may indefinitely postpone an attack of apoplexy, and finally die of some very different disease. Any man over fifty, whether he be short and thick, or tall and slim, is liable to an attack of apoplexy any day, if in his previous life he has studied hard and long, or studied severely for a short period, or has been engaged in great enterprises, or in weighty and responsible avocations, bringing a strong, steady, and protracted strain on the brain.

As apoplexy is almost always fatal, it will save a great deal of unnecessary trouble and apprehension to be able to decide at once, when a person suddenly becomes unconscious, whether it is apoplexy or not.

First. If it be preceded by an altered condition of the kidney or bladder, whereby the proper amount of urine has not been passed from the system, and has been reabsorbed to poison the blood and cause diseased conditions in various parts of the body, then the disease is not real apoplexy, but is uræmia, which means that the urine is mixed with the blood and caused the attack in question ; if, under such circumstances, attention is paid to the urinary organs the patient may soon get well, and permanently so.

Second. If the person is "dead drunk" the ailment is of alcoholic origin, known by the smell of the breath and other attendant circumstances, and hence is not really apopletic.

Third. There may be this "coma" or insensibility from narcotic poison, accidental or deliberate, which has been induced by taking laudanum, morphia, or kindred articles ; if that is the case the pupil of the eye is contracted ; if the attack has resulted from some other poisoning the pupils are on the contrary dilated ; in such cases, by using "antidotes" (which see), the person may recover in a short time, and by next day be as well as ever.

Fourth. Insensibility, coma, may result from a stroke on the head or a fall, which is to be determined by a history of the case or by appearances of things around the patient.

Fifth. It may be a common fainting-fit ; but in that case the lips are blue, the surface of the skin cold, there is no pulse, the breathing is interfered with, or there seems to be no breathing at all.

Sixth. If it is a sunstroke the pulse is feeble, skin dry and hot.

Seventh. If it is catalepsy the muscles are rigid, everything remains as at the instant of attack, the pulse is rapid, the attack soon passes off and returns again repeatedly, without any paralysis of any part. In short, apoplexy has a slow pulse, noisy breathing, and stupor. Epilepsy has a quick pulse and convulsive motion of the limbs.

Fainting has no pulse, no perceptible breathing, and a pale face.

TREATMENT.

In an attack of real apoplexy there is, not much to be done. The first thing is to send for a physician ; the next is to do what is possible to give temporary relief, but go about it with a certain degree of hopefulness and confidence, because if the person is thirty, or not much over, whatever may be the form of the apoplexy, he may get well, especially if the constitution be not broken.

The first thing to be done is to have the patient sit up, so as to allow the blood to fall down from the head by its own gravity; in addition, use more active means to draw the blood from the head, by putting large mustard plasters to the legs and back and belly, one after another; use a speedy "injection" (which see) during the attack, so as to unload the bowels, and as soon as possible afterwards give a dose of salts or castor-oil, so as to clear out the bowels. If there be much hair, cut or shave it off at once, and place a bag of pounded ice over the scalp, or keep cloths dipped in cold water, pressed out slightly so that the water shall not dribble on the clothing, applied to the scalp; renew these cloths every five minutes until the head seems to be of the natural warmth. In all cases administer an active purgative, one tablespoon of castor-oil every hour, or a tablespoon of salts every hour, until the bowels act freely.

But as apoplectic attacks are becoming so frequent, in comparison with past years, in consequence of a generally prevalent straining on the brain in conducting the affairs of life, every professional man after fifty, every man engaged in responsible employments, every student, every literary man, all sedentary persons, should consider themselves liable to apoplexy, either by acquired or hereditary conditions, and use those preventive measures habitually, systematically, and persistently which have been already stated, giving special prominence to—

First. Light and early suppers.

Second. One free, full evacuation of the bowels every twenty-four hours.

Third. Avoid the use of intoxicating drinks late at night.

Fourth. Avoid all sudden and violent outbursts of passion.

Fifth. Guard against hasty, violent, or long protracted exercise.

BROKEN BONES,

Or fractures, really come under the head of Accidents or Casualties. We are shocked at the idea of having a limb sawn off, but there is no more feeling in the bone itself than in a finger-nail while paring it; the actual pain is the mere feeling of a prick as the knife goes through the skin. Yet when a bone is broken the slightest motion of the broken ends gives great suffering, hence it is of the utmost importance in case any bone is broken to keep the person as perfectly quiet as possible. If the body, or any part of it, must be moved, it should be done slowly, gently, and with the greatest care.

But when the ends of the broken bone are united properly, and the body is healthy and strong enough to set up a healing process by sending out its own glue, as it were, called callus, to unite them again, then pain comes, steadily increasing; but if these ends are kept constantly in position, touching each other at the same spot, the process of reunion begins in a few hours. This is the reason why splints are used—long strips of wood on two sides of the limb—and strips of cloth wound around them and the limb. In this way everything is kept in place. The limbs of any of the domestic animals would reunite in a few days if it were possible to keep them still after the ends of the broken bones had been properly adjusted. Although the process of reunion commences rapidly it requires several weeks for completion, hence the greatest patience is required, the more trying because in all other respects the body is perfectly well. Even when there are indications that the bones have reunited, the greatest care should be taken in rising from the bed to favor the limb so as to force upon it the very slightest strain possible; and in the use of it great care should be observed to employ it gently, and have but a few steps or motions at a time, and then give abundant rest before used again. In all fractures of bones, until a perfect cure is effected, the general health should be maintained by eating regularly, moderately, no desserts, light suppers (which see, and also General Health), being careful to keep the bowels acting every day. A small amount of meat is allowable twice a day, eaten slowly and cut up fine. Oranges, lemons, apples, bananas, fruits, berries, tomatoes, with "coarse breads," should make a considerable part of breakfast and dinner, endeavoring all the time to bear with the pain, for it is the pain which causes an extra excitement, bringing an extra quantity of blood to the part, from which extra quantity the natural glue is made which is to bind the bones together quite as strong as they ever were before. If there were no pain or irritation there would be no healing. If the ends of the bones protrude through the skin, or if crushed like an egg shell pressed in the hand, the aid of an experienced surgeon is imperatively re-

quired ; but in simple fractures, a good way to tell whether a
limb is broken or not, is to ask the sufferer to raise or bend it,
and he will fail to do it.

IN SIMPLE FRACTURES

the things necessary to be done can be explained with sufficient
clearness to enable a person of ordinary intelligence to "set a
bone" successfully.

THE THIGH BONE

is generally broken about the middle or lower part, either square
across, called transversely, or obliquely ; the patient can't move the
limb, the foot is turned outwards, the limb seems to be shorter and
the lower end of the bone usually slides behind the upper end in
oblique fractures ; those straight across show no displacement usually, except to careful feeling.

Get a board which will reach from two inches above the lower
edge of the ribs to three or four inches beyond the sole of the foot,
broader at the thighs, tapering towards the ankle to three inches
broad, thick enough not to bend easily. There should be two
notches at the lower end to tie the end of the bandage, and two
holes in the upper end of this board ; put the patient on a firm bed
—a hair mattress is best ; the limb is now to be bandaged from
the toe upwards with a strip of cloth, some two inches wide, this
is to keep the limb from swelling ; now let one person gently and
steadily draw the foot downwards until it is as long as the other,
feeling at the same time with the finger at the broken part to
ascertain if the ends of the bone exactly correspond with each
other, that there is no ridge or offset or unevenness at the point of
fracture. Then put pads or cushions on the board to protect the
skin from injury, extend the limb on the board, take a " surgical
roller " (which see), and beginning above the knee, wrap it around
the limb and the splint down to the foot, and having turned round
the ankle, pass it through the notches and thus bind it firmly to
the splint.

Next make steady the upper end of the splint by a broad bandage around the lower portion of the body, and going downwards,
still including both the splint and the limb, until the other bandage is reached ; next fasten a broad bandage around the waist, to

bind the splint to the lower part of the waist; next pass a handkerchief over the groin and buttock, fastening its ends by means of the holes in the splint; by tightening this handkerchief the limb is extended, which should be done often to keep the limb straight.

A cure under favorable circumstances is effected in about six weeks, during which time the bandages should be renewed three times; but since the bony reunion has not in this time acquired its full strength, the whole weight of the body should not be thrown on this limb under any circumstances for a single instant, but use a crutch all the time for three or four months, and if the patient has a feeble constitution, the crutches should be used for a month or two longer, for if broken over again, the reunion is more slow, and attended with greater discomfort, and perfect convalescence is protracted for a wearisome time; be careful to protect the skin where the handkerchief passes under the groin, have it as smooth as possible, and let the ankles be carefully protected from chafing or abrasions, or painful pressure.

LEG FRACTURE.

The leg has two bones; the tibia, or shin-bone, and the fibula, which is behind it.

If the shin-bone is broken and the knee is bent, this bone sticks out at the upper part; roll a bandage from the toes upward. Have a splint to reach from the middle of the thigh to near the heel. Have a pasteboard splint for both sides, but a wooden splint, hollowed out some, to fit the limb, on which extend it, and apply a roller to inclose both limb and splints; care should be taken that all the splints should be properly adjusted, and have the roller applied so as to have them in their proper place; if it is not well done, try it again. Pads must be placed under the heel to keep it raised. Bands of strong linen an inch wide should be used to tie the lower end of the splint and limb together, in such a way as to have the knots on the outside.

The above are the directions when the shin-bone is broken near the knee; if it is broken near the ankle, there is great pain on the slightest movement, and the leg is helpless. The exact seat of fracture is easily ascertained by moving the finger along the shin-bone, as there is little but skin there, and a ridge is felt, or there is a grating noise if the ends of the bone are moved in opposite directions; have a pasteboard splint inside and outside from just below the knee to near the ankle, with cushions between the splints and the skin; then secure the whole by half a dozen broad tapes along the line of the splints, making them more or less tight, according to the needs of the case.

BOTH LEG BONES

are sometimes broken; they break not always in a line, but an inch or more apart, turning the foot out, bending and deforming the leg, until rectified. The favorite bandage for such a fracture is the

EIGHTEEN-TAILED BANDAGE,

made thus: take a piece of linen, three or four inches broad, and as long as the leg; take eighteen strips of the same width, and stitch them across the other at equal intervals; they should be long enough to go one and a half times around the limb; they should be stitched so as to cover each other about a third of their breadth.

Then set the bone by bending the knee a little and extending the limb, or draw it down until the ends of the bones come in contact, which may be known by the grating sound, if rubbed together, and having a padded splint ready, extending from above the knee a little beyond the ankle, let the bandage be placed under this splint, being very careful in transferring the limb from the pad to the splint that the ends of the bones shall be precisely in their places; now take the lowest tail and pass it obliquely across the leg to the opposite side, the other end of the same tail must then be similarly brought on the other side, so as to intersect the first; apply the other tails in the same way until the upper one is reached, carry them always under the limb; next place a soft pad on the upper part of the limb and on that a splint, then take half a dozen strips of linen or broad tape and tie around the whole, next make a frame for the limb by nailing boards together, inclining both ways down to the foot, in a pyramid form, with a board for the foot. The splints should be removed in six weeks, if things go on favorably; but the limb should be used lightly and with great care for several weeks longer, for, although the bones are knitted at the end of six weeks, additional time is required for them to have the firmness and solidity of texture requisite for free use.

FRACTURE OF COLLAR BONE.

This usually takes place about the centre; the exact spot can be ascertained by running the finger along the bone; the outward or shoulder end falls down; place the ends in contact by stretching the shoulders as far back as possible; then adjust the ends of the bone, keep them so by a suitable bandage, place the arm across the chest, fingers pointed towards the top of the other shoulder, fasten all in that position by a broad band around the chest; it is an addition to put a pad under the armpit in such a way as to assist in keeping the ends of the broken bones in more exact positions.

BROKEN RIBS.

This is a frequent accident. The remedy is to bind a broad bandage around the chest, the tighter the better, so that the ribs should move as little as possible in breathing; the patient should cultivate the habit of breathing with the muscles of the belly or abdomen as much as possible; this will be a great aid to a speedy restoration; if there is great pain, or restlessness, or anxiety, the patient may be bled to fainting; for several days the diet should be mainly of coarse breads, berries and fruits, and by all means keep the bowels free; the broad tight bandage about the chest may be best kept in its place by shoulder-straps made of strips of cloth.

BROKEN ARM

is known by its lying down helpless by the side of the patient; he has no control over it, and it is somewhat shorter than natural. Grasp the elbow with one hand, stretch the other end of the limb with the other hand until the ends of the bone are exactly opposite each other, and no ridge is felt where they adjoin; apply a strong pasteboard splint from the armpit to the elbow, and another on the opposite side, from the top of the shoulder beyond the elbow, first steeping them in hot water and softly padding the arm; if the splints are broad enough to almost envelop the arm it is better, so that on the subsidence of the swelling they should not overlap or even meet, for then they loosen; then apply a bandage that shall reach from the ends of the fingers, rolling it upwards until it reaches the elbow; it should be applied moderately tight, but not to interfere with the circulation. Apply a wooden splint on the outside of all this, but only until the pasteboard gets dry and forms a kind of case around the arm; the elbow should be carried at a right angle and the arm be well supported in a sling, adjusted in such a way as to aid in holding the ends of the fractured bone together. In about a week the swelling subsides. Look in under the edge of the pasteboard and see if the ends are still adjusted right; the bone usually begins to unite in seven days, to be completed in a month; but for a month after the arm should be carefully used, no straining, no lifting of weights or pulling.

FOREARM FRACTURES.

The forearm, like the leg, has two bones, the *ulna* and *radius;* the latter is oftenest broken, the nearer the wrist the greater is the distortion. The point of fracture can be ascertained by running the finger along the arm; it causes pain to turn around, and a grating noise will be heard if the ends of the bone are moved in opposite directions. When the *radius* or outer bone is fractured, the ulna or inner one keeps it in place. Have soft pads ready, then dip pasteboard splints in hot water, and have a roller to go round the whole; one splint should reach on the outside from above the elbow to the tips of the fingers, and another from the bend of the arm to the end of the palm of the hand. Place the arm in a sling, the palm of the hand lying flat on the breast, never moving the palm in any direction, because the slightest turn in it moves the bone at the point of union, and every such motion arrests healing.

If the ulna is broken, treat it as the other.

If both bones are broken, all use is lost of the hand, the arm swells, and it is considerably shortened. Extend the arm until the ends of the bone meet. Apply splints of pasteboard dipped in hot water, as before, using one wooden splint on the outside until the pasteboard is dry. If there is not much flesh on the arm a soft compress of lint should be placed between the bones of the arm first, serving to aid in keeping them apart, thus holding the broken ends in their exact position.

BROKEN FINGER.

Put a wooden splint along the back of the fingers, with a soft pad between, and bandage on to keep it in place.

JAW FRACTURE.

At whatever point broken, arrange so that all the teeth shall be in their natural positions, touching, with respect to one another; then secure the jaw, shutting the mouth by strips of adhesive-plaster of fine leather at least two inches wide, extending from the chin to the ear. Then make a bandage two yards long, two and a half inches wide; split this from each end to within six inches of the centre; make a hole in the centre for the chin, bring the two lower ends upwards over the head, and carry the two upper ends along over the jaw to the back of the neck, thence several turns over the head, fastening at the ends and crossings, to keep in position.

KNEE-PAN FRACTURE.

The upper part is drawn up, the patient cannot straighten the limb, and the fissure can be felt and seen. Have a stiff splint from the middle of the thigh to the lower end of the calf, binding it with a roller; if the breaking is across the knee-pan buckle above and below the fracture, around the limb, then, by other straps attached to them, draw on the buckles until the sides of the fracture are brought exactly together, for if this is not done, there will be no union by one bone growing to another, but only by ligaments.

If the fracture is up and down, a bandage around will bring the parts together, using compresses to keep the parts cool, and a splint to keep the leg extended and still.

DISLOCATION

is when a bone is removed from its place, or out of its socket, easily known by the protuberance on one side, and a hollow on the other, with more or less swelling, pain, heat, inflammation; if it has just occurred, it may be readily put in its place by gradually and steadily and gently drawing on the limb, until the patient has lost all power of resistance; as soon as the bulb of the bone comes to the edge of the cup or depression from which it has been carried, it pops in with a snap. If a week or two, or more, passes without replacement it will be a life-long disablement, for new attachments are made. If it was not possible to do anything for some hours or a day or two, and there is pain, inflammation, and swelling, dip several folds of flannel in hot water, and lay them on the spot, renewing every five minutes, or even less, if pain is great; after considerable relief, apply a warm poultice of milk and wheat bread, or of coarse meal of oats or corn, mixed with oil and vinegar half and half; when the pain and inflammation have subsided, set the bone as directed above; it may be necessary to bleed first.

After a dislocation has been remedied, and there is any pain or heat, or swelling, dip several folds of linen into spirits of camphor or vinegar, and lay on over the spot, renewing frequently, until the parts feel and seem comfortable. Use a sling, if the dislocation is in any part of the arm; if it is in the leg, it should be kept on a chair, extended on a level with the seat of the person.

If a limb is dislocated and broken at the same time, it may be best to heal the fracture first, if the dislocation cannot be remedied at too great a cost of suffering.

SHOULDER DISLOCATION

is generally downwards, and the head is in the arm-pit; the arm cannot be moved without great pain, and the arm is much shortened. Place the patient on a low seat; one person must hold the patient firmly, while the operator takes hold of the arm above the elbow, and gradually and steadily extends it; put a towel under the arm, and tie it around the operator's neck, and when the arm is pulled out far enough the operator must gently raise himself up, pulling the patient's arm upward with his neck, his assistants pulling on the patient's leg, while with his own hands he takes hold of the end of the bone and directs it to its place, into which it jerks with a snap; then use hot fomentations and camphorated cloths, until the heat and inflammation have subsided.

7

If there is swelling, pain, or inflammation, use leeches, fomentations, loosening medicines, and a cooling diet, until relief is afforded; castor oil (which see), may be used to keep the bowels free, and live on coarse bread, and fruits and vegetables.

DISLOCATED ELBOW.

One should hold the arm above and an other below the elbow, each pulling gently and steadily in opposite directions until the operator can, with his fingers, put the parts in their proper positions; keep the arm bent and cary it in a sling for some days, until there is a feeling of strength in the parts, keeping down heat and fever by poultices, compresses, or simply pouring water on the parts, or keeping them wound round with wet rags. Pretty much all dislocations are remedied in a similar manner, always taking care to keep the bowels regular and feeding lightly, as just named.

HIP-JOINT DISLOCATION.

Very many old persons have their hips dislocated by jostles and falls, and are made invalids or cripples in all after-life, but often it is a result of want of prompt treatment. If the dislocation is downwards, then one leg is longer than the other; if upwards, shorter; if downwards, the foot and knee are turned outwards; otherwise, inwards. If downwards, lay the patient on the back, to be held or strapped fast. Tie a cloth around above the knee, in such a way that a person can drag the limb downwards with this cloth until it is near its proper place, and then the operator can guide it with his fingers.

If an outward dislocation, lay the patient on the face, and while one person is drawing upon the limb, the operator must guide the head of the bone inwards until it gets to its proper place; then raise it upward, so as to help it into the socket.

As there must be more or less drawing in all dislocations, it must be remembered that the patient instinctively resists that drawing for fear of being hurt; but if this drawing is steadily persisted in, he presently loses all power of resistance, is perfectly helpless, and the limb is then comparatively easily adjusted.

JAW DISLOCATION

sometimes takes place from gaping immoderately, as well as by violent laughter or other means. Place the patient on a low stool; let one person hold his head firmly, while the operator gets behind, puts each thumb, covered with linen, to be protected from slipping or being bitten, into the mouth as far as he can, while the fingers are to be applied to the jaw outside; press the jaw steadily and strongly downwards and backwards, until it comes to its proper place with a snap. Then rest the jaw; avoid much talking, or gaping, or chewing anything hard, until it recovers its natural healthful tone.

DISLOCATED NECK

must be promptly relieved, or death will soon take place; but it can be remedied thus: If partially dislocated, the chin falls on the breast, preventing speech, swallowing, or motion; face is turned aside, countenance bloated, neck swollen, and there is no sensibility. Place the patient on his back, for there is not a moment to lose, the operator behind, so as to hold the head with both hands firmly; fixing his knees against the shoulders of the patient, pull the head with gradually increasing force, moving it from side to side until the bones of the neck drop into their place, known by the noise of a snap and returning breathing; then secure the head in its place by proper bandages; bathe the parts with cloths dipped in vinegar or spirits of camphor, put to bed, keep the bowels very free with cooling diet (which see). If the neck is completely dislocated, death ensues.

TYPHOID FEVER.

Typhus is a Greek word, meaning stupor, depression, a lack of sprightliness. Typhoid means similar to Typhus. It is better for all practical purposes to consider them as of the same nature, Typhoid being an aggravation, a worse form of Typhus.

CAUSE OF TYPHOID FEVER.

It arises from breathing the exhalations from what was once a part of animal bodies, especially of human bodies. If a great many persons are confined in a ship or room or prison, especially in warm weather, they will soon begin to have typhoid fever; if on shipboard, it is called the

SHIP FEVER.

If, on the other hand, it breaks out among prisoners, confined in narrow quarters, it is the

JAIL FEVER,

of which so much was written many years ago. It is emphatically a "catching" disease, as the common people express it. Medical men call it contagious, that is, easily taken by persons who come in contact or close association with the patients, it is not necessary to come into actual contact with them, to sleep in the same bed with them, nor to be in the same room with them, in order to take the disease. Striking examples of this are given in the author's book on *Sleep, or Hygiene of the Night.* A case is given where one of the cells in an English prison, a hundred years ago, was much crowded; the jailer and jailer's wife, whose business it was to furnish food, introduced it from a room above the cell, through a very small opening; they were soon taken sick. They represented that the stench which came up in their faces through the little trap-door was loathsome beyond degree; it was intolerable. They both died before any of the prisoners were seriously ill, because the most poisonous air in a warm crowded room ascends to the ceiling, hence the jailers breathed it in a more concentrated form than the prisoners themselves.

If a person having had typhoid fever goes with the same clothing, especially if woollen, into a room where there are others, the more delicate of them will be apt to take the fever. If the bedding or the clothing worn in sickness by a typhoid patient is packed in a trunk, and the trunk is closed for months, and is finally placed in a room and opened, the person sleeping a single night in the room is very liable to an attack.

It is not only the perspiration and fumes and odor coming from the bodies of living human beings crowded in a small, warm room which are capable of causing typhoid fever, the emanations of human and animal offal generate the disease with great rapidity, especially in persons of frail constitutions, or of sedentary or depraved habits of eating, drinking, carousing, and debauchery. A person with a debilitated constitution may have typhoid fever from a few times passing a place where animal offal is in a state of decay ; but robust constitutions may resist the daily breathing of it for some time, but must eventually yield to its deadly power. Hence all classes are liable to typhoid fever, the poor from crowding and filth, the rich and cultivated from having to pass filthy localities.

Whether the matter which causes typhoid fever is breathed into the lungs or is taken into the stomach through the water which is drunk, the effects are the same—to corrupt and poison the blood in a most malignant manner. Hence if families drink water from a well or spring which is near a privy or sink, or household drain, and these make their way into the fountain, especially in the summer-time, typhoid disease will soon appear.

A CASE.

A family of ten persons lived in a remarkably healthful locality ; they occupied a large house, built on an elevation ; for many years there had not occurred a single case of sickness in the house ; but all at once, one, then another, and another of the family were attacked with typhoid fever, to the wonderment of that whole section of country; more than half the family died, all were sick. On a thorough investigation suggested by the doctor, it was found that about a month before the fever appeared the pump was broken; and as water was almost as handy from a a stream near by, the family derived their supplies from it ; this stream flowed near several barn-yards and family out-houses, and not only received the washings of the same into them, but the soakings of all these places made their way also into the stream, and by the time the water reached the premises of the doomed family it was thoroughly impregnated with the poisonous material coming from human and animal offal; it indeed seemed sparkling and clear, but a proper examination showed that there was a visible sediment of human excrement. Three members of this family were not sick at all, apparently from the peculiarity of their circumstances, they did not in all that time use any of the water from the brook.

In a small village near New York City, during 1871, typhoid fever attacked a whole family with marked violence. On examination it was found that an old forgotten house-drain crossed the pipe which supplied the family hydrant with water, and that at that crossing there was a leak in the old sewer, and the matter of it made its way into the water-pipe at its imperfect joinings; this state of things was remedied, and the sickness at once abated and soon disappeared.

Some time ago in a part of Philadelphia where a large number of the poorer classes lived, supplied with drinking and cooking water from a spring which was at the lowest part of the settlement, as summer came on a variety of bowel disorders made their appearance, and various grades of typhoid fever. On its being pointed out that the spring was in a bottom, and that the drainings of all the outhouses would naturally make their way into it, although it was sparklingly clear, the use of the water was abandoned entirely, and the sickness at once disappeared and has not since returned.

It is well known that Prince Albert of England died of typhoid fever. He was a man who would have been thought to be the very last person to have a disease of that kind, because possessing a fine constitution, temperate in all his habits of life, systematic in exercise, regular in eating and free from every vice, all these considerations should have tended to length of days; but no constitution can survive the steady breathing day after day of a pernicious atmosphere. The London *Lancet*, the highest medical authority, states, that knowing there must be some specific cause somewhere, careful inquiry and investigation elicited the fact that an old drain from a village had been carried across the castle grounds before the buildings were erected, and that there was a break in this sewer, just under the library of the Prince, and as he spent a large portion of his time in that apartment, he necessarily breathed a great deal of the foul atmosphere which was there generated, and breathing it, died.

Very recently two British noblemen had to pass some yards for the preparation of manure; one of them having gone near twice was taken seriously ill next day; the other, with his servant, passed repeatedly in the course of a few weeks, and died after a few days' illness; the servant lingered longer, but followed his master, both being victims of typhoid fever from breathing the odors from decayed human excrement in course of preparation for the fields. Let it then be distinctly understood that where typhoid fever attacks a family, close examination will generally elicit facts to show that the cause is found in human excretions being taken into the body through the lungs or through the stomach; in the latter case by the water used, in the former by breathing air saturated with human effluvia.

Recently there was a flood in the river Ribble, which receives the sewage drains of the Swill Brook Mill at Preston, England. The contents of the sewers were thus dammed up, driving the odors into a room where eleven persons were at work, every one of whom became ill, and in a few days four died of marked typhoid fever; hence all offensive odors should be excluded from every human habitation. The worst forms of typhus fever are induced by breathing the odors of kitchen sinks, drains in the back-yard, open privy seats or doors, and of decaying rats behind base boards, ceilings, and other places. A barn-yard may be a mile distant on a higher piece of ground, and yet its drainage will make its way to some neighbor's spring lower down, to be taken into the stomach in the drinking-water and from the tea-kettle.

Two cases of diphtheria occurred in one family. On examination it was found that the lead pipe connected with the water-closet in the house was joined to the iron drain, but at the junction the iron had rusted and thus allowed the fumes of the drain to come into the house; and it may be safely said that where diphtheria, typhoid fever, and allied diseases appear in a family, the cause may be found in some deficiency connected with the channels which carry away the various offals of the house, although the disease has various other causes.

TREATMENT.

The diet should be milk, if it is palatable, two or three pints in twenty-four hours, beef soups and gruels.

If there is not one action of the bowels in twenty-four hours, use an injection or mild laxatives.

If there is much sickness at stomach an ipecac emetic is beneficial, relieving the nausea at once.

If there is a fast, strong pulse, it is calmed by taking, two or three times a day, small doses of tincture of aconite leaves, from fifteen to twenty-five drops, or about five drops of the root tincture.

In typhoid fever, the fever is continuous ; it seems to last all the time, and must increase that debility which is an invariable attendant of that disease, hence it is of considerable importance to abate it. This is often well done by giving about thirty drops of diluted hydrochloric acid every three hours in half a glass of sweetened water, to be continued day and night until the fever subsides.

If the bowels act more than once in twenty-four hours, or there is sleeplessness or disposition to delirium, all these are remedied by a dose of Dover's Powders, five to fifteen grains in water or syrup ; ten grains of this contain one grain of opium. Hence its tendency to give sleep and to calm the action of the bowels.

If the patient seems to be prostrated, about two grains of quinine in a table-spoonful of brandy every three or four hours gives strength and animation.

The things which distinguish typhoid from other fevers are mainly :

1. It comes on very gradually.

2. The fever seems never to leave the patient for a moment, although it is not a very high one.

3. Bleeding of the nose.

4. The bowels discharge a dirty yellow substance.

5. Abdominal symptoms ; the belly is drum-like, swollen and tight from gas in the bowels, causing tenderness on pressure and a kind of gurgling noise ; in most cases there is a weakening looseness of the bowels, which, if not controlled, begin to ulcerate, bleed, eat through, and death is inevitable.

6. Above all, there is a peculiar eruption of the skin in Typhoid Fever ; little spots appear separately over the belly, of a rose or pink color, so little elevated as to be noted only by the finger, not the eye ; of an oval form, and one or two lines broad. The redness of these patches disappears for a moment if pressed with the finger ; generally not more than eighteen or twenty of these rose-colored small spots can be seen on the whole surface of the belly, and sometimes not more than four or five. Now and then there may be a

great many spots, which may extend to the extremities; occasionally these spots are only to be found in the back; these spots die away and others come; after death they are not seen. They begin to appear usually during the third week of the disease. This eruption is not always present, especially in children; its presence or absence, its copiousness or scantiness does not measure the severity of the disease.

In this disease, as above stated, the pulse is always too frequent, and the more frequent it is the more likely the person is to die, because a quick pulse always wastes the strength, and want of strength is particularly present in typhoid fever. If the pulse on an average is under a hundred the chances are greatly in favor of recovery; if it beats a hundred and ten times in a minute or over, a fatal issue may be pretty certainly looked for.

If the pulse suddenly rises and continues ten, fifteen, or twenty beats faster, a very unfavorable change has taken place, and there is most likely inflammation of the lungs or bowels, this latter indicating approaching ulceration, perforation, and death.

As nations grow older with increasing civilization so-called, the tendency to typhoid diseases increases, in consequence, in part, of increased debility of constitution, induced by luxurious living and idleness and sedentary employments, and in other part by new habits of life, induced by wealth. For example, in cities especially, water-closets are found in almost every house, are liable to get out of order all the time; the pipes and drains connected with them are studiously kept out of sight, are covered up in the ground or are concealed in the plastering, so that they may get out of order in their joints and remain so for months and years with little probability of discovery, and all this time one by one of the household may be dying off as a direct effect of a defective house-pipe. Of late years in England typhoid diseases and spotted fevers, and diphtheria, have very largely increased in number, and so in the United States; hence too much pains will scarcely be taken by housekeepers to cultivate cleanliness, not only of clothing and person and chambers, but purity of air especially as impaired by defective pipes and drains.

Another cause of the increased frequency of typhoid fever is the vast increase of population, and this tends to the cities; this great increase involves greater crowding and a greater concentration of offals and human dejections in much more limited spaces.

Unless an increasing civilization and populousness of any locality or city or country is accompanied by increased cleanliness of habits and practices and homes, diseases of all kinds will become more frequent and more fatal.

BODILY HEAT.

If a thermometer is placed in the arm-pit of a man in health it raises the mercury to ninety-eight degrees. This is called blood-heat. In typhoid fever this rises in the first three days to one hundred and three; and if a greater increase is observed the symptom is proportionally unfavorable; for if it reaches one hundred and seven or eight in the morning, it means death. During the progress of the disease there is a variation of the heat, between morning and evening, of two or three degrees; but as a person is getting well this difference amounts to eight or ten degrees.

While a sudden and great rise of the pulse indicates a dangerous complication in the lungs or bowels, a sudden and great fall usually precedes bleeding from the bowels, which is also an unfavorable indication.

SYMPTOMS OF TYPHOID FEVER.

The patient begins to be dull, drooping, and drowsy in mind and body. This goes on increasing until it becomes a stupor; then a wandering condition of the mind; next a low muttering delirium, excessive bodily exhaustion. The body slides down to the foot of the bed; reddish spots appear on the skin; there is twitching of the muscles; blood comes from the bowels, or they are the seat of ulceration which eats through them, when death speedily follows, the disease running its course in about three weeks. If, however, in the course of the disease, the countenance brightens, the pulse grows stronger, the tongue cleans, and the appetite improves, restoration to usual health may be looked for, if there is no relapse, no "back set;" but the disease oftenest returns, and a relapse is death.

INJUDICIOUSNESS IN EATING.

The body has been greatly debilitated, and its cravings for food are sometimes almost irresistible. The appeals for this, that, and the other longed-for article are so pitiful that affection can scarcely resist them; the rule should be a little at a time, at three hours' interval; nothing between, because the stomach must have rest, must have time to prepare itself for the work of digesting another portion. The food should be light, easily digested, and such as the patient was accustomed to eat in health; it should be well cooked, cut up as fine as a pea, and chewed deliberately and well. A lady was recovering from a long and tedious attack which brought her to the very verge of the grave. She fairly yearned for a sweet-potato. She ate but a small part of one; it lay like a load in her stomach. She had a relapse, and died. The sweet-potato is a very compact food, as little fitted for absorbing the digestive fluids of the stomach as wax. Had she eaten toasted bread in its dry state the juices of the stomach would have been taken up into it as a sponge takes up water, and would have dissolved it at once. Hot loaf-bread and hot biscuit would have been as bad as the sweet-potato, for they are not much better than dough. Take a piece of hot bread or dough, make a little cake of it, and place it in a saucer of water, it will remain there for hours without taking up any of the water. Take a piece of stale bread and place it in a cup of water, and if well baked it will all fall apart in a few minutes. This is what is meant by light food; well-cooked meat which is tender, if chewed well, is also light food, and is very nutritious. In the absence of teeth to masticate it well, it may be beaten almost to a paste, and if thus eaten with its juice, a tablespoonful at a time, it is a "light" food. The patient should also be very careful not to expend his strength either of mind or body, unnecessarily; all study and worry and excitement should be carefully avoided; all bodily exercise should be gentle, deliberate, a little at a time; no hurry, no bustle, nothing that strains or is protracted. More can be done by judicious nursing than with medicine, although the aid of the latter can be called in with immense advantage at times. The great feature in typhoid fever is debility, prostration; hence to husband the strength and to increase it are the two main features of treatment. As to the former, the previous page makes general suggestions.

To give strength, the first step is to give good air to breathe, as it was breathing bad air which caused the sickness. See article, ". Ventilating Sick-Rooms." The room should contain a fire-place even in summer, and that should be kept open day and night, and if day and night, incessantly a lamp or candle were kept burning on the hearth near the back, in summer, and a light fire in cool weather, a permanent draught would be set up thereby, and to the fire-place all the out-door air would tend which comes in under the doors and at the window crevices, thus driving before it into the fire-place and up the chimney all the heaviest and worst gases and human exhalations; to promote this, an inner door, which is safer, or a window should allow some air to come in, but in such a way that the draught should not be upon the patient.　Next keep the skin clean by the use of sponges dipped in water of such a temperature as is most soothing and cooling to the patient; sometimes cold water is most refreshing, at others tepid or warm.

The condition of the bowels should be carefully watched, looseness is more to be guarded against than costiveness; for looseness weakens.　Aim to have one action every twenty-four hours.　If costive administer "injections" (which see), or use the mildest "Aperients."

If there is a tendency to looseness, to thin passages, use "rice" boiled (which see), or from five to twenty grains of

SUBNITRATE OF BISMUTH

(which see); this may be taken three or four times a day.　Great attention must be paid to the condition of the bowels, for that is the characteristic feature of typhoid fever, so much so, that eminent German writers have called it "abdominal typhus," our "belly" typhus; some of our own physicians term it "enteric fever," that is, fever of the bowels; these statements are made to impress upon the reader's mind that, as it is a disease of the bowels, so the greatest care should be taken to keep them in proper condition, and to avoid taking either food or medicine which would be calculated to irritate them, to aggravate any inflamed or ulcerous condition which may be present.

In the early stage of Typhus fever the belly is flat, with no tendency to loose bowels for two or three weeks; but as it runs into typhoid the belly swells in consequence of some of the "glands" of the small intestine becoming inflamed by the continuance of the disease, then ulcerated, swelling, and so distending the skin of the belly that there is a drum-like sound if stricken lightly with the finger.　This

SWELLING OF THE BOWELS

in typhoid fever, occasioned mainly by large quantities of wind, may be relieved more or less by "kneading the liver" (which see), or a long gutta-percha tube may be carefully introduced by the "rectum" (which see) or lower bowels. At other times

" FOMENTATIONS "

(which see), if hot, do a great deal of good.

The patient sometimes suffers greatly from burning hands or feet, or other local fevers; these may be relieved by inducing perspiration, in a gentle way, by wrapping up in bed and drinking largely of hot teas, or even hot water, which, however, is the safest, because it does not irritate nor excite either the stomach or the intestines.

During the first week the skin gets hotter, the pulse goes up to a hundred or more (see "Pulse"), with coated tongue; the sleep is short and less refreshing, great restlessness, pain in the small of the back and in the head; if the disease is progressing. The second week is marked by a tendency to diarrhœa, the belly swells; on the surface of it little rose-colored spots are seen, while on the chest and neck little pimples appear in drops almost as clear as if they were drops of sweat.

In any stage of the disease the fever may be abated by taking every hour, in a little sweetened water, from two to ten or fifteen drops of "veratrum viride" (which see); if the fever is kept down there is less of delirium, which rarely comes on in the first week; oftener in the second, but in the third week this symptom is decidedly manifest in three cases out of four. This delirium arises from weakness of mind, is most manifest in the night, and, if not watched, the patient gets up and dresses, or wanders about and out of the house, to the great waste of strength, hence the necessity of good, conscientious nurses; other things require watchfulness; in three cases out of four diarrhœa takes place; in many cases the patient, from indifference or inability to restrain, befouls the bed; and cleanliness is essential in the whole progress of the disease; if the discharges are involuntary or bloody, the danger is very great, and there is but little hope of recovery.

But it happens in typhoid fever, as in other ailments, that at the very point when all hope of recovery is abandoned, and skill and science stand helpless by the bedside, not even attempting to do anything but to alleviate, the symptoms change for the better; every few hours a further advance is made towards health, giving all new hope and heart, because, in some part of the body distant from the seat of life some swelling appears, increasing in size as the patient improves, to result in a few days in an ulceration or running sore, which, if allowed to remain, gradually runs itself dry, and the man is well; if this ulcer is tampered with and attempts are made to "heal it up," there will be a relapse which will end fatally. The course which typhoid fever ran in the case of the Prince of Wales in 1871, strikingly confirms the views and statements made above. From the verge of the grave, and when his attending physicians had abandoned all hope of his recovery, the civilized world heard with gladness that there was a pause in his disease. "He was no worse;" a few hours later the telegraph announced that he was "better," and the almost simultaneous "swelling" in the neighborhood of the left hip told the story that at a most critical juncture a swelling began to show itself in a spot which was in a sense far from the vital parts of the system, which drew away the disease from portions of the system which could bear no more, thus giving them relief and rest, and final life. It is useful to remark here, that life is often saved by this very process of nature in all forms of disease. Ulceration or abscess, internal or external, or even an ordinary boil, serves as a centre of attraction for all the diseased particles to run; or, in other terms, a drain is set up through which diseased, decaying, poisonous, and dead matters are carried out of the system.

A lady over sixty had a troublesome cough of some months' continuance; she and her friends apprehended consumptive disease, as, besides the cough, other symptoms were present: debility, feverishness, quick pulse, and night sweats; her alarm increased on the appearance of a sore at the edge of the nail of the big toe; yellow matter began to ooze out, and forebodings of an eating and fatal cancer were indulged. Her physician saw in this an effort of nature to cure herself. It was advised to promote the running by keeping the parts clean, and the application of soft poultices of milk and bread, to be renewed thrice a day, to keep down the inflammation; the bowels were made to act every day;

nourishing and plain food was eaten thrice a day without anything between; colds were avoided, and the sleeping apartments well ventilated; the result was that in a few weeks the cough left her, and she had good health thereafter, dying at the end of ten years, aged seventy-five.

AGUE,

FROM a Gothic word meaning to shake or tremble, that being the most characteristic and most striking symptom of the disease known usually as Intermittent Fever, Chill and Fever, and Fever and Ague; why it should be called Fever and Ague, when the Ague comes first, thus reversing the phenomena, is not known, unless it be for its easier designation of "Fevernager," that being the vulgar appellation, and which must have been invented "for short," by the man who was said to have been so lazy, that when he had the disease he wouldn't shake; it certainly takes all the energy out of a man, all his courage, all his ambition. The shaking of a regular Ague may be distinguished from a similar shaking from exposure to severe cold, the latter being, to some extent at least, controllable by force of the will, while no amount of mental effort can suppress the chill of Ague.

FEVER AND AGUE.

MANY thousand families are annually afflicted with this discouraging disease, which in many cases lays the foundation for tedious and even fatal maladies. When the results are not fatal, and the disease is imperfectly cured, it is liable to a return from very slight causes every spring and fall. For these reasons the article on Miasm should be read and studied by every intelligent parent, for this is the cause of fever and ague in all its varieties. This same miasm is also the prolific cause of the various grades and degrees and forms of diarrhœa, dysentery, bilious, dengue, yellow, and congestive fevers, and always and in all countries, wherever miasm is abundant, there cholera in its most deadly forms sweeps its multitudes into the remorseless grave.

MIASM

causes fever and ague by being introduced into the blood through the stomach and lungs, poisoning it, making it thick and black and heavy, so that it does not pass through the small blood-vessels or channels in various parts of the body, most noticeable in that portion of the system which from any cause is weaker than natural, giving names to disease according to the location; if for example the blood almost ceases to pass through the channels of the lungs, it is

PNEUMONIA;

if it dams up in the inner coating of the bowels it is

DYSENTERY;

but if this impaction or "congestion" (which specially see) takes place in the lungs and heart, or in all the terminal blood-vessels of the body, the phenomena of fever and ague may be manifested.

SYMPTOMS

of fever and ague are numerous; to detail them in all their minuteness would only confuse the mind of the reader, hence it is considered quite sufficient to say that there are four kinds.

First. Quotidian, or daily coming on with a chill in the forenoon, followed by a fever, then with a general perspiration; after that, for a few hours, the system seems to be in a natural condition, of a proper warmth; but this does not last long, for the natural heat begins to decline, and in proportion the blood becomes more sluggish, circulates with less freedom, until about the same time of day as in the preceding another chill takes place; and thus it may go on for weeks and months. This is the slightest form of fever and ague, and is more easily cured than the others; the "Tertian," for example, is more difficult of management; it comes on about noon, to be repeated in its heat and sweating and natural stages, to return with its chill at the end of forty-eight hours.

The "Quartan" has its ague fit in the afternoon, to return again in four days.

If the ague fits come earlier every day; it is an unfavorable sign; if they come later and later, or with less violence, it indicates a decline in the disease, and a looking forwards to a healthy termination. The

COLD STAGE

is attended with great thirst, as if nature knew that the blood was so thick it could not circulate, and that if it was diluted with water a remedy would be afforded ; at length, as if some desperate effort were seen to be needed, this same watchful nature appears to arouse herself to the necessity of forcing a more active circulation with a view of warming up the system, and so fever comes on, in proportion to the chill both in increase and duration ; this effort at length seems to weaken the whole body, and it relaxes; the fever subsides ; perspiration, the perspiration of relaxation, takes place ; then follows a season of apparent natural repose.

CURE OF FEVER AND AGUE.

In the cold stage hot drinks may be taken ; the patient may be put to bed with bottles of hot water to the back, arm-pits, and feet. In the hot stage cooling drinks may be used, acid beverages, and feet and hands and forehead may be wiped with a mixture of vinegar and water. But these are not advised ; in all sickness, rest is the one great and best medicine ; to be constantly doing something to a patient, requiring change of position, even to get up to take a drink of tea or water, does an injury, and much greater is the injury if this disturbance is associated with having to take some disagreeable physic ; the sick man should not even be talked to, much less questioned ; it is effort enough to have to listen to anything for politeness' sake, but to be required to give attention to a direct question and the instinctive effort necessary to give a correct answer is very often a waste of strength which the patient cannot afford. If conversation goes on in the sick-chamber at all it should be directed to other parties ; it should be cheerful or of interest, and in a distinct tone, so that every word can be heard without an effort. In fever and ague as well as in all other diseases, the idea should be always present that the invalid has no strength to spare, and that any exertion of that strength, physical or mental, which is not absolutely necessary, ought to be philosophically and conscientiously avoided.

Of all diseases in the world that very common and familiar one, fever and ague, most requires to be treated with medicine, and is least likely to be cured safely, radically, and lastingly by any other means than medicine.

The best time to begin to cure it is about two hours before the chill comes on. The object of any medicine in this case should be —First, to warm the system; Second, to thin the blood; Third, to unload it of its impurities. Therefore, about two hours before the expected chill, take two or more (See page 114) Pills; they begin to act on the system at once, and tend to warm it, and thus to prevent its falling into the low, cold state of ague or chill; at the end of two hours the calomel begins to act on the liver, either directly or indirectly, with the effect of drawing out of the blood that element which makes it thick and bad, and causing it to be passed off into the bowels and outwards; thus is the blood in fever and ague warmed, thinned, purified; but then it is necessary to keep up the circulation in order to prevent its falling again into the low, cold stage of ague. The best way to do this is to give quinine.

The tendency of the system in fever and ague is to run around, to pass through a process and to repeat itself, and, if you can interrupt that process, whether it be the cold or the hot stage, the habit of the disease is to that extent broken up; a single interruption will sometimes effect the object in mild cases. For example, a man was told that he could cure himself of fever and ague, from which he had suffered severely and long, if he would start soon after breakfast, run two miles, bore a hole in a tree, make a plug, and drive it into the hole with an axe, and then run back home; but he was not to stop an instant until his return. It was a perfect cure; because the exertion of the body and the interest of the mind, which was wholly absorbed in the novelty of the thing, forced up the circulation of the blood to an extent which made a chill impossible.

But as quinine acts upon the circulation of the blood in the same way, and with such certainty as to be considered "a specific" in that form of disease, meaning thereby a remedy which never fails; and as it is so much easier to swallow a few grains of quinine dissolved in water than to perform the feat above named, almost every one prefers to take the quinine, which, although it is made out of the bark of a tree growing in South America, discovered by an old negro, has made many persons invalids for life; for it is thought by too many that as it is a vegetable remedy it can do no harm, if it does no good. But a grain of strychnine or a drop of nicotine, both vegetable, can destroy life in an instant. This subject is specially alluded to here, because fever and ague is such a wide-spread disease, and quinine is such a common remedy, and is taken with such inconsiderate recklessness, that a public good may result from this extended treatment of the subjects connected with it.

It is generally supposed that to have the best effects of quinine on the system, to prevent the recurrence of fever and ague, it should be taken in doses large enough to cause a ringing in the ears, varying from five to fifty grains at a dose, according to the constitution, age, and habits of the person. But taken thus it has made many persons more or less deaf for life, and has originated headaches and other forms of brain-affections which have embittered the whole subsequent existence; and yet the author advises it in all cases of fever and ague, as it makes the cure certain and permanent in all curable cases, without any ill effects whatever in a single case ever yet known, in small doces.

If fever and ague is treated with quinine alone, it is liable to return in a week, a month, or a year, on the very first exposure of the body to any special cause of disease, as constipation, a bad cold or severe chill; it will break up the chill and fever to be sure, by waking up the circulation of the blood, warming it, and thus thinning it; but it does not rid the blood of those impurities, of those miasmatic particles which caused the disease; on the contrary, it puts the whole system to the dangerous strain of forcing through it this unnatural mass of blood, thick, impure, and excessive in quantity. No wonder, that in passing through the delicate organ of hearing it so frequently impairs that sense for life, if, indeed, it does not destroy it forever; but by giving the calomel first, the blood is not only diminished largely in amount, it is not only thinned, but warmed and restored almost to its natural and pure condition. Then comes in the timely and benign stimulus of the quinine, to keep it in circulation, and besides, to do somewhat in improving the appetite, as

" bitters " do, and promoting, aiding the digestion, by which nourishment is derived from the food, and carried into the circulation, to give the strength so much needed to build up the body after so many and large drafts have been made upon it.

The medical treatment which will cure all curable cases of fever and ague is as follows :

At bedtime take a pill made of five grains of calomel, one-sixth grain of tartar emetic, and one grain of gamboge; if it does not act on the bowels within twelve hours take one tablespoon of castor oil or Epsom salts every hour until the bowels do move, not eating any solid food during the day, except cold bread and butter, with tea, or bread-crust broken into any kind of soup, at five hours interval, and nothing whatever in the way of solid food between ; may take hot tea freely ; meanwhile take in the morning, at two o'clock, and at six o'clock of that day, and during breakfast, dinner, and supper each day thereafter, the following

FEVER-AND-AGUE DRAUGHT.

Put into a small bottle thirty grains of sulphate of quinine, add a tablespoonful of water and one teaspoonful of elixir vitriol, shake it well ; then add two tablespoonfuls of peppermint water; twelve ounces, that is, twenty-four tablespoonfuls of best brandy ; if not at hand, whiskey or gin or alcohol or spirits of wine ; then add one teaspoonful of capsicum, which is the best red pepper powdered, and is only to be had at the best drug stores under the name of capsicum. Shake this well and take one tablespoonful at a time in three or four tablespoons of water; in violent or long-continued cases two tablespoons may be taken at a time, especially at the morning dose. In milder cases, less than a tablespoon may be sufficient. As there is so much fever and ague all over the United States, especially in localities far removed from drug stores and physicians, thus throwing the treatment and its responsibility on persons not familiar with medicines and sickness, this article is more extended than it would be under other circumstances, in order to make the instructions more full, and to acquaint the reader with the reasons of the treatment, what a medicine is given for, what it is expected to accomplish, and the effects which that medicine is expected to manifest ; in this way it will be very satisfactory to the patient and friends to observe that the medicine is doing what it was expected to do, thus affording great encouragement and hope to all. Then again, there may be peculiar cases and constitutions upon which the medicine will have no effect whatever, when it would be useless to pursue it beyond a day or two. Then again, in a thinly settled country far away from civilization, one or two ingredients may not be had, and the person might therefore think that if all could not be had it might be better to take none of it. But if, on taking such of the ingredients as can be had, the desired effects follow, then the way is clear and open. Therefore, it is better to state the philosophy of the whole treatment. When persons have fever and ague for a long time a hard cake forms above the edge of the ribs on the left side, as large as a plate; this is commonly called an

AGUE CAKE,

and is known to be the result of the hardening and enlargement of the spleen, situated at that side of the body.

Physicians know that the spleen is the reservoir of the blood to supply it to the liver when wanted, and that all the blood of the body passes through the spleen into the liver, whose work is to withdraw from the blood all its impurities. These impurities we call

BILE.

These facts show that the spleen and liver are intimately and directly connected, consequently the disease of one is likely to be communicated to the other. The ague cake shows that in fever and ague the spleen becomes diseased; it is, then, a reasonable inference that in fever and ague the liver becomes diseased; if proof of this were wanting, it is in the fact that in very protracted cases of fever and ague the liver swells and hardens, and there is an ague cake on that side also. It is, then, clear that the seat of the disease in fever and ague is in the liver and spleen; the spleen, being the mere supplier of blood, is the passive; the liver, working up the blood, is the active agent, and consequently we must address the remedies to it. To determine what is the matter in the liver it is only necessary to notice, that as it and the spleen are liable to swell, to increase in size, and as that could not happen in any other way than by there being more blood in them than is natural, we conclude that the blood sent there from the spleen to be worked up, so as to have the bile taken out of it, is not worked up fast enough, consequently accumulates and accumulates until it is so engorged that it can't work; there is not room, as it were, for the little manufacturer of bile to turn around or move about, like a man in a dense crowd of people—he can't raise his hand to his head until by desperate exertions he forces a little room for freer movements. The thing to be done, then, in the present case is to stimulate the liver to extra exertions in order to enable it to work up the blood, and thus diminish the amount.

It is said in ordinary medical conversation, that calomel "acts" on the liver, that is, stimulates it to work. It is an undisputed fact, that if calomel is given, the liver is relieved; the way in which this is done need not be discussed here; it is sufficient to have the fact.

When persons die of torpid or diseased liver, and it is examined after death, a substance is often found which is described to be as

BLACK AS TAR.

Very often in liver-diseases when calomel is given it is followed within ten or a dozen hours by a discharge from the bowels as "black as tar," and in other respects just like that which is found in the liver after death. Putting these things together shows that calomel does bring this black matter from the liver into the bowels and out of the body. Hence it is said that in effect calomel "acts" on the liver, "stimulates" it, unloads it.

Besides this, calomel excites a kind of fever in the human body; this fever means a quicker and stronger circulation of the blood through the body; this fever, this quicker and stronger circulation, extends to the liver, helping it to make a more desperate effort to free itself from the crowd, or damming-up of the excess of blood within it; so calomel acts in two ways on the liver, directly or indirectly, the effect of both which is to relieve it of the load of accumulated blood.

But after the liver has been whipped up to this extra exertion to disencumber itself of the excess of blood and bile, the reaction comes, and it is by this extra exertion left weaker than it was before, so that at this point something must be done which is known to keep up the circulation—to excite, as it were, an artificial fever; and quinine, which is prepared from the bark of a tree, is known to do this almost infallibly. Hence after the calomel has unloaded the liver the quinine comes in to keep the passage clear, by forcibly hurrying the blood along all the blood-vessels everywhere, so as to make another accumulation impossible ; so a dose is taken, and before its effects have passed off another is taken, keeping up the circulation until a habit of it is established, and the man is permanently well. The cure of fever and ague consists, then, in two things :

The calomel purifies and thins the blood by helping the liver in some way to withdraw the bile from it, and in this thinner and purer condition it is easier to keep up its circulation along the blood-vessels than if it were as thick as mud.

Thus it is seen that in reality fever and ague is an effect of the accumulation of blood in the liver, of blood made thick and bad by the bile that is in it ; calomel purifies and thins that blood and makes it easy of circulation, which circulation quinine promotes and keeps up until it becomes natural and healthful.

CHILL AND FEVER,

or fever and ague, or intermittent fever, are one and the same, as stated before ; all showing that there are two conditions of the disease : fever, or an excited circulation, and a condition when the circulation is not excited. Fever is the highest stage of excitement, chill is the lowest or slowest stage of excitement, or rather circulation, and the system, like a pendulum, swings between the two; the highest point to which the pendulum rises is the highest point of fever or heat; the lowest point to which it falls is the lowest point of cold. Health is the equilibrium of these, a regular state of natural warmth.

In the cold stage of an attack Nature seems to be aware of the danger, for cold is death, and with an inherent instinct seems to feel the necessity of making a desperate effort for life, beginning at the heart, making it beat faster and stronger ; but by the time the accumulations are removed she seems to be left exhausted, and falls down to the cold, slow stage again ; but in getting down to that cold, slow stage she passes through the condition of health, for after each fever comes perspiration, but that is too much of a circulation for health ; hence the perspiration passes off and the natural condition of the body is resumed, and the patient feels almost well; but at this point the system has exhausted all its strength in keeping up the circulation, gets weaker and weaker every instant, cooler and cooler, until another chill comes on.

In view of all these statements, advantage may be taken of these different conditions of things to the effect of curing the disease more speedily and with less strain or shock to the system, thus—

About two hours before the expected time for the chill, which comes on about ten o'clock in the morning in ordinary fever and ague, which brings us to about eight o'clock, take on an empty stomach the pill named; it soon begins that excitement in the system which calomel induces, and by the time two hours have passed, this excitement is at its highest point, and it is time for the chill to take place, thus preventing the chill from coming on, or at least modifying it; hence an important step is taken towards keeping the circulation more equable; then about noon take a dose of quinine, keeping up the circulation, and repeat it at supper-time, which will keep it up well on towards morning; the whole treatment being to equalize the circulation, to prevent the system going down to the cold stage, and making it unnecessary to rise up to the stage of fever. Other things may do the same things which quinine does; high mental or moral or physical excitement coming on about two hours before the chill have accomplished the same thing; but as quinine is the most infallible and more convenient, physicians prefer the surest and easiest way.

Various things are advised in medical books for alleviating the different symptoms in the successive stages of an attack; as a warm bed, warm drinks, warm bottles to arm pits, back, and feet in the cold stage; cooling drinks, lemonade and similar things in the hot stage; but such things tend to weary the patient or oppress the stomach, hence, as a general rule, it is better to do nothing but give the calomel and quinine, and let the sufferer have all the rest possible.

The quinine alone in half a glass of water is all that is really necessary in composing the draught before named; yet each of the other ingredients have a separate advantage. The elixir vitriol, or sulphuric acid, or even vinegar, is added because it helps to dissolve the quinine more effectually, so that the same amount will do more good; the peppermint water is used to give an agreeable taste and smell; the brandy has its own stimulating effect, while the capsicum has a wonderfully warming power in the stomach and bowels, and also promotes the general circulation.

If the attacks come on every day, or every other day, or

every seventh, fourteenth, twenty-first, or twenty-eighth day, it is well to take the calomel pill about two hours before the expected time of chill. There is a tendency to periodicity in many diseases—a tendency to come on at certain hours of the twenty-four, or at intervals of twenty-four, thirty-six, or forty-eight hours, or at intervals of sevens of days, or once a month, or once a year, as hay fever, for example; but more than all others fever and ague tends to this periodicity, and advantage should be taken of this by beginning, as above directed, a while before the attack. Tartar emetic is put in the pill because it has a tendency to nauseate, to relax the system, and thus aids the action of the calomel in unlocking the bile. The gamboge is to make it more certain that the bowels shall act within twelve hours, for if there is a good action of the bowels within ten or twelve hours after it is taken salivation is almost impossible. Salivation is caused by the mercury remaining too long in the system before it is worked off; it is caused by a continuation of the action of the mercury; hence unless it is desired to produce salivation the pill above-mentioned should not be taken oftener than once in a week, and should be worked off with castor oil or Epsom salts within twelve hours after it has been taken; but if it acts itself within twelve hours neither the oil nor salts are necessary, and so with any other preparation of calomel or mercury. Neither castor-oil nor salts are essential; anything else may be taken which has the effect in the particular individual to move the bowels, such as the various spring waters sold at drug stores and other places.

It is bad practice, it is unwise, it is positively injurious to attempt the cure of fever and ague with quinine alone; the pernicious effects of such an endeavor are constantly narrated in medical publications. Sometimes it seems efficient, but sooner or later the attack returns, in a week or two, or month, or more; it is like cutting off a weed at the surface of the ground; but preceding the quinine with an efficient dose of calomel is digging it up by the roots.

When a person has succeeded in preventing a chill it is better to continue the quinine a week at least; then at the end of the week reduce the dose one-half; then for a week take it but twice a day; then only of mornings for a week; then omit altogether. In this way sure work will be made of it; otherwise it is likely to return, and thus hang on for weeks and months, baffling and discouraging the patient, if indeed it does not lay the foundation for dropsies and other chronic diseases more difficult of removal than the fever and ague.

In case the chills are not satisfactorily broken up after one pill, and after taking the quinine for two or three days, then double the dose, and take another pill in seven days after the first, and observation will show when the disease is eradicated.

Sometimes it is more efficient when the returns of the fever and ague are at the eve of the seventh, fourteenth, etc., days, to begin taking the quinine on the day preceding.

DIET IN FEVER AND AGUE.

The patient ought not to eat much for breakfast, because the digestion of the food draws a good deal of heat from the general system to the stomach, leaving the body colder than it would have been, thus intensifying the chill.

At noon, and for some hours after, the fever takes away the appetite generally, and it is always hurtful, even in health, to swallow a single mouthful without an appetite, for it will remain in the stomach unchanged, to oppress and worry for hours sometimes. But by supper-time the system gets into its natural condition generally, and having had little food, it is naturally very hungry; the multitude yield to this, make a hearty meal, have a bad night's rest, wake up in the morning unrefreshed, unstrengthened, with the result that disease is aided, aggravated, and kept in the system for a long time; the very mode of life antagonizes the efforts of nature to cure, and the wholesome effects of medicine. The general diet in fever and ague should be as follows:

During the day in which the pills are acting, eat thrice, with at least five hours interval, taking nothing but hot tea or soup, with the crust of cold bread broken into it, using as much red pepper as practicable, because it is warming; the best is that known in good drug stores as "capsicum," or Cayenne pepper. On other days, whether quinine is taken or not,

BREAKFAST

not later than seven o'clock, because a good warm meal rouses the circulation and increases the warmth, thus early begins to antagonize the cold stage which tends to come on at about ten. This breakfast should consist of some hot drink, with cold bread and butter, and some fresh meat, fish, or fowl, with plenty of capsicum; cut the meat up fine, chew it deliberately, and eat slowly, about half as much as you want, for if you fill the stomach it will be oppressed, and thus will the chill be increased. If you eat but half as much as you wanted, you will feel in half an hour that you have taken quite enough, and will be glad that you had not eaten more.

DINNER

same as breakfast, not sooner than one o'clock. One vegetable may be added, but no dessert whatever.

SUPPER

should be about sundown, aiming not to eat at shorter intervals than five or six hours, because it takes the stomach about five hours to "work up," to digest an ordinary meal, and it should be allowed some rest, otherwise it would soon be overworked, and would not digest anything well, healthfully, because it had not the strength; that is

DYSPEPSIA.

The best supper for the fever and ague patient is a cup of hot drink, some cold bread and butter, and nothing else whatever. Not anything afterwards until breakfast next morning. There are two things which the patient should watch against with great care—costiveness, and getting chilled.

COSTIVENESS.

To prevent costiveness, either use whatever remedy you are familiar with for that purpose, or common castor-oil (which see); take about a tablespoon, more or less, night and morning—just enough to cause the bowels to act once in twenty-four hours, for if that is not the case, quinine will injure the system, will do more harm than good.

Persons will always get well of fever and ague more rapidly by removing to another locality, either farther north or to a more hilly or mountainous section, where there is less liability to have stagnant water or sluggish streams.

If calomel and quinine cannot be had, or these medicines from some cause cannot be taken, another remedy is found sometimes efficient. After clearing out the bowels effectually, take four grains of alum, and three grains of sulphate of iron, made into pills, three times a day for ten or fifteen days; it certainly has, now and then, been exceedingly efficacious; at the same time, confidence is not imposed upon any other remedy than calomel and quinine.

A HOMŒOPATHIC REMEDY

is said to be found in filling an ounce-bottle half full of homœopathic arsenicum pellets, drop on them five drops of

FOWLER'S SOLUTION,

or arsenical solution, being a preparation of potash and arsenic; take ten of these pellets every four hours, putting them on the back part of the tongue, but be sure to keep the bowels acting freely all the time, at least once or twice a day; or, after the allopathic manner, take from three to ten drops three times a day, in one or two tablespoons of water. Arsenic is a poison, and thus taking it, it may disturb the stomach, constipate the bowels, causing headache, confusion of mind, dizziness, oppression, despondency; in such case leave off its use for a few days, and then begin again.

WATER-CURE TREATMENT

is often efficient when it is impossible to procure any medicine whatever, hence the usefulness of its being detailed here.

Begin by giving tepid injections to unload the bowels freely; if there is sickness of stomach, poor appetite or coated tongue, drink warm water freely until copious vomiting is induced, this brings up a large quantity of bile, and thus helps to unload the liver. Use the wet sheet, or in the last stage immersion is desirable; if there is headache, use the

HEAD BATH,

by folds of cloths dipped in cold water, placed on the head and renewed every five minutes, or a stream of water poured on the head with the face downwards, the head being held by an attendant over the side of the bed, protecting the bed by a sheet or blanket thrown over the patient's neck and shoulders, a tub being placed on the floor to receive the water. This water should be poured from a pitcher in a continuous stream until the head is cooled, that being the object; the water running down over the temples and cooling them off rapidly.

Or the patient may lie down on the floor in such a position, having a pillow or two under the shoulders, as to hold the head back in a basin of water several inches deep, thus keeping the scalp in the cold water all the time. When the fever is absent a hot bath might be taken, followed by a cold dripping sheet or shower bath, all the time keeping a cold-water bandage around the abdomen, covering the region of the liver; this opens the pores of the skin over the liver, and thus gives exit to disease-producing matters.

Slight attacks are cured by a few "packs" (which see, under head of bathing), or a single immersion in cold water; but if the system has been under the influence of these attacks for weeks and months, a patient treatment is necessary by gradually establishing the healthful natural action of the skin, spleen, and liver.

In connection with the above, the diet should be of bread made of the whole of the wheat grains, Graham bread or, cracked wheat made into a mush, with a little milk and sugar, to make it more palatable, with a moderate use of fresh, tender vegetables; apples baked, stewed, or raw; berries, grapes, tomatoes, prunes, and dried fruits of every description; or break into warm drinks the crust of light bread. Drink water freely, exercise in moderation, carefully avoid over-exertion; boating, horseback and carriage riding; so as to have the benefit of the out-door air without much fatigue; for over-exertion, great tiredness, may bring on an attack any day.

MIASM

MEANS emanation, a rising up from the surface of the earth; it is a result of the combination of three things : heat, moisture, and vegetation ; the three together give rise to decomposition, a destructive decay of vegetable matter, the product of which is " Miasm," the great commencing cause of fever and ague, and other more serious forms of fever. Whether miasm is a gas, an impure or poisonous air, holding in it a vegetable product or a living thing, animal in its nature, is not here discussed ; for whatever it may be, the laws which govern it are understood, and its effects towards originating various forms of disease are the same, while the vegetable material of leaves, grass, and wood is the thing from which miasm arises. There is one condition essential to its production,—this vegetable matter of leaves, grass, and wood must first decay ; but this decay cannot·take place without both moisture and heat acting on this dead vegetation, for the leaves and grass and wood must die first. If a piece of wood is kept under water it will not decay in a thousand years ; if it is always kept dry it will last always ; or if laid on an iceberg in Greenland it will endure for ages. Therefore, to cause fever and ague, vegetable matter must be decomposed, must be rotted by the application of moisture and a certain degree of heat, which, it has been observed, must be over eighty of Fahrenheit.

The farther north we go the less fever and ague there is, because it is too cold, there is not heat enough. In the great deserts of the world there is no fever and ague, because there is no moisture, and vegetation dries up. But where leaves and grass fall and die, and twigs and limbs and logs of wood float on our ponds and streams, acted upon by our summer suns, there fever and ague abounds, attacking individuals, striking down whole families, and afflicting extensive districts of country.

The localities most favorable for the production of miasm are swampy lands, flat river bottoms, mill ponds, and other stagnant bodies of water. The common observation of the people is, that such conditions cause fever and ague. Fever and ague, bilious, yellow, and congestive fevers are one and the same disease essentially, only different in degree ; the cause of them all, when they prevail among a whole community, is miasm more or less concentrated. An experiment has been tried, that if a barrel or two of the air of a miasmatic locality in the South is taken a thousand miles north, and placed in a room where a man is sleeping, the room kept closed and of a southern temperature, fever and ague will be caused in a day or two.

HOW MIASM OPERATES.

The above experiment shows that the thing in the miasmatic air which causes ague is taken into the system by being breathed into the lungs and swallowed into the stomach; in both ways passing directly into the blood, to corrupt and poison, making it bad blood; proven by the fact that the blood of such persons is thicker and blacker than is natural, growing thicker and blacker, to become bilious fever; but in congestive fevers it is seen in the most concentrated form, almost as black as tar in some parts of the body, and so thick with impurities sometimes, that if a lancet is run into a vein in the arm, the blood will not flow; called " congestive " from the very fact that the blood dams up to the extent of approaching a condition of solidity; these more fearful forms of fever are more common in the South, where it is warmer, where the flatness of the country favors stagnant waters, and where vegetation is so luxuriant that all the conditions of the miasmatic production are increased and intensified; thus miasm causes a third form of disease in the prairies of the Northwest, the fever and ague which rankles in the system for weeks and months and even years without producing fatal results. Along the stagnant bayous of the South, with surfaces covered with a green, bubbling, fermenting material, congestive fevers are generated which strike down the strongest constitutions, and the most stalwart and vigorous of men are laid stiff in death in a few hours.

PREVENTIVE MEASURES.

Although the heat of the summer's sun cannot be modified by any human agencies, yet much can be done by draining flat lands, by filling up low places and stagnant ponds and streams, and by the removal of undergrowths, and using all possible means for the promotion of cleanliness in all the surroundings of human habitations. But until communities can be educated to precautions like these, individuals will have to protect themselves by antagonizing the effects of miasm on their own persons and on the members of their household, and this is not difficult to be done, if the laws of miasm are well understood.

Fever and ague generally comes on in the fall of the year, although when a person has once had it, it often reappears in the spring; but a first attack is usually in the autumn, because the continuous warmth of the summer has heated the surface of the earth to the degree requisite for the decomposition of leaves, grass, and twigs. When the atmosphere is impregnated with miasm, its virulence changes several times during the twenty-four hours; at noon-day and at midnight it is least hurtful to breathe it. In the earlier years of the country, when Charleston in South Carolina was so frequently visited with the yellow and other malignant fevers, the merchants and others in the better walks of life arranged to live in the country in the summer-time; but as it was necessary to be at their business places in the city at least occasionally, common observation impressed the fact on the minds of observant persons, that those who rode to town in the heat of the day and returned in the heat of the day, escaped the fever; while those who came in the morning and returned late in the afternoon, when it was cool and comfortable, were sure to get sick, while it was almost certain death to remain in town all night.

In the early days of Californian gold discovery it was a received fact that persons who slept on the Isthmus at Panama usually died with fever in a few days. Such a result was so uniform that the commanders of vessels would never give the sailors permission to remain all night; it was imperative for them to return before sundown. An eminent Bishop, having occasion to go to California, was invited to perform a marriage ceremony at Panama. Notwithstanding the caution of the captain of the steamer to be sure and return to sleep on board, he decided after the ceremony that he would remain all night; he left early next morning; but the disease had entered his blood; he was taken sick the same day and died soon after.

Travellers who have occasion to cross the marshy country outside of modern Rome are invariably reminded of the almost fatal results of sleeping all night on the way.

Scientific observation has shown that these results are founded on the operation of certain physical laws as imperative as that of gravitation.

Heat rarefies the air on the surface of the earth and it ascends to the higher regions; cold causes its condensation, and it falls to the ground again. At midday in summer, at Charleston, the heat is such that the miasm is carried at once towards the clouds, while the atmosphere on the surface of the earth is so rarefied by the heat that it contains scarcely any miasm; as the sun goes down it becomes cooler, the air is condensed and falls to the surface of the earth, or so near it that it is readily breathed into the nostrils, is carried to the mouth, and with the saliva makes its way into the stomach, to be conveyed into the general circulation of the blood; as the air gets cooler towards midnight the miasm falls so near the surface that it is not breathed, hence is innocuous; but with the rising sun the air is warmed again, and the miasm ascends to a height to be readily breathed in; but by midday there is none left. This is the reason why persons in the country could come into Charleston at midday with impunity; they could have gone in at midnight also without harm, but by remaining all night the poisonous air of sunset and sunrise was taken into the system and death resulted.

It is seen, then, that it is the air about sunrise and sunset which causes the poison of fevers, of whatever grade; but to make that air innocuous, all that is necessary is to make it as warm as at midday, by kindling a bright blazing fire on the hearth in the family rooms at sunrise and sunset in miasmatic localities; and sit by that fire until breakfast has been taken in the morning, and supper has been taken at sundown. As long ago as eighteen hundred and twenty this precaution was taken by the more intelligent persons of the Western country, and with unfailing success, these families being exempt from fever and ague, while scarcely a house escaped where these precautions were disregarded.

The clear sharp rule is—

In all localities where fevers prevail, from June to frost, avoid going outside of the door until breakfast has been taken, and dress before a blazing fire. Go into the house before sundown, and remain in a room where there is a cheerful fire until after supper; after that there is no danger from being in the night air until sunrise, because the atmosphere is cold and heavy with its

9

load of miasm, and rests immediately on the surface of the earth.

The advantage of eating breakfast before going out of doors in the morning, and of taking supper at sundown is this, the breakfast warms and strengthens the stomach, which has taken nothing to sustain it for perhaps twelve hours, and the presence of food in it gives a vigor to the circulation which repels the attack of disease ; while supper tends to revive the body, weak and tired by the labors of the day.

It is certainly a very delightful thing after a hot summer day to sit in the porch or on the stoop or under a tree, before the door, and have the balmy breeze of a summer evening to cool the fevered face and brow ; but in southern countries, where epidemic fevers kill multitudes every day, it is a well-understood fact that the sundown breezes are indeed most delicious, yet they are but the prelude of greater fatalities for several days to come.

Within a very few years the heir to a European throne, while travelling in summer through a marshy flat country, expressed a wish to get up early in the morning and take a ride on horseback in the cool of the day ; his host represented to him that it was dangerous to do so, and urged him to take his breakfast before starting. The suggestion was disregarded, he was stricken down with the fever in a day or two, and soon thereafter died.

In all these cases where it seems imperative to go early into the morning air in summer, and a regular warm breakfast cannot be taken, the next best thing is to take some kind of hot drink, or a sandwich, or one or two apples, oranges, or plain cakes, something which will stimulate the stomach to that kind of activity which unquestionably has the effect to repel disease or nullify the causes of it with great uniformity.

The French and Spanish creoles of the South live long and healthfully ; they are proverbially exempt in a great measure from the ill effects of the fevers of the country. It is universal with them to have a cup of hot coffee brought to their bedsides before they get up in the morning, or arrange to have it on their tables ready for them as soon as dressed ; a custom taught by the common-sense observation of the people of the country, ignorant of the reason, but confirmed as to the facts of the case.

If a bundle of facts are thrown together there may seem at first to be no uniformity in the operation of miasmatic laws, but if these facts are analyzed and properly classed, they will be found to be beautifully simple.

A gentleman of wealth built for himself a handsome country seat, costing a large amount of money ; his calculation was to spend his summers there with his large family of growing daughters. The situation was splendid, for it overlooked the bay, and the sea and its pure breezes were relied upon to plant the rosy hue of health on every daughter's cheek. In a short time the coachman was taken with chills and fever ; soon afterwards another member of the family, and then another. Before the summer was over he abandoned the place, and by the next year had built another mansion in another locality ; for he saw that the prevailing winds blew over a sheet of stagnant water, in the direction of his house, but with their delicious coolness, morning and evening, they came heavily freighted with the deadly miasm of the pond. His nearest neighbor on the other side of the pond never had a case of chill and fever in his family. Lesson : in selecting a location for a house, make a note of the direction of the prevalent winds, that they be from the house towards miasmatic localities, and not from miasmatic localities towards the house.

A New Yorker, wishing to have more room and a purer air for his growing family, purchased a site further up-town, and erected a dwelling upon it, which cost him over a hundred thousand dollars. He moved into it, but within a few weeks several members of his family had intermittent fever, a mild form of fever and ague. He abandoned the house at once, because he found that it had been built upon a sunken lot, which had been filled up with every variety of city garbage, and kitchen offal, the bottom of the lot having been previously covered with water, and receiving the drainage of pastures and woodlands with their dead grass and leaves. For years the emanations of them came up through the cellars and crevices of the floors night and day. Many years ago the bed of a small stream was filled up in Rochester and a street made of it ; about that time the cholera made its second appearance in this country ; the street was dug up for the purpose of laying down water or gas pipes, thus allowing the accumulated miasms of years to rise and spread themselves along the whole line of the street, with the effect that scarcely a family or resident escaped the cholera, and along that street its most fearful ravages were made, showing that the elements of miasm may be covered up for years under many feet of earth, but on being allowed to escape, have their most malignant effects, teaching the lesson, " Never locate a dwelling over a sunken lot, or on the line of a filled-up drain or pond or running stream."

A well-to-do farmer had, in the course of years, made himself a splendid home, regarded as one of the most healthy locations in all that region of country. But in the fall of the year a servant was taken sick, then another, then a member of the family, until the handsome mansion became a hospital, and at length the whole neighborhood for miles became infected with various forms of disease, chiefly fever and ague. There had been a freshet in the spring, the mill-dam had been washed away, and left the black slimy bottom of the pond exposed to the hot sun. And as this dark mud was largely made up of the decomposition of leaves and grass and twigs and rotten logs, the accumulations of years, miasm was generated with great rapidity, and in its most concentrated and malignant form ; the remedy in this case was either to fill up with fresh earth, or with water a foot or two or more deep, for miasm does not rise through water, nor has it as yet been known to cross any rapid stream a mile wide, the presumption being that the water rapidly absorbs it and carries it away.

Some years ago there was a very unhealthy neighborhood of considerable extent along a valley, for the most part dry except a few months in winter ; agues and fevers and diarrhœas and dysenteries became increasingly frequent, until the discouragement of the people was such that they began to sell out for what prices they could get, and move away. The very next year there was scarcely a single case of sickness, and the remarkable healthfulness continued for several years, when it as suddenly returned. The reason was, that by the operation of the not uncommon " crevasses " of the Mississippi River, the surplus water found its way into this valley, covered its bottom with a running stream several feet deep. Later on, by another change, the stream of water ceased to flow through, having been diverted to another channel, and left the locality as " sickly " as before.

A neighborhood noted from time immemorial for its healthfulness, is desolated with a fatal disease in a single season. Multitudes of cases of this kind have occurred, because the sickness was preceded by the driest summer known within the memory of the "oldest inhabitant ;" that dry summer evaporated the water from the ponds and water-courses in all that section of the country, leaving muddy beds exposed to a summer sun.

Another time a section of country proverbially sickly escapes the annual visitation, while every one was looking forward to a season of greater sickliness than had ever been known; the reason was that the greater amount of rain had kept the beds of streams and shallow ponds so deeply covered with water that the sun could not act upon the matters fruitful of miasm. On one occasion a uniformly healthy section of country became suddenly sickly in the early part of August, becoming more and more virulent for a whole month, when it suddenly ceased, and everybody began to get well, from an inevitable law of miasm. Up to the first of July, there not only had been little or no rain, but the weather was fearfully and continuously warm; but the warmth and drought continuing, the disease at once abated, because the unusually warm and dry weather combined to empty the ponds and shallow streams of their water, leaving only their muddy beds, festering in the hot sun, engendering miasm in large quantities and of a most virulent character; but the heat continuing, and no rain falling, the bottoms of these springs and ponds and shallow streams became dried to powder, then there was no moisture, and where there is no moisture there can be no miasm.

Thus it is seen there is a beautiful uniformity in the law of miasm in all countries and in all seasons. Miasm and disease will always follow the exposure of the bottoms and edges of ponds, springs, and shallow streams to a hot sun; that disease will be promptly arrested when those bottoms are reduced to the dryness of powder, or are covered with a foot or two of water, especially running water.

Miasmatic diseases follow exposure to the cool air of morning and evening, about sunrise and sunset, especially when the stomach is empty or the body is weary, tired, exhausted, or the mind is harassed or distressed, because in any of these conditions miasmatic influences are unresisted, are taken into the stomach and lungs, absorbed into the blood, and rapidly corrupt and poison it; this poison giving rise, according to its virulence and the weakness of the constitution, to the various forms of autumnal disease, beginning with the mildest type of ague and fever, sometimes called fever and ague, or intermittent fever, bilious, congestive, and yellow fevers, as well as diarrhœa and dysentery. When the causes of miasm are general, miasmatic disease pervades whole neigh-borhoods ; when confined to circumscribed localities, only one or two families suffer, or single members of a family. It is impor-tant for useful, practical purposes, to give some facts on these points in order to impress the mind indelibly, and to be handed down from father to son.

Some years ago, on the eve of inaugurating a United States President, a large number of the inmates of a fashionable hotel of Washington City were taken ill; so many persons were so suddenly and alarmingly attacked with a variety of forms of sick-ness, that the impression was made throughout the whole country that it was the result of accidental poisoning; numbers died within a few days, some lingered on the borders of the grave for weeks and months, only to recover with a blasted constitution; others again never recovered. It was finally ascertained that the drains of the house had been obstructed to such an extent that when the privies were entered their contents spirted up between the joints of the floors; these contents were made up of what is ordinarily found in privies, together with the backwater of a slug-gish stream, the vicinity of which has been afflicted with the various grades of fever and ague for time immemorial. Persons who came to the hotel and took supper, and no other meal, were sometimes more affected than those who ate there all the time, for two reasons: First. The house was warmer at night, making the miasm more concentrated. Second. All men, especially travel-ers, are more wearied and exhausted at the close of the day, hence are more likely to suffer from the effects of bad air, especially of a miasmatic atmosphere. The ladies in the house, as permanent boarders, were less affected, as a general rule, than their hus-bands, who were away the greater part of the day. 1st. Because ladies generally rise late and come direct to the breakfast-table, thus "stay" their stomachs at once, and are not chilled by the cold air. 2d. They are for the greater part of the time in their rooms in the upper parts of the building, while gentlemen come home to tea weary and worn-out, and remain on the lower floors, where the noisome gases are more concentrated, which they breathe for several hours in succession; in the morning they rise earlier, go down-stairs to breathe the miasm in its concentrated forms and on an empty stomach. In all these statements the effects of miasm are various, but on close observation the laws of its action are as uniform as those which govern the motion of all worlds.

A family had lived for years on an elevated position, with a reputation for healthfulness which was the envy of many. But on one occasion the cook was taken sick, then the house-girl, and one by one the different members of the family, until nearly the whole household was seriously ill of a low form of fever. The investigation of the family physician pointed out the fact that some alterations had been made on the premises, and that a quantity of boards had been piled up not far from the kitchen door; on taking these down, a depression was found to have been made by having dug out some of the earth to make mortar; into this depression all the water and slops thrown from the kitchen door found their way, until a respectable little lake was formed, the whole dirty surface of it bubbling up with its decompositions of filthy ingredients. It was immediately drained, sprinkled all over the bottom with lime, filled to heaping with fresh earth, with the result that, from that very day, every member of the family began to improve in health; the result being that all were restored.

THE PRINCE OF WALES,

in the long and dangerous illness in the autumn of 1871, and which so excited the fears of the civilized world, by reason of what revolutions might follow his death, was for many days on the very verge of the grave from a low form of fever, with which he was attacked in common with his servant and a nobleman who had been with him some days; only the Prince survived. These three persons had to pass daily a certain yard where manure was manufactured; the inhalation of this offensive effluvia was so hurtful that the Duke of Beaufort, having had to pass it twice in one day, and once at another time, was taken seriously ill the same night. Thus it is that high and low are alike the victims of miasmatic influences, and will continue to be in the ages to come, unless a practical intelligence suggests measures which, in the light of miasmatic laws, shall prevent disease.

A certain room in the house of a family of means was renovated and set apart for the convenience and comfort of transient guests. It was summer-time. The first person who slept in it was taken ill next day; returned home and got well. Next, a member of the family had occasion to occupy it for a day or two, and became seriously ill; similar incidents were noticed for nearly a year, when at last the observation was made that every case of illness was preceded by the person having slept in that room. Beautiful and faultless as it was, it seemed impossible that the sickness could result from lodging in it; but the result was so uniform, the conclusion could no longer be resisted, that there was death somewhere in that room.   All at once it was remembered that it had been repapered.   The physician advised that all the new paper should be removed.   In one part of the wall it was found that several bricks had been removed, and in order to make the surface uniform and even, the upholsterer had filled up the hole with a mixture of paste and odd pieces of wall-paper, which in time began to decay and give out noisome exhalations, the paste being made of vegetable matter which soon began to decompose.

It is evident from the preceding facts in reference to miasm and its laws, and the sudden appearance of unusual sickness in a neighborhood, in a house, or in a single family, that the first effort should be to make a thorough investigation of the causes, and then remove them promptly; or if that cannot be done, to convey the patient to some distant and more salubrious locality.

Within the author's memory, Louisville, Kentucky, was one of the sickliest localities in all that portion of the western country. It abounded in stagnant ponds, the site originally having been very uneven.   Through the writings of several of the professors in the Medical Department of Transylvania University, men the most eminent of their time, to wit: Caldwell and Dudley and Yandall, and especially John Estin Cook, the giant of them all, every pond was drained, and the depressions filled up, with the result of an immediate improvement in the health of the people; and at the end of forty years, Louisville is now one of the healthiest, as well as one of the most beautiful and thriving cities of the whole Mississippi valley.

Many of our farmers, in all sections of the country, have sickness in their families for a greater part of every year, which could be escaped by simply draining their farms, or such portions of them as have too much water in the soil.

SITES FOR DWELLINGS

should be selected with an intelligent reference to the facts which have been stated; it is a sad thing, after the effort of a lifetime in getting a little ahead in the world, and to feel able to build a house to suit one's self, expecting it to be a home for life, to make an error in location, and find it to be so "sickly" as to enforce its abandonment, because the laws of miasm were either not understood or were disregarded.

ACID,

FROM a Latin word meaning sour, *acidus.* There are natural acids, as in the lemon; and artificial, as the common vinegar, under the name of acetic acid. Then there is a pyroligneous acid, meaning fire and wood, because it is made by destructive distillation, wood shavings put in water to be heated to a certain point. The vegetable acids are more natural and healthful than the artificial ; hence for all medicinal purposes, internally, the natural acids, as of fruits, are by far the most beneficial. The acids, vinegar especially, seem to have an action on food most like that liquid which the stomach generates to convert what we eat to a condition capable of imparting nutriment to the system, called gastric juice. Hence when there is a deficiency in the quantity of the gastric juice or in its strength, in dyspepsia, a tablespoonful or two of good vinegar promotes digestion.

AUSCULTATION

Is listening to the sounds given to the ear when it is laid on the chest, whether over the lungs or the heart, to ascertain whether they are in a healthy or diseased condition. To do this with advantage, the person must first know what are the natural, healthful sounds of these organs.

Something can be told by an experienced and quick medical ear, whether certain diseased conditions exist in the bowels, by placing the ear over the belly, and also, at certain stages, whether there is a living child in the womb.

But as actual heart-disease is comparatively rare, auscultation is mainly applied to the chest, to ascertain the condition of the lungs, whether they are consumptive or not. Consumption seldom exists on both sides of the lungs at the same time, hence if the sounds given out on corresponding spots of the chest are the same the presumption is that there is no consumptive decay.

Consumption nearly always commences at the top of the chest, immediately under the collar bone. If the sound given to the ear is precisely the same at corresponding parts, the presumption is there is no consumptive decay in either.

If in either of the above cases the pulse is uniformly about seventy beats in the minute, consumption is absolutely impossible.

When the air is drawn into the lungs in their healthy condition a distinct sound is given, something like the gentle moving of the air in the tops of the trees on a summer's day. This is not so distinct in health when it comes out.

If the sound is more distinct coming out than in going in, there is something wrong. If that sound is blowing, or like blowing into a wide-mouth vial, then there is a "cavity" in the lungs, which means that there is consumptive decay, which, if it could be seen, would be like a hole made in a cheese by mice eating into it; it would be an empty cavity.

But suppose in drawing in a breath, or in going out, a sound is heard as when blowing through a quill or other tube into a thick fluid, as syrup or molasses, that is proof that the lungs have decayed away at that spot, and that the cavity is partially filled with decaying lung-substance in the shape of thick, yellow matter, just like that which is spit out of mornings, or during the night, meaning that the person is in the last and hopeless stages of consumption.

There are cases in which the family or friends of the invalid must be thrown upon their own judgment, when it is indispensable that they should decide for themselves, as when a physician cannot be had, or implicit confidence cannot be imposed on him. It may be that the question is to be decided whether business should be given up, or serious sacrifices must be made to raise the means to take a long journey in search of health; or it may be a question of dying from home among strangers, or in the bosom of one's family. There are many cases of consumption where persons of ordinary intelligence can decide correctly themselves, thus : take a healthy man into a quiet room, throw back the collar of the coat, lay your ear flat on the vest, hold your own breath so as to make no noise, and listen to the sounds given out in a few inspirations and expirations ; then lay your ear on the breast, in the same way, and in the same spots, as in the healthy man ; if the sounds given out are pretty much the same in both persons at each point in the chest in front, or at the points of the shoulder blades in the rear or between the shoulder blades, where alone the lungs are fastened to the body, then, whatever may be the matter with the patient, there can be no consumptive decay. But if you hear the blubbering sound there is decay, there is a cavity, and that cavity is partly filled with yellow matter, the result of decayed lung-substance ; if with this the pulse is among the nineties or over, it is confirmed consumption in its last stages, and the man must die ; except that if there be very great energy of character or a great force of will, one in a thousand can live down the disease, and live on for a number of years, and finally die of some ordinary malady.

Sometimes in laying the ear on the chest there is no more sound than if it were laid against a wall; this means that the lungs at that point are solidified, that the little air-cells of the lungs, of various sizes, from a pin's head to a pea, are filled up with tubercles, which are the seeds of consumption ; or with blood, as in inflammation of the lungs, which is the same as

PNEUMONIA ;

or some other material, meaning in each case a dangerous condition of the lungs, always giving a symptom which is never by any possibility absent—shortness of breath.

In Asthma the sounds given out are of a wheezing, whistling character, or of a multitude of chirruping birds. There are other sounds given out by the lungs in different states of health and disease, but they are of minor importance, are not so appreciable by the inexperienced, nor can their meaning be decided upon except by those who have had large and long experience. These are omitted because they would rather confuse than profit the general reader ; only the obvious, unmistakable symptoms and indications have been stated.

ABSCISSION

Is the cutting out or off some useless or dead part from the body.

ABSINTHE

Is a new intoxicant, and a great favorite with the French of late years, especially of the Parisians, by whom its employment has become so general, and its observed effects so baleful and demonstrable, that the government has had its attention directed to the important subject of limiting its use. Kunsmuller, a German chemist, was the first to discover the peculiar qualities of Absinthin, which is from a Greek word meaning pleasurable, and which he obtained from our familiar plant

WORMWOOD,

or the Artemisia of the botanists ; this Absinthe is an intense bitter, which, modified by certain ingredients, is the basis of the modern French drink of Absinthe, against the employment of which in any form or in any quantity the reader is plainly warned, as it destroys the intellect, the morals, and the body of the man.

The leaves and flowers should be gathered in August and dried in the sun ; their medicinal properties are long preserved. As a medicine it may be used as other bitters ; it was so employed in fever and ague before quinine was discovered ; a dose of the powder was from twenty to forty grains ; or an ounce of the leaves and flowers in a pint of boiling water, dose when cooled, one or two teaspoonfuls several times a day at meals.

ABSORBENTS

"Suck up" every particle of matter in the human body which is in a liquid form, and pass it forward to one point, to be emptied into the heart and mixed with the blood.

There are two kinds of absorbents, Lacteals and Lymphatics. The

LACTEALS

are delicate little tubes connected with the alimentary canal. Their object is to take up the nutritious portion of the food as it

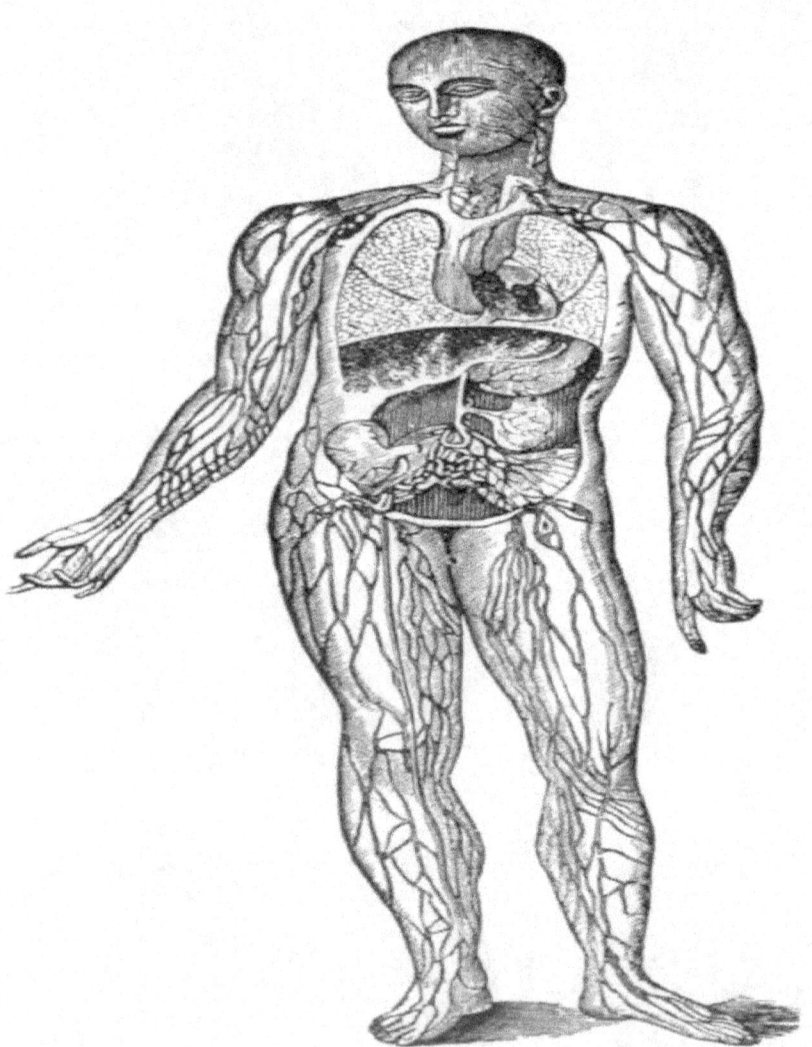

LYMPHATIC SYSTEM.

passes along the intestines; they constantly unite with one another, forming, as it were, larger branches or channels which become fewer and larger until they make one great branch or trunk, which passes up in front of the spine, and finally empties into a large vein which communicates directly with the heart. In this way all the nutritious portion of what we eat or drink is poured into the heart, where, meeting with the real blood of the body, it is instantly transformed into blood itself, to be made more perfect and pure, and to give more life when it enters the lungs.

As the fine roots of a plant suck up from the earth the nutrient material, and the finer roots lead into larger ones, until through one large root the juice of the plant is conveyed into the stock or tree, so the little lacteal fibres piercing through the intestines suck up little particles of nourishment from the whole mass of food as it passes along, so that when it gets to the lower part of the body, the intestinal canal, the rectum, there is no more nutriment in it and it is ready to be voided forth as of no further use to the body. These finer roots of lacteals join into larger ones until one large canal is made which empties itself into the heart, as named before. These lacteals take up particles which are not absolutely dissolved, as fats and oils. But there is another set of absorbents called

LYMPHATICS,

from their carrying a lymph or watery material from every portion of the human body, finally leading into one great duct or channel, which empties itself into the large vein as it enters the heart, like the lacteal system. This lymph or watery material consists mainly of all the waste matters of the system, matters which, having performed their part, subserved their uses, must be carried out of the system as the ashes are carried from a grate or stove or fireplace, otherwise there would be such an accumulation that no fire could be made. The human machine is like a clock which by long running wears away, and these worn-away particles must be removed, the watch must be cleaned or it will not run; only Nature has this advantage over art: the human machine is contrived with so much wisdom and beneficence, that it is made to clean itself, to carry out the waste particles as soon as they become waste and useless. This the lymphatics do to perfection, when in health, and thus keep the house we live in always "swept and garnished." In some parts of the body, near the surface, these lymphatics cross each other and form a kind of "bunch;" if by any means at this point the lymph which they are carrying is detained, is arrested, there is a kind of damming up, each little vessel becomes fuller and fuller, until the whole together presents the appearance of a "lump," more or less movable, more or less hard; sometimes a cold settles at one of these spots and causes a swelling, more likely to be in the groins, in the armpits, sides of the neck, and other places, and we call them

WAX KERNELS.

Sometimes these swellings are the result of inflammations, or bad feeding and other causes; many times they go away of themselves; at others, unless properly attended to, they inflame and break and cause running sores very difficult of cure. The first best step to be taken is to improve the

GENERAL HEALTH

(which article see); if the swelling does not subside in a week paint the part with a soft brush dipped into a strong tincture of iodine every other day, and patiently continue it for weeks and months if necessary, making it a point, at the same time, to eat nourishing food, meat and bread and fruits mainly, being out in the open air several hours every day in steady labor or pleasurable exertive exercise, by all means keeping the feet abundantly warm, dressing warm, and securing one regular daily action of the bowels, full and free. The importance of taking all this trouble to get rid of a simple swelling, which often gives no pain or other discomfort, is seen by considering the fact, that the lymphatics are employed as the scavengers of the system, carrying out of the body all that is dead or useless, which if not thus carried out must remain in the body, the further to clog it up, to derange its working, and finally to stop the whole machinery, and the man is dead. But a useful lesson of economy is taught us by the action of these same lymphatics: they do take up the waste matters of the system, but at these spots where the lymphatic vessels cross and inocculate with each other, making what is called a gland—and here lymphatic glands, this waste material is worked over again, and there is extracted from it a substance called fibrin, fibre-making, and being conveyed into the blood it helps to make flesh, and thus aids in supplying the waste of the system, which under ordinary circumstances is computed to be sixty grains every hour.

But these lymphatic vessels have another use, to convey water into the circulation; there is always water in the air we breathe, and this air comes in contact with the skin. If a man is very thirsty he will be appeased if he takes a bath. Sailors at sea in open boats have become drenched with rain, and the tormenting thirst has passed away. Narrations have been given to show that persons in an open boat at sea, without a particle of fresh water to drink, have had their thirst relieved by having sea-water poured over their clothing, these little vessels seeming almost to have an instinct that water was needed, hence they take up the water, but not a particle of the salt which it contains. Should the reader be so unfortunate as to be perishing with thirst, he can make use of these facts to great practical advantage. These little vessels should take up water and oils and fats, and not salt and other solid substances, because it is not their nature. A similar exhibition of selection is seen in filling a vessel half full of oil, then with water, stir it up, dip a piece of wick in oil, immerse one end in the mixture and set the other on fire, after a while all the oil will have been passed along the wick and consumed, the water left behind. It is not the nature of a wick to pass water any more than it is the nature of a lymphatic vessel or tube to pass some solid substances along it, and not to pass others.

Thus we see that the lacteals carry the nourishment which the food contains into the blood at the heart, while the lymphatics perform a similar office to the extent of utilizing the wastes of the system, so that

"NOTHING BE LOST."

When the lymphatic glands are very liable to swell and to ulcerate, there is a scrofulous condition of the system, and all such persons should make it a point to keep up the general health habitually, systematically, and thus prevent these glandular diseases, which, when they do break, should be treated as under the head of "Abscesses."

ANGINA PECTORIS

MEANS, literally, a kind of suffocation. There is a sudden and violent pain about the breastbone, extending towards the arms, indicating great and imminent danger; there is a cold-like sensation across the chest, great debility and alarm; it is a nervous affection, always, perhaps, depending on an organic disease of the heart, or the arteries leading to it, by which they become hardened, filled up with a kind of limy substance, as does the spout of a tea-kettle in limestone countries; the medical term is ossification. Gouty persons are most liable to it; it is almost peculiar to old men; women seldom have it. At first an attack goes off in a few minutes, hours, or days, with copious perspiration and urination, to be repeated with constantly shortening intervals until a fatal issue. At the same time persons subject to this affection have been known to live for many years.

To relieve an attack apply a mustard plaster to the chest and between the shoulders; this draws the blood away from the heart and lungs, and thus gives relief; at the same time put hot applications to the feet, wrap the patient warm in bed, drink hot teas of any kind, take three or four teaspoons of Hoffman's anodyne, or a teaspoonful of Warren's cordial in some hot water, or one or two tablespoons of brandy in a little water, repeated every half hour if necessary.

The real nature of the disease is that the blood cannot get to the heart, because the channels of the arteries which lead to it are nearly closed, and that very little blood passes, while there is damming up of the blood at the point where the ossification commences. One point to be accomplished is to draw away some of that accumulated blood to the surface by keeping it warm, and by the irritation of a mustard plaster, and then by the stimulants above-named to give more strength to the circulation for a short time, in order to force the blood through with a greater power and force and volume than Nature could do of herself; this gives the heart a little greater supply of blood, and the system generally becomes composed.

ANGINA ATTACKS PREVENTED.

If a person is subject to these distressing attacks, inasmuch as there is no cure, the effect should be to live in such a way as to prevent the attack coming on, simply by avoiding those things which are calculated to send the blood to the heart in greater quantities than is natural or usual, such as overstraining in any way, whether by heavy lifting, or running or other rapid exercise; or too protracted exertions of any kind; all violent emotions of the mind should be watched against, and in every way possible a calm, even, quiet mode of life should be cultivated, using all possible means to keep the general health in good condition, eating regularly of plain nutritious food, having a daily evacuation of the bowels and a free exposure to out-door air and sunshine.

ADDISON'S DISEASE,

So called from a physician of that name in Guy's Hospital, London, who in 1855 directed special attention to a malady known by the dark, dingy appearance of the skin, a kind of bloodlessness or want of natural nutrition, sooner or later always fatal. This bronzed appearance of the skin comes on very gradually, oftenest in bulky fat persons beyond middle life, and seems to be connected with a diseased condition of the

RENAL CAPSULES.

In many cases these capsules contain a creamy yellow matter, sometimes of a grayish appearance, which increases to the extent of destroying the organs.

Addison's disease proves fatal in from two months to two years, ending in diarrhœa, convulsions, or apoplexy; beyond attention to the general health there is, as yet, no cure for this kidney disease.

APHONIA

Is loss of voice, at least to the extent of not being able to speak above a whisper, and even then not without an effort, exhaustive and sometimes very painful; the first thing to be done in such cases is not to speak at all, in any strain, because the effort may snap the tender cords which form the voice, and thus lose that voice forever; even if this result does not follow, the effort to speak tends to increase the inflammation which causes the difficulty, and only protracts the cure.

10

The voice-making organs are at the top of the windpipe, two on each side, one above the other, the fraction of an inch apart; they are called vocal cords, being rather very thin membranes, which are made to vibrate by the air passing along, causing them to move; but if there is phlegm about them they will no more vibrate freely, will no more make a clear sound than would a fiddle-string or harp if encased in glue or mucilage. The reader has many a time felt a little "hoarse," the words would not come out clear and distinct, but by hemming or hacking up the phlegm in a forcible way he was able to speak with perfect distinctness.

In a common cold as it is getting well there is coughed up a yellowish or white-of-egg-like matter which comes from the lungs in consequence of their inflammation (which word see); this inflammation relieves itself by throwing off this matter until the health of the parts is restored, and the man is "well of his cold." This same process goes on in the voice-organs; they have been inflamed, this inflammation forms this gluey, mucilaginous phlegm, plasters it all over the vocal cords, or plates, above and below. Sometimes the inflammation is so great, or the cords are so loaded with this phlegm, that there is no power to move them, and there is no room for their vibration, no room for them to move an atom, or a line; in such cases there is complete voicelessness.

The remedy in such cases is the same as in a cold or as in asthma: something must be done to loosen the phlegm, preparatory to its being hawked or hemmed or coughed from the throat. Warmth on the outside has a tendency to do this by its opening the pores of the skin over the throat and neck; hence warm flannels are wrapped around the throat for "hoarseness," especially at night; more efficient in the night than in the daytime, because in the night the neck and head are more or less motionless, and the flannel is kept close to the skin, causing it to be continuously warm. In the daytime the head and neck are always in motion; every time the head is turned to one side, or the chin is elevated, as in looking to the top of a tree or house, a space is made between the skin and the flannel, the cold air rushes in, chills the parts, closes the pores, and gives a new cold, aggravates the hoarseness. To be benefited by muffling up the neck in any way, it must be done so as to keep the woollen flannel touching the skin all the time, otherwise harm is done and no good.

The phlegm may be diluted and loosened more speedily by flapping up hot water against the throat continuously for ten or fifteen minutes at a time, then very cold water for half a minute; this causes "reaction" (which word see), making the blood flow to the skin with great rapidity, and in such abundance as to cause considerable redness of the skin. A mustard plaster does the same thing (see "Derivation") by drawing the blood on the outside from the inside, thus cutting short the supply of material from which the phlegm is made; that is, phlegm is made out of the blood, and if you diminish the supply of blood in any way, there will be less phlegm made, less to be coughed away, making the cure more speedy. If moist warm air is breathed or drawn into the throat from the spout of a vessel filled with warm water, the phlegm is more or less loosened and diluted, as in asthma, bronchitis, and other affections of the air-passages. Nauseating remedies will do the same thing, as syrup of squills, wine of ipecac., and tincture of lobelia.

Swallowing small pieces of ice, or gargling freely with cold water, by cooling off the inflammation, affords grateful relief in some cases. But it is always important, in all forms of this disease, to keep the bowels acting freely once in every twenty-four hours, and eating regularly and in moderation.

Sometimes there is a loss of voice from certain derangements of the womanly functions, called

HYSTERICAL APHONIA,

which often passes off in a few hours or days of itself; sometimes it lasts for months, in consequence of a want of vigorous health; the only way to meet such cases efficiently is to use means to invigorate the body and the general constitution. The best are, regular bowels, exercising largely out of doors, or steady work in the open air for the greater part of daylight, until a good appetite and a vigorous digestion are secured, when the voice will return to its natural state. The above is voicelessness simply because there is functional derangement; all the machinery is there, but it is hampered, it is clogged, hence it does not work well; but there is

ORGANIC APHONIA,

where there is a cog missing or a wheel broken, and can never be repaired, because some ulcer has formed near or in the parts, and has eaten them away ; or some permanent tumor has grown in the vicinity which prevents healthful action ; these are to be determined by the personal inspection of an experienced physician. If there is actual ulceration the voice may never return, but the progress of that ulceration may be arrested by securing good "general health" (which see), and by the application of the nitrate of silver in such a way that it shall touch the ulcerous spot ; but as it is an exceedingly disagreeable operation, and the exact spot is often failed to be reached, and the healing would take place of itself by keeping up the general health, the application of the nitrate of silver is not advised, because it could not cure any case unless the general health were improved, and if that is done the ulceration would cease of itself, in all curable cases. The writer has seen no conclusive evidence that any throat ailment was ever permanently benefited by the application of the nitrate of silver alone. Some years ago almost every one was using it, now, almost no one, since the death of the introducer of it ; this simple fact ought to be an indication that it was not a valuable remedy in throat complaints. Electricity has sometimes been used for aphonia, and may be serviceable in hysterical or nervous cases, with this caution : if there is shortness of breath, or a shrill cough, electricity ought by no means to be used.

DYSPHONIA, ·

or difficulty in speaking, as in the case of clergymen and other public speakers, is of the same nature as aphonia, only less troublesome and more easy of cure. Very generally it arises from a wrong condition of the stomach (see "Throat Ail "), but there is a caution which is imperative, neglect has many a time proved fatal: Never make a public address when it requires an effort to speak clearly and distinctly ; one may almost as well put a razor to his throat. In such cases there must be absolute rest of the vocal organs, in reading, singing, or public speaking, followed up by recreation in travel, change of air and scene and habits of life and modes of preparing food, with a proper attention to the regulation of all the bodily functions. In many cases loss of voice to the extent of not being able to speak plainly or above a whisper, without considerable effort, becomes fatal within a few days ; thus a public speaker is hoarse ; he feels compelled to make an address; there is a large assemblage; he becomes excited, makes more of an effort than he is conscious of. In doing so the voice-organs and lungs have been overstrained, overheated; he goes into the open air, raw, damp, cold, and windy; in addition, perhaps, he walks against the wind to his home, or has to ride several miles; he gets thoroughly chilled, pneumonia sets in, and he dies within a week.

AMAUROSIS

Is an obscuring of the eyesight in consequence of some disease or injury done to the nerve of the eye, or of the brain near that point; it was formerly called gutta serena, from a misapprehension of the nature of the malady; it comes on by a very gradual diminution of the sight, the eye seeming for a long time to have nothing the matter with it; floating objects appear with variations of color; a kind of spectra, without any real existence; the pupil sometimes dilates, and the eye is insensible to the light. All these symptoms may be the result of a disordered condition of the liver or stomach, indicated by headache, bad taste in the mouth of mornings, not much relish for food; in such cases take three or four of Cook's pills at bedtime, living lightly (page 105 see); keep the bowels regular, exercise in the open air several hours every day, and keep the feet warm. If the symptoms do not improve in a week, if the spots or spectra do not disappear, and the sight does not become more natural, the presumption is that the nerve of the eye or some of its connections is in a diseased condition; in such case, if an oculist cannot be had, or a physician of experience is not at hand, until one can be secured, in addition to what has been advised above, the eye should be rested, there should be no reading or writing or sewing or any occupation which requires close observation of small things, doing everything in the mean time to promote the general health and build up the constitution.

Amaurosis is now used to imply defect of vision, and as this may arise from a great variety of causes—from nervousness, from uterine disturbances, from the striking in of any eruption on the skin, or the sudden stopping of any habitual discharge of any description—the point first to be ascertained is, is there anything the matter with the person but a disturbance of the vision, if so, and that is corrected, the sight will be restored; but when there is no other derangement, when there is nothing in the eye to all appearance indicating a diseased condition, then it may be decided positively that it is amaurosis, as a result of a diseased or injured condition of the nerve of the eye, and that there is no remedy, except in such treatment as some eminent oculist may designate. The cause of such injury most generally acts directly, as a stroke, a concussion, a gunshot wound, or straining the eye too much, as in habitually reading while lying down, or reading a great deal while riding in vehicles, as such exercise of the sight is particularly straining to the eye, as it is so baffled in adjusting the angle of vision to every motion of the vehicle.

Whenever persons discover a kind of hurting sensation behind the ball of the eye while reading or sewing or fixing the sight on any fine object, it is in many cases amaurosis in its forming stage, an amaurosis which affects the integrity of the structure of the eye and its nerves, and which, if allowed to go on, will prove certainly fatal, even before the eyesight is lost. Reading by artificial light is most particularly injurious in this connection.

Antiphlogistic is that kind of treatment of inflammatory diseases which is calculated to modify, to lessen, to dispel the inflammation.

Antidotes, as applied to disease, are those medicines which meet or arrest or destroy the effects of other medicines on the system, especially applied to poisons. Acids and alkalies are antidotes to each other; oils are antidotes of acids; strong coffee is an antidote of opium, whether in the form of laudanum, paregoric, or morphia. (See poisons.)

Alteratives in medicine are those remedies which change the condition of the system. Everything swallowed, whether fluid or solid, whether medicine or nourishment, is alterative; but as specially applied to the treatment of disease it means the changing of the character of the disease, so as to give a milder form of malady for a severer form; a safer form for a more dangerous one. You have a pain in the chest, or a sensation of smothering; a mustard plaster is applied, which, by drawing the blood to the skin from the ailing part, affords most speedy and gratifying relief.

In a past age salivation by calomel was the great favorite, universal alterative; only get the mouth to water and the patient was considered safe, because it drew the fluids from the suffering parts and gave exit to them through the mouth. The human body in disease is like a full barrel, tap it where you please and there is an outward flow which diminishes the bulk by that much. All ordinary diseases are the result of too much blood or other material at some one point; make an outlet at any point, and the surplus at any other point flows off to that outlet, and relief is almost inevitable. As soon as a boil or ulcer breaks a man begins to get better in various ways, whatever may have been the matter with him. This is the philosophy, the operation of issues, of blisters, of setons, of emetics, of purgative medicines. There is scarcely a disease known not connected with loose bowels, which is not more or less modified or lessened or made better by anything taken which promotes the action of the bowels.

ARNICA

Is the Arnica montana of botanists; its common name is Leopard's-bane; the leaves, flowers, and root are used medicinally, externally and internally; but as it irritates the stomach and bowels it is better employed as an external application in the effects of falls and bruises, on the nerves, brain, and muscles. Dose of the powdered flour about ten grains; powdered root, twenty grains; the essential oil, from one to ten drops.

Infusion, an ounce of the flowers or root soaked in a pint of water; dose, one tablespoonful every two or three hours. Often beneficial in headaches and nervous affections, especially those connected with the brain. Before taking the infusion as a medicine it should be strained through a linen rag, as there are little particles which would otherwise irritate the throat and cause troublesome coughing.

Tincture of Arnica is made by pouring alcohol or spirits of any kind on two or three ounces of the root or flowers; but it is better to obtain it from a good druggist under the name of Tincture of arnica, and keep a pint bottle of it in the house, marked poison, as if swallowed in that form it would produce instant and very dangerous effects; in such event swallow diluted vinegar or lemon juice, or suck lemons freely, until the effects subside.

ARNICA WASH

or lotion is made by adding one part of the tincture of arnica to six parts of water, to be used in every variety of wounds, as often and as freely as the case requires; when an eruption appears on the skin its use should be discontinued. If persons have a very irritable skin, or are subject to erysipelas, or are of an inflammatory constitution, or are excessively nervous, one part of arnica in twelve parts of water is strong enough; or one part in thirty for children under ten. This same preparation may be used to advantage as a gargle or wash for the gums, or the throat.

But if the external application of arnica in any form is too irritative, the next best substitute is calendula officinalis; no doubt it is more mild in its action, is very good to heal sores and ulcers which are sluggish, and often prevents the formation of scars after cuts or lacerated wounds, prepared with the same strength as tincture of arnica.

The preparations of arnica are used in amaurosis, typhus fever in its latter stages, hydrocephalus, and in various forms of paralysis. Dose of the tincture is thirty drops in water; of the extract from five to ten grains. It has been regarded as

A PANACEA

for all falls and blows, especially those causing concussion of the brain. That it acts specially on the brain and nerves is evident from the fact, that if taken in large doses it stimulates them very highly, even to the extent of difficult breathing, headache, convulsions and spasms of the limbs. As its effects are to stimulate the brain and nerves, and rouse them into action, it must be a valuable internal medicine, when taken under the eye and by the direction of a skilful physician; without that, the reader would do well to employ it only as an external application.

It is not well to be using remedies for every little ache and pain, otherwise the system soon begins to call for their employment, and a day will not pass without resort to them in some form or other. But in cases where it is important to relieve a person of a variety of symptoms, the tincture of arnica is beneficial in two ways—it stimulates the skin, and to that extent acts like a mustard plaster; it draws the blood to the surface, and relieves the deeper-seated trouble. Hence there is scarcely an ache or a pain which will not be more or less relieved by the arnica-wash. But it is also beneficial from the fact that the alcohol in it, which is needed to extract its peculiar virtues, is cleansing and cooling. In the first place, it removes all dirt or dust or oil from the surface of the skin; keeps the pores open, by which ill humors escape; and, in addition, by its volatile character (the more so the warmer the weather) its evaporating powers are very good; hence it carries the heat from an affected part with great rapidity, thus cooling off fevers and inflammations of a part, thus removing pain and soreness and other discomfort with remarkable promptness; hence the growing favor it has had among the people of late years, especially those who are friends to homœopathy, who employ it freely as a wash or ointment in all forms of bruises, swellings, contusions, dropsies, chills, unnatural perspirations, shiverings, hot flushings, eruptions, humors, pimples, scabs, ulcers, itchings, tingling, etc. But the intelligent reader should always bear in mind that all these sensations are more or less transitory, and necessarily pass off in a few moments; if they do not it is because their origin is in a diseased condition of the whole system, and that instead of seeking temporary relief by mere expedients, the wiser course by far, and the only radical and permanent remedy, is the improvement of the "general health" (which see) by means of plain and temperate living, spending a large portion of daylight in the open air, in such activities as enliven the mind and promote muscular exertion, thus waking up the circulation, working out of the body through the open pores of the skin these humors, these invisible particles which. being in the blood, poison it and keep the whole surface of the body, which the blood feeds and keeps alive, in a condition ready to take on diseased action from the slightest possible causes.

After all that has been said of the various uses of arnica, the judicious reader will not only confine himself to its employment externally, but will limit himself to the application of it to sudden requirements, such as cuts, bruises, and blows, and effects resulting therefrom.

ARNICA

is found growing in the mountainous parts of Europe and in some of the Western States of our own country. Water extracts its virtues, which are found in the whole plant, root, flower, and all. Arnica stimulates the brain and nervous system. It acts as an irritant to the stomach and bowels, often producing an emetic and cathartic effect, and is supposed by some to be diuretic, diaphoretic, and emmenagogue. It is much used by German and British physicians, who prescribe the flowers and roots with advantage in amaurosis, paralysis, and other nervous affections. It is very serviceable in that disordered condition of the system which succeeds concussion, falls, blows, etc. In bruises it is invaluable; and it is gratifying to know that in this plant we have a remedy of singular efficacy, applicable in all cases, from the most trifling to the most severe. Experience demonstrates it to be unapproached in power by any remedy, or combination of remedies whatever. Homœopathy has been honored as the introducer of this valuable plant; but this is a mistake, as it is an old popular remedy. To bruises, to allay the smarting of wounds after operations; to fractures, dislocations, and other similar injuries, it may be applied with implicit confidence in its power, to the exclusion of fomentations, cooling lotions, etc., etc. The only objection against its use is that it sometimes irritates the skin, but this proceeds from its being employed in too great strength or quantity; or it may be possible that there may be some peculiar idiosyncrasy which predisposes the skin of some persons to become irritated by it. It is an excellent remedy in bruises from blows, falls, and other accidents.

AORTA

Is the great canal or tube which carries the blood from the heart towards all parts of the body, and has three portions: first, the arch of the aorta, near the heart; then that branch of it which goes to the chest; and the third, which supplies the abdominal organs, or the belly. The arch of the aorta, near the heart, is liable to be filled up with a stony substance, making the patient subject to attacks of

ANGINA PECTORIS

(which see); the other two divisions are most liable to aneurisms, called aneurism of the thoracic aorta, and aneurism of the abdominal aorta.

ANEURISM

is simply a dilatation of an artery, made by the blood being sent with such force to the part as to distend it, make it swell out, or stretch until a kind of bulb or bulging is made, which gradually increases, and with this increase the sides get thinner and thinner, and weaker and weaker, just as happens in stretching a piece of india-rubber, until at length the weakness is such that the membrane bursts, because the force of the blood, its pulsation, is just as strong now as when the sides of the artery were manifold stronger; in such cases death follows in a few moments. Sometimes the blood in the veins distend in the same way, as seen in the legs of many old people, called varicose veins; rupture there is not dangerous; on the contrary, it gives relief. It then becomes a matter of life and death to know how to decide whether the bulging of a blood-vessel is in an artery or a vein: if in an artery, puncture is death; if in a vein, puncture is a relief. The difference is ascertained promptly, infallibly. If the enlargement or bulging is felt to throb or pulsate, especially if there is a thrill with it, it is the aneurism of an artery; if it has no more motion than a sac or bag of water, it is the enlargement of a vein.

Nothing can be done in either of the three divisions of aortic aneurism named towards effecting a cure; taking care of the "general health" (which see) sometimes retards the progress of the malady, and renders it less active, less severe, and less painful and distressing.

All aneurisms are benefited by limiting the amount of fluids drunk during twenty-four hours to a single half pint, as this materially diminishes the amount and volume of blood to be pressed along the aneurismal artery.

AIR,

OR the atmosphere we breathe, is, in its purity, composed of twenty-three parts of oxygen and seventy-seven parts of nitrogen, but it contains particles which do not naturally belong to it. In a damp day the air is so full of water or fog that a pint of it may not contain more than three-fourths of a pint of air, and as the atmosphere is the thing which acts directly on the blood in the lungs, to withdraw from it all the impurities which it contains, the purer the air is the more capable is it of absorbing the impurities of the blood in the lungs. Hence the purer the air the purer the blood, and the purer the blood the better health is enjoyed in all climes and countries. The purest air is out of doors. There is no pure air within any four walls of a house. You may go into any room, even if it is entirely empty, and a musty or close smell will be immediately observed. Much more will there be impurities in the air of our dwellings in proportion to the decaying or odorous things in it—as slops, food, fruits, flowers, and the like. That air is best for the health which has no perceptible " smell " about it. The fragrance of the rose and the pink are delicious ; but if a person were to sleep in a close room in which there were a great many pinks and roses he would be nearly dead next morning, because the nature of the flowers is such that they are throwing off a multitude of odorous particles every instant, and they being more material, more solid than the air, displace it, so that in every breath there is less air taken into the lungs and more of the substance of the flowers.

A breath of air taken into the lungs may be represented by a piece of fine sponge, from which the water has just been squeezed out ; put it into a vessel of dirty water ; it will take up more of that than if it was half full of water before it was put in. So a breath of pure air taken into the lungs will take up more of the impurities of the blood than it would have done if it had contained or absorbed a large amount of impurities before it went in. Hence the necessity of arranging habitually to breathe the purest air possible. The easiest way to do this is to spend as much of our time in the open air as practicable, and when we are indoors to make it a point to have fresh outdoor air coming into our houses all the time ; to have fire-place or door or window more or less open all the time, day and night, but in such a way as not to come in with a draught.

Other information can be obtained in reference to the air and its connection with health by referring to the articles on Miasm, and Typhoid Fever.

ATROPHY

MEANS without nourishment; the person or part of the person wastes away.

First, as a man would without food, or a flower without water.

Second, want of exercise, as some of the devotees of the far east, who consider it a religious merit to hold out or hold up an arm or other limb; for want of exercise the blood is not driven into it, and it suffers and wastes away until it becomes little more than skin and bone.

Third, if a tumor or other cause stops the blood in an artery leading to the brain, there is "softening of the brain."

Fourth, if, from similar or other causes, the flow of nervous influence is arrested and prevented from reaching a part, a limb for example, then there is paralysis, loss of motion in that part.

HYGIENE,

PRONOUNCE hygeene, with two syllables, is from the name of Hygieia, who was the daughter of Æsculapius. There were statues erected to her as the goddess of health. Her father, according to the mythology of the Greeks, was the god of health; he was the son of Apollo, who was the model of manly beauty, the god of medicine, music, poetry, and eloquence; he brought up his son to the study of medicine and to hunting. There was always a meaning in these old Greek legends, and the mind naturally connects hunting and its necessary activities in the open air, its exhilarations and its excitements, with health. Health without medicine, as if Apollo thought that if health could be maintained and regained without the use of medicine, it was the perfection of the healing art, and now, three thousand years later, the people think the same thing, and this is the idea connected with the word hygiene, the maintenance of health and a recovery from disease by other means than medicine, such as by judicious attention to air and exercise, to dress, clothing, eating, sleeping, and the general habits of life.

ACCIDENTS

MEAN, literally, falling to, or coming upon, by agencies beyond our control. The ancients regarded them as coming from heaven, and the idea has descended to modern times, and is expressed by the word providential.

PROVIDENTIALLY HINDERED

is a frequent phrase, but the accident which brings harm to a man's body will be found on investigation to be the result of ignorance, carelessness, or design on the part of the injured, or of some other person. It is called a railroad accident if a switch has been designedly misplaced; it is regarded as an accident if a person's clothing takes fire from the bursting of a

KEROSENE LAMP,

when in reality it resulted in the ignorance or carelessness of the person handling it, in great part, but not altogether; the man who supplied the oil is in part a criminal for supplying a burning-fluid which is dangerous, and which if honestly prepared would not have taken fire. It was his business to have ascertained by his own testing that the oil was safe, which he could have done without expense or trouble in five minutes, thus: fill a cup half full of water, pour on it one or two tablespoons of oil, apply a burning match or piece of paper; if a good quality of oil it will not take fire, if spurious it will.

In most accidents or casualties there are several things to be done at once, and in many cases these first things decide the issue of life and death.

First. Nine times in ten brandy or wine or other forms of stimulant are almost instinctively offered; if drink is asked for give cold water, if not asked for, wait.

Second. If anything is likely to obstruct the breathing, as tight clothing or mud or other thing about the face and nose, remove it and place the person in a reclining position, if the brain or head is not injured on the back; and beyond two, or at most three persons, keep every one away at least ten feet distant, and, a great deal better, out of the room altogether, for the very sight of many persons present tends to excite and alarm and discompose by the expression of their countenances alone. `In very many cases the injured person is more calm and self-possessed than any one present, and, for an additional reason, a crowd should be kept at a distance to allow abundant pure air to get to the sufferer.

Third. Before moving the person notice if any limb is broken, or if there is much blood flowing; if flowing in spirts or jets, an artery has been severed, and there is no time to be lost in moving, for the person may bleed to death in a few moments. (See Bleedings.) If there is not much blood discharged, and it comes out slowly, removal can take place; but then it is generally better to promote the bleeding by the use of a sponge and warm water, for in most accidents moderate bleeding unloads the system and tends to prevent inflammation and erysipelas from setting in.

Fourth. Do all that is possible to compose the patient, to give rest to the body, to each limb, and by all means to keep the clothing dry, and the body and extremities warm; this is always of consequence, always of vital importance. In addition, keep out of the sufferer's sight everything which might excite or discompose or discourage or alarm; remove everything bloody, everything soiled and torn.

Fifth. The persons around the patient should exhibit a quiet, confident, composed, assured air, so as to inspire the same in the mind of the sufferer.

Sixth. Avoid all sudden motions or starts or hurry; avoid noisy talking, especially all whispering, which is a pest to any chamber; do not allow the patient to observe you steadily gazing at him, and ask him as few questions as possible; try and find out what is wanting without inquiry.

Seventh. In all cases of injury by accidents send for the nearest physician without a moment's delay; if one cannot be had send for a nurse; if none at hand send for the woman nearest, who has had most experience in nursing the sick.

Eighth. Until a physician or other help arrives, have two basins of cold water and half a dozen soft rags; and wherever there is a wound or bruise or swelling apply the rags dipped in the water, sometimes dabbling them on the spot, at others laying them on the spot in four or five thicknesses, renewing every four or five minutes ; the object being to cool the parts, to keep down fever and inflammation, and to stop excessive bleeding ; for these purposes there is nothing better than cold water, proven by the experience of physicians and nurses of all ages and of all schools ; better than all the balsam and ointment ever made.　　Multitudes are impatient to apply something which has an ingredient which they suppose of special value ; but rest assured that pure water is the best, for all that is wanting is to cool and cleanse.　　Bear it in mind,

TO COOL AND TO CLEANSE

sometimes warm water is better than cold ; it does not give such a shock, to begin with ; but whether warm or cold, be careful to prevent the water from dribbling about on the clothing or bed, both of which should be kept perfectly dry.

If the person is in an insensible condition, apply camphor to the nostrils, and cloths dipped in hot water to the pit of the stomach ; rub the limbs vigorously with the hands or hot dry towels ; bathe the temples and forehead in water and vinegar, half and half ; a feather may be put up the nose ; or cold water may be dashed on the face.

A very efficient means is to have boiling water at hand, kept boiling all the time; dip into it a broad knife or spoon or anything having a broad, flat, metallic surface, then carry it at once to the sole of one foot for a second or two, then to the other sole, then to the pit of stomach, arms, calves, spine ; rapidly from one part to another, so as to feel at once for the place most susceptible of being waked up to life.　　In some cases the metal may remain two or three seconds, and having gone the rounds, dip into the boiling water again and go on again as before, in the hope of waking up to consciousness.　　If there is a burn of the skin it is over such a slight space that no harm can result, and a second application would be more efficient ; even the broad face of a common hammer may answer the purpose.　　Mustard plasters, blisters, cauteries, answer the purpose, but hot water and a spoon or knife may be always at hand.　　Or a burning candle may be held near the skin long enough to blister, or the actual cautery called

MOXA

may be applied thus: dip a piece of tinder, an inch across, into alcohol, set it on fire and hold it on the skin so as to make a blister.

BLEEDING WOUNDS,

or gashes: first wash the parts with cold water so as to remove all dirt or mud or foreign material, bits of clothes, hair, or anything else, and apply cold compresses; if the cut is slight and does not bleed much, dip a soft rag in cold water, lay it on the wound or cut, bind a silk handkerchief over it, and let it remain for a few hours, then renew; or instead of removing the moistened rag it is better, if the wound is jagged, made by a ball or slug, or by the stroke of a blunt instrument, simply sprinkle cold water on the rag every few minutes, or as often as it begins to get a very little dry; the point is, keep the soft rag wet all the time without binding it on with a silk handkerchief; if the cut is on the side of the face, or other inconvenient spot for keeping the rag to it, a little ingenuity will meet the requirements.

CUTS.

Such wounds as make gashes should first be washed out, then as soon as possible bring the edges in contact, and devise means for keeping them together; keep a cold wet cloth on, and it will grow together; always keeping an eye to one main point, keep the bowels acting very freely every twenty-four hours, and live quietly, regularly, eating mainly coarse breads, mush, hominy, cracked wheat, fruits, berries, melons, and the like, not much meat, and even that at the noon-day meal only.

In all cuts or gashes let the part wounded be so adjusted as to do most in keeping the sides of the wound together; if in the palm of the hand keep the hand closed; if on the back, keep the hand extended; if on the knee, keep the leg extended; if under the knee or inside of elbow, keep leg or arm bent; if on the neck, bend it towards the wounded side; and in all cases keep up the bend, for if the wound is allowed to gape open in the least

11

every now and then it cannot heal. In all cases, if there is a prospect of getting a physician soon, an attendant should keep the edges of the wound pressed together with the fingers.

In some wounds from a sharp instrument, a well-adjusted sticking plaster aids to keep the sides of the wound in contact.

In cases where the wound gapes wide open, and there is no prospect of a surgeon coming, it is not so fearful an operation as one might think, to take a fine needle, put a silk thread into it and sew up the wound with over stitches not too close to the edge of the skin, say an eighth of an inch, drawing the edges of the wound and skin slowly and closely together, aided by the pressure of the fingers of the assistant on each side of the wound. After being sewed up, the cold, wet application should be kept on, so as to keep down fever and inflammation, with cooling drink and food and free bowels.

In using adhesive plaster it should be cut into strips, and they should be placed at intervals of half an inch, so as to allow the escape of any blood or exudations. Sometimes it is necessary, in order to keep the parts of the wound close together, to make small rolls of linen as large as the finger, and place them each side of the wound, and wrap a compress around all, in such a way that the tendency of the pressure should be to keep the lips of the wound together. Having once adjusted it, it should not be disturbed ordinarily for about four days; then remove the bandage carefully, gently, slowly; the compresses or rollers often adhere, soak them in warm water until they fall off; in removing the plaster strips lift one end upwards very carefully, taking the precaution to press the wound with the fingers of the other hand together, else, in raising the strip of adhesive plaster perpendicularly, it might stick, so as to tear the wound apart; after the plaster strips have been removed sponge the parts gently with warm water, and when clean adjust new plasters with compress rollers, and bandage as before. If in any form of wounds the cold water cloths are not sufficient to keep down the inflammation apply leeches; being careful always to keep the bowels free, as just stated, and also to use a light diet, with no stimulating drinks whatever.

CONCUSSION OF THE BRAIN

may result from a violent shaking or fall or blow, or explosion of cannon or steam boiler, causing, if severe, a sudden loss of sense and motion, and death follows.

If slight, there is dizziness, sickness of stomach, more or less confusion of ideas, with only momentary loss of sense and motion ; the breathing is affected ; the more laborious it is the more dangerous the condition of the patient, especially if the feet are cold, the pulse weak and fitful ; great restlessness, irritability of temper, shiverings and delirium.

Apply tincture of arnica externally three or four times a day as a lotion, until the pain and swellings have disappeared.

Keep the patient well covered in bed ; do all that is possible to restore warmth to the extremities, especially the feet ; take pieces of flannel, dip in very hot water, wring them out, pour on them some spirits of turpentine and apply ; renew every ten minutes ; make the same application, without the turpentine, to the chest ; if these are not sufficient to restore warmth, use mustard plasters, and in proportion as the pulse rises and the extremities grow warmer, good is done.

To prevent inflammation of the brain, which is to be greatly dreaded, administer an injection at once, so as to unload the lower bowels and give three or four antibilious pills, the object being by clearing the liver to promote the freer circulation of the blood through the body, and in this way prevent an excess of blood going to the brain through the arteries, for this is

INFLAMMATION OF THE BRAIN.

At the same time additional safety will be found in taking a teacupful of blood ; if there is a tendency for the pulse to beat hard (see pulse) and the skin to become hot, drink hot teas or hot water very freely, and use all other means to cause perspiration. The diet should be light (see diet), of coarse bread, fruits, potatoes, oranges, lemons and the like, sago root, arrow root, and barley-water.

If inflammation of the brain is induced from any other cause, coming on suddenly or gradually, blood should not be taken unless advised by a physician, but the head should be elevated, and the general treatment above advised should be followed out. If the inflammation is sudden, a safe and speedy method of relief is to place the patient upright in a chair and let the blood flow from the arm until about to faint, or if there is actual fainting no harm is done.   In addition, shave the head and keep it cool by all means, by bags of pounded ice, or snow and salt, half and half.   If these are not at hand, dip cloths in a mixture of vinegar and water or spirits and water, half and half, and lay them four or five folds thick on the head, and renew every five or ten minutes.   If at the same time the feet up to the knees are immersed in hot water, kept hot by adding more hot water from time to time, or in a mustard bath, so much the better.

If actual blood-letting is objectionable in any particular case, apply twenty-five or thirty leeches to the nape of the neck ; great good will be done if the system can be kept nauseated.   Meanwhile, with a view to keep the skin moist,—because a moist skin most effectually draws inflammation from the head,—one of the simplest and most efficient means of doing this is to give a few drops of tinct. ipecac in a teaspoon of sweet spirits of nitre every hour or two, just as much of the ipecac as will sicken a little, but not gag or vomit.

The antibilious pills should be given every third day, if the bowels are not free, or at least every fifth day, the bowels being kept in daily action in the interval with castor-oil.   If there is not free urination, the water should be drawn three or four times a day by a catheter.

As the patient improves, the diet should be gradually more liberal ; avoid everything excitable, promote quiet and repose in every way possible, and if there is a tendency for the inflammation to return, better make sure work and place a seton in the neck, or cause a running sore or open blister ; the drink should be cold water, avoiding altogether the employment of spirits and strong teas of every description.

TEMPERATURE OF CHAMBER.

In all forms of accidents and hurtings the air of the sick-room should be pure ; that is the first essential.   A whole family living in a cabin with one room were taken ill in the winter time ; with the best medical care there seemed to be no adequate improvement, when one cold day, the family being poor, complained to the physician of their misfortune in having a glass broken, and their inability to procure another ; as his previous efforts to have them air their room had been unavailing, he suggested to them it would be better not to replace it for the present; from that day all the members began to improve and finally recovered. This shows the importance of a good ventilation, of a constant coming into a sick-room of the pure outdoor air to replace and drive up the chimney or out of some other opening the foul, poisonous air of the sick-bed.

In addition, it is greatly better to be sick in a cool room and be made comfortably warm with extra bed-covering, if necessary, than to have a warm room and light covering; for warm air, while it is generally impure in proportion to its warmth, is less nutritious than cool air, does not purify the blood so effectually, nor give as much life to the body as cold air; hence the most favorable condition for the sick is to be able to breathe a cool air, and yet have the body comfortably warm by extra clothing. This good ventilation and pure air are most easily supplied by having the fire-place kept open all the time, as also a door or window. If no fire-place, let the window be let down from the top and hoisted at bottom, yet, so as to prevent a draught upon the patient. If the window cannot be let down at the top, or in case a current of air will cross the bed, saw a board, two, three, or more inches broad, and just as long as the window-sash is broad, hoist the lower sash, introduce the board, thus filling up the space made by the hoisting; this elevates the sash in such a way, that at its joining with the upper sash an opening is made, by which the air is compelled to enter the room in a direction upwards, towards the ceiling, where it is warmed and makes its way towards the floor, thus airing the room without any draught whatever in the direction of the patient. The same convenient and safe arrangement may be made by any one who is compelled to sleep in a small room with no ventilation.

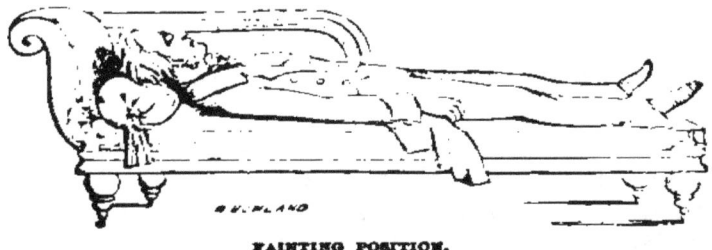

FAINTING POSITION.

If a person falls in a fit and begins to snore loudly, with very red face, it is apoplexy. Let him be seated so as to favor the blood going downward, away from the head; apply cold cloths to the head, or cushions of equal quantities of snow or pounded ice and common salt. If the person is perfectly still, face pale, and no perceptible breathing, it is a fit of fainting. Place him on his back instantly. Do not touch him, except to loosen the clothing; then keep off some five or ten feet distant, so as to allow the air to come in; make no noise; and there will very soon be a calm, quiet return to consciousness and life, for it is only a momentary cessation of the circulation of the blood to the head.

If in a sitting position, it is harder to throw the blood upwards to the head, which is higher than on the horizontal line of lying down.

But suppose there is a violent motion of the hands and feet, and all sorts of bodily contortions, it is epilepsy. Let the man contort until he is tired; you can't hold him still; all your efforts only tend to aggravate the trouble and to exhaust the strength; all that ought to be done is to keep the unfortunate man from hurting himself. There is no felt suffering, for as soon as he comes to, he will tell you that he remembers nothing whatever of what has passed, appears to be the only calm and self-possessed person in the whole crowd, and is apparently as perfectly well as before the occurrence. Dizziness often comes instantaneously, and we begin to reel before we know it. Shut the eyes, whether you are walking down the street, looking over a precipice, ascending a ladder, or climbing to a ship's mast-head; the fear or dizziness disappears instantly if you look upward.

MYSTERIOUS INFLUENCES.

PERSONS sometimes feel remarkably well, the appetite is voracious, eating is a joy, digestion vigorous, sleep sound, with an alacrity of body and an exhilaration of spirits which altogether throw a charm over life which makes them pleased with everybody and everything. Next week, to-morrow, in an hour, a marvellous change comes over the spirit of their dream; the sunshine has gone, clouds portend, and darkness covers the face of the great deep, and the whole man, body and soul, wilts away like a flower without water in midsummer.

If a bee has wandered far away from its hive on a beautiful June morning, every flower is unfolded, ready to yield all its treasures of sweetness; suddenly he speeds away towards his home with an arrow's swiftness, for a cloud has come between him and the sun, and forebodings come of ill; his little heart is just as full of hurried hasting for home, as but a moment before it was of hope to get its fill of honey.

Both bee and man are affected by changes in the condition of the atmosphere; many fly before an east wind as a bee before a cloud, the electrical conditions of the atmosphere having been changed in both cases.

When the weather is cool and clear and bracing, the atmosphere is full of electricity; when it is sultry and moist, and without sunshine, it holds but a small amount of electricity, comparatively speaking, and we have to give up what little we have, moisture being a good conductor; thus in giving up, instead of receiving more, as we would from the cool, pure air, the change is too great, and the whole man languishes. Many become uneasy under these circumstances; "they can't account for it;" they imagine that evil is impending, and resort at once to tonics and stimulants. The tonics only increase the appetite without imparting any additional power to work up the additional food, thus giving the system more work to do instead of less. Stimulants seem to give more strength; they wake up the circulation, but it is only temporarily, and unless a new supply is soon taken, the system runs further down than it would have done without the stimulant; hence it is in a worse condition than if none had been taken. The better course would be to rest, take nothing but cooling fruits and berries and lemons and some acid drink, when thirsty, adding if desired some cold bread and butter; the very next morning will bring a welcome change.

BRUISES

From blows, strikes, falling timbers, and the like, if slight, may be let alone; if severe, deep, or extensive, the swelling, blackness, and blood are all favorable, because they show that the blood comes outward ; while if it went inward, as to the brain, for example, death would ensue.

As the result of a bruise, the blood sometimes comes up to the skin without coming out, spreads like a sheet, and blackens ; this is called

EFFUSION.

Such wounds affect the muscles, the flesh, make them sore, painful, and weak, according to the severity of the injury.

Sometimes, if there be but little life in the system, the parts die, mortification ensues, and there is a

SLOUGHING,

either to be thrown off by nature, detached from the healthy parts, or must be cut out by the surgeon.

TREATMENT OF BRUISES.

First prevent inflammation, by having soft rags, five or six thicknesses ; lay them in ice-cold water, and spread over the bruise ; either remove every five minutes, to be replaced immediately by another always in readiness, or lay over the wet cloth a piece of oiled silk, extending over its edges about an inch, so as to keep in all the steam ; this causes a sweating, an evaporating process which carries off the extra heat rapidly, and this effectually prevents inflammation. If the frequent cold lotions are used, the extremities of the blood-vessels are congealed, and the bleeding also is arrested ; when these two conditions are secured, that is, the prevention of inflammation and the arrest of the bleeding, use warm poultices to keep up the evaporation and the coolness, and the parts will usually heal, if the bowels are kept acting freely every day, and the diet is cooling, that is, mainly of lean meat in small quantities, once a day, with coarse breads and fruits and lemons and melons.

COLD-WATER STREAM.

One of the very best remedies for bruises as well as sprains is to have a stream of cold water fall on the part until it almost aches with cold, then desist, and renew every third hour until the pain subsides ; a pitcher or tea-kettle or old coffee-pot can be used, but this requires the time of another person, which can be obviated by having a barrel of water higher than the head and attach to it an india-rubber tube, which can be stopped with a cork, or if there are water pipes in the house, have a tube large enough to go over the end of the faucet. Bruises are cured and the blood and other parts are absorbed by the application of a bandage, but this requires skill, hence it would be better to use the cold water in one of the ways named ; or employ washes or bathings of

TINCTURE OF ARNICA.

Apply it every hour or two, or keep a rag or lint, saturated, kept wet by it on the part until the symptoms have abated, and there is a feeling of quiet and comfort.

The concentrated tincture of *rhus tox.* may be employed to advantage when joints, tendons, and synovial membranes are injured ; but in all cases keep the bowels freely acting every day ; this is indispensable always.

Very painful wounds and bruises are often promptly relieved by taking a shovel of burning coals,—of wood is better, sprinkle common brown sugar on the coals, and hold the wounded part in the smoke ; in case of splinters or rusty rails piercing the flesh and causing pain, fever, and irritation, the discomfort is sometimes removed in fifteen minutes. Other

WOUNDS AND BRUISES

may be treated successfully in the same way.

Another method of allaying inflammation and modifying the ill effects of metals piercing the flesh, and thus preventing

LOCK-JAW,

mortification, and the necessity of amputation, is to unravel a piece of flannel or woollen stocking, or take common woollen yarn or much worn woollen fabrics, saturate them with sweet oil, hog's lard, or melted butter. Put them in a kettle, set them on fire so they shall smoke, without blazing ; hold the wound over the smoke, and cover the wounded part with a blanket so as to condense the smoke about the wound, doing all in such a way as not to smoke the sufferer or strangle him to death.

Another method, successfully adopted for many years, was

holding the wounded or bruised part over the smoke made of old shoes or any bits of leather made to burn without blazing, saturating the parts with the smoke; all these methods prevent the mortification of the living part, just as the old-fashioned smoke-houses of half a century ago prevented the hams, and sides, or middlings of pork from decaying. In all these cases we have the one thing, the condensed smoke as the curative agent, known in later years as

CREOSOTE,

which is really the essence of smoke or soot. Common tar is made by setting some kinds of wood on fire, covering it over with dust, so as to prevent it from burning, leaving the red solid wood in the shape of charcoal, while the other part, the tar, flows out, is gathered, and preserved for various uses. When this tar is distilled it yields creosote.

CARBOLIC ACID

is the tar of coal oil, which is found in that portion of coal tar which distils over under a heat of three or four hundred degrees; it is a colorless liquid, of an oily look, of a burning taste, and has something of the smell of soot; hence creosote and carbolic acid are of the same nature in some of their qualities, and in their effects on wounds resemble the details given of the smoke arising from burning leather, rags, etc. But in many places of accidents and burns, as on steamboats and railways, and in the interior of the country, where neither of them could be possibly obtained, some old woolen rags, or old shoes, could be got together, and the smoke of them concentrated on wounds, bruises, cuts, crushes, and burns, and be of inestimate value, all having the one effect of

COAGULATION.

By coagulating the blood it arrests bleeding; it also constringes the extreme ends of the smallest blood-vessels, and thus also arrests the flow of the vital liquid and heals every variety of wounds and hurts.

In addition, it prevents putrefaction; it averts mortification as well as prevents it; in addition, it takes away all ill odors, and keeps the parts in a cleanly, healthy condition.

One part of carbolic acid with forty parts of hot water, shaken well, and then strained or filtered, is an excellent wash for all sores, ulcers, bruises, and the like.

A horse was about dying of a festered wound; some old shoes were cut up in a hog trough, the pieces were set on fire under the swollen wound of the horse; in a few hours the swelling began to subside, and to discharge yellow matter, and the horse was saved. Another horse had been gored by a bull in the abdomen; nothing seemed to be of any avail; the smoke of leather was advised, and the horse got well.

A man's foot was cut with an axe, and while bleeding badly a lady seized hold of it, held it over the smoke of burning tag-locks, or scraps of leather; in a few moments the bleeding stopped, the wound never maturated, nor was there any pain, and it got well rapidly. The smoke which contains creosote or carbolic acid coagulates the albumen, and thus prevents putrefaction; it coagulates very rapidly, and thus arrests bleeding; hence smoke has a valuable healing power when applied to ulcers, sores, and man's skin diseases; but as carbolic acid contains the curative element in the smoke, or rather is itself the curative principle, every family would do well to have it always on hand. To further impress this on the mind of the reader, it is proper to state that a patent has been taken out in Paris for a new agent to stop bleeding, etc., in wounds. The French government has for many years been far in advance of all civilized nations in purchasing valuable secrets from persons who have discovered them, and then making them public to all the world. This new agent is made thus: take common

PETROLEUM,

And stir into it, cold, one-sixth of its weight of caustic soda; let it stand twelve hours; it will then be found to have separated into two layers; the lower one is

PHENATE OF SODA.

Run it off and keep in a glass bottle for use; if a cut, dip several folds of linen or muslin into it, and lay it on the cut; press it on the wound, and then with a rag apply more phenate on the compress; it causes no pain or irritation; then apply a second compress; wash it also with a rag dipped in the phenate; keep on applying a new compress saturated with the phenate until the bleeding stops; these compresses are applied one over the other, until the blood coagulates.

If a wound is made by a bullet, or sharp knife, or other instrument, inject the phenate into it several times, then saturate lint with the phenate, and fill the place with it. The operation of this valuable remedy is

GOOD.

It coagulates the blood. It renders the edges of the wound insensible. It causes the sides of the wound to contract by its constringent power. It contracts also the minute blood-vessels, causing them to send forward what blood they have, thus removing the congestion, and by diminishing their calibres on the same principle, prevents too much blood from coming into them and through them, to cause inflammation.

ALOES AND ALCOHOL.

Take one part of Socotrine aloes and two parts of alcohol, dip into this a soft rag, or lint, and lay it on any sore, such as bed sores, ulceration from burns, or other causes; it often heals without causing any scars. This preparation should be always kept in the house. Aloes is a common drug, a vegetable product, and is used largely in purgative preparations, so that there is no danger whatever in its employment externally.

THE MONTH MALIGN,

September, sheds its malignant rays over humanity, infusing the poison of hateful disease and sudden death on half the globe, especially in our latitudes, those of the United States, because mainly the weather has been hot for weeks, evaporating winter streams and fresh-water ponds, leaving exposed to the sun's rays their soft, wet, slimy bottoms, generating miasmatic influences, disease-engendering emanations which enter into the circulation through the stomach and lungs, poison the blood, thickening it, making it congest in the small terminal vessels, laying the foundation at once of diarrhœa, dysentery, and every class of fevers, from the comparatively undangerous ague to the malignant bilious, typhoid, and yellow jack.

One-half of all these diseases could be prevented at one swoop by cleanliness and scientific draining. Look at New Orleans, during the Federal occupation of the war. One party seemed to think that the merciful One had forsaken them, the other that they were the special favorites of heaven; both were equally wide of the mark; it simply was the secret of one intelligent mind, compelling clean streets, and what was equivalent to a constant drain.

Many a farm, with as rich a soil as the Delta of Egypt, cannot be sold at ten dollars an acre, because it is

A SICKLY HOLE,

fever and ague reigns rampant; with a proper draining it would be worth a hundred dollars an acre, the very first crop paying the expense of drainage.

But it is too late to talk of draining, when whole families are shaking with ague, others growing as yellow as pumpkins, others again sinking under typhoid.

All the ailments named are bilious ailments, are the result of an inactive liver; there is so much blood dammed up in it, that it has no room to work, to free itself, no more than a man can use his elbows for deliverance when urged onwards to the door of a building on fire, by the affrighted crowd around him. The physician understands what remedies are needed under the circumstances. The allopath is enthusiastic on his calomel; the water cures slosh away with might and main, inside and out, top and bottom, with a free through ticket thrown in, while the infinitesimal admirer gives a mite a month, throwing the whole responsibilities of the case upon the broad shoulders of his

OLD STAND-BY,

Doctor Nature, and in many cases that same old Doctor don't always come out second best; he has a way of his own and waddles long, as in the celebrated race between Messrs. Turtle and

Hare, a long time ago, in such a way as to come out half-a-neck ahead, colors flying.

It is very true that a pour bath of ice water, or even water just from the spring, will break up the chill, and cure the disease in many cases, but the remedy is little less than terrible ; few would submit to a second operation, and some have died in its progress. That mercury is the most infallible agency known to man is an accepted fact ; but many have a prejudice against its use ; meanwhile we will leave it to the tincture of time, and the little pellets to cure all who are suffering now, it being a main province of this book to prevent these diseases.

Places, neighborhoods, now under the bane of miasmatic emanations, should be drained before another season, ploughed over and put under cultivation, or filled up, after a winter and half summer exposure.

But a few practical facts in reference to the nature of miasm and its laws are worthy of repetition, until the people can be made to apprehend them and act intelligently in reference to them.

Miasm, the one great cause of prevalent epidemics, from the simplest fever or diarrhœa to malignant Asiatic cholera, is most pernicious, almost exclusively so for the hour including sunrise and sunset, there being a dampness, rawness, and heaviness in the atmosphere at such times, not found at mid-day or midnight, leading to the practice of intelligent families, where these autumnal diseases prevail, to have a blazing fire on the hearth at sunrise and sunset, in the family room where the family should be gathered, of course ; the cheery fire antagonizes the influences named, changes the physical condition and constitution of the atmosphere. But there is an additional precaution, and both together have amounted to a total exemption from the diseases in whole families, simply by arranging to take breakfast before going outside the door in the morning, and getting back into the house a little before sundown, and sit down to a hot supper as soon as reaching home, at least something hot enough to wake up the circulation of the body, and thus repel the influences of disease until the digestion of the sufferer commences to impart nutriment and strength to the system. It is peculiarly appropriate in the morning, where fever and ague and similar diseases prevail, to take something hot into the stomach, a cup of coffee or tea, or chocolate or broma; these are best, especially if a bit of cracker or bread is added. In many cases, one or two oranges or apples, or dry cracker or lemon are sufficient, because they excite the secretion of the stomach, warm it up, wake it into action, and thus prevent the absorption of poisonous gases, giving in their stead healthful nutriment to the blood, and not the baleful miasm.

------ ∞ ------

THE WARNING KNOCK.

NOT long ago a lady guest came down to the breakfast table, and in the course of conversation remarked in a very casual manner,—

"I was knocked up over early this morning."

"How's that?"

"I waked about daylight, and was thinking over the plans of the day, when such a crashing noise was heard at the head-board of the bed, I thought it was a pistol-shot; in one instant I was erect in bed, the next on the floor; but there was nothing there."

"Why, Miss Kate, you don't think it was a warning for you?"

"Oh no, indeed; but something's going to happen."

And something did happen; for that very night the sun set over the Jersey land-flats one minute later than it did the day before, and what's more, the moon did not make its appearance at the same moment next day.

In a few days after, the excellent lady sickened; and after a brief interval further, I stood by her grave in Greenwood, under the exceedingly impressive offices of the Rev. Mr. Haight.

The intelligent reader will see in this a mere coincidence. Cracks and noises in wooden furniture are a frequent result from incessant shrinkage and expansion; it is this which often makes the thunder of the avalanche, the iceberg, and the lava slide; bureaus, bedsteads, and tables are liable to these changing conditions from heat to cold, from dryness to moisture, and the reverse. Such occurrences have a very depressing influence on some minds, and in feeble conditions of the body may be the pivot of life or death, of recovery or the grave; and it is well that the reader should have a rational view of such things while in health, especially as the weakening influence of disease impairs the reasoning powers.

THE BRAIN-WORKER'S DOOM.

WHENEVER a thinker, or student, or scholar, gets into that condition when he feels very tired all over, at the close of the day, especially tired in the legs from the knees downwards, he ought to take heed of kindly Nature's warning; the brain is giving out; not that he is going crazy, but he is getting into that nervous condition which makes instant abandonment of all mental application most imperatively necessary; without such prompt action, the whole machinery of the nervous system may become disordered, and months and years may not suffice to repair the damage; it means that the nervous energy is so nearly exhausted that there is not vitality to send it to the extremities; these energies have got such a set toward the brain that their consumption is in that direction; the magnet is there, drawing all into itself. It is just at this point that the

MOVEMENT CURE

is most rational, most applicable, and most efficient, physical motion of the limbs, and little or no action of the brain, so as to change the current of nervous flow and set it in another direction to parts which most need it, and thus re-establish the equilibrium. It is wonderful to note the change which a single day's excursion to the country will make, especially if several hours are spent in walking, or on horseback. But if a man has been suffering with weak legs for months he cannot expect so prompt a change in his feelings.

If overworked, over-anxious wives have these feelings from the responsibilities of household cares, the generous husband will take them to the country right away, or if in the country already, will bring them to the city, that seeing its sights and walking its streets, the ruts of the nervous currents may be changed and the necessary repairs made, before sleepless nights' come on, or the lightning stroke of the palsy, or the sundering of the heart-strings close the history.

When persons feel this weakness and tiredness in the legs, inclining them to lie down all the time, if it is because there has been too much thinking or care or study, this tiredness will disappear if several hours are spent in out-door activities, because these compel the nervous influence in the direction of the limbs, while the brain is in a state of comparative rest, and will soon, by that very rest, be renovated.

HASTE HURTFUL.

A MAN of wealth was about stepping into the cars on his afternoon return to his country-seat ; the car was passing before him ; he made an effort to jump on to the step leading to the front platform, missed his footing, fell under the wheel, and was crushed in a moment. Had he waited sixty seconds he could as easily have made the attempt to jump on the rear platform, and missing his hold there, he would have had a fall and nothing more, for there would have been no wheels to run over him.

Very recently a distinguished professor in a Virginia University wanted to deposit a letter in the post-office on the other side of the railroad track. A locomotive was approaching ; he thought he could cross before the ponderous engine could come along. He miscalculated the speed. In another moment he was a shapeless mass. Had he waited two minutes, half a minute, the train would have passed along, and he could have leisurely deposited his letter.

A young lady wished to show her friends how easily she could cross in front of a locomotive ; she did cross, but her streaming dress caught in the passing wheel, drawing her back under its crushing weight.

One afternoon about sundown a young wife was looking out of the window of her beautiful country home for the return of her young husband from the city. For the six months just past of their married life they had been busily fixing up their country place ; both were young, both healthy ; the husband was in business on his own account, with every prospect of increasing success. She saw him get out of the cars, and passed down-stairs to

12

greet him at the door; but when she reached it, he was not there; she thought he was playing her a little trick; she called for him playfully, affectionately, but there was no answer; she saw a crowd of men approach the gate, open it, come up the path with her dead husband. He did alight from the cars, and safely stepped on the platform of the station house. There was a train coming in an opposite direction; he thought he had plenty of time to cross in front of it, and did cross, except by one single inch; the wheel struck the heel of his boot, wheeled him round under the cars, and all was over; one minute longer, and he could have crossed with the locomotive behind him.

Limbs are broken, lives are lost every year, in any large city, by attempting to cross in front of a moving horse or vehicle; an infatuation seems to come across many under such circumstances, as if they were willing to risk limb and life itself to save one single sixty seconds. The next day was

" CHRISTMAS."

A happy family of wife and five or six children, in Brooklyn, were looking for their father to come over from his business place in New York, to arrange for that mysterious visitor called Santa Claus and Khris Kringle. It was just dark; he was somewhat later than usual, but surely the next boat would bring him over; there it was at the wharf, for they could see it through the window, not a quarter of a mile away. Fast footsteps pattered along, on the pavement, coming nearer, coming opposite, passing along, and died in the distance; other footsteps approached, passed on, fewer and fewer all the time; and at length there was silence; father had not come, so they thought; but they were mistaken; he did cross in that boat, loaded with the most beautiful assortment of toys and sweetmeats, something even for the baby, just nine months old. In his hurry to meet the happy faces which he well knew were peering through the darkness at the window pane, he made an effort to step from the boat before she touched the platform; the distance was greater than he supposed; he fell half through into the water, his body caught between the timbers, and life was gone. Fifteen seconds more and he could have stepped on solid ground. To save a minute, a life was lost; just as in another direction we waste time and lose eternity; we spend our whole existence here, we hurry on in our own business for the accumulation of money, giving no thought of preparation for the great future which so nearly concerns us all, and in a moment to pass away, without any preparation whatever.

---—∞—---

HERNIA, OR RUPTURES.

SOMETIMES persons are born with them, at others they are induced by over-straining in lifting, or jumping down from a height and lighting on the heels. Ruptures occur generally at the lower part of the belly, where its walls are thin, an opening having been left for certain blood and other vessels to pass out, so that if there is any undue strain, that being the weakest spot, the parts give way by the whole mass of the bowels pressing downwards and forwards. After protrusion the muscles at the part sometimes spasmodically contract, and in a sense choke the rupture or hernia, so called from a Greek word meaning a branch, as it protrudes or branches off from the belly; this choked rupture is called strangulated hernia, and requires instant relief, as it stops all passage of the bowel contents and causes mortification and death; the opening must be enlarged by cutting it, so as to allow more room for the return of the bowel. As soon as a rupture is noticed, place the patient on his back, raising up the head and shoulders, bending the head forwards, and drawing the knees up, so as to relax the abdomen; then raise the clothing, return the protruded bowels with the balls of the fingers, for the nails may cut them, gently and adroitly pressing inwards and upwards; it may be known that it is in place by a peculiar gurgling sound on the instant of return within the walls of the belly; then a pressure should be made over the spot where the protrusion took place, to prevent its recurrence, this pressure should be made with a pad to which is attached an elastic spring, so as to have more or less give in it, in coughing, straining, lifting, or other motions; such a contrivance is called a

TRUSS,

which adapts itself to all the motions of the body; these trusses have generally to be worn for life. The rupture is told by the protrusion, sometimes tense, at others lank; the skin is not colored, but seems altogether natural; the swelling varies in size and tension according to the position of the body, smallest when lying down, largest if standing; coughing changes it very much; sometimes there is colic, constipation, or nausea and vomiting.

If, before the bowel is returned, there should be a spasmodic contraction of the muscles of the parts so as to act upon the protruded bowel like the drawing of a purse-string, it is called a

STRANGULATED HERNIA,

and as this prevents the passing along of the contents of the bowels, mortification and death will soon take place unless this spasmodic contraction is overcome by immediately placing the patient in warm water, which has a relaxing effect; if not sufficient, bleed the patient while in the bath until he faints or is about to do so. This relaxes the whole body, and the parts can be returned; still, it is always advisable to send for a physician promptly on the appearance of a rupture, especially if strangulated; the advice above given is to be followed when a doctor cannot be had; it is what a doctor would follow if he were present, and if he can't be got, some one must do it in his place. It requires a great deal of patience to push back the rupture; even if it takes half an hour, patience should not be lost, for it is often of critical importance.

Great care should be taken not to injure the intestines with the end of the finger-nails, hence some surgeons cover the hands with a thin cloth or glove. The pressure should be gentle, steady, firm, upwards and inwards. If the warm bath or bleeding does not relax the parts, some have dashed a bowl of cold water against the spot, as a last resort; it is a dangerous and desperate remedy, but has been effective.

LITERARY HUSBANDS

ARE certainly as capable of loving their wives as sincerely as other men love theirs; but so much of the nervous energy goes to the brain, that the heart is too often left to wither away; too much of that energy is expended on the intellectual faculties, too little on the emotional; it is an avoidable calamity.

THE ABDOMEN.

THIS plate represents the appearance from the navel down to the crotch, if the clothing, skin, and flesh were removed.

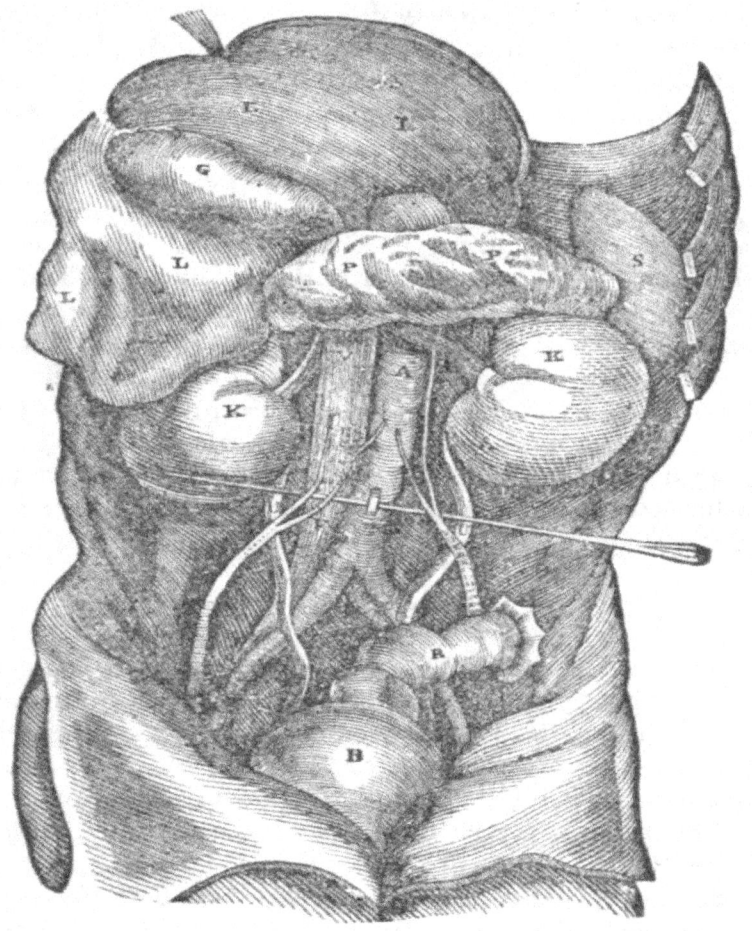

EXPLANATION OF THE PLATE.

A, the aorta which carries the blood from the heart down-wards, branching towards the bottom of the body to carry life and strength and health to each limb. By the side of the aorta is V, the vena cava, or great vein of the body, through which all the blood is brought from the lower extremities up into the heart again, to be sent on to the lungs, to be purified by the fresh air drawn into them and to be forwarded in its renovated state as before through the aorta. It will be seen that they both lie by the side of the backbone, or spinal column. Under the letters L and L, and in front of P P, was the stomach which is removed. One person eats a pound or two or more at a meal, including drink; the weight would be four or five pounds or more sometimes. It is easy to see that if, soon after eating, a person lies on the back, the whole weight of the stomach and its contents rests or presses on the great artery and vein, and their thin soft sides being yielding, the flow of blood would be stopped in the aorta, preventing the life-blood from going to the lower portion of the body, and would also prevent the blood from going towards the heart, hence there would be a double cause of stagnation, and stagnation of blood in the body means death; it is death in an instant, if in the brain; sleepless Nature takes alarm, fills the whole body with uneasiness, terrible dreams come to the disordered brain, an impending cala-mity is just upon us, a mad dog is at our heels, a lion is just about to spring at us, we are just upon the verge of an awful chasm, the man whom we promised to pay borrowed money is just coming across the street. Then comes the dreadful shriek. It is the

NIGHTMARE.

We lie down on our backs too soon after eating a hearty meal. The spasmodic jump, a single touch of some friendly finger at our side, sends the dammed-up blood bounding away again, and the wild cat is gone; we didn't owe the man anything, and we are saved, except that we are in a tremble or dripping perspiration.

But in that terrible struggle we feel that death is inevitable, and we roll over the precipice in utter horror and helplessness, but " catch ourselves " at the very last second. Some, however, do not catch themselves; they are dead in their beds next morning. "Died in a fit," some say; others, " of heart-disease," and others still of apoplexy. So the reader can see how near he has been to death more than once. The first time a youth touches the cheek of his sweetheart with the tip end of his finger a kind of an electric shock runs through his whole system, and the other one's too, wholly disproportioned to the force of the contact; so in nightmare, the gentlest shake of the arm, the slightest

POKE IN THE RIBS

sets the whole blood of the body in motion again, when the sharpest sound of the voice would have failed to do so. Hence the very instant you hear the dreadful moan of a nightmared person, and certainly it is dreadful to hear, touch him instantaneously, don't wait to speak to him, he can't hear you; better to give him a

QUICK KICK

outright, for every second is a second of agony, until the blood is set in motion. Surely no reader can ever forget the nature, cause, and remedy of the terrible nightmare, and it is hoped that ever hereafter, if he hears the sound, even although it may be in a distant part of the house, he will feel prompted in pity to run with all his might, to touch, or shake, or kick the sufferer at the earliest possible second; for a second later and he may be dead.

B indicates the position of the bladder. It will be seen that R, the rectum or lowest portion of the bowel, is immediately behind the

BLADDER.

In women the womb is between the bladder and the rectum, hence, in order to give more room for the passage of the infant, Nature is constantly prompting to urination, so that if labor pains come in an instant, as sometimes they do, the bladder may be empty, for if full it is pretty sure to be ruptured and death is inevitable. Hence the unwisdom, towards the close of gestation, of resisting the inclination to urination, or of complaining of the trouble of it, or of doing something, or wanting to take something, to prevent it.

Another important lesson is, that towards the close of gestation there should be secured by any and all means one full evacuation of the bowels, if not two—one in the morning and one at night— and few would fail of that, if the food were to consist mainly of coarse breads, fruits in great abundance, and vegetables. This practical suggestion can scarcely be underrated in importance.

G, the gall bladder.

K, the kidneys, which are situated immediately on each side of the backbone and close to the back, thickly enveloped in fat, as may be seen any time at a butcher's shop. All know the line of the lower edge of the ribs; the kidneys, as will be seen, are in the rear, about one part above the line named, and one part below.

L is the liver. P is the pancreas.

S, the spleen.

U, the ureters, or channels, which carry the urine from the kidneys into the bladder.

Abdomen, accent on the second syllable, which is pronounced like the word "dough," means to hide, or cover, as it does, like a curtain, all that has been explained.

The stomach is not seen in this plate; it was removed in order to show more fully the liver, pancreas or sweet bread, spleen, and kidneys.

In front of all these, like a veil, is the

PERITONÆUM,

a very thin membrane, which covers and lines externally, running down in between all the organs above named.

HICCOUGH

Is a nervous contraction of certain muscles connected in their motions with the stomach. It is a fatal sign in some forms of disease, while cases are on record where the hiccough was so persistent as to induce convulsions and death. The old cure was "nine swallows of water," which, by distending the stomach, gave relief in many cases. But it is always desirable that the memory be stored with a variety of remedies for an affection which is so common, and at times inconvenient, to say the least of it. A lump or two of sugar, dissolved in the mouth and swallowed, has sometimes relieved the most distressing cases, and comes within the meaning of "The Food Cure." Sometimes a few mouthfuls of food, or even a diversion of the mind, is all-sufficient.

DIABETES,

Or sweet water, as it is called by the common people, is attended with great thirst and large urination; a gallon of water has been drunk in a night and as much urinated. It may be months and even years before the disease reaches this extent of action; but whenever it is done, there is great debility of all the muscles of the body, a man "can't work." Sometimes there is general emaciation with distention of the belly, as if there were an immense tumor there; and yet the bowels may be regular and appetite good; still the great overshadowing symptom is present—an insufferable frequency of urination every few minutes, sometimes indeed at intervals of three and four hours or more, as in healthy persons.

Some persons discharge two or three gallons of water in the course of a long winter's night; under such large discharges, the cure, when possible, is necessarily slow, requiring weeks and months. From the numerous remedies which seem to have been successful, there can be no doubt that nature is sometimes her own best physician. For example, several persons have stated in print that they have been perfectly cured by drinking no other fluid but their own urine.

A reliable treatment under which persons who have been suffering many months, and have gained fifteen and twenty pounds in a few weeks is found in the use of tannic acid, opium and ergot, thus:

Take one hundred grains of tannic acid, ten grains of opium, and twenty grains of ipecac, make into twenty pills; take one at a time three times a day at six hours interval, the last on going to bed.

Take one teaspoonful of tincture of ergot in a little water, just before each meal.

Rub into the spine lightly and patiently, with the hand, night and morning, a quarter of a large teaspoonful of ointment made thus:

Sixty grains of poke-berry root, called American hellebore or veratrum viride, mixed well with a teaspoonful of hog's lard; the poke-root has a stimulating effect on the skin, the lard is cooling, and the frictions with the hand are very beneficial, and all together do a great deal of good.

The diet should be of vegetables, coarse bread, and fruits, drinking moderately of hot teas; the whole treatment to be persevered in until the flesh and strength return, and urination takes place on an average not oftener than at four hours interval. The cures which have followed this treatment have been permanent; which may be known by the urine having its natural saltish taste instead of sweet; it loses its violet or sweet milk smell; its excessive quantity, and dry skin; and emaciation and debility gradually disappear. This disease was first noticed by Celsus, a medical writer in the time of Augustus Cæsar, in the age of Virgil and Horace, and Cæsar and Cicero.

Diabetic urine in a summer temperature turns sour, sometimes ferments, and by adding a little yeast a vinous fermentation takes place. A gallon of this diabetic urine will average a pound of solid matter, if boiled down.

Diabetes is more common to men than women; to the old than the young; to the spare rather than the stout; it is inherited, but oftener is brought on by the use of liquor, its causes are all such as tend to throw more work than is natural on the kidneys. For example, in cold weather the kidneys have to do more work than in warm weather, because the surface of the body is more exposed to chilliness, and less water passes off in the form of perspiration; and as a certain amount must be passed out of the body during each twenty-four hours, in health, if less is passed off in perspiration, more must be passed off by the kidneys, hence it is that in damp and cold climates and localities, diabetes is more common than in high, warm situations; it is also brought on by frequent checking of perspiration, by the drying up suddenly of old sores or runnings or issues, or by the sudden driving in of any breakings out on the body, hence in all treatment of diabetes two things should be ever kept in sight: at least one full, free action of the bowels in every twenty-four hours, because the freer the bowels are, the more of the wastes of the system do they pass off, leaving less for the kidneys to do; and for the same reason persons ought to dress warm, and keep warm, so as to promote a soft perspiring condition of the pores of the skin, hence any medicines which tend to promote a soft moist condition of the skin, are very valuable, hence the value of large doses of opium. Sydenham found this out more than two hundred years ago. Opium, in large doses of half a grain at a time, does not have the constipating quality of small doses, as a general rule ; but if it does have that effect in any case, means must be taken to counteract the costiveness, such as oil, chewing rhubarb root, or the use of the dinner-pill, to the extent required. For the same reason moderate labor or exercise, continuous, but not carried to the extent of weariness at any time, especially if in the open air, promoting and causing perspiration, will always have to that extent a curative effect, if care is taken after the perspiration has been excited, that the system is not allowed to cool off too quickly.

Whatever medicines are taken to cure diabetes, three things must be done outside the use of medicine, or a cure need not be expected in any case.

First. Keep up the general health to the highest point all the time (which article see).

Second. Get up a good appetite and a vigorous digestion by means of exertive exercises in the open air. (See article on Air and Exercise.)

Third. Do all that is possible to diminish the amount of work done by the kidneys, by keeping the bowels free, and by promoting the vigorous action of the skin, washing the whole surface of the body twice a week with soap and warm water, and vigorous rubbing of the surface with the hands—not with sponge or harsh cloths, or brushes ; the object being to keep the skin soft and moist.

A great deal has been said about the appearance, color, etc., of the urine in this disease, but as few know what the urine should look like in health, and as its color and quantity are altered by so many circumstances of diet, exercise and weather, and as some persons are very imaginative, and really sensible people are occasionally drawn into the habit of forever inspecting the urine, it has been thought best to say nothing as to what it looks like in diabetes (see urination), and as soon as possible let any one having it apply to an educated physician.

Sometimes, when the discharges of water are very large, take one or two or three of the following pills every day, one at a time, to the extent of causing two full evacuations in every twenty-four hours : four grains of extract ox-gall, two grains of rhubarb, and one of aloes ; or, if the liquid form is preferred, four drachms of the inspissated extract of ox-gall in water, one dose three or four times a day, to the extent of causing two actions of the bowels daily.

There is too much sugar in the urine, hence food and drink should be used which furnish as little sweetness, as little sugar as possible, such as spinach, lettuce, cabbage, celery and onions, meats, eggs, butter, and jellies of any kind, made of animal product, using mainly bran-bread without any sweetening; if stimulants are needed, claret and sherry wines are best in small quantities.

Whenever a person has diabetes and is increasing in weight, he is to that extent certainly getting well, it is a more important symptom of improvement than the lessening sweet taste of the urine. Diabetes insipidus is an immense discharge of limpid water with inappeasable thirst and great debility; it is rare, and an improvement of the general health is the best means of cure.

This diabetes, "a running through," as the Greeks expressed it, as if the water taken into the stomach passed immediately onward through the system, is treated

HYDROPATHICALLY

by inviting the blood to the surface in all possible ways, frictions, bathings, rubbings, and fomentations; beginning with a tepid sheet bath, succeeded immediately by being placed in bed with a dry pack in a way to secure profuse perspiration, with a gradual cooling off and thorough rubbing of the whole skin with the hands, or warm flannels, or even cloths, whatever seems to aid most in keeping the skin soft and warm; water is allowed to be drank most freely; the diet is almost wholly of the meal of any kind of grain, with potatoes, and fruits, and berries as a dessert after each meal, even to drink freely bran tea, made by pouring hot water on bran, a pint to a pint, let it cool, and drink it as it is, or make a kind of lemonade out of it; the meals, thrice a day, to consist wholly of the meal or flour made of the whole grain, used as mush or Graham bread. The water used in quenching thirst should be rain or distilled water, or common water boiled, but this last is not as good as the others; better take pains to get the best.

ALIMENTARY CANAL.

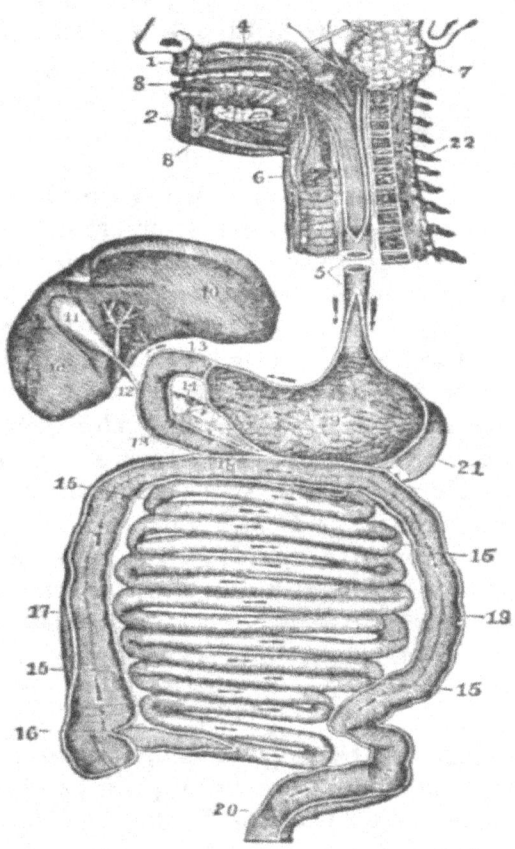

THE above cut is to show the progress of the food from the lips until it gets to the lower part of the body.

1 and 2, Upper and lower jaw.

3, Tongue.

4, Roof of the mouth.

5, Œsophagus, showing where the swallow, or throat proper, ends, and leads into a tube which is the channel for the food, into the stomach.

6, Trachea, or windpipe, which is in front of the "swallow," or œsophagus. It marks the point where Adam's apple is, made by the structure of the voice-making organs or larynx, the seat of laryngitis, or clergymen's sore throat.

8, Sublingual glands, that is, under the tongue.

9, Parotid glands. Both 8 and 9 manufacture the saliva to keep the mouth moist and to dilute the food, so that it can be swallowed more readily.

9, Stomach.

10, 10, Liver.

11, Gall-bladder.

12, Gall-duct which conveys the bile into the intestines, drop by drop, after eating chiefly, just below the stomach; but in heaving as in vomiting, the bile passes upwards into the stomach, causing deathly sickness, for that is not its proper place; but when it gets to where it belongs it causes no discomfort whatever, unless it has been kept in the gall-bladder too long, causing it to become concentrated and acrid, then it causes great burning or smarting or pain, or even cramps, as it passes along through the alimentary canal; hence, when there is griping after taking medicine, it is a favorable sign, as showing that the contents of the bowels are passing along downwards; and the griping shows how necessary it was that the bile should be carried away; when it is the result of liver medicines patients are very apt to attribute the griping pains to the harsh nature of the medicines, when it is really the bad, acrid bile, which the medicine is bringing away.

GALL-STONES.

It is at the point of the figure 12, where the gall-duct is the narrowest, that such insupportable pain is experienced when gall-stones are passing out of the gall-bladder into the intestines. Anything which causes deathly sickness relaxes this canal, allows it to stretch, and then the gall-stone passes more easily; but in passing, the inflammation which it causes is so great sometimes as to occasion death in a few days. These gall-stones form mainly because the liver does not carry off the bile, and then it crystallizes and forms into hard stones. Persons liable to gall-stones should eat no wheat, or bread made out of it, or any other grain (see article The Best Bread), because there is so much lime in wheat, as also in the water, but should drink milk, rain or snow water, or distilled water, and eat rice, sago, tapioca, fruits, berries, and lean meats and vegetables, for these have no lime in them.

13, 13, 14, Pancreas or sweet bread, the use of which gland has not yet been satisfactorily ascertained, but the fluids secreted or manufactured by it, aid in the promotion of digestion ; this gland is immediately behind the stomach, and lies right across the spinal column, a little to the right of the spleen, which is about the lower edge of the left ribs.

15, 15, 15, 15, is the small intestine ; the arrows show the direction which the food takes. One part of this intestine is called Colon, from a Greek word meaning to arrest, because it keeps the food so long in passing through it, that it may be said to arrest it, requiring from five to ten or fifteen or more hours in passing the whole distance of the intestines, some thirty feet from the stomach to the outlet. It will be seen that after the food passes from the stomach it crosses from one side of the body to the other a number of times on a descending plane until it gets to the bottom, then it ascends to near where it started, crosses again immediately under the stomach, and then descends to No. 20, where it enters the

RECTUM,

which is the largest intestine, and the lowest and last; it is the reservoir for the reception of that part of the food which is called waste, and of which no use can be made. It would not answer for these waste matters to be constantly passing from the body, any more than the urine, hence Nature has given the rectum a considerable capacity for holding; it gets fuller and fuller all the time, until the distention reaches a certain point, causing uneasiness and inclination to stool, when by an effort of the will, we open the outlet of the rectum, called the

ANUS,

which has muscles to close it, very much like the strings which by being drawn close a purse. The ordinary contents of the rectum are of the consistence of mortar, but if they remain there too long, heat or fever is generated, the more watery particles are evaporated, leaving the rest hard and so shrunk, that there is not distention enough to cause the inclination to discharge. This is called

COSTIVENESS,

if it continues for a day or two ; if for several days or a week, it becomes

CONSTIPATION.

Hence it happens, that when the bowels have been torpid for a day or two, not acting, the first that comes out is hard, sometimes in little balls. When an

ENEMA

or injection is used, the object of it is to supply fluid in the place of that which has been absorbed or dried up, with a view to obtain an amount of distention which will cause a desire for an evacuation. A great deal of mystery is occasioned sometimes by having this, that, or the other kind of injection; some want salt water, some want flaxseed tea; the principle of all is the same—an increase of bulk, so as to distend the rectum to an extent sufficient to create a desire to evacuate, and water is the simplest and best. When medicines are given to act on the bowels they simply come down to the rectum, and distend it, as castor oil; or they irritate the tender lining of the bowels and make them throw out water, as an irritated eyeball; salts do, or even common salt water.

When medicines are given to act on the liver, the bile in the liver is thrown out into the gall-bladder, thence into the intestines, and in such larger quantities than common that it irritates the bowels, causes more water to be thrown out, and the extra bile mixing with it makes it all look yellow or green or dark; whereas the water caused by salts is not specially colored; hence we speak of bilious discharges, which are always healthful; then persons should notice the color of the privy paper, which will enable them to know whether they are going to be better or not. It is the colorless or watery passages which make one weak and do not give promise of better health. Much has been said about

FIGS

being good to remove costiveness, and so they are, as well as tomatoes and

WHITE MUSTARD SEED.

The little seeds, in passing along this immense bowel tract or surface, irritate, cause watering, and really act on the same principle as drugs, only they are milder in their operation. It is believed that the reader has now a better and clearer idea of the philosophy of purgatives, enemas, or injections, which will be exceedingly satisfactory in after-life.

AGUE CAKE.

21 is the spleen. It is the swelling of this, and s hardening, which causes

AGUE CAKE.

The spleen is the reservoir of the liver, to keep it supplied with blood. Hence when the liver has been affected for a long time, as in fever and ague, the spleen becomes diseased also, because the liver is so congested, so full of blood, that it cannot receive the blood from the spleen; but as the heart is all the time driving the blood into the spleen, and the liver will not receive it, it becomes full, and swells and hardens, as the mother's breast hardens if the milk is not drawn from it fast enough. Hence, also, if the liver pains it soon passes over on the other side, and the spleen pains also—sometimes one side, then another; that is about the lower edge of the ribs. Persons are often annoyed by having pains along the edge of the ribs below, apprehending consumption; but the experienced physician always feels relieved when a patient complains of a pain at the right short ribs, especially if it goes over to the left side sometimes, for he knows it is too low down for the lungs; that it must be in the liver and spleen, hence is far less dangerous; in addition, the disease there tends to draw disease away from the lungs, is an actual protection, and if the pulse is not over seventy beats in a minute he is delighted, because when the lungs are consumptive, and no bleeding from them, the pulse keeps above eighty, and up and up over a hundred and still up, and the man dies.

16 is the opening into the large intestine.

22, Upper part of spinal column.

ALIMENTARY CANAL

includes the entire distance from the opening of the lips to the outer opening of the "rectum," for along this whole channel we find the aliment must pass, undergoing various changes at several different points. The lips open to receive it; at the very threshold the front teeth take hold of it to divide it, next the jaw teeth press it and grind it into a pulp, then the tongue pushes it to its back part to the top of the throat or œsophagus, which is called by some the swallow, through this it passes into the stomach, where it is detained several hours; during the whole of which time it is kept in motion, being carried round and round, under-going a process of dissolution, or melting, from without inwards until all solidity has disappeared, like stirring bits of ice with a spoon in a vessel of water, until all is water; then it is in a condi-tion to pass through the lower, right-hand portion of the stomach, called the

PYLORIC ORIFICE,

into the upper part of the bowels proper, along which it passes more or less slowly for twenty or thirty feet, when at the end of about twenty-four hours in ordinary health it reaches the rectum and is voided from the body; but from the time it enters the stomach until it reaches the rectum the food is constantly parting with more or less of its nutritious particles; a certain kind are ab-sorbed by the veins in the stomach, others are sucked up by the lacteals of the bowels, and by the time it gets into the rectum all the nutriment is absorbed, has been carried into the circulation, and nothing is left but useless waste matter, containing no sub-stance, no nutriment whatever, and this is called "dung," which nourishes, manures the ground, and makes it more productive of whatever may be put into it by the farmer or gardener, and thus it is that we feed upon the products of the earth, and the rem-nants go to enrich that earth again, making an eternal circuit to the end of time.

It is said that if the urine and excrement of a person were preserved for a year, and properly mixed with earth and spread over the ground, there would be enough to manure sixty-five acres of land, doubling the productiveness. At first thought this may seem very repulsive, but the blood and de-caying bodies and bones of thousands and thousands who have perished on the battle-field have enriched the soil for years and years afterwards, causing the most luxuriant crops of grain, which were just as sweet, just as perfect wheat and corn as if it had been raised from a virgin soil; the ablest chemist has never been able to find one atom of matter in one that was not found in the other, the products of both being perfect, as are all of Nature's works and processes.

Look again at No. 12. It is easy to see that if pressure was made on the gall-bladder, its contents would naturally run in a down-ward direction into the bowels. Its situation is at the edge of the ribs and a little above on the right side ; if, then, the ball of the thumb or hand is used by pressing it from the edge of the ribs downward, beginning at the hip-bone and extending around as far as the navel, and from the navel back to the hip-bone, the tendency of it would be to empty the gall-bladder, and make more room for bile to come into it from the liver, hence relieve the parts of the extra bile without medicine, that is, tend to cure all symptoms which arise from a torpid liver, that is, all the symptoms which arise from biliousness, such as poor appetite, foul tongue, yellow skin, yellow eyes, headache and cold feet, resulting from a torpid liver ; but they sometimes arise from very different causes. Hence this kneading of the liver five or ten minutes night and morning is a very valuable mechanical remedy for torpid liver, biliousness, wind on the stomach, indigestion, and other kindred symptoms. It is to be hoped that the reader will not allow the idea to be forgotten or to be unappreciated, because of its simplicity and availability and costlessness. There are persons who for a quarter of a century have used these kneadings for the various ailments named, have used no others, and have maintained their health, apparently, by these very same means. It requires patient persistence and the avoidance of colds, constipation, over-eating, and constant confinement in-doors. If these same kneadings are continued lower down, when there is wind in the stomach or bowels, it will be uniformly successful in pushing the wind downward and outward.

APPETITE

Is literally a seeking to or for, as a means of gratifying an inclination, and is most frequently applied in its relation to food. It is distinct from hunger, which may be painful in its extent ; it is Nature's intimation that something is wanting to supply the place of what has been used or taken away. Every motion of the body wears away some particles, and unless other particles are deposited in their places, the parts would be worn out or would lose their strength, and the machinery would cease to work ; the appetite is in the nature of an instinct, a faithful monitor, and will not cease its admonitions until the want is supplied, until something has been eaten.

The best and most healthy appetite is that which inclines us moderately to eat when the regular eating time comes. If the appetite is voracious day after day, it is the appetite of disease, and instead of gratifying it freely, it should be only partially done. The easiest way to correct a voracious appetite, such as is connected with dyspepsia, is to take half as much as usual, eat it slowly, and if in half an hour you feel as if you were not hungry at all and had eaten enough, then a persistence in this course will in a reasonable time break up the voraciousness. But if, when you have not eaten "half enough" according to your feelings, you continue to be tormented with hunger, it is most probably the result of the presence of a tape-worm (which see).

THE WANT OF AN APPETITE, CALLED ANOREXIA,

is the result of disease, generally of biliousness (which article see), and if the means there suggested are used, it will not be long before the appetite returns.

Perverted appetite is present in cases of chlorosis; the person wants to eat chalk, clay, slate pencils, dirt, or other things, indicating that the whole digestive function is in a diseased condition, although there may be no sign of disease.

MORBID APPETITE

is present in various forms of disease; it is of practical importance to know how to distinguish it, to know whether it is morbid or legitimate; it usually manifests itself in one or more of five different ways, each of which is opposed to a natural, healthy appetite.

First. It comes on suddenly, and often with very great violence, driving the person sometimes to feats of perfect desperation, seeming for the instant to quench the reasoning faculties, and to extinguish all fear of personal suffering or responsibility. A drunkard was once sentenced to the penitentiary, where no liquors were allowed, under any pretence whatever, unless by the express permission or prescription of the prison physician; on ordinary occasions he had resisted the desire. One day he came running towards the keeper, holding up one arm, all bleeding, frantically exclaiming, "Brandy! brandy! a bowl of brandy to stop the bleeding." In the confusion it was run for and handed to him; he thrust the stump of his arm into it and the next moment drank his fill with the eagerness of a famishing wild beast. He then explained that such a terrible desire for one more drink of brandy came over him like an avalanche, that it was perfectly irresistible; he felt that he would willingly give his life for one more drink, and instantly the expedient came to his mind, and was instantly adopted, to cut off his hand at the wrist and carry out the ruse as he did.

Sometimes persons, without any special indication of there being anything the matter with them, are suddenly seized with a fit of hunger; perhaps it may have been excited by the appearance of some unexpected dish, or the smell of soup or other things from the distant kitchen; this feeling may come on within an hour or two after a regular meal. It is a morbid appetite, and if indulged in is certain to be followed in a few hours, or before next morning, with some nausea, vomiting, cholera morbus, or some distressing ailment in connection with the alimentary canal (which see), while the gratification of this sudden appetite will greatly aggravate the disease which is about manifesting itself. Abstinence from this gratification may not be sufficient to prevent a modified attack; hence when this sudden feeling of hunger is noticed, it should be regarded as a friendly admonition of Nature to go out of doors immediately and walk briskly, or work an hour or two or more to the extent of getting up a gentle perspiration; cool off very slowly when returning to the house, and if after dinner, eat nothing whatever for the remainder of the day, or take a cup or two of hot tea; and a breakfast of cold bread and butter and a cup of hot drink and nothing else. In this way an attack of sickness will be certainly prevented; Nature will have time to regain a healthful condition of the system, and all will be well, and thus several days of troublesome sickness and loss of time may be avoided. If this sudden hunger should come on between breakfast and dinner, omit dinner altogether, and about 5 P.M. take a bowl of soup or hot tea with bread crust broken into it, and nothing else for that day, and aim to secure three or four hours in outdoor activities.

Second. A morbid appetite is insatiable, it wants more and more. However much a person relishes a good apple, a luscious peach, or a cooling water-melon, there will soon be a feeling of having had enough, and for five or six or more hours afterwards the sight of any one of these would not cause any desire for them.

But every drunkard knows that when he takes one drink, even if it be to the fill, in a very short time he will want it just as much as if he had not taken that fill.

Third. A morbid appetite seems to aggravate itself, as a fire in a large city, the more it burns, the more furious does it become.

Fourth. A morbid appetite destroys a natural appetite. A slave to tobacco or liquor becomes more and more subject to its tyranny, and in proportion loses his appetite for everthing else; the same is the case with the slavish use of tea and coffee; after a while nothing else is wanted, until the end is reached to drink and drink and die.

Fifth. A morbid appetite wants one thing; the whiskey-drinker wants whiskey and nothing else; the man who chews tobacco comes to the point at last when he must have it in his mouth all the time; the appetite for food in both cases becoming less and less, the flesh becomes thinner and thinner, the legs become mere spindles, and the whole man is a skeleton, a shadow, mere skin and bone; so it is precisely in the excessive use of any stimulant. It should be borne in mind, then, that the appetite is morbid, and disease and premature death will certainly follow when that appetite is sudden or insatiable, or constantly increases or destroys desire for other things, or wants more and more the one thing. The natural appetite is the reverse of all these; it comes on slowly, it is moderate, it is satiated, it is appeased by eating any one of a dozen "good things;" however satisfied with one thing to-day, it will be satisfied with almost any other the day following, while the poor drunkard calls out for whiskey yesterday, to-day, and forever, with louder and louder cries, until body and soul are ruined for time and for eternity.

Then there is the fitful or fanciful appetite of pregnancy; things are wanted which are out of season; this want increases the more it is thought about, until it amounts to an unappeasable longing; the popular prejudice being, that if it is not gratified some "mark" will be the result; it is well to endeavor to satisfy these desires as soon as possible; to take pains and to spare no expense to appease the desires on her part, whose condition appeals to all the best feelings and sympathies of our nature.

Then there is the variable appetite of childhood; at one time eating most voraciously, at another eating almost nothing at all; if the sleep in such cases is disturbed, the face pale, and more or less gnawing in the stomach or bowels, especially if there be itchings about the anus, then worm medicines should be tried without delay.

The simple

WANT OF AN APPETITE,

unconnected with any special disease, means that the body is too full, has too much in it, is clogged, and is not ready to receive any more; to force the appetite under such circumstances is suicidal ; its tendency is to destroy the body. The very first thing to be done, and which is of essential importance, is to diminish this fulness, to work off this excess of material which is clogging the wheels of life and prevents the human machine from its proper working.

When this want of appetite is present, the whole body seems to be out of order, there is a general feeling of discomfort everywhere, the body is indisposed to exertion, there is no elasticity, no vigor, the mind itself is depressed, the spirits are dull, and the whole man is out of order without there being any actual disease. But notwithstanding this indisposition to go out of doors, to dress and take a walk, only if the person does so, he at once begins to feel the better for it, simply because every step he takes wears out and off from the system both solid particles and those more fluid and gaseous in the perspiration, and if the walking is continued long enough to get up a good perspiration so as to carry off some of the load, the man feels actually less tired than when he took the first step. If such a person is in a great hurry to get an appetite, it will expedite matters to take three of Cook's pills at bedtime on a light supper, and next day to take nothing but soup or tea with bread crust broken into them, at intervals of five hours and only thrice in the twenty-four ; but after that, eat regularly, at regular meals, nothing between, no dessert at dinner and only one cup of tea and a piece of cold bread and butter for supper, but walking or working steadily for about two hours in the forenoon and two hours in the afternoon; and if this is judiciously done, and kept up, there will be appetite enough in less than ten days, especially if the two hours in the forenoon and afternoon are extended to four each, and the simple walk becomes steady, useful work. When Nature's machinery is clogged up with waste and useless and dead particles, she takes away the appetite purposely, for every mouthful swallowed under such circumstances only increases the clogging; first work off the surplus instead of adopting a universal yet ruinous course of " taking something," bitter tonics and the long list of appetizers; for it is simply fighting against Nature, it is endeavoring to compel her to take into the system that which will only oppress it more and more, and might weigh it down into the grave, to say nothing of the danger of getting into the habit of taking bitters, of getting up a taste for them which may lead to a drunkard's grave, and which has done so in hundreds of thousands of cases of persons who felt perfectly assured that there was no danger of their learning to drink, and would almost feel insulted at the most remote intimation of such a thing, for let it be remembered that " bitters " means nothing more than disguised alcohol in all cases.

THE INSTINCT OF APPETITE.

Chemical analysis and physiological research have established, beyond dispute, that every article of food and drink is composed of elements differing in quantity or quality. It is equally true that the various parts of the human frame are different in their composition—as the bone, the flesh, the nerve, the tendon, etc. But there is no element in the human body which is not found in some article of food or drink. A certain normal proportion of these elements, properly distributed, constitutes vigorous health, and forms a perfect body. If one of these elements be in excess, certain forms of disease manifest themselves; if there is not enough, some other malady affects the frame. When the blood contains less than its healthful amount of iron, it is poor, watery, and comparatively colorless; the muscles are flabby, the face pale, the eyes sunken, the whole body weak, the mind listless and sad. If the bones have not enough lime, they have no strength, are easily bent, and the patient is rickety; if there is too much lime, then the bones are brittle, and are broken by the slightest fall or unusual strain. The highest skill of the physician in these cases consists in determining the excess or deficit of any element, and in supplying such food or drug as will meet the case; when the medical attendant cannot determine what is wanting nor furnish the supply, Nature is often loud enough in her calls, through the tastes or appetites, to indicate very clearly what item of food or drink contains the needed elements; this is the " Instinct of

Appetite." Chemistry is unable to say of but one article of food, that it contains all the constituents necessary to supply the human body with every element requisite for its welfare, and that is pure milk, as supplied by the mother of the new being; but after the first years of life the body demands new elements, in order to enable it to meet the duties which increasing age imposes; hence Nature dries up this spring, as being no longer adequate, and compels the search for other kinds of sustenance, showing that milk is a proper, sole food for the young ones; but healthy grown persons who live upon it mainly, will always become invalids.

All kinds of life, whether vegetable or animal, have within them a principle of preservation, as well as of perpetuity; were that not the case all that breathes or grows would die; this principle or quality is common to man and beast, and all that springs from root or seed; it is named "Instinct." It is instinct which calls, by thirst, for water, when there is not fluid enough in the system. It is instinct which calls for food, by hunger, when a man is weak and needs renovation. It is curious and practically valuable as a means for the removal of disease, to notice the working of this instinct, for it seems to be almost possessed with a discriminating intelligence; certain it is that standard medical publications give well-authenticated facts, showing that following the cravings of the appetite the animal instinct has accomplished far more than the physician's skill was able to do; has saved life in multitudes of cases, when science has done its best, but in vain.

Some years ago the little daughter of a farmer on the Hudson river had a fall, which induced a long, painful, and dangerous illness, ending in blindness; medication availed nothing. By accident a switch containing maple-buds was placed in her hands, when she began to eat them, and called earnestly for more, and continued to eat them with avidity, improving, meanwhile, in her general health for some fifteen days or more, when this particular relish left her, and she called for candy, and, as in the case of the buds, ate nothing else for two weeks, when this also was dropped; a more natural taste returning with returning eyesight and usual health. This was instinct calling for those articles of food which contained the elements the want of which lay between disease and recovery.

A gentleman, aged thirty-six, seemed to be in the last stages of consumptive disease, when he was seized with an uncontrollable desire for common table-salt; he spread it in thick layers over his meat, and over his bread and butter; he carried it in his vest pocket, which was daily emptied by eating a pinch at a time. He regained his health, and remained well for years afterwards.

More recently, a case occurred in England of a child gradually declining in health, in spite of all that could be done by a remarkably shrewd and observant physician. On one of his visits he found the father sipping a glass of toddy. The thought occurred to the doctor to offer some of it to the child, who took it with great satisfaction. The hint was improved; more was given, and more; and for two months this child of two years old lived almost wholly on whiskey-toddy, when the desire declined, a more natural appetite returned, the health improving every hour, and was eventually entirely restored; but ever thereafter the child loathed the very smell or even sight of whiskey-toddy.

A similar case is reported where a sick child took a pint of ale daily, and nothing else for many days, ultimately recovering, when the sight of an ale-bottle could not be endured. The child of a New Yorker was supposed to be dying of the "summer complaint." As a last and desperate resort it was hurried off to Rockaway in August, having the (usually considered fatal) hiccup when it started. Immediately on its arrival—on a cold, raw, chilly evening, about an hour after sundown—some fresh milk from the cow was instantly boiled and offered to it. It was with difficulty that the bowl could be withdrawn from its poor emaciated fingers. After an hour's interval more milk was given, and nothing else, for a number of days. That child is now one of the heartiest, healthiest girls in New York!

In the cases above given, the children could not name their cravings; but accident threw in their way what the instincts required. Grown persons can express their cravings. There are many persons who can record, from their own personal experience, the beginning of a return to health from gratifying some insatiate desire. The celebrated Professor Charles Caldwell was fond of relating in his lectures that a young lady, abandoned to die, called for some pound-cake, which "science" would have pronounced a deadly dose; but as her case was considered hopeless she was gratified, and recovered, living in good health afterwards. But in some forms of dyspepsia to follow the cravings is to aggravate the disease; life is made intolerable, and suicide closes the scene.

In low fevers, typhoid, yielding to the cravings is certain death.

To know when and how to follow the instinct of appetite, to gratify the cravings of nature, is of inestimable value. There is a rule which is always safe, and will save life in multitudes of cases, where the most skilfully "exhibited" drugs have been entirely unavailing. Partake at first of what nature seems to crave, in very small quantities; if no uncomfortable feeling follows, gradually increase the amount, until no more is called for. These suggestions and facts find confirmation in the large experience of that now beautiful and revered name, Florence Nightingale, whose memory will go down with blessing and honor side by side with that of the immortal John Howard to remotest time. She says:— "I have seen, not by ones or tens, but by hundreds, cases where the stomach not only craves, but digests things which have never been laid down in any dietary for the sick, especially for the sick whose diseases were produced by bad food. Fruit, pickles, jams, gingerbread, fat of ham, of bacon, suet, cheese, buttermilk, etc., were administered freely, with happy results, simply because the sick *craved* them."

But as instincts sometimes mislead, it is better to give but a very little of the craved thing at a time at first, then a little more in five or six hours, and thus feel the way along to the right course.

ASTHMA

Is laborious breathing; the need of breath is such that there is an instinctive feeling, that if you were to stop long enough to say a single word you would suffocate; you imperiously wave a person away who is approaching you, as if you felt he would keep the air from coming to you.

There are two kinds of asthma; one is spasmodic, coming on instantly sometimes, without any premonition; it is more correctly a nervous asthma, as it arises from an unnatural condition of the

PNEUMOGASTRIC NERVE,

that is, the lung-stomach nerve, which so connects the lungs and stomach, that if the part connected with the stomach is irritated or in any way disturbed, the lungs are implicated in that disturbance. Hence, if a person has an attack of indigestion from over-eating, or from having taken something which does not agree with the stomach, an attack of this nervous or spasmodic asthma may be brought on ; great emotions of the mind can do the same thing, the mind being connected with the nervous system ; in either of these cases the nerves act in such a way as to contract the air-passages, the branches of the windpipe, or may prevent the air-cells from working naturally ; thus it is that anything that sickens the stomach may relieve, for nausea relaxes ; on the other hand, anything that antagonizes indigestion, that corrects acidity, may bring relief in an attack ; therefore it is that alkalies in any form, soda, potash, and the like, may act efficiently. In this connection it is useful to state, that wherever there is a wood fire the means are at hand to give relief in an attack of nervous asthma, by pouring hot water on a handful of fresh ashes of wood, stir it ; when settled pour it off, and if not too strong, swallow it down after it has cooled a little ; or common ley, diluted with water, is a substitute, this being the foundation of potash ; for if ley, or the water of the ashes, is boiled it is converted finally into a solid material potash, which is an alkali, and when purified and whitened makes saleratus ; thus a little saleratus dissolved in water sometimes is a grateful relief in an attack of nervous or spasmodic asthma arising from indigestion or a sour stomach.

The common form of asthma is that which is really

FUNCTIONAL ASTHMA,

the lungs not being able to work well in consequence of the bronchial tubes, that is, the branches of the windpipe, which convey the air to the lungs, being plugged up with a tough phlegm, as hereafter explained. This common asthma comes on about two o'clock in the morning, sometimes so suddenly, that the patient bolts upright in bed from a sound sleep, draws up the knees, lays his arms across them and leans his head forward on his arms, this position being more favorable for easy breathing. After several hours of torture the system becomes relieved, the breathing becomes easier, and about daylight sleep gives the sufferer rest. The essential nature of this form of asthma, as just stated, is the prevention of the air from getting out or getting into the lungs by a plug of phlegm forming ; and before mid-day the patient feels, in many cases, as well as he ever was in his life, except the debility, only to go through the same process the next day and the next for weeks and even months, unless proper remedies are used; this is the humid asthma, the other is the dry, the spasmodic form. Persons seldom die in a fit of asthma. The great preacher, George Whitefield, did so in Newburyport, Massachusetts, in 1770, aged only fifty-six, whereas asthmatics generally live to sixty or seventy. Asthma is antagonistic of consumption. The great overshadowing symptom of each is difficult breathing, greatly increased by exercise, but this difficult breathing in consumption is always present in rapid movements and in ascents; in asthma it is only present during an attack, while absent in the intervals of attacks. The labored breathing of asthma distends the air-cells, makes them capable of receiving more air, while the essence of consumption is the inability of the lungs to receive into them air enough for the wants of the system. Hence a person who has consumptive symptoms is cured by the disease changing to an asthmatic form, for the more air the lungs are made capable of receiving, the more perfectly is the blood purified, and improved health follows necessarily, other things being equal. Relief in common or humid asthma is the most urgent demand, and can be had safely in only one way, softening or diluting the tough tenacious phlegm in the branches of the windpipe; until that is done, the distressing anxious imploring look of the sufferer becomes more and more dreadful to witness. A large mustard plaster (which see) all over the chest, or between the shoulder-blades behind, will give more or less immediate relief; but the exposure of the skin to the air is calculated to aggravate the trouble, hence it is better to do all that is possible to keep the skin of the whole body warm, or get it into a perspiration by tucking in the bed-clothing in a warm bed; drinking any kind of hot drinks, perhaps water is best, although not so palatable; bottles of hot water to the feet and under the arms, or along the spine; for whatever induces perspiration on the outside has a similar effect at least in among the lungs, diluting and loosening the phlegm as before stated. Another method is to take syrup of squills or tincture of ipecac (which see), to the extent of causing decided nausea, which it is known causes the mouth to water, and this watering extends to the lungs and branches of the windpipe and dilutes the tough phlegm, loosens it, so that it may be brought away with a slight cough.

The various preparations of opium give relief in asthma, only at the cost of leaving the patient in a more suffering condition than before, because they have a tendency to dry up, to close the mouths of those little vessels, which nauseating medicines open.

A very eminent clergyman was suffering from asthma, brought on by long confinement to a damp apartment. He alleviated his agonies from time to time with chloroform; it gave such prompt, such a delightful relief, that he exclaimed, with a feeling of gratitude that he had it to take, "A vial of it is worth a farm." But each dose, as in opiates, makes every succeeding one more necessary, until, as in his case, death is inevitable. Hence the aim should always be, during an attack of asthma, to get up a cough, for a cough is the result of loosening phlegm, and the phlegm is to be loosened by warmth, by nauseants, and sometimes by breathing the steam of pretty warm water from the spout of a teapot, taking care not to draw in the steam with such strength as to draw the hot water with it and scald the throat.

A lady, suffering under an attack of asthma, seemed to be at the last extremity; it was night; a powder was left to be taken at intervals. Said an attendant, "But what if the powder does not give relief?" "It must give relief," said the doctor, seeming to mean thereby that if she did not get relief she must die. It was Dover's powder, containing opium. It quieted the little cough she had, and her suffering increased every moment. The writer was called at midnight. Nauseants were given freely; in the course of an hour she coughed once; the next cough was waited for with great solicitude; it came in less than an hour; by daylight there were several coughs during the hour, then phlegm began to come, and she was saved, dying twenty-five years later of a wholly different disease. This is given to impress the mind with the importance of cultivating a cough in an asthmatic attack, instead of repressing it. Nothing that eases the patient's breathing in asthma does any real good, but actual and dangerous harm, except in so far as it loosens the phlegm, and increases the cough, for that cough helps to dislodge the phlegm, to bring it up out of the branches of the windpipe, it unplugs them, and to that extent makes way for the free passage of the air into and out of the lungs, and that is the only true cure.

Paper is sometimes soaked in water in which saltpetre has been dissolved, then dried and burned in the room or made into cigars and smoked. The dried leaves of the mullen leaf are sometimes smoked, and a great many other remedies are advised from time to time; but all relief is dangerous, unless it is the result of loosening phlegm, and increasing cough; for it is the tough, dry phlegm in the lungs and branches of the windpipe which causes the agonizing breathing, and gasping, and sense of impending suffocation in asthma, and nothing can do any real good which does not have a tendency to loosen that phlegm and bring it away. But after all, the wisest plan in those subject to attacks of asthma is not to have an attack, which is easier of prevention than of removal and cure. An attack never comes on of itself; it is always caused by something; these causes are different in different individuals, and every one who is subject to attacks of asthma, should notice for himself what brings them on to him, and this, to him, is

THE CAUSE OF ASTHMA.

No attack of ordinary asthma comes on except it is preceded by one of three things—

A cold,
Constipation,
Biliousness.

And as a cold is naturally the cause of the last two, it may be safely asserted, that if a person never took cold, even a person subject to attacks of asthma, such attacks would not be repeated. (See article, "Checking Perspiration.") If the principles involved in this article were intelligently practised, a cold need not be taken for many months together.

Persons liable to attacks of asthma should make it a point of study—of daily practical attention—to watch against constipation (which article see), and the very hour it is observed that the bowels have not acted, means should be taken to secure that action, and to keep up a natural, healthful, daily motion.

If a cold has been taken, means should be adopted within the hour to arrest that cold, to cut it short off, and be done with it. (See article "Colds.")

If biliousness is present, remove it in the way named in that article. Biliousness causes, brings on, aggravates costiveness, and colds bring on and aggravate biliousness, which has one never-absent symptom—no natural appetite; manifesting itself in various ways—the appetite is fickle in some, voracious in others; while many have not only no appetite, but a positive disrelish, and even an aversion to food. Sometimes the whites of the eyes are yellow, or there is sickness at stomach; tongue coated with an ugly yellow covering, bad taste in the mouth of mornings, and a general feeling of despondency and miserableness.

This biliousness is caused by a torpid, non-acting liver, which calomel pills, or blue mass will rectify. When the liver is thus torpid, the blood becomes thicker, more impure, hence attacks of asthma are often preceded by symptoms which give notice of its coming, and which, if heeded, would ward off the attack, would either modify it greatly, or prevent it altogether; these symptoms are drowsiness, wakefulness, headache, rumbling in the bowels, eructations, or other symptoms of indigestion.

It may be always known that the patient suffering under an asthmatic attack is going to get better, if, laying the ear on the chest, there is heard a vast multitude of varying little sounds as of the singing of a thousand tiny birds, because it shows that the phlegm is in various stages of softening at different parts and points preparatory to coming away in a short time.

An attack of ordinary asthma passes off in a few minutes sometimes; at others, hours pass before there is any striking relief; or it may keep up, at varying intervals, for weeks and months even, but most likely to come on between one and three o'clock in the morning.

It may be said truthfully that there is no medicinal cure for asthma. It cures consumption, it keeps it at bay indefinitely long; and sometimes it cures itself, that is, it sometimes disappears at the changes of life. A child may inherit asthma from a parent, and have an attack of it whenever a cold is taken; but at the seventh year it often disappears, never to be heard of more, especially if pains be taken to expose such children to the outdoor air a great deal every sunshiny day, to dress them loosely and warm; to keep their arms and legs and feet always warmly clad, to attend to the daily regulating of the bowels; regular eating at home, nothing whatever between the regular meals, early retiring to bed, and abundant sleep.

At the change of life asthmatic women lose their liability to their attacks, but nearly always it is because some other more dangerous and threatening disease is forming in the system, such as internal cancers, ulceration of the womb, and similar maladies.

Persons sometimes lose their liability to asthmatic attacks on the appearance of an ulcerous sore in any part of the body, such as a sore leg, a white swelling, or king's evil.

Sometimes a severe attack of small-pox breaks up the asthmatic tendency for life. The same thing is done in many cases by a great change in the daily habits or occupation or callings in life; if a merchant becomes a ploughman, a banker a drover, a clerk a railway conductor.

At other times habits of asthma are broken up by a change of residence from a flat locality to a mountain top, from a prairie to a forest home, from city to country, and the opposite of all these. A London gentleman could always get relief within the hour, by going into the country. Sometimes a damp locality, at others a dry place of residence breaks up the habit of asthma.

But in the absence of all these, when a person has become subject to asthmatic attacks, there is no absolute, permanent cure this side the grave, but there is a mode of securing permanent exemption from attacks, by avoiding colds, constipation, indigestion, and biliousness, as before named.

There is another form of the disease altogether more unmanageable; it is called

SYMPTOMATIC ASTHMA,

that is, it is a symptom or sign indicating that the structure of the breathing organ has undergone some change for which there is no remedy, but in the mode of amelioration already referred to.

HEREDITARY ASTHMA

is the more frequent of all causes; it may come on at any age, or it may be brought about by some constricting influence of gases, or fog, or smoke. The smell of particular things seems to cause an attack.

Powdered ipecac will bring on all the symptoms of catarrh or bronchitis, makes the nose run, the eyes water, the lids inflamed within an hour; some persons have it in the haying time of year, as if there floated from the hay some perfume or more solid par-

14

ticles, calculated to bring on an attack, causing the common people to give it the name of

HAY ASTHMA,

but it may be observed that if such persons, at the specified time of year, will go to a place where a blade of hay never grew, the attack comes on all the same.

There is a feeling instilled, brought down to us from childhood, that it is natural to be sick once a year. Our mothers used to give us various unwelcome doses in the spring; one would give us sassafras tea, another egg-shells pulverized and mixed with honey. Still, it is true that different persons become ailing at certain seasons of the year, some early in the spring, others later in May or June, while a third with a more vigorous constitution may keep the enemy at bay, and does not become bilious until August or haying time; and when a man is bilious, he is a hundred-fold more susceptible to cold from slight causes than when he is not bilious, a cold is taken at last and settles at once in the eyes and nose, with everlasting waterings and sneezings and nose-wipings, keeping one person all the time busy in washing pocket-handkerchiefs. But suppose such a person, although a sufferer for twenty years, should, at that particular season or a little before, be called to some great change in life, to some great trouble, to some absorbing enterprise involving incessant and laborious travel day and night, by rail, steamboat, stage, horseback, footways, over untrodden hills, and dangerous valleys and impenetrable wildernesses, it is pretty certain that there would be no attack of hay asthma that year anyhow, simply because these unaccustomed exertions worked all the extra bile out of the system, and by giving a good appetite, a vigorous digestion and glorious sleep, a newer and purer blood has been supplied, dashing through the remotest veins with a power and life which repels all disease and has made the man over again.

Whatever may be the immediately exciting cause of an attack of asthma, there is in the constitution a tendency to asthma, either hereditary or acquired, just as there is in some persons a tendency to take cold, or a tendency to biliousness, implying that there exists a bilious constitution, an asthmatic constitution. Whether the attacks come on in the early morning, for a day or two or more, and may not come again for weeks or months, as in ordinary asthma, or whether it be dyspeptic asthma, arising from an attack of indigestion as a result of over-eating, or injudicious feeding; or from costiveness, or from simple nervousness, the sufferer should observe what is the cause of an attack,—for asthma can never come on without a cause,—and then make it a point, habitually, systematically, persistently to watch against those causes, then by greater and greater care, a longer and longer time may elapse between the attacks, until the habit of attack may be broken up and the person may thus "grow out of it."

But if the whole study is to find out what will merely give relief during an attack, and call that a "cure," the susceptibility will increase; the attacks will become more and more frequent, until existence is nothing more nor less than a protracted agony. It is greatly better to turn all the energies towards preventing attacks, guarding against the cause of them. The causes of asthma are very capricious; some things bring it on in one man, and the same things remove it in another. But wherever a man is most exempt from it, that is the place for him to live. A habit of life or an emotion may bring on an attack; one man is relieved by sleeping near the ground, another by having his bed in the garret or highest room in the house. Sometimes sleeping on the north side of the house, where no sunshine comes into the room, invites an asthmatic attack, when removal to a southern exposure, drying, warming and purifying the air, causes it to disappear as if by magic.

Some persons have hay fever, or asthmatic attacks, regularly once a year, the same month, same day, and almost the same hour. Now and then such attacks may be escaped by snuffing up into the nostrils, several times a day, a "saturated solution" of common sulphate of quinine; but this endangers some more critical internal suffering. But if there be some urgent necessity for this expedient, the precaution should be taken to take some medicine at the same time which will act freely on the bowels, so as to carry off those matters in that direction, which nature was seeking to carry off through the nose, but which were officiously repelled and driven inwards.

Also keep the bowels acting freely, eat plainly, temperately, and regularly, while using any means to ameliorate an attack, whether by smoking the leaves of stramonium, which some call thorn-apple, others Jamestown weed, by the use of chloral, or laughing gas, musk, or hyoscyamus, or any of the hundred and one remedies called "cures," when they only alleviate, and even that at the expense, many times, of greater evils in another direction.

In consumption we cannot get air enough in the lungs to sustain life ; in asthma we cannot get enough out, and what is in must get out before any more fresh air can get in. There is a great nerve, one branch of which goes to the stomach, another to the lungs and throat, and if that nerve is irritated or becomes diseased at a point before the branching takes place, the ill effect may be felt in the stomach, or it may be felt in the lungs, or in both places. One effect of the irritation of this nerve, called "pneumogastric," or lung-stomach nerve, is to contract the lungs, to lessen their capacity, so that the air cannot get out with natural rapidity, causing a terrible feeling of tightness across the chest in the act of breathing, especially in expiration, breathing out. Under this effect of irritation, the lungs contract like a squeezed sponge, and as long as that contraction is present, the difficult breathing of asthma continues.

Violent coughing or excessive laughter is accomplished by driving air out of the lungs, and these, in persons subject to asthma, sometimes bring on an attack, because the air is so nearly exhausted that the lungs have lost their spring, as it were—their power to expand—that is "constriction ;" hence persons have died from fits of coughing and from excessive laughter ; the lungs lost their power of distention, no air could get in or out, and there was strangulation.

Whatever tends to relax, tends to relieve this form of asthma ; nauseating medicines relax ; a bleeding from the arm will relax ; the vapors of various vegetable substances, as before stated, will relax, such as the fumes of saltpetred paper, or tobacco, or stramonium—which is the thorn-apple, or Jamestown weed ; but none of these are curative, they merely give present relief. It is because the irritation of the stomach-branch of the nerve is occasioned sometimes by indigestion, that over-eating, or eating something which is indigestible, may affect the lung-branch of it, and give a tickling in the throat, or a cough, or difficult breathing. Hence it is, too, that consumptives and other persons sometimes eat a late, hearty supper, go to bed, begin to cough, and cough for hours together ; at last vomiting comes on, the whole meal is thrown up, the stomach is emptied, sleep comes within a few minutes, to be continued until the morning.

Many a troublesome cough, after getting into bed, is modified the next night by taking little or no supper, or, to be more specific, take only a cup of hot drink and some cold bread and butter. For it may sometimes happen, that if nothing is eaten, there may be such a feeling of hunger as to prevent refreshing sleep, or a feeling of debility may be induced, which may aid the nervous affection, in a way to increase or continue the contraction of asthma.

It is clear, then, why so many things, vastly different, benefit or relieve asthma; for if the attack comes from the stomach-branch of the nerve, medicines addressed to the stomach will do good; if the lung branch is affected, then applications made to the lungs, or the nervous system, or remedies which affect these, as fumes, smokes, etc., will do good.

If a gouty person has asthmatic attacks, relief is to be found in the use of arsenical preparations, sulphur, iodide of potash, and other alkalies. But in all forms of asthma, permanent relief and an indefinite postponement of attacks must be looked for only in the use of remedies which keep the liver in healthful action, and regulate the bowels to a free and full daily motion, adding thereto an avoidance of colds.

The homœopathic remedies are ipecacuanha, when there is constriction; arsenicum, when in great distress for breath; bryonia, when towards morning there is difficulty in breathing, with cough, more or less dry and ineffectual; nux vomica, when there is great tightness; pulsatilla, if there is constriction, or rattling in the chest; antimonium tart., if a great deal of phlegm comes up.

SPITTING BLOOD

Is always observed with a shock to the whole system, as if it were the knell of death, which it nearly always is as to men. In women it is rarely observed except in connection with some form of suppression; then it is a vicarious action, and always does good; it is Nature endeavoring to get rid of a surplus in another than natural way.

When a man spits blood, there is an amazing tendency to attribute it to any other cause than the real one; that it is from the throat ; that it is from the gums, that it came down from the head, or from a defective tooth, or from the stomach.   In rare cases it does come from some of these sources ; but in nine cases out of ten it would not be just to the reader to allow an impression so wide of the truth.   In ninety-nine cases out of a hundred, the man who spits up a very few drops of bright-red blood, either clear or mixed with phlegm or saliva, is in the forming stages of consumptive disease, and will certainly die of it, within three years, on an average, unless he changes the whole course of his life to an active out-door occupation, which will keep him out of doors in the open air for a great part of all of daylight.   The very celebrated writer N. P. Willis was attacked with severe

HEMORRHAGE OF THE LUNGS.

With great judgment and decision he immediately went to the country, purchased some wild land which nobody seemed to think worth anything, but which, in his far-seeing eye, could be made one of the most beautiful places on the Continent.   He sat down and built him .

IDLEWILD,

on the Hudson, now so notable.   By means of personal supervision and horseback exercise daily, and frequent going back and forth between his beautiful home and New York, sixty miles away, he managed to protract his life many long years, although during the time he had a number of alarming bleedings, a pint or more at a time.   Let it be noted that on every occasion of his being induced by friendly counsels to try this, that, and the other, that was never known to hurt any one, but on the contrary had been known to effect very remarkable cures, he not only failed to derive any benefit, but in several cases nearly killed himself ; but promptly recuperated when he relied exclusively on out-door air, the saddle, and abundance of plain, nutritious food, at regular times.   These statements are made at length to impress the reader with the importance to health and life, to steadily resist all advice from other than educated medical men of acknowledged repute and of high standing among the people with whom they have lived for some years.   Always inquire if the wonderful cure was the case of a woman ; if so, it will certainly do a man no good,

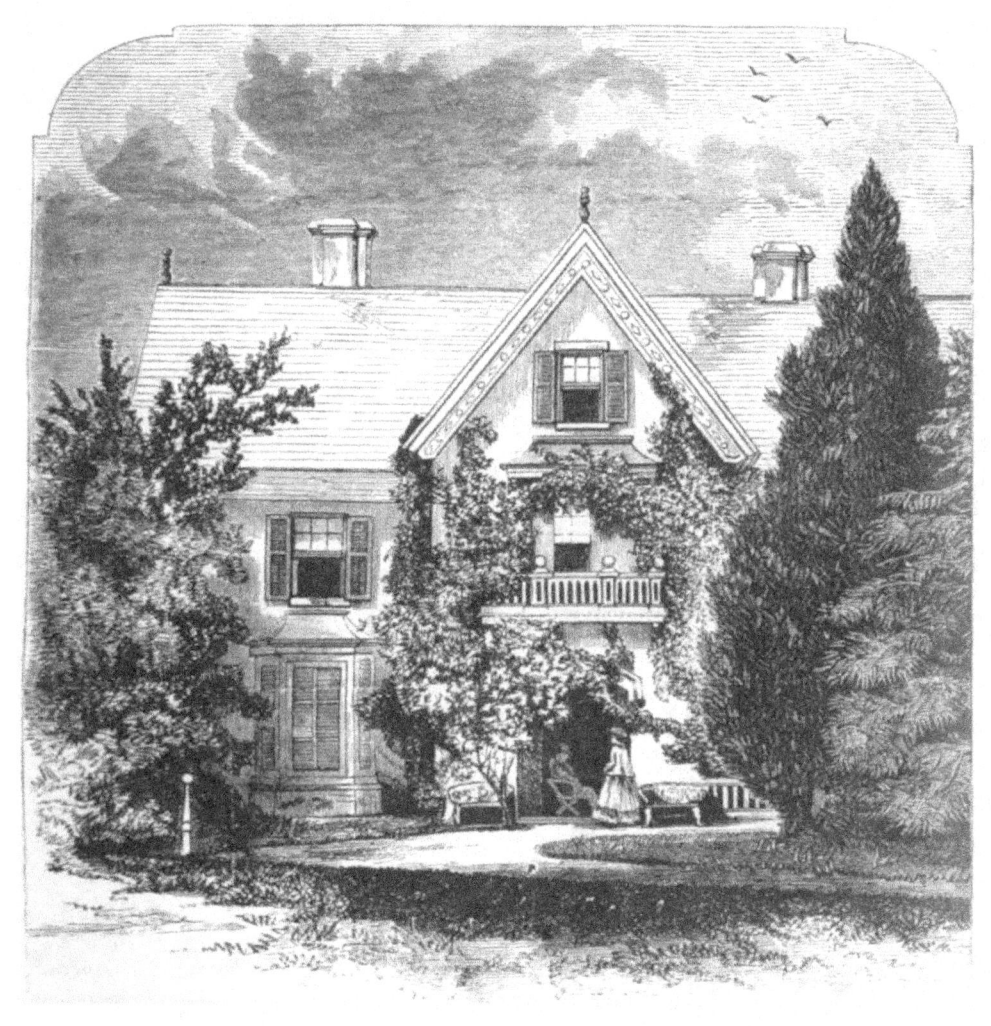

because the woman's bleeding was vicarious, and stopped of itself as soon as the system was relieved of its burden.

Besides, bleeding is a positive benefit when the lungs are affected in all cases, and unless it is beyond a tablespoonful, should not be arrested, if it could be done, for it is a great benefit to the lungs. It gives freer breathing, and is a very great relief to the cough; it is a known fact that persons who are consumptive, and have frequent little bleedings, live several years longer on an average, and do not cough half as much as those who do not bleed at all.

When a bleeding is excessive, or the patient becomes nervous or excited, the best plan is to go to bed, or lie down on a sofa and eat common salt freely; this excites thirst in the interior vessels, or in some way absorbs or attracts the more watery particles of the blood, thus diminishing its bulk and thereby relieves the over-distended blood-vessels in the lungs, which were pouring it out because they were too full to hold it.

Twenty grains of alum, dissolved in a teacup of water, taken every two hours, a swallow or two at a time, has been efficient.

Many other things are advised which do good by amusing the patient by doing something, but it is most probable that nothing taken has any effect towards stopping the bleeding; besides, if the blood is in among the lungs, when it has once left the blood-vessels, it is better out than in, immeasurably better.

The reason that spitting of blood, with a pulse uniformly above eighty beats in a minute, is an indication of consumption of the lungs, is, that there is congestion, that is, the small blood-vessels are "filled to overflowing" with blood, so full, that more being forced in, by every beat of the heart, the delicate sides of these channels or canals burst, and the blood pours out among the lungs, causing that same kind of a tickling in the throat occasioned by a little water or crumb going the wrong way, that is, passing down the windpipe into the lungs instead of down the throat into the stomach. These small blood-vessels are thus overcharged with blood, because it is obstructed; it not only is thick with impurities, and thus does not flow freely, but there are tubercles in the lungs, little lumps of a hard growth the size of a pin-head, more or less, and they, pressing against the yielding side of a vein, very naturally diminish the internal calibre, thus intercepting the flow.

When consumptive persons spit larger quantities, of a tablespoon or more to half a pint, it is because these tubercles are softening, decaying, and in that decay eat into the lungs as mice eat into a cheese; when a large blood-vessel is come to, it also is eaten into, as a rat eats into a lead pipe, and the contents escape; but, inasmuch as this escaped blood is among the lungs, if kept there, would soon occasion a dangerous inflammation, it must come away; hence the only thing to be done is to cough it up until it is all got rid of; but prevent any more from leaking out into the congested blood-vessels, by diminishing the amount of blood in the use of salt, as before named. In this connection it may be stated that cases are given in medical books where persons appearing to be consumptive have taken a great fancy to eat salt, would carry it in their vest-pocket, and take it a pinch at a time during the day, as much as a tablespoonful or more a day; and of others who by force of circumstances were compelled to live on salted food altogether for some weeks, having been cast away at sea in open boats. In these cases, the good effects of breathing a pure air night and day, and not having the opportunity of over-eating, ought to have credit for a part of the improvement in health.

In one case of protracted bleeding at the lungs the bleeding ceased by forcibly drawing into the lungs every hour half a teaspoonful of the impalpable powder of persulphate of iron, but then the bleeding might have stopped without the powder.

The homœopathic remedies are pulsatilla and sulphur. If the blood is of a bright red, rhus; and if continued, acid sulph. In very severe cases, arsenicum is used; nux vomica to the intemperate; and to restore the strength, china is the best remedy, with quietude of body and mind.

BITES AND STINGS

OF all animals and insects which are considered poisonous, injure the system by their acid character. The remedy is to apply an alkali; the strongest known is hartshorn; hence bathe the part with it as soon as possible; the best way is to use a soft rag or sponge in the way denominated dabbling; keep applying it all the time until discomfort ceases, and in addition saturate a linen cloth of four or five thicknesses, lay it over the wound ; lay a larger piece of silk or india-rubber over the linen, or another dry cloth, so as prevent evaporation. If no hartshorn is at hand, pour boiling water on a pint of wood ashes, stir it, let it settle, and as soon as cool enough apply as above, this product being an alkali. Benzine is also good. As these are remedies always at hand, and as the principle of cure is to antagonize an acid with an alkali, this may be considered applicable to every form of bite or sting from any animal or insect known, snakes and mad dogs included. Yet strong acids are also available sometimes, as will be seen.

The cobra of India kills in a few minutes by its bite. A few drops of its gall is said to be an instantaneous cure; as also for other snake-bites less terribly fatal. Possibly the gall of any poisonous creature would be an antidote to its poison ; possibly of a mad dog also, if he could be caught and cut open soon enough, and thus prevent

HYDROPHOBIA,

which means literally a fear of water; there seems to be an instinctive shuddering at the very sight of it sometimes. This terrible malady follows the bites of cats, and other animals at times, but the disease does not follow a bite necessarily. The great Dr. John Hunter found that the bite proves poisonous in one case in twenty ; that is, if a mad dog bites twenty persons, only one on an average will become hydrophobic, showing that there must be a certain condition of the system which makes it susceptible of the poison, and if that condition is not present, the poison will not take. Hence the numberless reported cures for the disease. If one only of Hunter's twenty men had died, and nineteen different remedies had been applied to the other nineteen persons, each of these remedies would be published by the persons using them as a certain preventive and cure of hydrophobia, such as large draughts of whiskey. A bite on the hand or face, a mere scratch may take effect, when a bite through the clothing down to the bone might not, the poison being wiped off by the clothing or absorbed by it. A good plan would be to wash the part with brown or black soap and water, make the suds very strong indeed, the soap, by the way, being made of the alkali, the lye or **ley** of wood-ashes, may antagonize the poison, if applied instantly. It is said that if a vaccined arm is well washed at the point of vaccination within half an hour after the operation, it will not take. It will be more efficient to rub a stick of caustic potash on the bite, or rather sharpen it and run it down into the wound made by the tooth, hold it there for fifteen or twenty seconds, however it may hurt.

The nitrate of silver or lunar caustic has been recommended; if none at hand, drop a little aquafortis into the place of the bite, or paint it over a scratch or abrasion with a pencil or bit of wood, the end of which has been chewed a little to make the fibres brushlike.

It is unquestionably true that hydrophobia is also a disease of the imagination; hence if a person is bitten by a dog, imagined to be mad, he would have the disease, but if it was ascertained satisfactorily that he was not mad, the disease would not be manifested; hence by no means kill a dog which has bitten a person. On the contrary, confine him in a room, out of which he cannot get; leave him to quiet, repose, and sleep; after a few hours put something in the room quietly which he can eat, then introduce a pan of milk or water, do this from day to day; if he was really mad he will certainly die within a week, if not mad he will get well.

The author knew a case where a friend's gardener was bitten by a dog. A year later the gardener was informed by a neighboring servant that a dog had bit a person a day or two before, and that after suffering terribly the person died. The gardener carried his hand to the part which had been bitten a year before, exclaimed that it hurt him, and making a noise something like a bark, so described, he went to his room and died within a few days, with the ordinary convulsions and terrible sufferings of those who are the victims of the malady.

A person not having a sore on the lip or tongue could suck a wound, and if it were full of poison and went into the stomach it could not injure, and might save the bitten man. In fact persons bitten, who have sucked the wounds themselves, have escaped madness.

Several weeks may pass after the bite, which may have healed over, leaving only a little pimple or pustule; if it becomes in the very slightest degree painful, it is on the point of disseminating the poison through the system; if at that time, or any time before, a piece of caustic nitrate of silver is introduced and held there, it is believed to be a certain preventive of the malady, and can be implicitly relied upon.

THE MAD STONE

is said to be a sure cure for a mad-dog bite, if pressed firmly on the wounded part for a few moments and allowed to remain until it falls. There are several of these in different parts of the country; they are of different sizes, shapes, and colors, but they are all porous, and are thus capable of absorbing or sucking any liquid like a sponge; such a thing is possible as their absorbing the poison. It ought to be tried whenever possible. Homœopathy advises for hydrophobia excision, or the application of a red-hot iron, or live coal, or cigar, whichever can be most instantaneously applied over as small a surface as possible, merely to the point of the wound; keep oil or grease or saliva around the wound to protect the skin from any loose virus. If after a week a vesicle should appear under the tongue, open it and rinse the mouth well with milk or water, meanwhile administer belladonna, lachesis; or if there are convulsions, hyoscyamus; stramonium, if the eye becomes fixed and brilliant, and a vapor bath of a hundred and six degrees, especially during convulsions, and until they cease. In insect bites camphor, aconite, and arnica applied to the wound are favorite remedies.

DEATH-RATE AND SICKNESS.

THE healthiest people in the world, of which there is a statistical record, are the Orkney Islanders, where the Shetland ponies come from, off the north coast of Scotland, in latitude 59° north. Of 1,000 men, women, and children, 12 die every year. With this as a starting-point, the intelligent reader will be greatly interested to know the death-rate of the principal cities of the world, by which it will be seen that figures make New York City and Montreal, Canada, the sickliest cities in the world in the year 1870. New York ought to be among the very healthiest of the larger cities of the globe, because it lies in the fork of two rivers which empty into the sea, while Broadway leads into Fifth avenue at Twenty-third street on a ridge, declining towards the rivers, thus allowing the rains to give a good washing at every shower; but these advantages are more than antagonized by so many people living in cellars, and a still larger number crowded into single houses, instead of each family occupying a house to itself as ought to be the case. Nearly one-half of the population of New York lives in tenement-houses,—that is, houses in which several families live,—in some of them there are scores of families. Over seventy-five per cent. of the deaths are among the tenement population. Where one person dies in a house on Fifth avenue, Madison avenue, or along the line of the broad streets, such as Thirty-fourth, three die in houses in which more than one family lives. These statements are made to admonish the reader that it is healthier to live in a two-roomed cabin of his own than in a brown-stone with others. On the same principle, the larger the rooms of a building, and especially the chambers, which should be the most commodious in the house, the healthier will be the occupants. And yet there is a very general impression that any room is good enough to sleep in, however small.

	Population.	Deaths, 1870.	Death-Rate per 1000.
New York	942,252	27,175	28.8
Philadelphia	674,022	15,317	22.73
Brooklyn	396,105	9,546	24.
St. Louis	312,963	6,670	21.3
Chicago	299,319	7,342	24.5
Baltimore	283,070	7,262	25.65
Boston	250,526	6,098	24.33
Cincinnati	216,239	3,978	18.39
New Orleans	191,512	6,942	27.58
San Francisco	150,351	3,293	21.57
Montreal	127,826	3,994	31.5
London	3,214,707	77,278	24.
Bombay	816,562	14,888	18.2
Vienna	622,087	18,518	29.8
Liverpool	517,567	16,094	31.1
Manchester	374,993	10,428	27.8
Edinburgh	178,970	4,706	26.3
Paris	2,000,000	42,900	——

In the same connection it may be interesting to know what are the most fatal diseases in a great city; in New York, for example, for one single quarter of a year, from January 1st, 1872, to April 1st, 1872:—

Spotted fever	69	Small-pox	320
Typhoid	96	Developmental	477
Measles	106	Consumption	1,155
Diarrhœa	227	Other lung diseases	1,256
Whooping-cough	247	Constitutional	1,652
Diphtheria and Cronp	294	Zymotic	2,009
Scarlatina	301	Local	3,005

In England for every person who dies in a year, twenty-eight are sick, equal to two years' sickness of one person.

Taking the whole population of England and the United States, town and country, the death-rate of England is twenty-two in every thousand each year; of the United States, twenty-four.

It is certainly true, at a very low estimate, to say that not half as many should die as do; not half as many should be sick—that is, half the sickness and death in the land is avoidable, could be prevented if the people could be induced to act wisely as to eating, drinking, exercise, sleep, and rest.

MORTALITY.

A comparison of the bills of mortality of Paris, London, and New York, for a single week in May, gives the following result:

With a population of 3,251,800, the British metropolitan district counts for 1,268 deaths; with a population of 1,980,000, Paris shows the record of 812; and with a population of 942,300, New York has 646 deaths. These figures show an alarming preponderance of the death-rate in the American metropolis over the two great cities of Europe. During the week ending May 18th, 39 people died in London out of every 100,000 of the population. During the week ending May 25th, 42 people died in Paris out of every 100,000; and during the same week the rate in New York was 68 deaths out of every 100,000.

·CONSUMPTION.

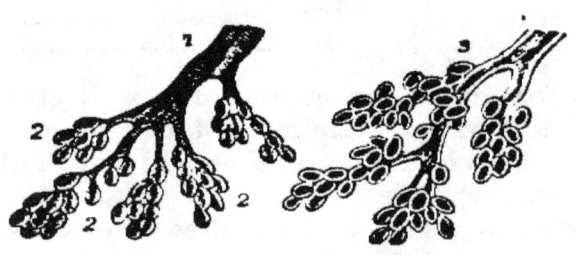

BRONCHIAL TUBE AND AIR-CELLS.

1 is a bronchus, or branch of the windpipe, growing smaller at each division until they are not larger than a hair, but are hollow, and through them the air is conveyed to 2, 2, which are the air-cells or the actual lungs, as buds are at the extreme ends of the twigs. The air comes into these cells or little bladders loaded with its proper amount of oxygen, then returns, leaving all its oxygen behind to purify the blood, taking out, however, in the place of this oxygen, carbonic acid, or the useless, waste, or poisonous matters which the blood washed out before it as it came from all parts of the body through the veins into the heart, which sent it to the lungs.

Nearly three hundred cubic feet of air goes into the lungs of a good-sized man every day, and comes out again, leaving in the lungs thirty-seven ounces of oxygen, nearly two pounds and a half, and taking out of the blood fourteen ounces of carbon, nearly one pound, this carbon being made up of the wastes of the system. Let it be noted here, how infinite is the importance of breathing a pure atmosphere; as every breath carries in more life, every breath brings out less death, for if the air is loaded with impurities when it goes in, it not only has that much less of oxygen, but, in a sense, has that much less capacity to bring outside of the body the impurities which were in the lungs; thus is the breathing of a pure air doubly healthy, and the breathing of an impure air doubly deathly. In a common breath we take in a pint of air, or twenty cubic inches at a time, although the lungs of a middle-sized man will hold twelve pints, or a gallon and a half; hence the lungs are nearly full of air all the time, and it is this residuary air which keeps us alive if breathing is prevented for a minute or so, as in suffocation from drowning or smoke or other causes.

The bronchial tubes are the seat of bronchitis, which is inflammation of these tubes, as is a common cold, which, continued for months, becomes bronchitis. The cells or little bladders which hold the air in the lungs brought to them through the bronchial tubes, they being supplied from the windpipe, are the seat of

CONSUMPTION,

which destroys them as mice eat into a cheese; the cells being destroyed, there is less room for air; hence the infallible result that in all cases of consumption the breathing is shorter and shorter, becomes more and more difficult. It is easy to see, then, that as in consumption the less air the lungs receive, the more important is it that it should be the purest possible; hence the fundamental truth in the treatment of every case of consumption, the chance of cure is increased in proportion as the person is out of doors, day and night, and in all weathers. Thus it is that in the most remarkable cases of recovery from consumption, the parties were exposed to the out-door air in all weathers and at all times of the day or night. Hence it has been repeatedly found that a consumptive going to sea as a cabin passenger dies; while the same man, who would take a whaling voyage round the Capes to the most northern latitudes, as a common sailor, for a three or four years' cruise, gets well; and so with consumptives who take long journeys on horseback, get well. See the author's book on "Coughs and Colds."

Consumption sometimes cures itself spontaneously, as does cancer. It is cured at other times by pregnancy. Persons also recover by some running sore breaking out in some part of the body spontaneously, although an artificial sore made by a seton or issue always fails of any permanent good effect in real consumption. On the same principle, if any permanent rash or tetter breaks out on the skin in consumption, the disease is either cured or is indefinitely postponed.

In June, 1848, a merchant aged twenty-five called on the author in New Orleans; measure six feet, best weight 160 pounds, then 118; pulse 100 a minute, breathing 25; drenching night-sweats, constant cough, with an incessant pain at the hinder part of one lung, which prevented him from lying down in any natural position. He had piles badly. He literally staggered when he attempted to cross the floor. He was advised to go to Canada at once, and practise horseback-riding extensively. By extraordinary exposures in going up the Mississippi river he became rapidly worse, but he pushed on to Canada; on reaching there a leg was fractured by the kick of a horse. With the views of other physicians that it was a hopeless case of consumption, and that he could not live six months, he wrote: " I hope to spend the few days I shall live out here in making a perfect preparation for that place where our state is invariably and forever fixed."

But he began to improve, and twenty-four years later, to wit, in June, 1872, he called on the author in Broadway, New York, on a trip of pleasure to his native Scotland. Age, 52; pulse, 76; weight, 152. His lung measure, or vital capacity, in 1848 was 172 cubic inches; in 1872 was 250; he had got a wife, eight children, all living, and had made a fortune besides.

He stated that his health was best when a rash was most extensive, which had been coming out upon him at intervals for the last five years. Hence hopeless cases of consumption do sometimes recover by keeping up the general health as directed in that article, and living largely out of doors. It is the belief of educated medical men throughout the world, that the medicine is yet to be found which has any curative effect in common consumption of the lungs, although almost every year finds a new cure and loses an old one, most of them failing to survive a few months' trial.

With these views it only remains to ascertain the signs by which a man of ordinary intelligence may ascertain for himself, with reasonable certainty.

Consumption generally comes on with a slight dry cough in the morning, then on going to bed, getting more and more frequent, with more and more phlegm to the last.

If any one has a cough, more or less, on retiring and rising, with an increasing debility, thinness of flesh, shortness of breath and quickening pulse, that is consumption always; but if there are occasional bleedings from the lungs, that keeps down the pulse, even to its natural standard sometimes. A natural pulse averages seventy beats of the heart in a minute; as the consumptive gets worse the pulse goes up to eighty, ninety, a hundred, a hundred and ten, a hundred and twenty, and he dies. A daily cough with a pulse almost always among the nineties and over, with steady falling away in flesh, is to all intents, a proof of the latter stages of consumption. Hence any one may safely conclude that consumption is steadily progressing with an increase of pulse, debility, short breath, and falling away.

Let the reader feel assured that the essential elements of cure in consumption are always a vigorous digestion and an active out-door life; without these no human means have ever availed; with them, permanent cures are effected.

AILMENTS DURING GESTATION.

IT is of great importance to avoid medicine as much as possible during pregnancy; therefore endeavor to relieve the varied ailments by external appliances and natural means.

Breathing is sometimes oppressed; if from a full stomach, especially after eating, eat less and keep bowels free; if from other causes cultivate quietude, avoid fast work or strains, or heavy lifting; let all bodily motions be deliberate.

Cramps: rub the limb with a cold wet cloth, and then apply vigorous and hard friction until the pain ceases.

Constipation: use castor-oil, as named under that heading, or enemas, provided the use of fruits, berries, and cracked wheat as the chief items of food have failed.

Convulsions: use warm bath, enemas, and frictions, and avoid their return by the use of the special fruit diet, so as to keep the bowels acting every day.

Diarrhœa: hip-baths, enemas of cold water, and a diet of boiled rice and milk chiefly; walk as little as possible, keep on a sofa or bed, and have the abdomen bound around with a woollen bandage fourteen inches wide.

Heartburn arises from taking too much food, gives cold feet and constipation; keep the bowels free, eat regularly, and in great

15

moderation of such plain nourishing food, in such small amounts as will not be followed by acidity.

Headaches arise almost always from cold feet, costiveness, or over-eating. If it is sick headache, carry out the same plan, only take a thorough warm-water emetic.

Longings: gratify them when practicable; but it is better to divert the mind, and regulate the eating to a special fruit diet, regular bowels, and more time in the open air.

Morning sickness: take nothing at all for supper but a cup of tea or some coarse dry bread, not both of these but one of them; notice which most abates the sickness; or take nothing later than four P.M.

Pain in the side: see that the bowels are free, feet warm; then use compresses bound on the side, covered with oiled silk, and renew until relieved. Sometimes warm fomentations are better. Use a special fruit diet.

Piles are sometimes very troublesome; keep the bowels free; use cold injections after each stool, and sitz-baths two or three times a day of the most agreeable temperature.

Pains in the breasts: if the pain is steady use cold cloths, frequently renewed; if irregular and darting, employ warm fomentations.

Pruritus, excessive itching about the organs of reproduction: use cold injections; sometimes warm are more efficient and agreeable.

Sleeplessness: soothe the system by hip-baths; if the head is hot apply cold cloths, and keep the feet warm; eat less, live on a special fruit diet, and avoid sleeping in the afternoon.

Sick headache: if a fruit diet does not remove it, with warm feet and regular bowels, take a liver pill.

Toothache is almost always neuralgia, and is removed by warm feet, open bowels, and a fruit diet for a few days, and an hour or two out of doors.

Urination: if frequent and scant, drink lemonade freely, or buttermilk when thirsty, or flaxseed tea made into a lemonade. If there is actual retention, a catheter should be used; if it cannot be overcome by warm foot-baths, use cold hip-baths.

Vomiting is sometimes very troublesome during pregnancy, generally due to over-eating. If the bowels are free, and feet warm, live on fruits, berries, fresh or stewed, and coarse breads for a few days; if not relieved, take a liver pill. Sometimes drinking ice-cold water freely is beneficial.

Varicose veins: take moderate exercise, fruit diet, and free bowels, or apply a judicious bandage.

Ventilation is second to nothing else in preserving the health and lives of infants, hence it ought to be the constant study of every intelligent and conscientious mother; it should be a subject of watchful care for every hour of the day, and should be provided for during the night, the last thing before retiring. A canary-bird will die before the morning if hung up in a curtained bed where two persons are sleeping. At all seasons of the year let the fire-place be open day and night where an infant lives and sleeps; let some fresh air be all the time coming in at an inner door or outer window. Without an abundant supply of out-door air no infant can live; for want of it, multitudes perish every year.

A mother should never nurse her child within an hour of any great mental excitement of fear, alarm, anxiety, anger, indignation or excessive nervousness, for the tendency is to throw the child into convulsions. Household solicitudes and responsibilities, continued from day to day, rob the mother's milk of its nutriment, and gives the infant diarrhœa and wasting, and if persisted in, death will follow.

MARRYING WELL.

A REAL wife is a "help-meet," an assistant suitable for her husband; a woman who adapts herself to the situation, circumstances, and position of the man who has engaged to provide her with a house and home, and to defend and protect her until she dies. It would not be just to say that no girl educated in a boarding-school ever became a good wife; but that boarding-school girls, as a class, make the worst of wives, is the impression of many a poor fellow who has had experience in that direction.

The very first care of a young man who is about to marry, should be to select a woman of vigorous health, from among those of his own religion, of his own neighborhood, and of his own grade in society. If he is of no account, he deserves nothing higher; if he is of sterling worth, he will elevate her from that hour toward the position which he himself merits, with the happy result, that as he rises she will rise with him, become proud of him, while he will have reason to be proud of himself, and in time will carry with him that presence and that bearing which belong to the self-reliant and to those who have a consciousness of ability and moral worth.

An important advantage in marrying from among one's neighbors is, that each party knows the social " status" of the other in a manner more perfect than is otherwise possible, and thus will all impositions be avoided ; for there are multitudes of persons whose inveterate aim is to impress those whom they have married with the idea of their position, their birth, and their blood, the more so as these are all questionable. The truly well-born never speak of these things voluntarily. It is not likely that William B. Astor or the Duke of Devonshire would proffer to any man the information that he was rich. A lady does not dress in violent colors ; her maid monopolizes these.

To enjoy religion more and more as we get older is the true ambition, aim, and end of life ; to do this to the fullest extent, there should be as few points of divergence and diversion as possible, whether in sentiment, in habit, or in practice. It is a sweet thing in declining years for husband and wife to sit together and read and sing and listen to the hymns which were familiar to them from childhood ; to talk about the same ministers, the members of the same church, of mutual friends and neighbors, and of common schoolmates. The truth is, the more two old people have in common, the sweeter will be their intercommunions until they die. With considerable opportunities of observation over many degrees of latitude and longitude, the impression has been deepening for many years, that for domestic peace and happiness, and for the luscious communings of pious hearts, it is best, as a very general rule, the exceptions being rare, that the young should marry in their own neighborhood, their own circle, their·own church, and their own State. A Southerner will always despise what is called the " picayunishness " of the North ; while the free and hearty abandon of the South, the Northerner can never reconcile himself to. The North is a precise old maid. The South is a reckless dare-devil. The North has not the power of accommodation. The South has wonderful facilities of adaptation.

The Northerner must have everything just so, or he is in a living purgatory. The Southerner readily conforms himself to privation and laughs at what a Northerner would cry over. Within a year a young lady of Brooklyn picked up a foreign husband at Newport; later on, she appeared at her father's door, a refugee from the intolerable treatment of her "lord," whom she had left in Italy; she was a Quakeress by education, and married out of her sphere.

In countless instances, "educated" women have made miserable wives. The fact is, in multitudes of cases, the wife is a slave, and, like any other slave, the less she knows as an intellectual being the less galling will the yoke matrimonial be, and the more likely will she be to discharge satisfactorily the material duties of a wife, which are the ordering of the household so that it shall be the haven and the heaven of the toiling husband, and the nestling, cozy refuge of the children. The truth is, the whole system of female fashionable education is an abortion and a curse. Our daughters are not trained for wives, in the true sense of the word; but for ladies, for puppets, for dolls, for playthings. Although John Bull has a high character for doing things in the right way, in respect to the girls born to him he is as unwise as Jonathan. In the European orphan schools and asylums of Calcutta and Madras, the children of soldiers are, with great liberality, taken to be educated, especially the daughters of soldiers and officers who have died in their country's service; but in place of being taught needlework, cookery, reading, writing, and arithmetic, and in the domestic duties of wife and mother, they are instructed in subjects that might be expected in a London boarding-school, and hence Dr. Mouat says he has often heard steady soldiers declare that they preferred an uneducated native wife to the best of the inmates of the institutions above mentioned, because the former was gentle, quiet, obedient, fond of staying at home, careful and tender of the children, and anxious to minister to the comfort and happiness of the husband; whereas the latter was far too often a fine lady, alike regardless and ignorant of domestic duties, fond of gossip and flirtation, and altogether ill calculated to maintain happiness in her husband's household. It is precisely this that is operating in New York and Philadelphia and Boston, and other large cities, and extending even to small towns and the country also, to diminish the number of marriages, leaving the most beautiful blossoms to be ungathered, while the bar-room, the coffee-house, and the club are more and more crowded, and the home of honorable wedlock is replaced by dangerous liaisons in New York, and the "furnished chambers" of New Orleans.

In short, there is reason to fear that unless greater attention is paid to the education of the heart in both the principles and practice of evangelical religion in our female schools, the time is not far distant when it may be said of the United States, as of the most corrupt capitals of Europe, that every third child is the offspring of shame. Let the thoughtful mature the subject well.

DEATH'S WEAPONS.

The higher the state of civilization, the more attention is paid by nations towards ascertaining the causes of disease and death, with kindred subjects, the object being to exercise that parental care and authority which becomes a beneficent government. The glorious English nation is pre-eminent in these regards, our own being too young to have inaugurated any system commensurate with the importance of the subject. In one year fifty thousand persons died of consumption in England and Wales. It is particularly noteworthy that the mortality from this disease in the city of London bore about the same proportion as that of hilly Wales. And it is not a new remark, that, as cities grow older, consumption diminishes; in consequence, no doubt, of the greater intelligence of the people and the greater conveniences and comforts of life. Another fact protrudes itself, and that is, that the doctors do not kill everybody. In Wales, twelve of every hundred persons dying had no medical attendant. In one district in England one person out of every ten had no doctor to help them over the bridge of sighs. Half of all who died were under seventeen years of age. This fearful truth will come more directly home, to parents at least, by saying: "Half of your children will die before entering their eighteenth year!" And why? Because it is natural that they should die thus early? Because they were not made to live longer? Because there is a necessity that it should be so? No; none of these. Nor is it because, inheriting a weakly constitution, they were born diseased. A wise care will overcome these disadvantages in a vast majority of cases. One of the greatest sovereigns in the world was born so decidedly scrofulous as to be threatened with a life-long deformity; and yet, of a houseful of children, not one has died, several have grown up to majority, and all are in high health, and by virtue, too, of a systematic and persistent attention to the laws of hygiene. It clearly follows that half of our children die before they become of age, because they are not properly taken care of, watched over, and instructed as to the means of preserving their health; they are not told by their parents how to avoid disease. This is certainly a fearful reflection, and yet it is undeniably true.

WHAT MOTHERS CAN DO.

FORTY-TWO years ago there was born to the wife of a poor and obscure blacksmith, a son. The father died, and, soon after, the mother; and their history and memory perished from before men. The infant child was left to the care of whomsoever might take a fancy to it; but as months passed, then years, one friend took it up and then another; and how, he could scarcely tell himself, he obtained a collegiate education and found his way into the ministry; when, one day, a thousand miles away from the play-grounds of his childhood, after preaching to a large and attentive audience, an old lady met him at the foot of the pulpit-stairs and said: "I was present at your birth: I knew your mother well, and I do not wonder you have risen to be a minister of the Gospel, for it was her habit to give you to the Lord in prayer before you were born." Blessed mother! unknown to the rich and great of her time, known, perhaps, even to her neighbors only as the "blacksmith's wife," she worked and lived and loved and prayed in her poor little obscure sphere, until it was her Master's will that she should go up higher; and she went early, because she was early ready; but her works follow after and upward unto heaven, as one by one souls saved by her son's instrumentality cross over Jordan, and meeting her with other angels bright on the better bank, they join hand to hand and file away upward to the Father's bosom, chanting in glory: "Saved by grace through her prayers."

More than a hundred years ago there lived in London the wife of a sea-captain : who were her ancestors, where she was born, or what of her life, no one knows or ever will know now. She was early left a widow with a fatherless child ; but she feared God and felt her responsibilities to the child of her love. But in spite of a mother's teachings he went to sea and became one of the most profligate of young men ; but never, in all his wanderings and dissipations, could he rid himself of the remembrance of the sad, pale, and sweet face of his mother, nor her earnest, patient, and loving teachings. She died, but her prayers bound him fast to the throne of God, and John Newton became one of the best of men. His pious conversation was the means of converting Dr. Buchanan, whose work, *Star in the East,* led Adoniram Judson to the Saviour, converted Dr. Scott, the commentator ; Cowper's piety was deepened, Wilberforce became a changed man, and wrote a Practical View of Christianity, which converted Leigh Richmond, who wrote the *Dairyman's Daughter,* and how many souls that book has awakened and led to the Saviour, and will continue to do, only the records of eternity can tell. Mothers ! however poor and obscure and unknown, look upon your boy-child, and remembering what God hath wrought through such as you, take courage, and pray in faith that the same he can do by you.

These are deeply impressive examples of the influence which the predominant states of mind of the mother during gestation has on the character of the child in after-life. If, however, the state of mind of the mother during gestation and nursing are vicious, the child is not relieved from moral accountability, on the ground that it had no agency in the formation of his own character, any more than all mankind is thus relieved from the consequences of the fall of Adam. The point which presses on us, is the fact that pregnant and nursing mothers do give shape and coloring to the physical and moral traits of their offspring, and that it is an imperative duty to act in the light of these high responsibilities.

ACNE,

Meaning " vigor," is a term applied to those little hard pimples which appear on the forehead, temples, and skin of young persons of both sexes; after a while they turn red, then become a little yellow, and eventually disappear, sometimes in the course of a few weeks, at others, they remain many months, to the great annoyance of the person having them, as they are at times very unsightly; most so, on the faces of young men; they indicate a gross habit and bad blood, as in high livers; sometimes hereditary. It is not known that there is any cure for them. They generally disappear of themselves after marriage, or when the period of youth is passed. Few have them after thirty. As they arise from grossness of blood, it is hurtful and is useless to do anything for them by application to the pimples themselves; but they may be modified and sometimes are dispersed by keeping the skin clean, eating regularly, with nothing between meals, taking care always to have a full and free action of the bowels every day; an active employment out of doors greatly hastens their dispersion. Benefit is derived from rubbing flowers of sulphur well into the parts twice a day with the fingers after washing in the morning and at bed-time, then brush off any loose particles of sulphur with a light cloth. When the face is simply rough, without any insects in the pimples, dissolve an ounce of borax in a quart of water, and apply it to the face with a fine sponge or cloth night and morning; this sometimes removes them effectually if persevered in.

BURYING ALIVE.

MANY persons have a great horror of being put into the ground before they are really dead; it is a very rare occurrence as a result of sickness. In a town in Germany it is the custom to place the person in church with a bell-rope hanging just above the breast, where it can be easily reached should the person come to life. It has not been rung once in a hundred years.

There is an aversion to wounding the body. A deep cut across the arm with a lancet or other sharp instrument would be very apt to wake to life again, if not really dead. It was the great fear of General Washington's life that he might be buried before dead; the very last words he ever spoke were in reference to that subject. If a lighted candle is held to the skin there will be a blister:

if on sticking a needle into it, a fluid escapes, there is life; if only air, death is there certainly, because in the latter case it shows that the blood is congealed.

NOSE-BLEED,

If not over a tablespoonful, ought never to be interfered with, for it shows that Nature is endeavoring to relieve herself of an excess of blood in the head; apoplexy is always the result of this excess; sometimes this spontaneous nose-bleeding is a great relief to a cold in the head. But when the bleeding is larger than the above, it may be arrested by plugging up one or both nostrils with cotton or wool or a bit of dough; this causes coagulation which blocks up the blood.

Sometimes the nose bleeds because the blood is poor, or from some disease existing in the system. The bleeding will often cease if both hands are held above the head for some time; this diminishes the flow towards the head. Apply ice-water, or a cushion of powdered ice to the head. Wash the face in cold water, or dip a towel in cold water and apply it between the shoulder-blades; sometimes snuffing up powdered alum into the nostrils, or the fine dust at the bottom of a tea-box, answers the purpose; so does pulverized gum arabic; pressure with the back of the forefinger up against the nose, between the lip and the upper gums, is effectual, as the same operation is in preventing an approaching sneeze; or press the finger steadily against the artery at the side of the nose.

Any kind of cold metal thrust down between the skin and clothing is sometimes beneficial; or

Put the hands in warm water into which ground mustard has been stirred; at same time have ice-cold vinegar and water kept on top of the head and forehead, in an erect position; stooping over a basin aggravates the bleeding.

Nose bleed in old persons and in heavy feeders indicates a tendency to apoplexy, and lighter living and freer bowels are absolutely necessary; a fruit and bread diet.

In extreme cases, where it must be stopped, and other means fail, put two grains of sugar of lead in two tablespoons of water, a teaspoonful of vinegar, five drops of laudanum, or even ten, a teaspoonful of honey or molasses ; take this every three hours until relieved ; but not more than ten grains of the sugar of lead in twenty-four hours ; or

Try fifteen drops of laudanum, one teaspoonful of tincture of myrrh, and one ounce of camphor-water.

TEMPERATE LIVING.

BREAKFAST a single cup of hot drink, some cold bread and butter, and a piece of meat, nothing else.

Dinner at noon, same, adding one vegetable, nothing else, unless, as a dessert, one kind of fruit or berry, ripe, raw, and perfect and in its natural state ; nothing else.

Supper about sundown ; a cup of hot drink and piece of cold bread and butter ; nothing else whatever, and nothing between meals, unless an orange or half a lemon.

FRUIT DIET.

Breakfast, cracked wheat (which see), with sugar or salt or butter over it, and after that one kind of fruit or berry or melon, as much as you want, ripe, raw, perfect, in the natural state, nothing else ; nothing whatever between meals.

Same for dinner, with any kind of lean meat or poultry or fish.

Supper, the cracked wheat alone.

Between each meal an orange or a lemon may be taken, alternately ; these, with the fruits and berries, have an acid quality which has the effect to cool the system, to clear it of its extra bile, and to keep the bowels free.

Such a diet as the above, with outdoor activities (which see) of two hours in the forenoon, and two in the afternoon, cannot fail in any case, where any human means are available, to bring about an improvement in any case of ordinary sickness. To give it a fair trial it should be followed up for a week. When fresh fruit or berries cannot be had, dried and stewed are the next best substitute.

MALARIA and MIASM. All the ordinary forms of fever, bilious, remittent, intermittent, congestive, and yellow fever, all grades of diarrhœa and dysentery, from the mildest forms of loose bowels to the most malignant types of Asiatic cholera, are caused by miasm or malaria; moisture and warmth acting on vegetable matter, causing impure, black, thick blood, congesting it in the liver, damming it up there to an extent of crowding it, so that it cannot work. The cause, then, is one—miasm, so acting on the blood as to produce the one effect of a torpid liver, requiring the one remedy which will act upon it, so as to remedy the congestion; this is done by calomel, or any other remedy which affects the liver, such as the extract of dandelion, called taraxacum, or in the form of coffee drunk at each meal, made of the root of the plant, cut in small slices, parched brown, and ground like common coffee; a heaping tablespoon of it for each person; or the extract of the bark of the black walnut-tree, or the extract of the beautiful tomato, or the powdered root of the May-apple, called by some mandrake, by others podophyllin; any one of these well prepared, freshly made, and judiciously administered, would act on the liver, and to that extent would cure either of the diseases named, and any other curable liver-disease.

If any one medicine, different from either named, was introduced for the first time and was found to be efficient in all those forms of sickness, it would at first sight be considered as a wonderful remedy; but when it is taken into account that they all originated in a torpid liver, and that the medicine acted upon the liver, stimulated it to work, and caused the accumulated blood there to flow on, it appears to be a plain and simple thing, easy to comprehend.

But calomel is preferable to all of them because, First. Its bulk is so small, less than the half of what would lie on a nickel cent. Second. It has no taste, hence is easily taken. Third. When once swallowed it will inevitably remain in the stomach, even when cold water or a cup of tea would be rejected. Fourth. Its virtues are not deteriorated by age, hence can always be relied upon for these reasons, none of which either of the other liver medicines meet. The

LIVER PILL,

whose efficient constituent is calomel, and which is so frequently advised in this book, is the best combination of drugs ever devised

in so small a compass. Hence the oneness of disease, the oneness of its cause, and the oneness of the remedy.

But it has a still wider application. The observant reader
knows that a

BAD COLD

affects different persons differently. In one case it will settle in
the head and give catarrh; in another in the throat, and give
hoarseness; in a third in the throat, causing croup; in a fifth it
occasions bronchitis by spending its force on the branches of
the windpipe; on the lungs, causing pneumonia; on the covering
of the lungs, inducing pleurisy; on the bowels, exciting diarrhœa;
on the stomach, giving rise to a form of dyspepsia affecting the
nervous system. But a bad cold causes congestion of the liver to a
greater or less extent in all cases, hence a liver pill will cure all
these forms of disease if promptly and judiciously taken, because
it removes the congestion of the liver, hence it cures all fevers
and all colds, that is, it is the best remedy for all these, and will
cure them when they can be cured by any human instrumentality.
But constipation, and costiveness, and sick headache, and bilious
colic, and a great variety of the minor forms of disease are directly owing to a congested liver, while a large class of other diseases are more or less directly associated with this same unnatural
condition of the liver, and which the liver pill will rectify.
Hence the liver pill may well be considered as deserving the
name of

CURE ALL,

as calculated to benefit the person who takes it for a greater variety of human ailments than any other remedy yet known.
How to prepare it, how to take it to the best advantage, and
under what circumstances, see " Liver Pill."

But simple as it is, so easily taken, so reliable, so certain in its
action, and so adapted to almost every form of ordinary sickness,
it is not advised in any one single case unless there is great urgency, because it is better to get well without medicine, incomparably better, leaving the medicine as something to fall back upon
in the severe cases where all other remedies fail. All medicines
are in the nature of a poison; they all impart more or less of a
shock to the system, the shock falling on that part on which the

medicine is said to act. It is better in all ordinary cases to employ first the natural agencies of rest, warmth, cleanliness, and abstinence from food, and here a remark is about to be made which is of more importance than any other in connection with human diseases. All ordinary sickness is the result of bad blood, and too much of it in the place affected, whether it be the head, lungs, stomach, liver, bowels, or kidneys.

But all blood is made out of the food eaten, and can come from no other source. Hence in any form of sickness thus induced, the first step to be taken is to make no more blood, for there is too much already, hence cease to eat on the spot, at least until next day, say for eighteen hours, and keep warm in bed, drinking as much hot water, or to make it more agreeable, as much hot tea of any kind as is pleasant to the taste, or eat lumps of ice, crushing them between the teeth until the thirst is fully satisfied.

If at the end of eighteen hours you are not better, which will be known by your being more or less hungry, then take a liver pill. But suppose you do not feel any better, you do not appear to yourself any better, you are better for all that—

If you have less thirst.

If you feel more like eating something.

If you are even a little stronger.

If you have had a good sleep in the mean time.

But you are better even if only you are hungry, if you feel that you would relish a nice bit of broiled chicken, or beef steak, or bread and butter and a cup of tea.

If then, after a fast of eighteen hours, with rest, and warmth, and sleep, you are hungry, take only a piece of cold bread and butter, a cup of tea, and some fresh berries, or ripe fruit, in its natural state, either raw or cooked, or if dried, stewed. It is not likely you will have appetite enough to eat so much of these as to oppress the stomach.

At the end of five hours, for Nature requires that time to pass an ordinary meal out of the stomach, and not having eaten an atom between, unless about half-way an apple, orange, or lemon, or plate of ice-cream, make another meal, adding to the first a piece of lean meat of any kind, beef, mutton, fish, or poultry. This will make two meals for that day. But if after the second has been taken, and five hours have elapsed, and it is still an hour or two to bedtime, and not having taken anything since the second meal, except an apple, orange, or lemon, then take a single cup of weak tea and a thin slice of cold bread and butter. On the next day eat moderately thrice a day, nothing between meals, except an apple, orange, or lemon, with a supper of bread and butter and a cup of tea.

Two additional things would expedite the restoration greatly; first, soak the feet in hot water, and then rub the body all over, well, with a cloth dipped in warm water and squeezed out so as not to dribble; this is to cleanse the feet and the skin, and to open their pores, or, better still, if practicable, a warm bath. There is one other thing of greater importance far than the warm bath; if, at the time of going to bed for rest, and warmth, and abstinence, there had been no action of the bowels within eighteen hours, or at most for twenty-four or more, either take an enema of warm water, or a tablespoonful of castor-oil every two hours until the bowels have acted, or some other remedy which will have the effect to move the bowels within twelve hours. If any parent or other person at the head of a household would carry out this course of treatment, carry it out well, in one single case of ordinary ailment, such a person would be so much gratified at the result, that it would be repeated during the whole of life thereafter, every additional repetition being but an additional proof of the value of the plan. And it would not be long before such a person would be considered

A PRETTY GOOD DOCTOR,

and could very well "set up shop" for himself as a neighborhood physician, because of the great variety of cases in which the treatment would be applicable and do a safe good. But if at the end of eighteen hours the patient had no appetite, was no stronger, had a "furred tongue" (which article see), although there might be no pain, no fever, no suffering, then take a liver pill, according to the instructions given under that heading.

CASTOR-OIL TREATMENT.

In very many cases where the sickness is not very decided, not enough to unfit for business, after abstaining from all food, from dinner at noon until next morning, take a tablespoonful of castor oil at bedtime, and on rising in the morning, and repeat night and morning, taking more or less, so as to ensure one full passage every twenty-four hours, then gradually diminish the amount until it can be left off altogether ; let the habit of eating be according to the article headed " Temperate Living." This treatment would be effectual in a great variety of cases of sickness connected with colds, fevers, and costiveness. Castor-oil, called oleum ricini, is obtained from the seeds of the palma Christi plant, known as the castor bean. The plant grows to forty feet in Africa. The oil expressed from these seeds needs no description ; it is a mild and speedy cathartic. The dose is two tablespoonfuls for an adult, two or three teaspoonfuls for an infant. If a full dose is taken, it passes through the bowels in two or three hours, carrying all before it ; hence in some cases it is an invaluable remedy. But when taken in full doses it often gripes, causes several passages, and leaves the bowels costive. If an immediate action is not essential it is greatly better to take half a tablespoon night and morning, a little more or less, so as to secure one full, free evacuation once in every twenty-four hours, gradually diminishing the amount until it can be left off altogether. If the object is simply to secure a daily action of the bowels, and it is managed in this way, it is an invaluable remedy, and would, thus taken, cure a great many obscure diseases, besides a number of common ailments. It is the quickest cure in the world for a common cold, if given in full dose within twenty-four hours after the cold has been taken. There are two objections to it ; it is so common, and so disagreeable to take. The latter objection is obviated by a little care. Pour the dose into the middle of a glass or cup of cold water, put the edge of the cup as far back on the tongue as you can, hold the breath, or what is the same thing, hold the nose, toss up the cup quickly, swallow without closing the lips, or without allowing them to touch the oil, and there is no more taste in it than water. It is drawing the breath, and allowing it to touch the lips that makes it at all disagreeable. Coffee or spirits may be used as a vehicle, but nothing is half as good as the coldest water you can get, taking care simply to pour it in the centre of the water, and not allowing the oil to touch the lips. With such a use of castor-oil it is one of the best things known to move the bowels, for it is cheap, is always at hand, always sure.

CARBUNCLE

Is known from a boil by being more flat and having a honey-combed appearance ; cut clear across it, and push into the wound some lint or cotton saturated with carbolic acid, and then paint the whole surface with the acid. Live on fruits and coarse bread, lean meat once a day, and take a liver pill weekly, making the bowels act thrice in every two days with castor oil.

If there is redness or inflammation, or much heat, apply wet compresses to the fullest extent necessary and as often as it is necessary.

If there is no heat, then warm fomentations applied persistently will be of great service. To keep cool during the night, a poultice made of Goulard water and bread crumbs is excellent.

When the heads of the carbuncle begin to soften it means its death, make two cuts crossways, completely across the carbuncle, even a little beyond it, and then press out the pieces and keep on poultices to relieve of any fever or pain. A common yeast poultice is as good as anything else, to be changed four times every day. When the dead parts are out, and the cavity begins to heal up, wash it once a day with a solution of ten grains of lunar caustic in an ounce of rain-water.

BURNS AND SCALDS

Are of four kinds, according to their severity.

First. When so superficial that there is only a redness, with more or less swelling, pain, and heat, continuing for an hour or more, or a day or two.

Second. When the outside skin rises into little blisters, which if broken or pierced pour out a little whitish, thickish juice.

Third. When the real skin is burnt off, the surface is soft or of a yellowish watery appearance ; or the burning may have been so severe as to leave the part dry, black, and burned.

Fourth. When the burning has extended down to the flesh or even bone, to inflame or mortify, unless prevented, the pain and

16

suffering in these cases is less than in more superficial injuries, because there is less sensibility than in the skin. In cutting off a limb, for the same reason, the most suffering is at the instant the instrument is passing through the skin.

The greater the surface implicated, the greater the danger to life, indicated by the patient complaining of being cold. There is a shivering all over, the pulse is very weak and can scarcely be felt, stupor comes on, followed apace by insensibility and death, this insensibility seeming to be mercifully sent to save the unfortunate from unendurable suffering.

TREATMENT OF BURNS.

If the clothing is on fire throw the person instantly on the floor, and cover with a rug, carpet, blanket, shawl, overcoat, or any other woollen material at hand; this smothers the fire, while the prone position prevents the flames from rising to the face and being breathed into the lungs which destroys life. If the legs or feet are burned or scalded, drawing off the stockings often brings the flesh along with them, therefore slit them up instantly with scissors or a penknife.

The first thing to be done in all cases is to exclude the air, for it is that which causes the pain; the first and easiest thing is to put the part in cold water, this relieves the pain perfectly and instantly, and gives time to think what had best to be next done, and also allows the patient to be composed and calm, and thus the better able to co-operate with the nurse in the employment of the means to be used.

If the burned surface is so large that there is a feeling of chilliness, then the application of cold water is injurious, and the parts should be sprinkled over with flour until no more will stick on; this forms a coating which is impervious to air, and in the slighter forms of burning, which allow immersion in cold water, the flour may be applied and nothing more need be done; have cooling diet and free bowels. After a day or two or more the flour will cake off and a beautiful new skin will be seen under it, but avoid picking off any of the cakes; tepid water should be applied until they are softened so that they will fall off themselves, as the new skin is necessarily very tender and frail. Cold applications should never be employed to the breast, belly, or any part of the trunk or body, because the unavoidable dribbling of the water, and the exposure to the air tend to induce chilliness, which should by all means be always guarded against. If the legs or feet, or hands and arms only are burned, then put them in cold water instantly, shoes, stockings, everything on; this may prevent blistering, and will allow time to think what had best be done next. If there are blisters puncture them, wash off the parts and then apply the flour.

CHARCOAL

laid flat, while cold, on a burn causes the pain to abate immediately; by leaving it on for an hour the burn seems almost healed when the injury is superficial.

CHERRY-LAUREL WATER,

eight parts, with a hundred parts of gum-syrup, made of equal parts of common syrup and mucilage of gum tragacanth, is very efficient by dipping two or three thicknesses of linen or muslin in the mixture; lay it on the burn, renew the application night and morning, but moisten it before attempting to take it off.

A PAINT IS

made of linseed oil and vinegar, equal parts, then powdered chalk stirred into it until of the consistence of thick paint, lay it on with a brush; as fast as it dries put on another coat, until all discomfort is gone; this is on the principle of other applications, and keeps the air out.

After all, the speediest remedy and oftenest on hand is cold-water immersion of the part.

--------- ∞ ---------

CHILBLAINS

ARE very troublesome, especially in scrofulous and old and feeble persons, caused by the cold inflaming the skin, which assumes a leaden or purple hue. They would never follow cold hands or feet, unless they were put in hot water, or held too near the fire. Better to warm them very gradually, by first putting them in cold water, then in water of sixty degrees for five minutes, then rub with the warm hands until they are comfortably warm, using your own hands or those of a more vigorous person.

When a chilblain is once formed, take thirty grains of sulphate of copper, called blue vitriol, dissolve it in three tablespoonfuls of water, and wash the parts well three times a day. Some prefer a wash made of 2 oz. of oil of turpentine and three drachms of spirits of camphor.

If the blains are not broken, apply a mixture of four tablespoons of sweet oil, white wax two drachms, melt them, add one drachm of balsam of Peru, and one drachm of hydrochloric acid, wash several times a day.

If the blains are broken or ulcerated, apply bread-and-milk poultice for two or three days, and paint them with iodine tincture made by dissolving a drachm of iodine in three ounces of alcohol, use only once a day, with a soft brush. To prevent chilblains, bathe the hands and feet in warm salt water every morning and night during cold weather.

§

CORNS.

THE leaf of the ground-ivy, bruised and applied to a hard corn, is said to be a speedy cure for the common corns on our toes. Instead of burdening the memory with a variety of intricate preparations, it is easier to remember the principles involved. First, remove the pressure or friction of the shoe which occasioned the corn. Second, keep it moist long enough, and it will drop out of itself, or can be easily picked out with the finger-nail; if it ever comes again, repeat the process. Lock-jaw has frequently followed cutting hard corns; at other times, convulsions and death. This risk ought never to be run as long as a bit of cotton saturated with water or sweet oil, or, better still, glycerine, which is the essential element of sweet oil, is a safe, certain, and efficient cure for hard corns, if kept constantly applied for a day or two, and no shoe is worn.

A certain mode of removing all corns is to bathe the feet in quite warm water every night, for fifteen minutes. Take one or two or more thicknesses of buckskin, according to the elevation of the corn; cut a hole in the centre of the buckskin so as to receive the corn; this guards the corn against any pressure; if any kind of ointment or pain-killer is used to fill up the spaces around the corn the softening would be facilitated. In a few days the corn will fall out, or may be picked out with the finger-nail. As often as the corn returns renew the treatment; it would not return if the shoes were not too tight nor too loose. There is no hard corn which cannot be safely and effectually got rid of in this way.

If pared closely and kept covered with a bit of india-rubber cloth the corn will disappear; but there is danger in the paring. A simple shield of buckskin made to receive the corn, so as to keep off pressure, is second to no other remedy.

Or paint the corn twice a day with strong vinegar or nitric acid.

Soft corns are always cured by warm-water bathings and buckskin protectors, and no parings are necessary.

BUNIONS

are caused by the pressure or friction of the shoe; the irritation makes the skin swell. Sometimes it is removed in the beginning by keeping a strip of adhesive plaster applied to it as long as there is any discomfort. If inflamed, apply a bread-and-milk poultice, or water compresses, until relieved. Or rub into the bunion, twice a day, patiently, some ointment made by mixing half an ounce of lard with fifteen grains of iodine, and wear a loose shoe. These bunions generally come on the ball of the great toe, or the inside of the first joint of that toe, or the little toe, or on the instep, caused by too narrow shoes and high heels; hence at once put on a loose slipper without any heels. Cover the bunion with a piece of oiled silk covered with some pain-killer or other ointment. Take a larger piece of buckskin, cut a hole in it large enough to receive the bunion; then another piece of oiled silk over that; in this way the bunion is relieved from the pressure which caused it. Rub the ointment first named on the bunion, twice or thrice a day, patiently and well, with the finger.

When these simple methods of curing

Hard corns,

Soft corns, and
Bunions,
are sufficient, and so available to all, it is scarcely worth while to encumber the page with the thousand and one cures advised by the multitude.

BRONCHOCELE

Is a swelling of the glands of the neck. Take two and a half drachms of iodide of potassium, one and a half drachms of iodine, and three ounces of water. Put some of this in a small vial, and take ten drops in a tablespoonful of water before each meal, and from the other portion of the mixture wet the whole skin, where swollen, three times a day with a feather, or camel's-hair pencil, until the swelling has subsided; keep the bowels freely acting every day. This affection sometimes prevails in certain localities, supposed to arise from the character of the water; hence it is worth the experiment to move to a distant part of the country with a different water.

SPRAINS

Of all the joints become painful immediately, in consequence of the inflammation. There is one direction applicable to them all: keep down the inflammation by allowing cold water to fall upon it in a constant stream until relief is obtained; as soon as the pain returns repeat the pouring; the colder the water, the better; ice-water, or salt water which is colder than common water. If it be the ankle, let it be in a horizontal position, so as to favor a return of the blood. If the wrist, keep it elevated a little higher than the elbow, take at night a liver pill, and keep the bowels acting very freely.

ZYMOTIC DISEASES

Are such as result from: 1st, bad food; 2d, bad air; 3d, filth; 4th, contagion. As the word "zymotic," introduced within a few years, is so commonly employed in medical reports, especially those connected with cities and large towns, persons of cultivation and intelligence would do well to obtain a comprehensive and accurate knowledge of the meaning of the word, and fix it in the memory; it is from a Greek word which means to ferment; there can be no fermentation where there are not three conditions:—

1st. There must be moisture.

2d. There must be heat.

3d. There must be some growth which can decay.

If either one of these be absent, there can be no fermentation, which word may be considered in this connection equivalent to rotting, putrefying, decaying, decomposition; all these terms bring to our mind the idea of filth and dirt. The fundamental meaning, then, of the word zymotic, is filth; and all diseases arising from filth are diseases of zymotic origin. But different kinds of filth, which is really absence of cleanliness, cause different kinds of diseases. If a man has a house near a pond, and there are a great many leaves in it and about it, and logs of wood, and there is a hot sun, these are the three conditions; and in a short time the persons living near that pond will be attacked with fever, dysentery, diarrhœa, running through the whole neighborhood.

If a man has small-pox, ship fever, jail fever, the emanations from his body and his breath fill the air around him; any one coming within a few feet of him will take the disease because of the filthiness of the atmosphere; in a measure, you come in contact with him; hence these diseases are called contagious.

If you sleep with a man who has the itch, or sleep in a bed which he has just occupied, there is an idea of filthiness in the mind; there is a general feeling that people who have the itch are dirty people; hence itch is classed among zymotic diseases, and is also a contagious disease, because if you come in contact with such a person you will have the itch too, not directly from filth itself, but from that which is dependent on what we call filth, to wit: insects or growth of some kind; hence this kind of zymotic disease arises from parasites, and may be called parasitic disease, of which there are now supposed to be other kinds than that of common itch.

Zymotic diseases, then, are those which result from a want of cleanliness of person or habitation, and are avoidable. But the deaths from zymotic diseases, avoidable diseases, diseases which arise from filth, occurring in Philadelphia, for the week ending February 10th, 1872, were two hundred and ten out of five hundred and ten; that is, two-fifths of all the deaths in so pleasant a city as Philadelphia result from the want of cleanliness. If these statements have the effect on men of intelligence and influence to inquire more particularly into the connection between filth and death, it may lead to results ultimately which will benefit and bless all of human kind.

PREVENTING SUFFERING.

MANY of what are called the "accidents" of life could be guarded against by the exercise of a very small amount of care or reflection. "I might have known better if I had only thought a moment," is a frequent expression of hair-brained people. If this chapter were read to a family once a year many a calamity would be prevented, many a life saved, and many a home made happy. This annual reading might be made a source of amusement as well as profit, by asking for reasons for some of the suggestions, or for suggestions as to what should be done under certain circumstances, in addition to what was named. This would impress the precepts on the mind more deeply, they would be longer remembered, and would be made available in emergencies.

1. Never go anybody's security unless you have the money already in bank to remain there until the time has expired, for the Bible says, "He that hateth suretyship is sure."

2. Don't delay insuring your house or life until one is on fire and the other lost.

3. Avoid debt as you would fire and brimstone, for out of debt out of danger.

4. Before you go to bed turn off the gas *fully*, instead of blowing it out.

5. Don't change to a lighter garment on Sunday; because you might become chilly in church, and would not like to get up and go out to rectify your mistake.

6. Before going to your chamber, if you are a housekeeper, see that all the fires are secure, and that no lights are burning, especially near window curtains with an open window.

7. In freezing weather take very short steps and slow. If a mad bull is after you, run.

8. Keep matches in metal cases.

9. Never throw a burning match on the floor. It cost Portland ten millions of dollars.

10. Never trim or fill a lamp except in the daytime and out of doors. This would save a hundred lives every year and prevent many a house from being burned to the ground.

11. Don't handle powder after night or near a fire; it sometimes goes off, when you go up.

12. If you take a horseback ride in freezing weather, have the shoes roughened.

13. If you are sick go to bed and rest from motion and food; many persons, women especially, in their ambition to do up the work, have reduced their strength so low that nature had no power to rise evermore.

14. Never put on a new shoe on going to church or on a journey; you might want to change it and couldn't.

15. Never throw broken glass into the street; it may cause painful wounds to the shoeless poor.

16. Never give a positive promise to make a friendly call; say, "I will endeavor to do so," or "It would afford me pleasure to make you a visit," that is, if you really think so.

17. Never use an empty bottle, nor drink from a full one unless its contents are marked. A gentleman just married built him a country-seat at a cost of over sixty thousand dollars. Shortly after its completion he made some cider and filled some empty bottles, which he had sent to town to sell; but as he could not get as much for them as he thought they were worth, he had them brought home and filled as above. In a few days a bottle of cider was required to be placed on the table; both the gentleman and his young wife drank of it. He died in a few days, she lingered a year or more, and died also; their splendid place was sold for twenty-five thousand dollars, one of the handsomest in New England to-day. The bottle had contained corrosive sublimate to kill bed-bugs; it had dried to the bottom of the bottle.

18. Never wake up any one suddenly, especially a child; convulsions have been induced thereby.

19. Never walk lengthways on a railroad track, a locomotive might overtake you; does overtake hundreds every year, and then the sexton has to undertake them.

20. Never throw an orange-peel or any other peel on the pavement.

21. When crossing the street look both ways and in front at the same time, and don't stop for an instant.

22. Never carry an umbrella or cane under your arm, for stopping suddenly, a person behind you may have his eye poked out.

23. If in a vehicle, never have an arm or elbow or head outside.

24. If your horses run away with the carriage and you in it, stay there; or if you must leave, drop yourself out from behind.

25. If your hat is blown off and is turning various somersets before the wind, let somebody else run after it; "they" will be sure to do it and save you the trouble.

26. When about getting out of a car, let it stop before you start, and be sure to get out at the rear door.

27. Never attempt to cross a street before a horse or vehicle; they will pass you in thirty seconds; better lose them than limb or life.

28. Be very cautious in promising anything to anybody; always leave a place to creep out at.

29. Walk to a skating pond and run from it, so as not to be overheated when you get there, and to warm yourself up gradually, when you are coming away. Riding from the ice has allowed many a person to get into a chill which never was removed.

30. Never step from the right path, for it goes farther away forever.

31. If you see a puddle don't put your foot in it, for the bottom may be spilled out; this precept has a wide application in the experiences of life.

32. Never speak of your father as "the governor," or "the old man," nor of her who bore you as "the old woman;" for "mother" is the sweetest sound in the language, and it is the last that is remembered.

33. If it lightens, let it lighten; it never hurts those who see it. At the same time the safest place, if in a house, is the middle of the room or tub of water. The cellar is no safer than the attic, for the thunderbolt comes out of the ground as well as from the

sky. A man lay down on a railroad track to avoid the lightning. It found him out and killed him; the rails attracted it. A woman got between two feather beds and the bolt followed her, because the post had an iron rod on the top to hold the canopy. Get as far from everything metallic as possible.

34. If caught in a shower or tumbled into a mill pond, go ahead, keep moving rapidly until you get home or to the nearest house, then drink a pint of something hot, preferring red pepper or ginger tea, next to that strong common tea, but it is better to drink hot water than to wait five minutes; drink it before undressing, which do quickly, put on dry clothing and take another hot drink. If in cold weather go to the nearest house, for it would be impossible to walk fast enough to keep off a feeling of chilliness.

35. Never perpetrate a practical joke, for no good ever comes of fooling.

36. Never reprove in the presence of a third person, for it is sure to wound or enrage.

37. Never speak harshly to the little ones at bedtime; let the last act of the day be a loving kiss, the last word full of the mother. The terrible croup may make it an angel before the morning light.

38. Never attempt to scare a child, nor to leave it while in a state of alarm, especially on putting it to bed. If you know your child is in terror, if left to go to sleep in the dark it is an unmitigated cruelty to call it "nonsense," and take away the light; that word demonstrates nothing, convinces nobody; would it convince you? If the little one is happier to have a light burning while it is going to sleep, by all means gratify it, or leave the door open, or do any other thing which would enable it to go to sleep with a feeling of safety and a quiet mind.

39. If you have inadvertently or otherwise swallowed a deadly poison, if it burns the throat swallow instantly the whites of several eggs, or rather than lose time take the whole egg, except the shell; it is the white, the albuminous part, which does the good, the yellow does no harm. A substitute for an egg is some flour stirred in cold water, drunk quickly.

40. If a poison has been swallowed which does not burn the throat, especially laudanum or morphine in any of their forms, the best plan is to get them out of the stomach as soon as possible, by taking a large tablespoon of common salt and as much ground

mustard, stir them quickly in a glass of water or a half pint, in a bowl or tin cup, and toss it down; on the instant of its reaching the stomach, it irritates it to such an extent, that it gives a convulsive heave, and casts out all that was in it; then take a drink of strong coffee, having already sent for the doctor, in either case.

41. Never go into a vault or deep well or cave; see if a lighted candle will burn, or a newspaper, or bunch of straw, hay, or shavings; if the flame goes out it is deadly. If a person is already in, and is in danger, pour a bucket or tub of fresh cold water into the well; this antagonizes or absorbs the bad air.

42. Never go to sleep out of doors in cold weather if you are benumbed with cold or feel drowsy, else you will freeze to death, and wake never more.

THE EYE.

CINDERS, specks of dirt, or other hard substances usually get in under the upper eyelid, and find a lodgment in a kind of groove or channel there provided to convey the tears or extra water away from the eye towards or into the nose; thus persons who begin to cry commence at once to blow the nose, to clear it of the water thus brought into it through a tube which runs from the inner corner of the lower lid into the nostril. In many persons this canal becomes inflamed and closes up permanently, causing the water to come out of the eye over the rim of the lid, out upon the cheek, causing a great inconvenience of wiping.

When anything gets into the eye, the first instinct is to put up the fingers and rub it; but as the parts there are very soft, this rubbing and pressure have the effect to imbed the particle more firmly, and cause greater difficulty in the removal, causing intense pain sometimes to last for hours or a whole day, as in railcar travel, when there are no conveniences for relief.

If, therefore, anything gets into the eye take hold of the upper lid with the thumb and finger of the right hand, turn the face in such a direction that gravity will aid in carrying it towards the nostril, draw the lid out from the eyeball and work it up and down over the ball; this excites additional water in the eye, and helps greatly in washing the offending particle out at the corner.

In case, however, of failure when the substance is hard or heavy, as a cinder, which will not float on water, being really a little stone, put your lead pencil horizontally over the eyelid, near half an inch from the edge, draw out the eyelid, turn it over the edge of the pencil; the speck will be seen at once, when a friend can remove it with the corner of a handkerchief turned over the fore-finger; then bathe the eye freely in cold water, or keep it resolutely closed from the light for an hour or two until there is a sense of relief.

In case it is a particle of iron or steel, as in workshops, a pocket magnet is the most efficient application.

When the eyes are weak, and persons find themselves frequently winking them, close them at once and keep them closed for ten or fifteen minutes, and then go at something which does not require such a close use of the eye as do reading and sewing.

It is not as great a strain on the eye to write as to read. If the eyes have been used in reading or sewing at night, it will be a great relief before going to bed to flap up warm water against them so as not to touch them with the fingers, carry the water up with the palm of the hand over the eyes, the fingers touching the nose; then apply cold water in the same way, and once or twice open the eyes in the cold water for as long a time as the breath can be held; it is very cooling to a fevered eye, and affords great relief.

But the eye is such a valuable organ that every one ought to be exceedingly cautious against putting anything into it, or upon it, in any way whatever. A friend of the author, a lady of educa-tion, wealth, and high social position, was advised to apply to her eyes, for a single night, a poultice made of rotten apple; it seemed very simple; everybody knew what a rotten apple was, and it could do no harm, even if it did not do any good; the person advising it knew a case where its application had been of wonderful ad-vantage. The next morning the lady waked up in darkness; she never saw again; the weight of the poultice and its being bound too tightly had done the mischief.

It is safe to say, that if rest and bathing in tepid water, do not relieve the eye, nothing should be done to it except by the advice of a physician; an oculist is still better.

All persons owe it to themselves to avoid reading or sewing at night or by twilight, as much as possible; the rule should be, unless there is a clear necessity for it, not to read or sew a moment after sundown, until the gas or candle or lamps are lighted.

Never read or sew by one candle; its unsteady flame or flickering is a great strain on the eye.

It is ruinous to read while on horseback or while riding in a vehicle, because every jolt or jar alters the focus of sight, and the eye is instinctively endeavoring all the time to adjust it, the effort to do which is perfectly exhausting, and is a permanent injury to the optic nerve; in fact, it often brings on

AMAUROSIS,

one of the most incurable and fatal of all maladies.

Reading while upon the back tends rapidly to the same disease, but to read on the back by candle or gas light, as some do, to read themselves to sleep, is a criminality, is murderous.

Avoid reading or sewing while facing a window or open door, the glare of the light is trying to the sight; better let the light fall on the page over the left shoulder.

CHILDREN'S EYES

are often weakened for life by learning their lessons after dark. It ought never to be allowed for a single night if possible. It is ten thousand times better to compel them to go to bed an hour after sundown, and rise the earlier in the morning, but on no account to use the eyes before the sun is up.

Sometimes when the eyes feel weak, as in reading or sewing, or in looking at near or small objects, it is a great rest to them to look for a while at something in the distance, half a mile away or more. Sailors' eyes are proverbially better than those of landsmen. A sailor is seldom seen with glasses; it is from the habit of looking out for things at a distance, for ships a mile away, and for the land.

Sometimes the eyes are "matted" in the morning, or after sleeping. The hard matter should never be picked off with the finger-nails, and yet it is often done, so uniformly and so invariably causing inflammation, that it has become a saying, in connection also with that the finger-nails are poisonous. When infants' eyes are glued together, they should be patiently bathed in tepid water; or the saliva of the mother applied with the ball of the finger, rubbing it along the eyelashes, is the best thing in the world, for this fluid is the softest and most penetrating in nature, in this connection; and for the same reasons grown persons with matted eyes in the morning should make the same application, instead of straining the roots of the eyelashes, and inflaming them by dragging on them. Next best is to have a basin of warm water, or make your way to the wash-room with the eyes shut, and open them with the face in the warm water and remove the matter, not with the finger and thumb nail, but with the ball of the finger, ending with flapping cold water over the closed eye or opening the eyes in cold water as above directed.

FROST BITE.

A young lady, after skating some time, complained of one foot being very cold. She was advised by the young gentleman who attended her to put it in warm water as soon as she got home. She did so. The foot inflamed, mortified, and had to be taken off.

It should be remembered that the injury done to a part by burning or freezing is pretty much the same, and is caused by the rapidity of the passage of the particles of caloric, or heat, inwards or outwards. The change should be gradually made; hence if there is a burn, not deep, it is cured by holding the part near the fire, which is said to draw out the heat. The meaning is, that it is very gradually relieved of the extra heat of the burning. So in frost-bite; go to a room where there is no fire, and rub the frozen parts with snow or cold water, almost ice-cold, then rub with flannels, and then with the hands, patiently and rapidly. If a limb is frozen, put it in cold water. A frozen part is whitened, hence the cold applications should be made until the color begins to appear. Ice is very brittle, so is anything frozen, the flesh as well, hence a part is easily broken off; therefore handle a frozen part with great delicacy, tenderness, and care.

CHILBLAINS

are milder forms of freezing, caused by sudden alternation of heat and cold to toes or fingers. There is more itching than pain. Children and old persons—those who are scrofulous or have a feeble circulation—are most subject to them. Bathe the feet in tepid salt-water every night. After every washing of the hands wipe them and then rub into them oatmeal or Indian meal, so as effectually to dry them. This course of treating the feet and hands tends to keep off chilblains from those who are subject to them.

When present wash them well three times a day with alcohol or other spirits, or spirits of camphor, rubbing the hands one in another very freely many times a day. A better plan is to take two drachms each of alum and sulphate of zinc to half a pint of water, then add one ounce of spirits of camphor; rub this while warm well into the hands three times a day. If they are broken the ulcers must be treated differently; then use cold water compresses every hour, or every five minutes, until all the inflammation is gone. If there is proud flesh use ointment of red precipitate.

TURKISH BATHS

And Russian baths are very much the same, and, except on very special occasions and under an experienced medical eye, are unnatural and dangerous, they are applicable for a cold within twenty-four hours after having been taken; in cases where all remedies have failed to remove a harsh, hot, dry state of the skin, if in connection there was constipation; in some forms of rheumatism accompanied with great suffering; but there are so many safer and more available means which can be employed without danger, that it would be better if there were no such baths in existence in this country, unless the proprietor of such bath was an educated physician of professional ability, and who superintended each case himself personally. The Turks, as a people, especially the higher classes, who alone can afford the national bath, are lazy, idle, effeminate, lecherous, and short-lived, proving that their baths are not promotive of health and longevity, if indeed they do not tend to shorten life by the great loss of power and elasticity which every bath must occasion. To breathe such a hot air in the lungs cannot but be exceedingly injurious, unless exceeding carefulness is observed in going into a cooler, especially an outdoor air, from October to May. Several persons, in the author's observation, have been brought to death's door, and some have died, as a result clearly traceable to a Turkish bath.

Miss Lillie Peckham, a young lady of great promise, and of unusual talents and ability, took a Turkish bath at Milwaukee, and was so debilitated that she died in a few days. Dr. Trall, one of the most able hydropathists, says that more than twenty seriously injurious or fatal cases have come to his personal knowledge, not from the dangerous nature of the baths themselves, but from their injudicious administration by the hands of ignorant hirelings.

Turkish baths may be good for filthy persons, such as have not had a good cleaning off in a year; but we never could imagine the utility of putting a decent man into a steam-boiler hot enough to skin a lobster, and then filing off all his hide to the very quick, by kneadings and remorseless scrubbings.

LOCK-JAW,

Or tetanus, is a cramp of the muscles of the face, and of the whole body, sometimes coming on with a difficulty in turning the head or moving the jaws, with difficult swallowing and pain darting from the breast towards the back. Swallow or breathe chloroform or ether, next administer a warm water enema; let attendants rub different parts of the body rapidly with the hand. Apply spirits of turpentine freely to the neck and face; sometimes a very warm bath relaxes the whole body; but as it is seldom immediately fatal, time is given to call a physician. In lock-jaw

17

the sufferings are terrible, face pale, brow contracted, forehead wrinkled, eyes fixed and prominent, nostrils dilated, corners of mouth drawn in, giving a kind of grin to the face, intense thirst, anguished breathing. It is brought on by cold and damp, or by cuts, laceration or punctures, such as the running of a· rusty nail into the foot; exposures of the wounded on the battle-field, coming on in three or four days or weeks. Laudanum is given in doses of from thirty to sixty drops every half hour. Turpentine friction along the spine, a stream of cold water on the head from a height of five or six feet. Inhale chloroform freely; or inject watery solution of aloes, or Indian hemp.

Homœopathists use belladonna, sometimes alternated with lachesis, or with cicuta virosa. In the worst forms arnica montana is taken. If opium is given, take hyoscyamus in six hours after the last dose of opium. Rhus tox., alternated with ignatia, is a favorite remedy. If there is inflammation take mercurius. In all forms administer enemas freely as may be desirable. Cases have sometimes recovered by taking a tablespoonful of brandy, and in an hour a grain of opium, in another hour a tablespoonful of brandy or whiskey, and so on until relief is obtained.

Chloral has been successfully used by different physicians.

------------◦◦◦------------

ANÆSTHESIA,

From two Greek words, meaning without feeling, is given to such substances as may be taken into the lungs by breathing, or swallowed into the stomach, with the effect of rendering a person insensible to pain and suffering. Oxygen gas is one of these; for if taken into the lungs, a skillful dentist can extract several teeth without the person having a particle of pain. This is the Nitrous Oxide, or Laughing Gas, which in its application for causing insensibility to pain, seems to have been the discovery of Dr. Horace Wells, a dentist of Hartford, Conn., on the tenth of December, 1844, Dr. J. Q. Colton being present, whose intelligence and persevering industry has since made painless tooth-drawing under the influence of Nitrous Oxide a common operation, and so safe, that in ten years not a single death has resulted. As a warning to the reader against the use of this and other similar articles as a stimulant or sedative, it may be well to state that Dr. Wells was a portly, noble-looking man, and from seeing the effects of ether when taken by others in relieving them from suffering, whether from bodily pain or mental depression, he fell into the habit of taking ether himself, and it grew upon him to such an extent that, being on a visit to the city of New York, and having used it too freely, he became so excited that he was for a while literally beside himself; went into the street after night, and began throwing oil of vitriol on the dresses of the women of the town whenever he met one. For this he was arrested and conveyed to the Tombs. On recovering his senses, he became so disgusted with himself that he resolved on suicide, and saturating his handkerchief with the oblivious ingredient, tied it over his mouth, threw himself back upon his prison-cot, and with one tremendous stroke of a razor cut his thigh, cut it to the bone, dividing one of the largest arteries of the body, and died immediately. This was the statement of a personal friend of Dr. Wells, who saw the body a very few moments after the wound was inflicted. Such was the sad fate of a man whose experiments have given one of the greatest boons to humanity. About the same time, Mr. Waldie, a Scotch chemist and bookseller, one day left a saucer half full of chloroform on the floor, and soon after a little dog was lying at the side of it, apparently dead; but after a while began to move one limb, then another, regained consciousness, and frisked away as if nothing was the matter. The chemist, thinking he had made a discovery, administered the chloroform to some cats with a similar result, confirming his belief. He went to Edinburgh, and communicated the facts to Dr. James Simpson, who made some experiments, all proving that breathing the fumes of chloroform had the effect of causing insensibility to pain and suffering, even of the drawing of a tooth or the sawing off a limb. And finally it was ascertained that the most painful surgical operations could be performed without consciousness of any suffering whatever. Prof. Simpson first published these results in 1857. The name given this remarkable agent was terchloride of formyl, which was soon shortened into the present designation,

CHLOROFORM.

Three parts of chlorine gas, and one part of formyl, taking their names thus; chlorine is from the Greek for green, that being the color of the gas, and more appropriate, too, from its being largely derived from substances taken from the sea, its plants and salts.

RED ANTS,

if made angry, discharge a very pungent acid substance called formic acid, "*formica*" being the word for ant. If these ants are distilled, a substance is produced so burning, that if it is dropped on the skin, it eats into it like fire. It is also derived from the stinging nettle.

PATENT MEDICINES

ARE those remedies for sickness and disease whose constituents are unknown, except to the maker of them, who is said to be the "proprietor." There is really no "patent" medicine in the United States, in the sense in which that expression is used; for, in the first place, the getting a "patent" for it at Washington would reveal its constituents, and the public would soon know that cough medicines were nothing more than the various preparations of morphia, and that the "Universal Disease Eradicator" was nothing but bread pills made up with the tincture of t(hy)ime; that is, if you are sick, take time, wait awhile, and you will get better, in very many cases indeed.

But "patent," as applied to medicines, ought to come from some word which means to cover, to hide, to keep secret; they are secret medicines; secret, because their constituents are not made public. That all such medicines do immeasurably more harm than good can scarcely be denied. Many of them are perfectly inert; but while the misguided taker is waiting for the good effects, the disease may be spreading in the body and eating out its life.

If, on the other hand, a patent medicine is really efficient, it is liable, as some of them certainly are, to place the system in a condition which impels their use for a lifetime; or, in some other cases, poison it by slow degrees, and eventually destroy life.

It may be safe to say, that any man who habitually takes any medicine, the constituents of which are unknown to him or his medical adviser, acts most unwisely, and endangers his own life.

The French are an age or two ahead of us in this respect. No man is allowed, under very severe penalties, to sell any medicine without having all the constituents and their proportions printed on what contains it. New York State, after the pattern of Illinois, has under consideration a similar law, and it is to be hoped that it will not fail of enactment. The sale of patent medicines is the greatest cruelty and the greatest swindle of the age; for patronized, as they mainly are, by the poor, who are not able to pay for competent medical advice, and are not disposed to apply to a hospital or dispensary for free aid, are the chief sufferers, because the effect is as if they threw their hard earnings into the sea, for the reasons above named.

It is not by any means claimed that patent medicines never do any good, for in reality most of them are the prescriptions of eminent medical men, and were adapted to special cases; but to apply them indiscriminately to a variety of forms of disease, and to do it for the sake of a little money, when such great risks are run as have already been referred to, merits the indignation and contempt of every intelligent mind. " Give me a dollar for my medicine or die," is the summing up of the character of every man who sells a secret cure for disease.

HOW LONG TO STARVE.

A MAN will die for want of air in five minutes, for want of sleep in ten days, for want of water in a week, for want of food at varying intervals, dependent on constitution, habits of life, and the circumstances of the occasion. Instances have been given where persons have been said to live many weeks without eating a particle of food; but when opportunities have been offered for a fair investigation of the case, it has been invariably found that a weak and wicked fraud has been at the bottom of it.

On the 28th of August the captain of a Boston whaler was wrecked. For eight days he could not get a drop of water, nor a particle of food. On the day of the wreck he weighed one hundred and ninety pounds ; when rescued he weighed one hundred pounds. A teaspoonful of brandy was given to each sailor ; but before they could be taken aboard the vessel which saved them, they became unconscious, and remained so for two days, but all eventually recovered. Many persons have been killed by eating too much after having fasted for a long time ; the safe plan of procedure, and which every reader should bear in mind, is to feel the way along, as persons who are travelling in the dark and fear a precipice ahead ; there can be no one rule given, because there are so many modifying circumstances. Give a teaspoonful of hot drink at a time, and if no ill result, repeat in five minutes, and the same amount of soft food, boiled rice or softened bread, or soup, or gruel ; for the stomach is itself as weak as the sufferer in proportion, and can only manage a very small amount of food.

Wading in water, or keeping the clothing saturated with water, even if it is sea-water, sensibly abates the horrors of thirst.

THE GREATEST DOCTOR

Is Nature ; just let her have her way, and she will cure three-fourths of all ordinary sickness without the cost of a dollar. In one important respect the human machine, built by Infinite power and wisdom and benevolence, passes any structure of human hands by a distance immeasurable,—it mends itself, it repairs the injuries received from outsiders with wonderful promptitude and perfectness. Cut a gash in the arm ; let it alone and it will get well. Let a man make a fool of himself by getting drunk or eating twice as much as he ought to have done, and although Nature has been outraged, the body shattered, the mind befuddled, and the man degraded, just give Nature a chance at him with a ten hours' sleep, and she will make it

"ALL RIGHT IN THE MORNING."

But man is so inconsiderate that instead of letting "the great doctor" have his way he takes to "arguing the case," when he gets sick, and thus reasons : "When I was well I could eat heart-fly ; now if I can only eat heartily I shall be well ; " and right away he orders a splendid dinner, and to give him an appetite he drinks brandy first, peppers his vegetables, plasters his meats with mustard, fills his plate with Worcester sauce, and " tops off " with absinthe, champagne, or " rot-gut whiskey." No wonder people die at forty-five instead of a hundred years.

The fact should be borne in mind by every reader of cultivation and intelligence, that three-fourths of the ordinary sickness of men would be safely, promptly, and efficiently cured by rest in a warm bed, in a cool room, with a clean skin, and eating only when really hungry ; eating in the daytime, at six hours' intervals, of two or three kinds of the plainest food, in small quantities, for a day or two.

But if the bowels are costive, if a day has passed without an action, the restoration to health would be greatly expedited if an enema were taken, or, what is better, a brisk walk in the open air until there is some considerable fatigue, then next morning the bowels will be pretty sure to act.

SUMMER EXCURSIONS.

MANY annually form plans for spending the summer. It is of secondary importance to decide where to go. The chief point is to go somewhere, north, south, east, or west. It is the change that does the good,—change of air, change of scene, change of food, of the mode of its preparation, change of associations, so as to have some new kind of excitement ; such a change as will bring into requisition a different set of muscles, of mental faculties, of moral qualities, of social and domestic enjoyments ; leaving at home, as far as possible, business cares, plans, schemes, labors, solicitudes.

There is some choice in localities : the hill country is better than the prairie ; the mountain top better than the valley.

The kind of occupation is important ; it is the out-door life that does most of the good—the sunshine and the breeze. If a person goes to the country to eat and sleep and lounge about the house, but little benefit can be expected ; but if nearly the whole time from after breakfast until sundown is spent in excursions on foot, on horse, in country wagons,—going every day to some point of interest, instructive and new, raising the spirits, stimulating inquiry, cultivating the better qualities of our nature, social, moral, and domestic,—then will benefit be derived ; a marked and enduring benefit to mind and heart and body. Those who have any ailment of the throat or lungs should keep away from lake and sea-shore and prairie, because dangerous, raw, bleak, piercing, chilling winds follow the rains even of summer ; besides, there is something in the sundown dampness of the sea-shore which is hurtful to weak lungs.

If persons are confined to the house, home is the best place for every sickness ; there is no good result under any hired or stranger's roof which can compensate for the quiet and freedom and roominess of one's own home; for the tender and sympathetic ministrations of friends and kindred. The risk is terrible,—the risk of dying among strangers. It is a beautiful parting prayer of one of the Eastern nations, "May you die among your kindred."

Change is the great health-principle involved, and the more complete that change the better,—change of air, of scene, of occupation, of food, of mode of preparation, of associations ; hence the people of the city should go into the country, the deeper into its recesses the better; and persons from the country cannot do better than to spend a month or two or three in the city during warm weather. The city ways would be a constant source of interesting observation and study ; would be a means of elevation, of expansion ; would give a greater breadth of view of things. Under ordinary favorable circumstances, a man becomes more of a man, and a woman more of a woman, by the contemplation of, and mingling with city life; their views of things become greatly enlarged, while the conduct and the manners are elevated and improved. As a matter of economy to those coming from the country, it is largely in favor of the city, as compared with the sea-side, the watering places, and other fashionable resorts ; for at all of these the charges vary from two to six dollars a day, which, with inevitable "extras," is increased · by fifty per cent., and all this for rooms often so small, that for toilet purposes one must remain in bed or leave the house until the other is dressed ; rooms with rickety "cottage furniture," soiled carpets, cloddy beds, bad attendance, and everlasting din and dust and dirt everywhere. In New York City, in any summer, large, elegant rooms, in com-

modious brown-stone houses, with all the appointments of cultivated life, in or near the best streets, can be had for ten dollars a
week easily.   A ride to and through the Central Park and return
home costs less than half a dollar; for half that amount a person
can go to the Park and return from any part of New York, and
can spend an hour or two there without any expense, with new
faces, and new equipages, and new views, every day and every
hour.   For a dollar one may take an omnibus to South Ferry, go
on a boat down the bay, in sight of the sea, spend a few hours
on shore on Staten Island, take a picnic, and return by the time
of the setting sun.   Between sunrise and dark an excursion can
be made to Long Branch, with sea-bathing, a delicious dinner,
and a movable, changing, splendid panorama of elegant men, of
handsome women, of beautiful equipages; returning to spend the
night in large and airy chambers, with no mosquitoes, no drunken
revelry, nor dice, nor cards, nor thimble-riggery, nor noisy halls,
nor degrading gallantries.

Then the promenades in Broadway or on Fifth Avenue are a
source of never-failing pleasure, amusement, and health; the
sidewalks are always dry, and in the hottest days there is a shady
side to every street, and a saunter can be made for minutes or
for hours; every step something new to meet the eye, something
lively to attract the attention.   In addition to these are city
preaching, lectures, libraries, and reading-rooms.

DANGERS OF KEROSENE.

Kerosene oil can be made which will not explode, and any one
with two ideas can find out whether it is fit to be used in a lamp
or not.   Take a saucer of warm water, say a hundred degrees,
that is not hotter than a healthy heat, pour some of the oil on the
water, and apply a flame to it; if the flame sets it on fire, it is
not safe; if it does not set it on fire, it is safe, and you should
tell every friend and neighbor where they can purchase kerosene
oil which cannot blow them up, burn them to death, or scare
them out of their wits.   If the clothing should take fire, lie down
instantly and roll yourself up in a carpet, blanket, or anything

else at hand.   If you stand up while the clothes are on fire, the
flame rises about the head and face, and breathing it in is certain
death.   If you lie down, the flame goes upward, and the face is
untouched.   Rolling yourself in a carpet or blanket smothers the
fire, as in the cut which follows.

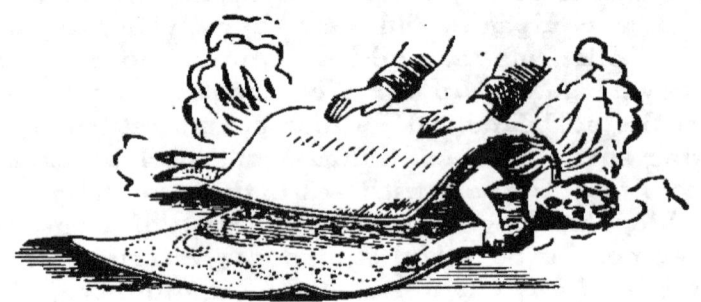

FOUR INDEPENDENCES.—To do without liquor.   To do without
tobacco.   To do without warm water in shaving.   To do without
going in debt.   Happy and great is the man who has force of will
enough to put his foot on the ground and say, "It shall be done."

A pig would not get drunk twice ; he who goes in debt sells his
independence and his manhood, and is only fit to be under a despot's rule.   As to the use of tobacco, it is so filthy, so disgusting,
so beastly, that it is really a wonder that any gentleman could
condescend to employ it either in chewing, snuffing, or smoking ;
and yet there are good men who are content to live under these
slaveries.   It has been said that a man may rid himself of the vice
of chewing by taking, after each meal, coarsely ground gentian
root, chew it well, and swallow the saliva, for a few weeks.

CHANGE OF CLOTHING.

IN March and early April the fitful weather is often more trying to the constitution than the steady and severe cold of mid-
winter, resulting in the death of many from pneumonia, that is,
inflammation of the lungs.   Such results are forwarded sometimes
by changing the warm winter clothing for a lighter kind.   Many
lives might be saved every year if no winter garment was laid
aside before May.   It is always safer to be dressed too warmly
than to have so little clothing as to allow the body to become

chilly. The rule should be to dress abundantly warm, at least until the spring weather has become more settled.

Colds may often be avoided, if, when there is a feeling of even slight chilliness, a brisk walk were taken and continued until a pleasant glow is felt all over the body ; for the want of this, or its equivalent in some form of exercise or work, the chilliness has continued and increased until a cold has been taken which it may require weeks to cure.

If persons can manage to keep the feet and hands naturally and comfortably warm, such a thing as a bad cold would seldom be taken. It is through cold feet and cold hands that troublesome diseases come to multitudes.

DROWNING

Is death by smothering. No air can get to the lungs, any more than when a pillow is pressed over the face, or a rope around the neck, closing the windpipe. The very first thing to be done is to send for a physician. The next, right on the shore, to take off all the clothing, wipe dry, wrap up the body in a blanket, and as quick as possible clear out the nose and mouth of any water or other obstruction there, and take means to get all the water you can out of the lungs, so that the air can take its place. While some are doing this, let others get bottles of hot water to put under the arm-pits and to the feet, so as to invite back warmth.

Turn the face downwards, with one arm supporting the forehead, so as to keep the nose and mouth from being buried in the sand or dust or mattress, or whatever else the person is lying upon. This also enables the tongue to fall forward, leaving the windpipe free, and the water falls naturally out of the mouth when any comes up from the lungs.

If breathing begins, assist the circulation of the blood by putting the hands under the blanket, and rubbing upwards, so as to keep the blood along towards the heart and lungs, where it will be warmed. Hot flannels and hot bricks should be applied, or hot sand in bags, to the soles of the feet, to the thighs, pit of stomach, as well as in the arm-pits. If now the patient can be got into the house, put him in the airiest, dryest, warmest room, windows open, giving every five minutes at first a teaspoonful of spirits, or a tablespoon of wine, or hot tea or coffee. Keep in bed, and encourage sleep as much as possible.

But if there is little or no breathing turn the patient on one side,—the right is better,—put snuff or hartshorn to the nose, or tickle it with a feather, or put the feather down the throat, for it excites cough, which helps to clear the lungs. Dash hot water, then cold water, on face and chest, and repeat from time to time with scarcely an appreciable interval for the first minute or two, but desist as soon as a convulsive attempt at breathing is noticed. If this does not seem to avail, put the patient on his face again, supporting the forehead with his arm as before ; a folded coat or pillow or any bundle, even a log or a stone under his belly, turn him gently on one side, then rapidly on his face ; repeat this as rapidly as you can, at least fifteen times in a minute, keeping a firm pressure all the while between the shoulder-blades, behind and below them. The object of all this is to bring about something like the artificial mode of breathing, for when the patient is on his side the air will enter the lungs ; when on his face it naturally comes out. While all this is going on, apply well-warmed flannels to feet and hands, and keep them dry, because dampness, by evaporation, carries heat away from the system rapidly, while the object should be to keep in it every atom of heat possible.

If this does not answer within five minutes, try another plan : Put the patient on his back, a small pillow or other bundle under his shoulders. Draw out the tongue, and run a string around it, so as to keep it out, thus leaving the windpipe uncovered. Take the arms above the elbows and draw them up steadily above the head. Keep them there two seconds. This expands the chest, and the air rushes into the lungs. Then draw the arms down to the sides, and close to them, pressing them against the sides of the chest for two seconds. This presses the air out of the chest. If this operation can be performed about fifteen times in a minute, the greatest chances are offered for a restoration of the breathing. The instant that is noticed, apply heat and warmth as quickly as possible, as above named. Bear in mind, in all efforts to restore drowned persons, *First.*—No time is to be lost, hence make the efforts immediately on the shore, unless it is cold enough to cause chilliness. *Second.*—The patient wants air in the lungs instead of water, hence get all the water out as quick as possible, and clear away everything from the mouth, throat, and nose, calculated to hinder breathing. *Third.*—All the motions intended to imitate the breathing operation should be quickly done as we breathe in health ; about 18 times in a minute.

If the person has been in the water for some time, or there are wounds or bruises ; if the eyelids are half closed, and the pupils are larger than natural, the skin getting paler and colder, life may sometimes be restored after twenty minutes' apparent cessation of breathing. In one case, a patient came to life after eight hours were spent in the treatment. If there is the slightest lividity of the face, or a twitching of one of its muscles, or a convulsive movement in any limb or other part of the body, it is a sign of life still existing, and it may be invited back.

All intelligent persons, especially heads of families, owe it to themselves to read these instructions over and over again, until they are most thoroughly understood and remembered, with the reason for everything firmly fixed in the mind. It would not be out of the way to practise the motions on the living body, for any day and any hour there may be the sad occasion for using them on the body of some child or brother or sister or friend.

A small dog was put into a tub of water. The instant the head went under a rapid inspiration of water was taken, and then a jerking expiration, which carried out a considerable amount of air. Thus the water took the place of the air in the lungs. No further effort to breathe was noticed, and in less than five minutes

THE DOG WAS DEAD.

The lips were closed, the top of the windpipe shut, and very little water was found in the branches of the windpipe.

A man fell into a well, and went under the water. He had his senses all about him, and he found himself trying to breathe out all the air he could, and aiming to prevent himself from swallowing water ; for the next relief to getting fresh air into the lungs is that of getting the old air—that which has been used and is foul—out. Soon after his recovery he vomited sand and mud. A young girl who was in the well with him used no precautions, and convulsively sucked muddy sand into her lungs, which inflamed them, and for several days she was spitting up sandy mud from time to time.

These things show that death by drowning is simply a suffocation. The water in the windpipe is that taken in by the first convulsive effort at drawing in the breath; the lungs, being supplied with no new air, cease to act; the pulse ceases to beat; the heart stops, and the man is dead.   This mode of death is called

ASPHYXIA,

which means, literally, " without pulse."

Sometimes it is a matter of very great consequence to identify a dead body, and to this end it is necessary, if the features are changed, to restore them as much as possible to what they were at the instant of death.   This is done in a measure, sometimes, thus : Cover the cleansed body in water ; pass through it a stream of chlorine gas.   This whitens the skin, improved by adding some common salt to the water, and injecting tincture of steel into some of the blood-vessels of the face.

As lives are lost every summer at watering-places, these suggestions are seasonable, and ought to be kept about the person, or within convenient reach.

If a person is struggling in the water, approach him if possible from behind, and raise the head only out of the water by the hair ; and as the body loses a third or more of its weight when it is in the water, it requires but little strength to keep the head out of water, and to drag the body to the shore.   For the same reason it does not hurt the person much who is thus held up and dragged.

The grasp of a drowning person is so unreasoning and so convulsive, that every effort should be made by the rescuer to escape his clutches.

Persons in the water who cannot swim, can keep their heads above the surface for a considerable time by commencing at once a vigorous and quick treading operation, with both arms extended, and the palms of the hands resting on the water, for, small as they are, some support is afforded.

At other times, a person who has some presence of mind can support himself for half an hour in the water, and even longer, by throwing himself on his back, clasping both hands under him, throwing his face upward upon the water, his feet extended, so that the nose only is out of the water.   He can thus float for a considerable time without the expenditure of much strength.

If a person breaks through the ice, as in

SKATING,

or in any other way, help is best given, and with greatest safety, by pushing a long rail or board or log of wood on the ice, until it reaches over the edge where it is broken, up to the person in the water, who can hold on to the end, and by this assistance can crawl out upon the edge of the ice, which might not be strong enough to bear both the rescued and the rescuer. If no bit of wood is at hand, then the rescuer might lie down on the ice, flat on his belly, and crawl towards the edge, keeping as large a part of the body on the ice as possible, for the strain on the ice is less in proportion to the surface to be supported. If more than one person is present to help save, let one go forward as before, and the next one hold on to his heel.

These things should be thought over carefully by all, that when there is occasion for them, the mind should feel at home in directing their execution.

WORMS.

ABOUT thirty kinds in all have been found in the human body. As there are three descriptions of living things which infest the skin of man, the head-louse, the crab-louse, and the body-louse; so there are three kinds of living things which find their dwelling and feeding places in the interior, in the alimentary canal: the pin-worm, the fish-worm, and the tape-worm.

THE FISH-WORM,

so called from its resemblance in shape, size, and color to the worm used for baiting hooks to catch fish, and which appears in such numbers when the ground is turned up in the garden for spring plantings, called technically *Ascaris lumbricoides*, or round worm, mostly found in the small intestines, but sometimes makes its way into the large intestines and into the stomach, even coming up into the throat and out of the mouth, and sometimes it has been half a foot to half a yard long, and as large round as a gold guinea. It is only when a good many are together that any special harm may be done. These worms get into the body by drinking water from shallow wells or muddy streams. Sometimes in adults they cause nausea, vomiting, and various symptoms of indigestion for weeks together, until they are vomited or voided. There is no symptom or set of symptoms which certainly indicate the presence of worms in adults or children, except the type of the worm itself after it leaves the body, although in children they may be suspected when they are observed to pick the nose, grind the teeth in sleep, complain of itching at the lower outlet of the bowels, swollen belly, irregular appetite, and sometimes convulsions; but one or all of these symptoms may arise from several other ailments. So there is no really certain proof that an infant, child, or adult "has worms," except the sight of one expelled.

PIN-WORMS

are sometimes a source of intolerable discomfort, by causing an inappeasable itching at the exit of the rectum, especially when getting a little warm after first going to bed. They are called pin-worms by the common people, because they are almost as slender as a pin, and short, from a twelfth to half an inch long; sometimes they come away in incredible quantities; besides the itching, they sometimes cause a great deal of nervous irritation, and keep the whole system in a debilitated condition. Inject a teaspoonful or two of camphor water, made by putting a piece of camphor into a small bottle and adding a teaspoonful of water, shake it and use it; the water may be added from time to time until the camphor has disappeared. Or take a teaspoonful of the tincture of *Cocculus Indicus* to a teacup half full of common water, and use it as an injection alone, or with the camphor water, but either may be stronger. Sometimes an injection of lime-water, as obtained from a druggist, answers the purpose; or press mercurial ointment into the part, and retain it over night; or take twelve grains of santonine, and thin it with cocoa butter, enough to make four rolls an inch long, cone-shaped, and near as large as the little finger; introduce one of these into the rectum on going to bed every night. This is a valuable remedy, and seldom fails.

TAPE-WORMS

have no sex originally, but if one of them gets into the human body in such a way that it can get some air, as in the alimentary canal, then it takes on sex, and reproduces itself. It has a head, with a short neck, to which is appended a kind of flat link; then comes another link, another and another, growing in length all the time, until there is a chain of three or four hundred links or more. The links at the end of the tail are cast off, sometimes six or eight a day; the whole animal may be some thirty feet long. There are no symptoms certainly indicating their presence, except seeing one or more of these links in the dejections. When one or more of these segments have been observed, it will be found that certain symptoms have been more or less present, such as irregular appetite, disturbed sleep, despondency, sadness, dyspepsia, itching of the nose, and general nervous irritation. Not long since an apparatus was devised for fishing it out through the throat. Eating largely of

PUMPKIN SEEDS

has the credit of having cured several serious cases of tape-worm. Gourd seeds peeled and made into a paste with honey, about two hundred at a time, taken fasting, as the pumpkin seeds are, have been efficient in a number of cases.

These remedies are more efficient if nothing has been eaten for twenty or twenty-four hours; this causes the worm to be ravenously hungry, and thus to take into its stomach what its instincts would otherwise forbid. Or make a strong tea of pumpkin or gourd seed, drink it at bed-time plentifully, not having eaten anything whatever since breakfast; the next morning a strong cathartic will bring away the entire worm, dead or alive. In one case this brought a worm away, twenty-five feet long.

HOUSE POISONS.

MANY persons have sickened and died after moving into new houses; others, after sleeping for a few nights, or even a single night, in the "spare room" of a friend. A few years ago four children in one family sickened and died, one after another. In 1860 a woman sickened in Boston, manifesting all the symptoms of having been poisoned; she recovered to a certain extent, but never regained her health. In the case of the four children, the paper on the wall was found to contain three grains of arsenic in every square foot; in the case of the woman, a removal of the paper on the wall was followed with improvement in her health.

In all cases of pining sickness, when there is no appreciable reason for it, two things ought to be promptly done: change the room and the water; live all the time in an apartment without paper on the walls, or curtains about the windows, or any green color in the carpets; in addition, use water which is obtained from the roof of the house, and no other; or obtain water which is at least half a mile away, from a spring or well, many feet higher than the usual supplies, because the water may be poisoned by the lead pipes in the house, or more likely by the drainage of barn-yards, pig-pens, hen houses, and privies finding its way into the well or spring lower down than those which supply the family. As to curtains, carpets, and wall paper having a green color, it may be regarded as a certainty that the color is produced by the use of arsenic; and the glazing material, of whatever color, is mainly composed of a poisonous preparation of lead.

Precaution should be taken to exclude all green candies, all green toys, all glazed materials, even visiting cards, for a little child died recently by chewing a visiting card; it had a sweetish taste, having a glaze made of sugar of lead. In a toy box of water-colors, one block of green paint, weighing forty grains, contained ten grains of arsenic; the green in lamp shades contains a large amount of arsenic, as do also the green papers which envelop the bon-bons of the confectioner. A tarlatan dress contained eight grains of white arsenic to every square foot of the material. Chemists are of the opinion that the dust of the arsenic is detached from these various objects by the moving air, or by handling, and is thus taken directly into the lungs, thence introduced into the blood. If any material supposed to contain arsenic is put into a small amount of hartshorn, spirits of ammonia, if white arsenic is present the liquid will have a bluish tint; if further proof is desired, pour a little of this bluish liquid on crystals of nitrate of silver; if arsenic is present, there will be a yellowish deposit on the crystals.

But these things are not new, only disregarded; for a hundred years ago a law was passed in France forbidding the use of arsenic in making any colors for domestic uses; but its employment was so profitable in coloring many things, vases, artificial flowers, and the like, that the law was gradually more and more disregarded; and when its re-enactment was proposed the shopkeepers rose in opposition, and declared it would ruin their business. Within a few years, in England, a paper-maker declared that he used four thousand pounds of arsenic every week in his workshops for the purpose of coloring and sizing.

A preparation for destroying vermin about houses is made largely of arsenic, called by various names; the most common is

SCHEELE'S GREEN,

being the arsenite of copper, the aceto-arsenite of copper, or

STEINFURT GREEN,

all dangerous to health and life, and should be sedulously excluded from every dwelling-house.

GENERAL HEALTH.

THERE are various forms of sickness and suffering which cannot be directly reached by medicine or medical or surgical appliances, and can only be benefited and cured by obtaining and maintaining a high state of general health for weeks and months, and even years in some cases, thus wearing the disease out of the system, "growing out of it," as children sometimes do.

A BEAUTIFUL LITTLE GIRL

of two years old, mother dead, was noticed to stand with her legs crossed, and would not change her position, holding to a chair, which she would continue to do, unless forcibly removed; if not removed the body would gradually settle down until it nearly touched the floor; the face meanwhile became motionless, a blank expression; her hands rigid and cold; she would then gradually regain her self-possession; nothing seemed to be the matter with her; she said it did not hurt her, and that she could not help it;

18

one person suggested worms; some worm-medicine was given, and brought some away; but the habit remained unchanged. These occurrences would take place, at several hours' intervals, several times a day; then none for several days. Physicians were consulted far and near; nothing whatever seemed to make any impression on the case. One thought it was epileptic; another, a vagary of the reproductive function, only to be relieved by a surgical operation, to be nothing for life thereafter. When she indulged in the habit most freely, she was pale, peevish, and fretful. She was an only child, and the father, a merchant of high position, was very greatly concerned; for if epileptic, the mind would eventually give way, and if of the other nature, there were very great professional objections to such an operation. It is always difficult to get little children to take medicine. The author gave it as his opinion that it was not epileptic, not an organic malady, that no such such fearful operation was necessary, that there was no abnormal action of the reproductive functions; in short that it originated from a deranged condition of the stomach, liver, and bowels, and that she could be cured without any medicine whatever. She was perfectly cured within two months, and remains cured to this day. The advice given is here detailed at length, with a view to stating some practical suggestions at the close of this article.

First. Send her to the country; it was summer.

Second. Let her be under the eye of some relative, who feels a personal interest in her.

Third. Let it be in a family where there are several other children of her age and a little older, so that playing with them may give her free employment.

Fourth. Encourage her to be out of doors in the open air from morning to night.

Fifth. Let her eat three times a day, with all the fruit, berries, and melons she can eat as dessert after breakfast and dinner, at regular hours, and nothing whatever between meals.

Sixth. See to it that there should be one or two actions of the bowels every day; if not that much, take enough castor oil, night and morning, to cause that effect without fail.

Seldom has a father been relieved of a greater burden when he saw his little daughter the happiest and the healthiest child in all that part of the country. The lesson to be learned is:—

When anything is the matter with a little child, or even a grown person, and the nature of it is obscure in the judgment of all, before any medicine is given, carry out the principles involved in the above treatment; at least for a week or two notice the points involved in the case.

First. She was sent to the country for the benefit of its pure air.

Second. She was to eat regularly, in order to give the stomach some chance to rest, and get a little strength to digest the next meal.

Third. She was to be with children of her own age, to amuse her, to be a temptation to keep out of doors, for every breath of such air drawn in went out of the body loaded with the impurities abstracted from the blood, leaving behind its pure oxygen to impart its life to the system.

Fourth. By having children to play with she was amused—she was tempted to run about pleasurably, every step she took helping to wear out of the system some of its useless particles.

Fifth. A plentiful supply of berries and fruits, the acid of which cooled off the system; kept it free from fever, kept the bowels open, without the need of medicine, all combining to bring about abundant agreeable exercise in the open air and a free state of the bowels.

There is no disease known to men which can be benefited or cured by any means, which such things will not benefit or cure in proportion as they are carried out.

This case proves conclusively the truth of the opening statement: that some ailments can be eradicated, when all other means have failed, simply by keeping up the general health.

There is another case in the author's hands now, which, if benefited at all, giving a little start with a dose or two of medicine, will be benefited by keeping up the general health.

Three years ago a young lady received, by the merest accident, a very violent blow upon her closed mouth, nearer the chin than the nose. She became insensible, and so remained for many days, with an attack of brain-fever. She has been entirely deaf ever since; scarcely any circulation below the knees; the feet always icy cold.

Incessant pain in the head.

Steady pain in the throat; can't see well enough to go anywhere after dark. Pains all the time at the top of the lungs.

Great shortness of breath on slight exertion.

Can't read or sew.

Bowels regular, appetite always ravenous, bad taste in the morning, and tongue always coated; better in summer than in winter. Sleep pretty good; very chilly.

This excellent lady can have better health, and eventually may grow out of her ailments, for she is only twenty-two. This opinion is given because being better in summer than winter shows that the open pores of the skin allow the escape of more bad matters than in winter, and if this escape could be increased she would necessarily be better in proportion; the fruit diet, the outdoor exercise, with the extra drains from the system, by a little medicine once a week, must necessarily be followed by encouraging results, if the feet can be kept warm, to draw the excess of blood from the head, which causes the pains and deafness there. A single liver pill once a week will greatly expedite her improvement, if the feet are kept warm, and the bowels very free every day.

Hence it is so frequently advised, in these pages, to keep up the general health, which involves two things,—a plentiful supply, at regular hours, of plain, nourishing food; abundant exercise of a pleasurable character in the open air every day, with a full, free action of the bowels every twenty-four hours, without medicine if possible, but the free use of it to cause that effect certainly if necessary; the only expense of the whole being a bottle of castor-oil, or its equivalent. There are internal maladies which can neither be seen nor reached, but may be cured certainly and permanently.

Long running sores can very readily be made to heal up by local applications; but the diseased conditions of the blood which caused them must be corrected by improving the general health, purifying the blood, otherwise the sore which seemed to be cured will attack some more vital part, to ruin and destroy.

A man is in good general health when the bowels act regularly every day.

When there is no bad taste in the mouth of mornings; when there is regularly a good relish for breakfast, a vigorous appetite for dinner at noon, and hunger enough for supper to make plain bread and butter and a cup of tea very acceptable, with no unpleasant reminder whatever after eating.

When the feet are always comfortably warm.

When the sleep is always sound and refreshing.

When the pulse is not over seventy beats in a minute midway between meals, and after having sat quietly for a quarter of an hour, for eating always excites the pulse for an hour or more after a regular meal.

When there is a general feeling of wellness, with a cheerful, lively, genial disposition.

But a man may be said to have good general health if the following conditions are uniformly present:

1. A regular good appetite.
2. No unpleasant reminders after eating.
3. A daily action of the bowels.
4. A pulse not over seventy.
5. Feet all the time comfortably warm.
6. Sound, refreshing sleep.

These six things show that the main bodily functions are in healthful working order, and that the blood is pure and good. To bring about the six conditions named, three things are necessary, and this is still further reduced to two points.

To eat properly.

To exercise judiciously.

By doing these two things habitually, three out of four of all ordinary ailments, acute or chronic, could be promptly cured; they will cure more maladies than medicine; they will cure many which medicine fails to reach.

Begin thus. At bedtime of a day, during which since noon dinner nothing has been eaten, take a good warm bath in a warm room, with plenty of white soap and water, and give the whole body, in every part of it, a most thorough scrubbing, washing, and rinsing. Take a liver pill according to the directions under that heading. For breakfast next morning, as soon as you feel a little hungry, take a single cup of hot drink and some cold bread and butter. Not sooner than five hours after take a bowl of any kind of soup, with the crust of cold bread broken into it, or in its place a bowl of oatmeal gruel, or a plate of cracked wheat. For supper take the same as at breakfast. Eat nothing whatever between meals.

The more you can be out in the open air from breakfast to sundown the better. The more lively the exercise, or the more interested you are in your work, the better; only one thing is to be guarded against, do not carry the exercise to fatigue, always stop

before you are much tired. All these things have been advised
to favor the action of the pill, which is to give you a good start
by clearing out the liver; this is aided by drinking abundantly of
cold water, if thirsty between meals, but none within half an hour
of eating. On the day after the liver pill has ceased its action,
no passage from the bowels is needed, that is, if you take a pill
on Saturday night, it acts during Sunday more than once, you
need no action on Monday, and so whenever you take one of
these pills, with these exceptions, you should arrange that the
bowels should act every day afterwards in one of three ways:

By an enema.

By medicine.

By the character of your food; this last is best, because it is a
natural remedy, is always safe, and when it is efficient is more
permanently so.

The first thing to be done, by each one for himself, is to
notice what kind of food or drink tends to loosen his bowels,
and use that more freely. If your attention has not been directed
to that point use the experiences of others, and on trial yours may
coincide with theirs. Some will tell you that they regulate their
bowels by going to the privy at a regular hour every morning
after breakfast, and, in the absence of any inclination, solicit
nature; do not be hurried away by your business; haste and
anxiety tend to drive off inclination; rather than strain it is better
to divert the mind by reading a newspaper or a book.

Others will say that a glass or two of cold water or of salt
water, on rising, is efficient.

A third says that making breakfast entirely of oatmeal gruel
or of cracked wheat is good in his case. And although what is
availing in one case may not be in another, yet by inquiry it is
quite certain that good suggestions will be had by comparing
ideas.

If the bowels are very stubborn at first, and if it is a defect in
your case, has been a prominent one for some time, weeks and
this time will be saved by taking an enema; and as soon as
is a regular action for a few days, omit it. Or medicines
taken. See the article "Castor-Oil." Take just as
no more, night and morning, as will secure one free
d when that has been secured for several days, begin to
the amount. Omit one of the doses, and after a while

the other; if the oil cannot be taken, then try Epsom salts night and morning, just enough to produce the desired effect, and leave it off as soon as you can; or a dinner pill may be tried for a while. But during all this time be making a steady effort to find out some kind of food which has a loosening tendency, such as stewed fruits, prunes, dried figs, tomatoes. If none of these avail, you must get out of the way of taking medicine to keep the bowels regular, for as a habit it is exceedingly mischievous. When other things fail, resort to a

FRUIT AND COARSE BREAD DIET.

For breakfast, take cracked wheat, thoroughly boiled until quite soft; put on it some sugar or salt or butter; make your entire breakfast of that, except that, as a dessert, take one or two oranges or apples, or a saucer of fresh, ripe berries, in their natural state; or one or two baked apples, or some stewed fruit. This last may be taken with the wheat, if the others, which are better, cannot be obtained, either preserved, canned, or fresh.

Dinner—Graham bread, or bread made of the whole grain of wheat, one vegetable, and any kind of lean meat, with a dessert of fruits or berries, as at breakfast, as many as can be eaten in their natural state, as if picked by yourself from the bushes. If sugar or milk or cream, or any other artificial sweet is used with berries, except currants, the cooling, opening, liver-acting effect of the natural acid is to that extent antagonized. No fluid should be taken with the berries, as it tends to make them sour on the stomach, and also dilutes that acid which gives them their cooling, healthful, opening qualities.

SUPPER.

The last meal of the day should be taken about sundown, and should be made of coarse bread and stewed fruits, or berries, raw or preserved, and nothing else. Nothing whatever should be taken between meals, so as to allow the stomach some time to rest; for it is frequent eating, giving no opportunity for repose, which makes half the miserable dyspeptics in the land. No body, no part of the system can work incessantly; even the busy heart is quiet one-third of the time.

EXERCISE,

by which is meant riding, walking, or working, or active engage-
ments in business, more completely expressed by the term of

MUSCULAR ACTIVITIES

in the open air, is essential to good general health. Sedentary
persons should spend two or three hours in the forenoon out of
doors, and one or two in the afternoon, from April to December;
and two or three hours in the middle of the day, for the remainder of the year. That exercise most avails which is taken,

RAIN OR SHINE,

not when the rain is falling; but it seldom happens that it does
so for twelve or fifteen hours in succession. There are intervals
of which advantage should be taken. If one thing is allowed as
an excuse one day, then other excuses will prevent other days.
The only safe plan is to make exercise in the open air every day,
for several hours, imperative, for two very strong reasons—first,
the fresh, pure air is needed just as much one day as another;
and the worse the weather, the heavier and the damper it is, the
more do we need the purest air, which is always to be had out of
doors; for, under all circumstances, the indoor air is the out-
door air tainted with the emanations from food, from the persons of the inmates, from their breathing, and from the dust from
carpets, curtains, and other hangings, given off at every touch,
and every breath of wind through door or window. Hence out-
door air is more needed in bad weather than good.

Second.—Food is as much needed when it rains all day as if it
were perfectly clear and sunshiny. We eat quite as much; that
food is to be digested. The very object of the outdoor air is to
promote digestion; and if it is promoted only in good weather,
then the blood it makes is bad, and corrupts the whole mass of
blood in the body, for it is all mixed together; thus the want of
exercise for one day corrupts the whole blood of the body, requiring a week often to rectify it. Hence the loss of time in
losing one day's outdoor exercise in the pursuit of a high state
of general health.

If, however, the person is actually sick, or if it should storm the whole day, eat nothing after breakfast until dinner-time, then take nothing but a single cup of tea, a single piece of bread and butter, and some stewed or raw fruit; for supper, some cold bread and butter, and a cup of tea and nothing else whatever, for the stomach may digest well this small amount of food, where it would not digest a large amount.

Most persons have observed how dull and stupid and inactive they feel when kept in the house all day; why, by the time night comes they are perfectly miserable; it is because they have eaten as much, if not more, than if engaged in active business; but food is needed in proportion to the exercise taken; hence, if as much is eaten on a day in which nothing is done, the result is that the food is not made into good blood, and more blood is made than there was need for, therefore the body is oppressed with an excess of blood, and with the pound or two of waste matters which remain in the system, but which would have been worked out of it had the usual outdoor exercise been taken, thus leaving the system oppressed, not only with the pound or more of waste matter, not worked out of it, but with the additional weight of the food eaten that day; no wonder that persons feel dull and stupid from remaining indoors all day, with these several pounds of extra matter oppressing the system.

These remarks are applicable to professional men, mothers and daughters and students, who are necessarily indoors a greater part of the time.

But many persons have no available method of outdoor exercise but walking (which article see); others have not the strength to walk half an hour; but they will soon have the strength, if a systematic and persistent effort is made to carry out the spirit of the suggestions made. Walk a block or a hundred yards and return home, lie down and rest, and in another hour repeat the walk, and so on, every hour of the day from breakfast to sundown. In less than a week you will be less fatigued in walking two hundred yards than the first hundred the first day; in this manner feel your way along, always stopping short of actual fatigue, and in the intervals, if very weak, have absolute rest on a sofa or bed. Keep these two ideas always in view, stop before much tired, and have perfect and plentiful rest between. But remember there is a time when all must die; that event is foreshadowed to you only if, after exercise, you feel worse than you did before, more weary, more tired than when you started out, for the presumption is that a dangerous disease is impending, or that the powers of life are failing. When you really cannot take exercise out of doors you are dying, and should have medical attendance. But, on the other hand, if you feel all the better for outdoor exercise when it has not been carried to fatigue, then it is pretty certain that you have vitality enough to be well again. Thus it is that in the management of disease, especially in those forms of it which are rather obscure or altogether inexplicable, the improvement of the general health is found to be

THE GREAT CURE-ALL,

and that is to be secured : First, By a clean skin. Second, By plain, nourishing food, mainly coarse breads and fruits. Third, A great part of every day to be spent in pleasurable activities in the open air. Fourth, A full and free action of the bowels every twenty-four hours, without medicine if possible, if not, then have that action by any means in your power. Castor-oil or salts, which articles see, are the most familiar and simple, or the liver pill twice a month.

SIMPLICITY OF MEDICAL PRACTICE.

FIVE classes of disease comprehend nearly all human maladies. Two medical principles are adapted to the cure of all those that are curable :—

First. Lessening the amount of the blood.

Second. Getting out of the system whatever is useless and hurtful.

Then Nature comes in to restore vigor to the system and health and life to the whole organization.

In a few hours' reading and mental application the whole system of medical practice and hygiene can be made as plain and simple and comprehensive as one of the most familiar demonstrations of Euclid.

The inflammations or the "Phlegmasiæ," as physicians like to term them, comprehend at once a large class of ordinary maladies. Inflammation means "flame-like," which we know is reddish, or the color of flame. If we see a red eye, we say it is inflamed. If we look at the edges of a sore, we observe that it is of an angry red color; we speak of it, also, as being inflamed. Medical writers have a very convenient way of classifying and distinguishing diseases of this character by attaching the word "itis" to the end of the name of a part, and that signifies that such a part is inflamed, "itis" meaning "flaming."

There are no less than eighteen common diseases included in this list, and one medicine is more or less applicable to their cure, in some one stage or other, and that medicine is the Liver Pill. The name of branches of the windpipe is Bronchi, add "itis" to that, and leave out one "i," and we have the very familiar name of

BRONCHITIS.

The name of the outer covering of the lungs is Pleura; add "itis" to that, and leave out the "a," and we have the common name of

PLEURITIS,

or Pleurisy. Such is the beautiful simplicity of medical nomenclature; simply adding "itis" to the Greek or Latin name of a part means that the part is in a state of inflammation. The part is inflamed, is red because the blood makes it so, for the blood is red, and there is more blood there than is natural, hence it is redder than natural.

But more, we know that this is arterial blood, for that is the reddest; we also know that this arterial blood is confined in the little arteries, that they are fuller of blood than natural, and being fuller, these little vessels distend, swell out, like a bladder, take up more room than they are entitled to, and, doing so, press against some other part, which must necessarily have less room than it is entitled to, hence it complains, as certainly as a man complains when he is crowded by his neighbor on the same seat, monopolizing more than his share of room. The next neighbor to every artery is a nerve, and this nerve being pressed, complains, as witness the slightest touch of the nerve of a tooth with the tiniest point of a needle or bit of softest wood; hence in all inflammations there is not only redness, but each artery is distended; hence there must be swelling, and, as just seen, pain; but as the blood is warm, the natural supply brings the natural amount of warmth, but there being more blood there than is natural, there is more heat there than is natural, and we call it fever; hence in all inflammations there are four things—

Redness,   Pain,
Swelling,   Heat.

All this is induced by overfulness of the arteries.   They are

CONGESTED.

But the veins are as numerous as the arteries, and are capable of the same overfulness, the same congestions, inducing by such congestions a still larger class of maladies; these are called

ZYMOSES,

or zymotic diseases, from a word meaning filth, which, entering the stomach by swallowing and the lungs by breathing, makes its way direct into the blood, makes it impure, unhealthy, poisonous, changing its color from red to dark, or even black, and its consistency to that of tar in some forms of sickness; so thick sometimes that when a lancet is introduced it will not flow out; in this condition it distends the veins of the part, not necessarily giving pain, and if it does it is not the sharp pain which is occasioned by the bounding blood of the arteries, where sometimes every throb is an agony; but if pain at all, it is a dull hurting, a grumbling. All forms of fever, all epidemic diseases, all contagious diseases, plagues and pestilences are zymotic diseases, originating in impurities in the atmosphere breathed; when, for example, a person goes to the bedside of a man who has the small-pox, if he has not been vaccinated, he will take the small-pox, even although he may not have touched the patient; it is because minute particles of matter and odors from the sick man were in the air around him, and this was taken direct into the lungs. Many a person has taken the small-pox from passing one who has it in the street.

A SUPPOSITION.

All the great northern lakes from Superior to Ontario are reservoirs of water, and are connected together in such a manner, that if the latter was emptied in whole or in part, all the other lakes would have their supplies of water diminished in the same proportion. If a clock in good running order is stopped, and any one wheel is started, the whole clock, every wheel in it, is started also.

There are a number of glands in the human system, which may be called reservoirs, or wheels, or manufactories—the liver manufactures bile, the kidneys water, and so on; but they are so connected that they make a grand machine, which is disordered in its workings in all forms of disease, but if you start one wheel, the whole will soon be in motion. Thus, in bilious fever, if the liver can be made to act properly the man gets well; in cholera, if the kidneys can be made to do their work and send urine into the bladder, we know that the disease is conquered when urination returns.

All these glands are reservoirs of blood, hold large quantities of it; the liver being the largest, holds the most at one time. But in disease the liver is congested, it is altogether too full of blood; but if you diminish the amount of blood in it you diminish the amount of blood in every other reservoir in the body, in every vein, in every artery, hence there is not an ache or a pain in any part of the system which will not be lessened in proportion as the liver has its supply of blood lessened; for when it loses its blood the blood of the other parts of the body flows towards it, in a sense to fill up the vacuum, as the upper lakes send their waters towards Lake Ontario, if any part of its water is drawn off. It will be readily seen, however, that the water in Lake Erie would fall sooner than that of Lake Huron or Michigan, and it would be a considerable time before Superior would be reached, because that body of water is so remote from the lowest lake. Thus it is, that in relieving the liver of a part of its excess of blood, immediate relief from pain or other suffering would be experienced in those parts of the body which are more directly connected with it, while it might be a long time before remote ailments, or those deep-seated, could be reached. Hence, in some ailments, the liver pill, which will always act on the liver, will always modify some sufferings within a few hours, while it might require days to reach those which exist by reason of congestion in very remote parts, in the very extremities of the blood-vessels. These comparisons are not literally true or exact, but they are sufficiently so to express the idea, the general principle of medical action and medical practice; the prime fact being that this liver pill, or any other medicine which so affects the liver directly or indirectly as to lessen the amount of blood in it, is

"GOOD FOR"

a hundred or more different diseases; is curative of them; the chief of which are

THE INFLAMMATIONS.

Bronchitis—Branches of the windpipe.
Cerebritis—Brain.
Dysenteritis—Dysentery.
Endocarditis—In the heart.
Enteritis—The bowels.
Gastritis—Stomach.
Hepatitis—Liver.
Laryngitis—Larynx or voice-making organs.
Meningitis—Membranes of the brain.
Myelitis—Spinal marrow.
Nephritis—Kidneys.
Pericarditis—About the heart.
Peritonitis—About the abdomen.
Pharyngitis—The throat or swallow.
Pleuritis or pleurisy—About the lungs.
Pneumonitis, or pneumonia—The lungs.
Stomatitis—The mouth.
Trachitis—The windpipe or croup.

The way to read the above is stomatitis, or inflammation of the mouth, because stoma means mouth; but to see what a wide range of ailments the above eighteen diseases include, it is only necessary to state that in stomatitis are included not merely an inflammation of the tongue, such as would be caused by drinking anything too hot; but 2, aphthæ, those little ulcers, with whitish surfaces, which are so often seen in the mouths of infants; 3, thrush, where there are a number of small whitish points within the mouth, which, joining, form little curd-like patches or exudations; 4, canker, or ulceration on the inner side of the cheeks, on the gums or the lining of the lips; 5, gangrene, when any ulcerations mortify; 6, mercurial sore mouth, as in salivation; 7, nurses' sore mouth. Here are seven forms of disease connected with inflammation of the mouth, hence the eighteen inflammations above-mentioned would include at least a hundred different ailments, every one of which, in some of its stages, would be benefited by any remedy which would act on the liver, which would have the effect to lessen the quantity of blood there.

The following is an enumeration of the various ailments which may arise from

VENOUS CONGESTIONS,

including all the forms of sickness which owe their origin more or less directly to filth, that is, a bad atmosphere, consequently are avoidable ; let this in passing be impressed on the reader's mind. All zymotic diseases, those arising from a want of cleanliness in person, habitation and atmosphere, are unnecessary, can be avoided, and the individual suffering from them is responsible for them, more or less directly :

Cerebro-spinal fever.	Measles.	Typhus.
Cholera.	Mumps.	Yellow fever.
Diphtheria.	Plague.	Variola.
Diarrhœa.	Pestilence.	Varioloid.
Erysipelas.	Puerperal fever.	Varicella.
Gonorrhœa.	Scarlatina.	Vaccine.
Hydrophobia.	Syphilis.	Whooping-cough.
Influenza.	Typhoid fever.	

In short, all contagious diseases, and the great variety of fevers, intermittent, remittent, relapsing, pernicious, dengue, or break-bone fever.

All the above diseases would be favorably affected by any agent which would have the effect to cause the liver to part with its excess of blood, which would remove its congestion, and which would cure if administered in the early stages; although in reference to some of them, a medicine which would do good in the first stages, might injure at a later period ; just as it often happens, when the physician has employed all the resources of art and science, without seeming good effect, he is compelled as a last resort to withdraw, to be a mere looker-on, a watcher, and

LEAVE IT TO NATURE.

Here comes in one of the most important general principles of the scientific practice of medicine. The great point in almost all dis-

19

eases is to diminish the amount of blood in the liver; the first step in so doing is to make no more blood, by ceasing to eat; all sick animals adopt this method instinctively, and so would man, if his will, or the power of his appetite, did not override instinct. Man is the only animal in the universe who forces his food, who eats when he does not feel like it; who, because when he is well he eats heartily, concludes that if he can only eat heartily he will get well.

When an animal, a pig, is sick he lies down, he rests; if he can, he will get into the warmest place, in the sun, and what is more, he seems to know that it is warmer against something than in an open space; hence he lies up against the side of a house or board fence, or rock, or mud-bank.

Thus, instinct leads the brute creation to adopt the first three requisites to the recovery of the health:—

Abstinence,

Rest,

Warmth.

Reason adds one more, to hasten restoration by using artificial means to hurry out of the system that which oppresses it; to wit, useless waste and poisonous matters, by employing remedies which, acting upon the liver, cause it to convert its excess of blood into bile, which bile is made up of those very particles which were oppressing and poisoning the system.

If these things were done, no more need be done in nine out of ten of all ordinary ailments; hence, those who are by any means thrown on their own resources in the treatment of common sickness, such as is usually incident to ordinary families, could very well get along with having no other medicine in the house than the three kinds of pills already named: the liver pill, the purgative pill, and the laxative pill; in fact, the first-named is a very good substitute for the others, will do all they possibly could do, and would reach many cases and conditions which they could not; hence instead of burdening the memory and confusing the mind with innumerable prescriptions, and the names and details of the symptoms of a great variety of diseases, a simpler, safer, and in the end a generally more efficient practice would be, wherever anything at all is the matter, adopt promptly the first three measures, and if special relief was not obtained within twelve or fifteen hours, then take a liver pill, which will give relief in two or three hours by its general effect on the system, and within ten hours more will so act on the stomach, liver, and bowels as to carry before it a large amount of liquid and solid matters, amounting in all, by the time it has done operating, to several pounds, when the most decided relief will be very generally experienced.

The animal would have been compelled to wait for this general cleaning out for a day or two longer, and for a day or two longer would have been compelled to suffer, and in this is seen the value of medicine. Let the reader bear in mind that in a very large class of ailments, whether the names of them are known or not, whether they be fevers, or rashes, or what are called

CATCHING DISEASES,

as measles, mumps, whooping-cough, and the like, the above treatment without the liver pill would lead to a safe recovery, especially if in the matter of

EATING

good judgment were used. After a liver pill the appetite begins to return generally within a few hours following its action. It is the rule in all cases when purgative or loosening medicines have been taken, to eat moderately.for the first day, that is, be content with taking, at five hours' interval, some bread and butter and hot tea of any kind, or soup with stale or crust bread, or crackers broken into it. If so simple a rule as this was observed after taking purgative medicines of any sort, an incalculable benefit would be derived, not only in preventing relapses, but in the prevention of suffering, and in saving time.

After the day succeeding the first twenty-four hours from taking the pill, the following regulation should be observed in taking food, until the usual health is restored, and may be designated as the

SPECIAL FRUIT DIET.

Breakfast, some cracked wheat, with butter, salt, or sugar on it, followed by fruits, berries, currants, cherries, or melons, in their natural ripe, raw, fresh state, a very little sugar may be added, but better without, so as to have the full force of the natural acids, which have such an admirable effect in cooling off the system; absolutely nothing else for breakfast, or the first meal of the day, fluid or solid.   If the invalid does not relish such a breakfast, nor a bowl of good, hot, well-seasoned soup of any kind, or oatmeal gruel, then he does not need any food, and should wait until he does relish it, until he feels that it would taste really good.

Not sooner than five hours take the same cracked wheat, or wheaten grits, or coarse Graham, or Indian (corn) bread, some lean meat or poultry or fish, and one vegetable, let this be tomatoes when they can be had, followed by the same dessert as at breakfast.   If fresh fruits or berries cannot be had, use such as are canned or dried or preserved, with a small amount of sweetening, the less the better, for in sickness all sweets are " feverish."

At supper a bowl of porridge or oatmeal gruel, or mush made of cornmeal, with a little salt or butter on it, and if to be had, a saucer of ripe berries of some kind, nothing else, liquid or solid. Not a particle of food between meals, but may drink as much water as wanted, but not within half an hour of eating, because any kind of fluid taken into the stomach with fruits or berries, causes more or less acidity, unless a person is in vigorous health, and many times even then.

It will be noticed that the meat should be lean, and but once a day; also, that there is no limit as to quantity of any of the articles of food named.   The rule should be, not take enough of any one thing to cause a feeling of discomfort afterwards, any feeling whatever which will attract the attention unpleasantly.

In bilious fever, the liver pill may have to be repeated in five or six days, and in other cases at intervals of a week or fortnight, or a month, for a short time, until the patient feels well; and when well enough to go to business or to work, meat may be allowed at breakfast as well as at dinner; and when the health is fully established, then eat as other people, but at regular times only, making the last meal of the day about sundown, strictly of a bowl of mush or oatmeal gruel or porridge, or a cup of hot drink, with some cold bread and butter.

The intelligent reader is urgently requested, especially if a parent or one who has the control of many persons, to try the above plan fairly, once or twice, and if he is not charmed with its efficiency it will be one of the marvels of the time.   Reference has been made to

CRACKED WHEAT,

or wheaten grits, which is simply common wheat grains broken up into several small pieces may be boiled slowly for hours until very soft, then strained of the water and placed on the table, to be eaten with butter or salt or sugar. It is wheat hominy, and is very generally kept in provision stores in paper bags, with directions how to prepare it for the table. Any one can crack the wheat for himself with a pestle and mortar, or by running it through a coarse coffee mill. This mode of using wheat as food has two immeasurable advantages. First. The whole nutriment of the wheat grain is saved; at least one-fifth of it is lost in converting wheat into common flour—the most nutritious part, that which gives strength to the bones, beauty and durability to the teeth, and food for the brain. Second. Many persons who use no other form of bread than wheaten grits, especially if ripe raw fruits or berries are taken afterwards as dessert, have been permanently cured of distressing

CONSTIPATION.

Any reader who is troubled with costive bowels is urged to try, for a single week, an exclusive diet of cracked wheat, and raw or stewed fruits or berries; it will be especially successful if an active walk of an hour or two is taken every day in the open air.

In the beginning of this chapter it was stated that all diseases were included in five classes. Two were mentioned; inflammatory and filthy. There is a third class, the

CACHEXIÆ;

literally, a "bad habit" of body, a falling away of flesh and strength as in consumption, a general wasting of the system. The cachectic diseases are

1. Addison's Disease. The supra-renal capsules are affected, the skin becomes colored like a dark bronze, and death is inevitable in the course of years.

2. Chlorosis is a poverty of blood in young girls, indicated by a peculiar sallowness of the skin, a pale, mushy, or bloated look, with a perverted appetite for clay, charcoal, lead pencils, etc., in some cases. This will generally be cured by the special fruit diet, a large amount of outdoor activities, and a liver pill two or three

times a month, provided the feet are kept uniformly warm, and the bowels are made to act every day.

3. **Diabetes,** is an excessive urination of a sweetish taste. Twice as many men have it as women; most common at thirty, rare after fifty-five; more common in the city than the country; caused by exposure to wet and cold; drinking cold water when overheated; by too much sweet food, intemperance, and by injuries of the brain and spinal cord. It begins with a slight loss of flesh, a general feeling of discomfort, thirst, variable appetite, and excessive urination; the sexual and mental powers gradually fail, often ending in consumption. The liver is at fault in this disease, making too much sugar, which has to be eliminated by the kidneys. It is usually a fatal disease; the true remedy has not yet been discovered. To ameliorate it, keep the bowels acting regularly, and have a moderate amount of exercise every day, with a liver pill twice a month, if its use seems to be beneficial.

4. **Hemorrhagic Disposition.** A tendency to various kinds of bleeding from different parts of the body; the best treatment of which consists in the special fruit diet, liver pill, and outdoor activities.

5. **Lithiasis,** or a tendency to form stone or gravel in the bladder, kidneys, and gall-ducts. To break up such tendencies a liver pill thrice a month, discarding water altogether, and all food made out of the grains, all forms of wheat and corn bread, using in their place milk, fruits, rice, sago, tapioca, berries, melons, oranges, lemons, lean meats, poultry, and fish.

6. **Leucocythæmia,** a diseased condition of the blood; very rare and not understood.

7. **Melanæmia** is also a blood-disease in severe forms of fever, induced by bad air, when the "congestion" (which article see) is so great that the coloring matter of the blood oozes through the sides of the vessels and is deposited in the liver and other glands. The treatment is the liver pill and special fruit diet.

8. **Mucous Disease.** 9. **Tuberculosis** or consumption. 10. **Syphilis.** 11. **Scurvy.** 12. **Spanæmia** or bloodlessness, that is poor blood, cured by exercise and nourishing food. Besides these there are other wasting diseases, such as Bright's disease of the kidneys, cancer, gout, rheumatism.

NEUROSES,

or nervous diseases, embrace

Angina Pectoris,	Hysteria,
Apoplexy,	Insanity,
Asthma,	Laryngismus,
Catalepsy,	Mania,
Chorea,	Monomania,
Convulsions,	Melancholy,
Delirium Tremens,	Paralysis,
Dementia,	Tetanus.
Epilepsy,	

The fifth class of diseases are those which cannot be well classified, embracing

Cholera,	Dropsies,
Colic,	Hemorrhages,
Diarrhœa,	Jaundice,
Dyspepsia,	Worms, etc.

In addition to all these there are half a hundred

SKIN-DISEASES,

manifested by various forms of eruptions, breakings out, varying in size, shape, and color to a remarkable extent, all of which are referable to the impurity of the blood; and in proportion to its impurity, it does not flow naturally, is congested either in the skin or in the liver, hence every form of skin-disease is cured by the liver pill and by the special fruit diet, with a reasonable attention to personal cleanliness, pure air, and moderate exercise. The reader will therefore see distinctly in reading the article on " The Simplicity of Medical Practice," " Preliminaries " on page ten, " Congestion " on page twenty-one, also the Oneness of Disease, that there is a beautiful simplicity in the practice of medicine; that the general principles are clear in character and few in number; that three-fourths of all ordinary diseases may be treated successfully by the administration of a single medicine, the

LIVER PILL,

conjoined with warmth, rest, and a system of eating laid down in the article headed

SPECIAL FRUIT DIET.

When the patient is able to leave the house, then the cure is to be completed by those judicious out-door activities which are so frequently referred to in these pages.

There is another general principle in treating all external ailments affecting the skin, which is of an importance, not too strongly expressed by the word vital, for literally life has been lost in multitudes of cases by neglect or ignorance.

ERUPTIONS.

Whenever there is a breaking out on the skin, it is perfectly certain that both the liver and the stomach are disordered, and that a liver pill is. appropriate, when it is not of insect origin, as in itch ; and that life is endangered if anything is done to drive it in. Nothing can be safely done to any breaking out of the body, as an external application, except with a view to cool the part and to keep the skin soft, moist, and with open pores, so as to admit of the freest passing out possible of all internal impurities called humors. These external applications are of three characters, washes, poultices, and ointments. The washes may be applied in the form of baths, compresses, or applying the liquid with the hand ; it may be cold or hot, it may be milk or water or spirits.

Compresses are simply several folds of woven material, woollen, silk, cotton, or linen, dipped in cold, warm, or hot liquids ; they should be of several thicknesses and thin ; two or three of them— one on the part affected, two in the basin of liquid, so that when one is taken off another is ready, while the other is cooling or warming.

If the parts are hot and painful, there is more or less inflammation, apply cold, by means of compresses, or cooling lotions ; if there is no pain or redness, then warm compresses or poultices, or spirit applications are better ; any form of spirits, or preparations containing spirits, called

TINCTURES,

such as tincture of camphor, tincture of arnica. Whiskey is a tincture ; so is rum, brandy, or gin ; it is almost instinctive to apply these to hurts and pains, simply because they evaporate rapidly, and carry away the extra heat in large quantities; alcohol does the same thing. Smear a little on the arm or face and a cooling sensation is felt instantly; hence all these washes are said to be cooling.

But spirits are not good for inflammations, because they tend to irritate the skin, and to that extent increase the inflammation, by attracting the arterial blood to the little vessels which already are too full. For the same reason hot water is not applicable in inflammatory cases; it is capable of causing inflammation. But warm water and spirits do two things: first they diminish the blood, the congestion of the parts, by evaporation; and in addition they excite the activity of the congested vessels, causing them to send on their fluid contents. Hence, the two great general principles of external applications: cold water where there is inflammation and pain; warm water or spirits or tinctures where there is congestion of the veins, as seen in bruises, where there is discoloration or swelling, without heat; and more of a hurting than pain; a dull sensation rather than acute. The advantage which

POULTICES

have over washings or compresses is, that they need not be so often reapplied; they are better for the night; instead of being changed every two or five or ten minutes, they can remain an hour or two or more, or half a day or all night.

Those poultices are best which are least weighty, and which remain moist the longest. A great ado is often made about the particular sort of poultice to be used; one advises to take the entrails of a live chicken and apply at once, but the entrails of a

DEAD DOG,

if just killed, would be just as efficacious, for both are moist and warm, and would remain moist and warm for several hours.

A scraped potato, or scraped apple, or scraped turnip, or scraped anything else are great remedies in the hands of some for preventing lock-jaw, resulting from a nail or other metallic point running into the foot or hand. It is the moisture and the compactness of the scraped material; if bruised, the effect would be the same; the scraping is applied, a bandage is put over it, it soon gets warm, remains warm and moist for hours. But in all these cases

whether cold or warm, are better, because they are lighter and stop up the pores of the skin less; but they dry earlier than poultices unless applied properly. The hydropathists accomplish almost miraculous results, sometimes, by the judicious and patient application of water to diseased subjects; the proper plan is thus: have four, five, or six folds of Irish linen which has been softened by wear. For this reason old linen handkerchiefs and sheets and shirts should be always laid away by a careful housekeeper, to be ready in cases of sickness and wounds, more valuable then than their weight in silver. By there being several folds the warmth and dampness are continued longer, and air being between, it does not lie so heavily on the injured part.

It is better to press out the water a little to prevent its dribbling on the clothing or bedding, lay it smoothly over the ailing part, and spread over it a piece of oiled silk, or other dry cloth if there is no silk at hand; but the silk is better because it is more impervious to air, and besides keeps the warm steam in better, and thus insures a softer, moister condition of the skin; this oiled silk should, for the same reason, extend about an inch beyond the edges of the wetted cloth, as by its pressure on the skin it prevents air from coming in and drying the compress. In this way a

WATER POULTICE

may be kept wet enough for hours, without the necessity of change. Remember that poultices do no good unless they are kept moist. There is another important first principle in the treatment of diseases besides the liver pill, and the special fruit diet, and the cold applications to fevered and inflamed parts, and water dressings, and spirit lotions to bruises and sluggish sores. There are ailments which give pain, more or less excessive; the may be of so prominent a feature that its relief is imperative anything else can be done. The first most available thing

MUSTARD PLASTER.

Mix ground mustard with vinegar, or, if none at hand, water; some add flour. This diminishes the strength, hence its efficacy. Vinegar is better and is more cooling. Spread it over a linen or cotton cloth to within an inch of the edge; this prevents its getting on the clothing and staining it. Then spread on the skin a piece of dampened paper, but very thin muslin is preferable, the thinner the better, the object being to prevent the mustard from blistering the skin, which it does without diminishing the efficacy. As the mustard soon loses its strength, it is rather better to let it remain; if, however, it cannot be endured, remove it after it has begun to burn considerably. This mustard plaster need not be placed immediately over the painful part—that may be sometimes impracticable—it may be placed several inches away. This mustard plaster relieves by drawing the blood to the surface, thus relieving the ailing part from the excess of blood which causes the pain. A mustard plaster is necessarily a temporary remedy; it is to give time for more efficient and radical and permanent means of relief. Suppose, for example, a patient is taken with great nausea at the stomach and vomiting, as from a bilious condition of the system; spread a mustard plaster over the abdomen or stomach, and the nausea will be relieved almost instantaneously, then give a liver pill, keeping the patient warm in bed; or suppose there are colicky pains, proceed in the same manner.

But there may be pains in parts too deep-seated, or too inconvenient for a mustard poultice, then a liniment may be used; but it is so powerful in its operation that it should be kept on hand as a last resort:

CHLOROFORM

liniment, made by putting equal parts of chloroform, sweet oil, and spirits of camphor in a bottle, shake it rapidly, pour some of it in a small saucer, dip in three or four folds of linen, muslin, or flannel, one or two inches across, lay it over the spot, cover it with a folded handkerchief and let it remain a quarter or half a minute, not longer, as the skin may be blistered; from the shaking of the bottle to laying it on the skin the least time possible should be spent, as the chloroform and other ethereal ingredients rapidly disappear. The bottle should have a ground-glass stopper, and even it should have some oiled silk or india-rubber tied over it, to prevent evaporation; but such a bottle of liniment should be kept in every family. Thus it will be seen, if the reader will turn to the article on poisons, that every ordinary sickness and pain can be relieved or cured by having in the house four things—

First. A box of liver pills.

Second. A box of kitchen mustard.

Third. A bottle of chloroform liniment.

Fourth. A bottle of linseed oil.

With these in the application of the doctrine of

CONGESTION,

there is no human malady which cannot be alleviated or cured, if curable at all; there is no human pain which cannot be mitigated, if mitigation is possible; the relief to be completed by keeping up the general health, according to the principles laid down in that article with the aid of

SPECIAL FRUIT DIET.

If the intelligent reader will turn to any book which has attached to it the name of

MEDICAL PRACTICE,

whether for family use or professional readers; whether in allopathy, homœopathy, or hydropathy; or if he will go to any physician of high repute and honorable standing among his brethren, it will be always found that there are a few favorite remedies upon which most reliance is to be placed to do the real hard work. In Congress, in any legislative assembly, in any political gathering, in all church judicatories, it will never fail to be found that a very few men do all the real work, that which is most important. Less than half a dozen men made the two great branches of the Presbyterian Church one; less than half a dozen men, in the Methodist Church, induced a million of people to assent to lay delegation; less than half a dozen men rule the whole continent of Europe; less than half a dozen men hold in their hands the destinies of the many millions of the British empire.

The greatest and most successful surgeon of modern times did everything for half a century, from the reduction of a joint, the extraction of a stone, the curing of a fracture, to the cutting off of a man's head, with three things: a vial of tartar emetic, a razor-edged knife, and a strip of muslin twenty feet long,—Professor B. W. Dudley, of Transylvania University in its palmiest days; sometimes he called in the assistance of warm water and boiled turnips, with brown bread.

Another man, with a logic that never was refuted, John Esten Cook, practised medicine triumphantly for fifty years, his whole stock in trade consisting of one pound each of calomel, aloes, and rhubarb; a pill, containing two grains of each, mixed up with cold water, was his great stand-by; he usually gave two or three at a time; if these did not act, gave six; and so on doubling at each failure of action. He was a perfect Boanerges in his way, and lived and died in honor and success.

No Allopathic physician could get along without his calomel and tartar emetic. Hahnemann himself would have died long before he got a name, had it not been for acon., ars., bell., and bry. An Eclectic could not keep his shop open a week without podophyllin, the May-apple root.

And Hydropathy would founder any day without a wet pack or a sitz-bath. All these things are so because the fundamental principles of successful medical practice are few and simple. When the body is weary, rest it. When burning up, cool it. When racked with pain, soothe it. When pressed to death's door by morbid and excessive accumulations, put no more into it, empty it—all to be done by going to bed, abstaining from food, and purgation; then to build up, not by tonics, not by spirits, not by bitters, but by out-door air, by moderate activities, and a nutritious diet of coarse bread, ripe fruits, lean meats, and garden vegetables.

The reader may rest assured that what these fail to do in ordinary diseases everything else will fail to do, and that, on the whole, the million and one fiddling prescriptions with which our medical books abound do more harm than good, by their everlasting annoyance of the patient, waking him out of his sleep, outraging his mouth with villanous tastes, filling the stomach with successive poisons one after another, sometimes half a dozen in a day. The truth is, Nature herself cures half the ordinary sicknesses that are cured, and time cures many. Sometimes a less active medi- cine will accomplish the desired result in a given case, or a more palatable one may be desired; but for all that, calomel, tartar em- etic, and opium were the great stand-bys of educated medical practitioners of a past age, are now, and possibly will be, until men have learned the lesson not to get sick. A few have learned it and lived long, healthily, happily, and successfully as far as use- fulness and influence and money are concerned; and there is no necessary reason why the number should not be indefinitely enlarg- ed, on the old-fashioned principles that "what was done once can be done again," "what ought to be, can be," "what Peter has done, Paul can do."

CHOKING.

It is best to prevent it by cutting up every particle of food, especially meats, as fine as a pea, to eat slowly, not put much in the mouth at a time, and always swallow deliberately.

In the case of children a good stroke in the back or shoulders with the palm of the hand is very effective.

If a pin or fishbone or similar thing has stuck in the pas- sage, be composed, and let some one equally composed at least, look down into the throat; it may be seen and caught with the fingers or a pair of pincers or tongs, if nothing smaller is at hand.

If there is a soft obstacle, as a piece of meat or bread, or any- thing which could not hurt the stomach, push it down with the handle of a knife or fork or spoon, with a roll or two of cloth over it to make a bunch, or place five or six grains of tartar emetic on the back of the tongue, or a level teaspoonful of ipecac powder; as they dissolve, the system is nauseated, and there is a relaxation of the parts.

If anything hard or insoluble has been swallowed, patiently wait until Nature carries it through by her own operations.

If a hair or string lodges in the throat, it is more promptly carried downwards by swallowing a mouthful of bread or pud- ding, than by drinking water.

ABSCESSES.

Abscess is a "departure" or "leaving," and means a coming from or separation; as applied to the human body, it is a yellow matter detaching itself from the body, a part of the substance of which it was. Abscesses are internal and external; there is abscess of the liver, abscess of the lungs; or they may be on the outside, on the surface of the body.

Abscesses are acute or chronic; the acute get well in a few days; the chronic remain for weeks or months or years, even for a lifetime.

Abscesses, like all ordinary diseases, such as cough, dysentery, diarrhœa, catarrh, and hundreds of other forms of human maladies, are indications that something wrong is going on in the system, that Nature is endeavoring to relieve and cure herself by detaching something from the body which is now foreign to it, and of which she seeks to rid herself.

The body is life, every atom of it is living, and when an atom by any means is alive no longer, it is no longer a part of the human frame; it becomes an incumbrance, nature takes alarm lest it might clog her machinery, and seeks by all the means in her power to pass it out, to convey it away from the body, as the bees of a hive will kill and carry out any intruder on their premises.

In the working of all machinery there is friction, and friction makes waste inevitably, and if continued the machine eventually wears out. This process of friction and waste is constantly going on in the body, which is as constantly conveying it out of itself, because all its workings are to push outwards. There is a groove or curve about the eye along which all the dust which strikes against the ball is washed out by the fluids, which in excess are called tears, and which convey this dust and other foreign matters out at the corners of the eye or through an inner passage into the nose; when nature cannot pass foreign, or dead, or waste matters out of the body fast enough by the ordinary processes, an extra effort is made to accomplish the object; that effort is self-operating, is instinctive, wholly outside of voluntary human control; for example, if too much dust gets into the eye, or if a hard particle is driven into it, as a cinder from a locomotive, nature makes an extra amount of water out of the blood, and we say the eye waters; this water is made out of the blood, is a part of the blood; in fact, a large portion of the blood is water, so constituted, that when extra water is needed for any purpose, as in this very washing of the eye, in diarrhœa, and in other forms of disease, there may be a reservoir of it in the blood. To withdraw the water out of the blood, there is in the eye and·in the bowels a machinery in operation which accomplishes the object; this machinery is the action of what are called glands, or manufactories, which are located in every part of the body; some to take water from the blood as in the eye and the kidneys; the liver is a gland, many times larger than any other in the system; its business is to withdraw, to secern the bile from the blood; if it does not do this fast enough the blood has too much bile in it; so much as to tinge it yellow, which is the natural color of healthy bile, and we recognize it, first in the whites of the eye, which are seen to be yellowish.

But if more water is wanted in any part of the body than is natural, if an extra supply is needed, inasmuch as the water is taken from the blood, then there must be an extra supply of blood. But nature fails not to send that extra supply through the arteries, and sends it so fast and in such increased quantities to the part which needs the extra water, that it becomes redder than natural, just as the eye becomes more yellow than natural when there is an unusual amount of bile in the blood. This abnormally increased amount of blood in a part we call

INFLAMMATION.

Thus it is seen that inflammation is curative. Now, as applied to Abscesses, they come on by an increased redness of the part. If superficial, this redness increases steadily, damming up, and swelling, and reddening, and distending, pushing the yielding skin upwards, causing intense pain.

But this increasing quantity of blood is not to bring an increased amount of water to that part, but it is freighted, loaded with waste, dead, impure, and diseased particles which it has washed out before it from the most remote parts of the body, and when it gets to the locality of the abscess the diseased and dead particles are separated from the blood, and are there deposited and collected in the shape of yellow matter which constantly accumulates and dams up, until the skin being unable any longer to hold it, parts, is said to "break," as in the case of a boil : the yellow matter, the impurities of the whole body are poured out of it, and the person begins to get well; feels better than he ever did in his life before. His friends confirm it by saying he never looked better. This is because the impurities have been taken from the system, leaving it supplied with a healthy, life-giving blood. Thus it is that an Abscess was said to be curative. In the same connection, and for the same reason, although not an exact statement, there is a common saying that " Boils are healthy." An abscess, like a boil, is a means of health ; leaves the body in a more healthy condition, but at the same time proves that it had been in a diseased state, and the abscess, like the boil, was an instrumentality by which Nature cured herself. A boil or an abscess may appear at any part of the body, but it always determines itself to that part which is the weakest ; made weakest by an accidental bruise, or puncture, or wound, or other cause.

A man of wealth was one day stepping into his carriage ; his foot slipped in such a way that a considerable portion of the skin was scraped from the shin bone ; it became inflamed, a running sore was set up, and immense amounts of yellow matter were discharged ; he was ill for a long time, and finally died. He drank liquor largely, never drunk, but always full ; the whole system was so clogged with impurities, that before it could clear itself he became exhausted in the effort, the work of cleansing was not completed, and the man died.

Running sores, boils, abscesses, are essentially one and the same thing ; they are evidences of a diseased condition of the whole body, of bad blood. Nature, in the way described, seeks to relieve, to purify herself ; hence the treatment of abscesses should be such as will help Nature, by promoting the running of the matter. But they are all painful, troublesome, more or less disgusting, and it is very natural that the persons thus afflicted should want them cured, that is, healed up ; and following the well-meant advice of friends, or of any benevolent stranger meaning well, means are too often taken to heal them up, and they are delighted with the result thus far, but not a little later.

Anne D., a Christian lady of great worth, aged seventy-five, had been a long time troubled with a running sore on the leg. A person in the neighborhood, who had the reputation of curing ugly sores, was sent to her by a friend to cure her sore. In a comparatively short time the sore ceased running, healed up " beautifully." In three days after, she died. Nature had been thwarted, the poisonous matter which she was throwing out of the system was shut in, to rankle, to corrupt, to stagnate, to clog, and the wheels of life were stopped forever.

These statements have been made thus at length to impress on the mind several most important truths, of a specially practical nature, because they are at the very foundation of all true, safe medical practice.

1. All symptoms, all pain, all that is abnormal, unusual, unnatural in the system, should be regarded as an effort of Nature to free the body from actual or impending evil.

2. The operations of nature should not be interfered with, except in rare cases, and by special intelligent medical advice.

3. The effort in every disease should be to know what is the matter, what Nature is doing, and to what extent, and how best to help her. Some first general principles will be found running through every page of this volume, for the treatment of every form of disease, and are purposely brought forward in the first important article in the book so as to give the reader the earliest opportunities of impressing his mind with these general principles, which are fundamental in their nature, which are far-reaching in their scope, and almost of universal application.

SYMPTOMS OF ABSCESS.

Acute Abscess shows redness, if superficial; with increasing redness comes pain, at first sharp, which becomes dull and throbbing as the swelling increases, and the yellow matter begins to form in a little conical point at first, growing in quantity until it is sometimes felt to fluctuate ; all along there has been more or less fever, local and general ; now there are little chills and shiverings. There is general uneasiness in the whole person ; the skin bursts, the matter escapes, and the process is completed.

Chronic Abscess goes on more slowly ; for some time there is nothing much out of the way to all appearance, until a swelling is observed. Matter slowly forms, but it is thin and flaky, like curds. If there is vigor in the system, the cavity left by the emptying of the abscess is gradually filled up by the deposit of healthy particles from a pure blood, which becomes purified at the instant, and is formed into solid flesh.

If, however, the person is weak, is old, or has a feeble constitution, the cavity does not fill up, because flesh particles are not deposited; there is rather sinking; there is no power of healing; there is not life enough in the blood to give life to the deposited particles, which instead begin to decay, and often form an ill-swelling, bloody-like matter to be discharged in large quantities for months and years, unless a more healthful condition is brought about, or the ugly matter is reabsorbed into the system, goes back into the blood, poisons it, gives the hectic hue to the cheek, the friendly warning of a certain and speedy death.

THE TREATMENT of Acute Abscess, as in boils and kindred affections, most generally advised, is to let them alone, unless their spread is likely to reach parts which, if injured, may result in serious harm; then it may be well to use a lancet, and let the matter out; but as a general rule, it is better to let Nature accomplish the object in her own way, which is to divide the skin when everything is ripe.

If, however, the abscess is very painful, dip several folds of cloths in warm water, to be placed on the part, and frequently renew until relief is experienced. A poultice of milk and bread applied to the part, to be softened or moistened with warm water from time to time, tends to take off the heat and fever and pain, which, indeed, is sometimes necessary in order to afford sleep. See under head of POULTICES.

In chronic abscesses the yellow matter should not be allowed to accumulate, but should be let out from time to time, otherwise it may be absorbed into the system, poisoning it, and leading to the fatal results before named. Sometimes abscesses heal up of themselves before the matter has been entirely removed; in such cases new issues should be made by using blister plasters near the spot, so as to cause an artificial running. But the rule should be always, if the abscess does not discharge itself, to let out the matter so as to prevent any large accumulation, to avoid the dangers above referred to.

Constitutional Treatment.—That is, what can be done in an

indirect way through the functions of the body, whether by medicine, air, exercise, diet, or otherwise. This principle of constitutional treatment so often comes into requisition in the treatment of disease, that it is most important to understand the philosophy of it most thoroughly; in truth, it is at the very foundation of the true system of medication, to act upon disease through the general system.

ABSCESS OF THE LIVER

is not an uncommon disease; it is out of sight, and cannot be reached directly; to cut into it with a knife would kill in nearly all cases, so abscess of the liver should be treated "Constitutionally," by remedies which act upon the general system, thus: an abscess, boil, "imposthume," as Washington used to call a boil, carbuncle, or any other "sore" which delivers yellow matter, is proof that the blood is in an impure, in a diseased condition, and that the system, or Nature, is endeavoring to pass the impurities out of the body through the abscess. The aim of constitutional treatment is to supply to the body healthful particles to take the place of the diseased or poisonous or waste particles which are passing out through the sore in the form of matter, generally yellow, at other times mingled with blood or watery portions; for if this substitution is not made, the body is wasting, is losing its strength. The uninformed soon see this, and begin at once to take means to "keep up the strength," some by eating more when they do not digest what they already eat; because the stomach is weak, like the body, in general because of its taking on its proportionate share of debility, by which it is not able to get out of the food the nourishment which it contains; under such circumstances, to eat more food, to crowd more into the stomach, when what is already there is not properly managed, is like increasing the load of an already overburdened animal as a means of aiding it in doing its work.

In this blind effort many eat when they do not feel like it; eat without an appetite, force the food on the stomach, giving as a reason they cannot get strong unless they eat, and that unless they get more strength they will certainly grow weaker, and will soon have to go to bed. Others resort to the use of porter, ale, beer, and the stronger preparations of alcohol, to give them strength to digest their food; with the inevitable effect of making them worse, for two reasons.

First. Alcohol does not give one atom of strength to the body; a man feels stronger after taking a drink, but it is only because he takes the strength of the next half hour, and with the strength of the present he seems to be twice as strong as he was before, and he really is; but in half an hour after, he will be twice as weak as he would have been had he not taken the spirits. If a man has a sum of money in bank, and draws a certain amount a day for the day's expenses, he may live more liberally to-day if he draws to-day's allowance and to-morrow's also, but then to-morrow he has nothing whatever to live upon. This is the ground of all that deceptiveness connected with the almost universal notion that drinking liquor increases the strength.

Second. There is another fallacy connected with this habit of drinking spirits to keep up the strength when a person is getting weak through the effects of a running sore; the liquor immediately increases the circulation, sends more blood to the abscess, making more matter to be discharged; thus ultimately increasing the debility; and not only this: it increases the inflammation, and this increases the pain.

The strength wasted by running sores cannot be increased by forcing food into the stomach, by eating without an appetite, nor by drinking liquor; both these positively increase the debility; the same truth applies to all forms of debility, to all forms of wasting disease. To increase the strength in such cases is absolutely necessary to a cure, but there is only one way of doing it.

First, Husband the strength by rest and sleep.

Second, Add to it by improving the digestion, and by increasing the appetite, which must be appeased by eating the best food prepared in the best manner; that is, in a way to retain the most of its natural juices and qualities, as more fully shown in the author's book entitled "Health by Good Living."

Under the heading of "Dyspeptics," details are given which, if carried out with judgment and discretion, will greatly aid in improving the digestion and increasing the appetite.

Acute abscesses begin to discharge in about three weeks, lasting a month or two ; before or at the time of their beginning to discharge, the fever or inflammation and pain often take away the appetite ; this is Nature's first instinctive effort to a cure, for in the preparation to discharge, there is a certain commotion in the system, such a summoning up of strength for an effort, that it would be out of place to burden it with the digestion of large amounts of food ; but when the discharge begins to take place, then means should be used to increase the strength so as to enable the constitution more completely to throw off all the poisonous and impure particles which disease the body.

Chronic abscesses, which are often internal, such as in the liver, womb, or other interior localities, continue for months, the time depending on the extent of the diseased condition, on the vitality of the patient—that is, his strength of constitution—and the character of the remedial means used. The various kinds of abscesses derive their name from their locality : if in the lungs, it is called " Empyema ; " if in the flesh, " Boils ; " if in the fingers, " Whitlow ; " if in the loins, " Lumbar Abscess ; " if in the neck, " King's Evil ; " if in the knee-joint, " White Swelling," etc.

The Allopathic or Old School treatment of acute abscesses consists in the application of cold cloths and poultices to keep the parts moist, so as to lessen the heat of the part by the constant evaporation going on ; eating plain food in small quantities, and at regular intervals, not less than five hours apart generally, but oftener and in smaller quantities if there is great debility ; in regulating the bowels to one full, free daily action.

In external chronic abscesses, cold applications should be made, with a liberal diet of plain, nourishing food, and regular bowels, acting daily ; if the strength is not satisfactory, use any one of the remedies known under the head of Tonics, which seem to have the most desirable effects.

IRRITABLE ULCERS.

Sometimes the edges of abscesses become hard, red, and painful ; foment them with cloths dipped in warm water, changing them frequently until relief is given, and renew as often as there is occasion.

INDOLENT ULCERS.

Sometimes there is so little vitality that an ulcered abscess will not heal, and extra growths spring up; these and the hard edges, after being softened with fomentations as above, may be removed by some of the " Caustics," which see; burnt alum powdered, often answers every purpose.

In the treatment of abscesses and all forms of ulcers, boils, etc., both Allopathists, Homœopathists, and Hydropathists, with minor distinctive differences of action, urge their respective constitutional treatment as being specially applicable. This is described under the head of "General Health."

ACIDITY, called by some Heart-Burn, and by others " Sour Stomach," has its seat in the stomach, but is felt in the throat, about the little hollow at the bottom of the neck, as a smarting or burning; sometimes there is a burning or scalding feeling extending from the stomach upwards to the throat. These sensations are also occasioned by a bad cold, but when arising from the condition of the stomach, they are felt in connection with eating from a few minutes to an hour or more, after a regular meal. In aggravated cases, this acidity is so great as to disturb the stomach, and cause a liquor to be belched or gulped up, which sometimes takes the skin off the tongue, but more generally it is the acrid gases which come up from the stomach; but whether the burning, smarting, or scalding be present, the cause is the same—Indigestion, which see. This indigestion is inability of the stomach to manage the food eaten, healthfully, it decays, it decomposes, rots, giving rise to fermentation.

The only safe and healthful method of curing acidity is in the proper digestion of the food, by the following general rules:

1st. Eat at three regular times every day.

2d. There should be not less than five hours between each meal.

3d. Eat nothing whatever between meals.

4th. Take no desserts.

5th. Drink nothing cold at meal time, or within half an hour of eating; at other times drink as much cold water as is wanted.

6th. If any liquid is taken at meal times, it should be hot, and not more than a common teacupful.

7th. The last meal of the day should consist of a piece of cold bread and butter, and a cup of hot drink.

Sometimes acidity is caused by taking any liquid at meals. Each must observe for himself, and experiment on himself. It can be easily done, and safely ascertained, thus: if there is any acidity after a meal, drink less and less fluid after such meal; if the acidity is lessened by so doing, then it is an indication that either no fluid should be taken, or only so much as will not be followed by any acidity. Many cases occur to experienced physicians in large cities, where acidity comes on regularly after supper, causing eructations, belchings, rumblings in the bowels, and general disturbance, but on ceasing to use tea for supper, all the symptoms disappear after following it up for a few days.

On other occasions, when persons have taken only tea and toast for supper, it was the toasted bread which occasioned the acidity; and on its disuse, and the employment of common cold light bread and butter, prompt relief was obtained. The same principles apply to eating, acidity being caused by eating too much, or by a certain kind of food; but by far the greater number of cases result from the quantity taken, rather than the quality.

The first step to be taken is to cease taking any liquid whatever at meals. Second, diminish the quantity by one quarter the first time. If the acidity is less, keep on diminishing until there is no acidity at all. Continue this amount for some days, and then increase the quantity of food by slow degrees if there is an appetite for it. If, however, it is found that a less and less quantity of food does not materially abate the acidity, it may be taken for granted that the disturbance is caused by the quality of the food. Then, first leave off one thing, next another, exercising acute and judicious observation the whole time, and be governed accordingly.

There are a variety of medicines which " cure " acidity, using the word in the common acceptation of the term among unintelligent persons, a disappearance of the symptoms being considered by them a cure. It is not intended here to name the various remedies which are employed to cure acidity in this meaning of the word; for it would only be putting it in the power of the reader to injure himself. Besides, there is many an intelligent man who would commit an indiscretion in eating when he knew that he had at hand a certain, agreeable, and speedy remedy for the acidity; whereas if no such remedy were known he would fear to indulge.

There are, however, two remedies, simple, always at hand, costing little or nothing, and promptly efficacious—powdered charcoal, and saleratus. Every one knows what these are. A common wood fire in the kitchen or parlor affords both in abundance; for a bit of charcoal needs only to be powdered into dust, stirred into half a glass of water, and swallowed down. It affords relief by its capability of absorbing a hundred times its bulk of gas or wind in the stomach or bowels.

Saleratus is found in abundance on the kitchen shelf; half a teaspoonful of it, more or less, stirred in a glass of water and drank down, is considered a simple, certain, and speedy "cure" for acidity.

This is as good a place as any in a book like this, intended for the reader's instruction and real good, to show an important practical truth in reference to that large class of remedies which are familiar, "simple," and can "do no harm, if they do no good;" "simple" being the designation of anything which is familiar, known, seen, or handled every day.

If you have no saleratus in the house, take a pint of common wood ashes from the fireplace, stir in a pint or more of water; pour off the liquid next day, and boil it until it is as thick as molasses; let it dry. That is saleratus. Nothing but the strength which water draws out of wood ashes; nothing could be more simple.

SODA.

Soda will answer the same purpose, for it is the same thing, only that saleratus is made of the ashes of wood, and soda is made of the ashes of seaweed.

A gentleman in London was advised to take some soda every day for a troublesome acidity. He did so; it acted like a charm, instantaneously; but, like most remedies, it was necessary that it should be taken oftener—that is, after each meal, instead of after dinner. It was next observed that it required a larger quantity to effect full relief and a perfect "cure." He was perfectly delighted with the remedy, and took occasion to recommend it to every friend, acquaintance, or stranger who happened to complain of "Acidity" in his presence; in fact, he thought it was a humanity to disseminate a piece of information which was of such general and frequent application.

One beautiful spring morning he called at the house of a newly married daughter in London, and while conversing with her pleasantly at the garden gate, he dropped down dead. On examining the body for the purpose of ascertaining the cause of his death, several ounces of saleratus were found to have been impacted in a solid, heavy lump in his bowels, in such a location as to cause the result.

Saleratus, like sugar or salt stirred in a cup of water, seems to disappear and be all liquid; but if the cup is set away long enough to allow the water to be evaporated, the full amount of these articles is found at the bottom of the cup. The saleratus was taken into the stomach in the form of a liquid, but when it reached the bowels, the liquid portion was taken up by appropriate vessels of the body, but the solid parts could not be taken up and accumulated with the results named.

Precisely the same processes go on in the use of

POWDERED CHARCOAL.

As an antacid, it will absorb twelve per cent of moisture, and a very great amount of gas in the stomach and intestines; and in this way is said to purify the breath. Some use it for pain in the stomach and

HEART-BURN,

in doses of from one to four teaspoonfuls at a time. In doses of a tablespoon every half hour, it sometimes has a remarkable effect in removing obstinate

CONSTIPATION.

But "simple" as it is, powdered charcoal has been known to accumulate in large quantities in the intestines, and become an impacted mass, causing very great discomfort; even in the small quantities used for

TOOTH POWDERS,

careful and judicious dentists are averse to its employment, as it tends to insinuate itself under the gums, separating them from the teeth, and thus rendering them liable to decay.

These remarks have been made in reference to Antacids in general, to show the people plainly that they never eradicate a complaint, while they do have dangerous and even fatal effects when used largely. All the good they do is to alleviate for the present, leaving the causes of the symptoms, which they are taken to relieve or remove, still in operation. A wiser plan is to use all possible means to avoid the causes of the symptoms for which they are taken. See articles on DYSPEPSIA.

THE HAIR

grows by projecting itself longitudinally, like the finger nail. If it is drawn between the thumb and finger from the root to the other end, it is smooth to the feel; but if in the opposite direction, it is rough; showing what is the fact, that each hair is covered, and protected with its own feathers or scales. Every hair rises from a little bulb just under the upper layer of skin; this bulb, which can be seen by pulling out a hair " by the roots," contains a pulpy substance, which is the food of each hair; if this pulpy substance is fully supplied to the bulb, the hair grows, and if not, it dies; this pulp, as it gets upward, is converted into hair, and pushes all before it, even if the hair is a yard long.

Sometimes, from fever or other causes, this pulpy matter is not supplied, or only partially so, and the hair falls out for want of nourishment; but often in such cases, as the scalp becomes more healthy, the capsule or bulb becomes full again, and the hair grows as before, sometimes more rapidly; all hair-oils ever sold have obtained their reputation by their having been applied just at that juncture when Nature was resuming her healthful action.

These bulbs are roundish on the scalp, but of an oval form in the eyebrows. Within the bulb each hair has three fibres or roots, uniting at the surface to make one body, or the hair itself.

The thickness of the human hair varies from the two-hundred-and-fiftieth to the six-hundredth part of an inch. The silk-worm web is the five-thousandth part of an inch thick; the spider's web is only the thirty-thousandth part of an inch in thickness; that is, two hundred and fifty human hairs, laid side by side, make an inch in breadth; to cover that same space with a spider's web, it would take thirty thousand strands.

A patient, learned German professor, in taking four heads of hair of equal weight, ascertained the number of hairs in each, in round numbers:

Red hairs	90,000
Black	103,000
Brown	109,000
Blonde	140,000

Agreeing with the received impression, that blonde hair is the finest and most silken. The average weight of a woman's hair is fourteen ounces, or six-sevenths of a pound.

A very good head of hair weighs about two pounds, bought originally for half a dollars' worth of trinkets or gaudy ornaments, and sold at wholesale for two dollars; if it is fine and glossy it brings four dollars at the polling. An Illinois lady sold her head of blonde hair for eighty-five dollars. A woman's hair averages nearly two feet; sometimes it is a yard long; there are cases when it has been long enough to reach the floor when the wearer was standing. To be of good strength and texture it ought not to be longer than two feet.

In the Industrial Exhibition in England specimens of hair were on exhibition from the heads of English, French, and Italian ladies; the English was jet black, and measured seventy-four inches.

BALDNESS

is sometimes hereditary, at others is occasioned by sickness, especially ailments which affect the head; it is of two kinds, curable and incurable. That which follows sickness will usually cure itself, if the scalp is kept clean, washed with cold water several times a day with plentiful frictions of the bald parts, with a coarse cloth first and then with the ends of the fingers and palms of the hands. If this does not promote the growth of the hair, nothing else will. Millions of dollars are expended every year for preparations which are said to promote the growth of the hair. What cleanliness and the frictions named do not accomplish in that direction, nothing else will. There are some preparations which may stimulate the scalp to a certain extent, but time would have done the same thing better, so that nothing is gained in the long run.

If the scalp is covered with a furze, the hair will grow again. If it is shiny, nothing can make it grow, because the roots of the hair are gone ; in that case it is as impossible for the hair to grow as it would for a flower to grow after it had been pulled up by the roots and thrown away, for the hair grows from a root straggling in various directions, as the root of a blade of grass spreads out at the ground end of it, these roots bringing nourishment to it from all quarters ; and no amount of manuring can make that same root grow again when it is thoroughly dead.

Keeping the head too much enveloped with a hat causes the hair to fall out prematurely, because the hat keeps the scalp too warm and prevents the air from getting at each root. Women who wear caps all their days do not generally become bald ; the cap is thin, and the air gets to the roots of the hair, thus preventing an overheating of the head.

But a

GOOD HEAD OF HAIR,

as it is termed, is as much a matter of inheritance as a fine beard, or a black eye, or a Roman nose ; nor is it connected with a good or bad constitution, nor a healthy or sickly body, necessarily. Many consumptives have immense masses of hair, giving rise in the minds of some to the belief that all the strength of the body, all the vitality, goes out through the hair. The best answer that can be given to the question, what is

GOOD FOR THE HAIR?

is cleanliness of the scalp—such cleanliness as results from frequent bathing the whole scalp in cold water, and plentiful frictions to the bald parts with the ends of the fingers and the palms of the hands. When the hair is long, as in women, the best treatment is the plentiful use of the comb and brush ; a fine-toothed comb should be very carefully used once a week only, pushing it along the scalp slowly, in a slanting direction, at an angle of not more than thirty degrees, so as not to drive it into the scalp and wound it ; it should be always in the direction of the growth of the hair ; then the brush should be used well once or twice every day. If the hair is short, as in the case of children and men, it may expedite matters, after having used a fine-toothed comb, to brush the hair quickly back and forth and in every direction, so as not to miss a pin point of the scalp; after this brushing is over, hold the head forward, in such a manner that the light may be thrown on the little specks loosened by the brush, and which are detached from the hair by flirting both hands back and forth among the hair, as if to shake off all the dust that might be upon it; keep this up until nothing can be seen to fall. This is the scurf called

DANDRUFF.

It is not a disease at any time. Any one can see flakes fall from the body in the sunlight, made by rubbing the hands rapidly over the skin; these flakes are the scales of the skin, which having answered their original purpose, like the scales of a fish, or the feathers of a bird, or the first teeth of children, are pushed out—are shed, to make room for new ones; but the hair prevents them from falling off the scalp; and in addition, they are matted to it by the perspiration, which is constantly escaping from the pores of the scalp; hence, dandruff is really a mixture of perspiration, skin, scales, and dust, which settle on the head, and is no more the result of disease than that which falls from a curry-comb when cleaning off a horse; and as a horse looks sleek and shiny if he is well groomed every day, so if the scalp is taken care of in such a manner as to keep the skin free from all unnatural accumulations, and has the free access of the air, it will aid very much in keeping the hair glossy and attractive, without the help of artificial applications.

The more hair is oiled the more will it be required; serving to keep an impacted layer of dust and scales and grease all over the scalp, so as to prevent a particle of air coming to the roots, thus depriving them of their vitality.

Nothing should be allowed to touch the

HAIR OF CHILDREN,

except pure, soft water; and if it were regularly cut every month, from three years of age to fourteen, not allowing during all that time a longer growth than two or three inches, keeping the scalp clean all the while, as above directed, the growth of the hair would be strengthened, its life invigorated, so that girls at twenty would have healthy, glossy, abundant hair of their own, to be kept, generally, until middle life, and thus avoid the necessity of loading the scalp so unnaturally as is now the custom, keeping it too warm, obstructing the circulation of the blood, and putting such a strain upon it with pins, and by various

CONTORTIONS AND DISTORTIONS,

greatly injure the quality and impair the life of what little they have. To such an extent are these unwise practices carried, and the proper treatment of the hair neglected, that a great number of our young, unmarried ladies, if divested of all that does not belong to them, have hair no longer and no more abundant than the opposite sex; and considering that the hair of a woman adds more to her native attractiveness than anything else, the teeth not excepted, it is greatly to be regretted that more attention is not paid to it in childhood than is done; for

BEAUTIFUL HAIR AND TEETH

can make any woman attractive, if they are all her own. All

HAIR-DYES

are a hypocrisy; nine out of ten of them are poisonous to the extent of endangering life. To want the hair of a different color than Nature gives, is proof of a weak mind. No man or woman of a lofty nature could ever stoop to such a deception. The nitrate of silver is a favorite ingredient for turning the hair dark or black; it always makes the hair harsh, injures the roots, or causes disagreeable and troublesome nervous affections. All these objections apply to the use of these compounds, as well to the hair as to the

BEARD AND MUSTACHE.

Nearly all hair-dyes contain acetate of lead, a virulent poison instantly inflaming the blood, combining with it and by its unhealthful agencies irritating the nerves, causing convulsions, and in many cases permanent paralysis and inability of motion of the parts implicated; this is the case as a result of the vigorous rubbing in the dye on the hair, or in the beard of the face, the frictions irritating the skin causing it to absorb the poisonous ingredient with greater activity; each manufacturer assures the purchaser that there is no such element in his mixture, but the only safe plan is to use no dyes whatever, unless the person using them knows the nature of each ingredient and mixes them himself.

A young man residing in Chester, Pa., was terribly poisoned by a species of hair-dye in common use among barbers everywhere. While coloring his mustache, the barber suffered a drop of the dye to fall upon his lower lip, which was slightly chapped. In a short time after, the part began to swell, became inflamed to an enormous size, and his whole face presented a shocking appearance. Convulsion after convulsion followed, and for some time his life was in great jeopardy. Within a day or two, however, the swelling subsided, and he recovered.

Hair-dyes, if used at all, should be made by the direction of the person using them, in order to know certainly what their composition is; that made of the nitrate of silver turns the hair black; that made of lead and sulphur, mainly, frequently restores the hair to its natural color.

Mix one ounce of nitrate of silver with six ounces of distilled water, or rain or snow water. Wet the hair first with a wash of one ounce of sulphuret of potassium dissolved in six ounces of rain-water; then paint the hair with the nitrate of silver mixture; but if this falls on the skin, it leaves an ugly stain for some time; yet it does turn the hair black in five minutes. But this sulphur preparation has a very disagreeable odor; hence some prefer a mixture without an odor. Add to the above nitrate of silver and rain-water mixture, some spirits of hartshorn; stir it in slowly with a stick or bone. It soon becomes cloudy; continue to add the hartshorn until it clears again. But before the hair is touched with this, it should be washed with a mixture made by dissolving in eight ounces of rose-water, one dram of pyrogallic acid, enough to dampen the hair; do not allow either of the preparations to touch the skin or fall on the clothing.

HAIR-OILS

are nearly every one of them made with hog's lard as the chief ingredient; but they are all fatty, and gather dust and dirt and soil the clothing. If, however, in certain cases, the hair is so dry or stubborn that it will not lie any way wanted, the least objectionable preparation is made of common castor-oil, two tablespoonfuls (one ounce) in a pint of good alcohol, as strong as ninety-five per cent. No better hair-oil than this can be made; it may be scented or colored, but the pure preparation alone is the best.

Many persons prefer the

GLYCERINE HAIR DRESSING,

as the glycerine retains its moisture longer than most other fluids. Dissolve four ounces of pure glycerine in twelve ounces of rain-water.

One of the most efficient and harmless washes to clean the scalp effectually, is

POWDERED BORAX.

Put a heaping teaspoonful into a teacupful of warm water; stir it up and pour it into a basin with a rounding bottom; wet the whole scalp with warm water, hold the face over the basin, keep the eyes shut, dip the ends of the fingers into the borax water, and rub it patiently and well into the scalp; bear almost as hard as you can; if done properly, the whole head will be covered with a white foam as if it were soap-suds, and is just as cleansing as soap, not having its harshness; after having rubbed the whole scalp into a lather, wash it off with fresh water; renew the water until the hair feels natural, as if all the lather were gone; then wipe dry with a soft towel; but do not comb the hair out until it is entirely dry when it will be found to be as fine and clean as the softest silk. One such a cleaning every month would never fail to keep the collars of the coats of gentlemen free from that very ugly and disagreeably suggestive sight of dandruff, for it means filth and neglect, worse even than

THE BLACK RIM

around the ends of the finger nails. The most healthful method of

WEARING THE HAIR

so as to promote its growth and beauty, is to let it fall as near as possible in its natural direction. Never allow it to be on

21

any more strain than by its natural weight, to that extent it may be parted in the front ; but as to ladies, the exact line of parting should be changed once a month, even if it be but a very slight deviation ; the neglect of this occasions that ugly,

BROAD PATCH OF SKULL

so often seen, instead of the deep, delicate, rich, and almost imperceptible line which is observed where there is a wealth of hair.

It would be well if the hair were worn, until married, falling down the back ; not plaited, nor twisted ; but just as loosely as will be allowed, by a silk cord between the ears behind, so as to keep it from falling forward, in the form of an oblong hoop. The almost universal fashion of drawing it upwards from the nape of the neck to near the top of the head is as injurious as it is unnatural and absurd. When not allowed to fall down between the shoulders, it should be gathered into a loose knot or twist, resting on the nape of the neck or very little higher ; the one object in all these adjustments being to prevent any one single hair from being on any strain beyond that of its own weight, as Nature doubtless intended.

Two or three times every day a lady's hair should be opened with a coarse comb drawn slowly and easily from the scalp to the ends of the hair, for the express purpose of cooling the scalp and letting the pure air get to each hair, down to the very root of it.

One of the most beautiful heads of hair known in history was that of an educated monk, who seemed to take great delight, for hours at a time every day, in gently combing out his locks to the farthest extremity.

If there should be a time to any one when there was an adequate reason for stimulating the growth of the hair, take one ounce each of glycerine, spirit of rosemary, and the aromatic spirit of hartshorn, four drams of the tincture of Cantharides, and five ounces of rose-water ; mix it well, and apply a tablespoonful night and morning. Or,

Two drams each of the balsam of Tolu, tincture of Cantharides, and castor-oil, two tablespoonfuls of lard, and half a teaspoonful or thirty drops of oil of rosemary ; mix well, and use it as a pomade every morning.

A more simple and convenient preparation is formed by mixing two ounces of spirits of hartshorn and twelve ounces of pure, white hog's lard; mix it well, and keep it tightly stopped, or the hartshorn will evaporate; a glass stopper will prevent this.

OILS ARE USELESS

to make the hair grow, because the hair is made almost entirely of nitrogen, of which no oil known contains a single atom; but hartshorn contains a considerable amount of nitrogen, and being mixed with lard, it is a means of conveying the nitrogen to the root of each hair, and keeping it there for absorption as long as the lard remains to prevent dryness. Hence oils only act as a polish for the hair. A good

HARTSHORN POMADE

is prepared thus : one quarter of a pound of almond oil, half an ounce of white wax, three ounces of clarified hog's lard, a quarter of an ounce of fluid hartshorn, one dram each of otto of lavender, and cloves. Put the oil, wax, and lard into a glass jar, set it in boiling water; when all is well melted, let it cool a little, and before it becomes hard, stir in the hartshorn and perfumes; put into small jars, and keep in a cool, dry place, to be used at night only; use the comb lightly and a soft hair-brush while this is going on. If persons are resolved to do something for the

CURE OF BALDNESS,

take several large handfuls of the common garden box, boil in three pints of water, in a closed vessel, for a quarter of an hour pour it into an earthen jar, and let it stand until next day. Strain this liquid, and add three or four tablespoons of cologne water; wash the whole scalp with this, and do it well every morning, until the hair grows or does not grow; then stop.

FALLING HAIR

is sometimes occasioned by the too free and constant use of oils, or ill-health; in such cases, a remedy is sometimes found in a mixture of half a pint each of sherry wine and elder water, tincture of arnica half an ounce, of strong spirits of hartshorn one teaspoonful. Apply this to the hair with a sponge every night, so as to wet it well. Keep the mixture in a bottle, wash the whole scalp twice a week with warm water, and use only the softest brushes while the hair is growing.

Pour boiling water on sage leaves, and let stand near a stove, or fire, half a day or longer; wash the whole scalp with this every day; in some cases this seems to benefit the hair.

It is repeated, in order to make a strong and an abiding impression. At the bottom of each hair is a little bulb containing what is called the hair pulp, which makes the hair grow and which colors it; this is the food, the manna of the hair: but if these pulps die or are plucked out, or otherwise destroyed, the roots of the hair are gone, leaving the scalp smooth and shiny, and so it will remain forever. But if not shiny, if there is a frizzy appearance, the hair has disappeared from accidental causes, and will return sooner or later; if any good can be done in the way of hastening its growth, the following may be tried. Take one quarter of an ounce each of fluid potash and oil of sweet almonds, rose-water two ounces, and fourteen ounces of rain or distilled water. Rub a little of this into the skin, with the ends of the fingers, at least five minutes at a time, twice a day. The cheapest and best

HAIR PRESERVER AND RESTORATIVE

in the world is soft water. Wash the hair well twice a week in pure, soft, rain, snow, or distilled, water, using daily a comb with no sharp points, moving it through the hair so gently, slowly, and easily as not to wound the scalp or break any of the hairs, or tear them out by the roots.

If the whole hair and scalp are washed well in pure, soft water every day, there is slight liability to any form of disease prevailing at the time, especially in crowded houses, hospitals, ships, and soldiers' barracks; there should be a complete immersion of the head in cold water every day, winter or summer.

HAIR OF CHILDREN

uld never be plaited; it strains them, impedes the healthful ibution of nutriment, hence checks the healthy growth.

The hair of girls should be kept cut short until fourteen, allowing to curl prettily over the head; after that it should be twisted very lightly into a loose coil; the ends, if tied, should be fastened loosely with a soft ribbon. Nothing but pure, soft water should ever be applied to the hair of children.

On looking at a single hair with a good microscope, it will be seen to be made of successive layers or overlapping cells, like the scales of a fish, each scale tapering to the thinned, infinitesimal point or cone; the edge of each scale serrated like the teeth of a saw. Each hair is marked by many transverse and irregularly crooked lines. Hog's bristles are more like the human hair than any other animal's.

MEN'S HAIR,

when it begins to fall out, may be saved sometimes by keeping it cut very short; brush it well when quite dry; this loosens the dandruff if the brush is moderately stiff. Then wash with warm soap-suds rubbed well into the scalp with the balls of the fingers, so that each particular root may be reached. Next, wipe the whole hair with a soft towel; then in the same manner rub into the scalp and roots of the hair some of the hartshorn washes previously named, or a little bay rum, brandy, or other spirits. This should be done twice a month. The scalp may be brushed well two or three times a week to advantage.

HAIR PHYSIOGNOMY.

The character of persons is sometimes foreshadowed by the color of the hair.

The bilious temperament, black hair, and dark skin are usually found together; there is strength of character and sensuality.

Fine hair and dark skin show purity, goodness, and strong mind.

Stiff, straight, and abundant black hair and beard are combined with a character which is straightforward, unyielding, strong, and rather bluff.

There is exquisite sensibility in fine brown hair, with a strong will for what is good and right, if not perverted.

If the hair is straight, lies flat on the head, there is melancholy; but you may safely rely on that person, be it man or woman.

If the hair is coarse, black, and sticks up, there is not much talking, and much that is stubborn, sour, and harsh, unless modified by grace.

There is fiery animosity in coarse red hair, with unusual firmness of purpose and strength of character.

Auburn hair, from the Latin "alburnus,"Ger."brennen," to burn, means reddish, like flame, or giving a golden hue, having a yellowish tinge; with a florid face gives purity, intensity, and great capacity for enjoyment or suffering.

Fine, silky, pliable hair, easily dressed, indicates delicacy, sensitiveness, and goodness.

Hasty, impetuous, rash people have curly, crisp hair; but if it is straight and smooth and even and glossy, there is a warm heart, a clear head, and superior talents.

White hair, as a general rule, indicates a good, easy, lazy fellow.

A red head is furiously passionate; there is sulphur there which takes fire in an instant.   Black hair has but little sulphur and a great deal of carbon or charcoal.

The hair naturally parting in the middle and falling on either side indicates womanly refinement, purity, and delicacy.   Thus, the old painters represented the poets and artists of their day— Homer, Virgil, Shakespeare, Milton, Dante, Raphael, Chaucer, and very many others.   This represents the feature of Him whose Name is above every name.   When the hair comes out and lies on the forehead in rings, it indicates a frank, open, genial nature.

The dark-haired races, the Spaniard, the Malay, the Mexican, the Indian, and the Negro, have physical strength, endurance, robustness in body.

The light-haired races are the thinkers of the world, the poets and the artists.

Dark-brown hair combines the two, and is the most desirable.

To sum up the whole matter:

Black hair is associated with bodily strength.

White hair with mental vigor.

Red hair is fiery in temperament, passion, and devotion.

Wavy hair is pliable, yielding, accommodating.

Straight, stuck-up hair is stubbornness and fidelity.

Very smooth, coarse-lying hair is oily gammon.

CURIOSITIES OF HAIR.

Wigs were worn three thousand years ago. One was found in a good state of preservation in a temple at Thebes, and is now to be seen in the British Museum.

The most perfect method of making wigs now, is to thread each hair and pass the needle through the imitation skin, as near the direction that the hair should lie as possible, with every hair having its bulb in the artificial wig, and not top end downwards.

All hair is very thoroughly boiled in water, most effectually killing everything that lives in it; hence, all the stories are without any foundation which intimate that those who purchase false hair are liable to be infected with vermin. The object of the boiling is to cleanse the hair most thoroughly : to make it as clean as silk ; otherwise it would rot and become unsalable.

The hair taken from the head of a diseased or a dead person is itself dead, is instantly detected by the purchaser, and the mere offer to sell it would subject him to loss of name as an honorable dealer; it would not be bought at any price.

In order to make hair curl and seem natural and remain so, the locks are wound around earthen rollers and stewed for two hours. This alone would kill any insect. It is then made into a literal pie, with the crust, and baked in an oven, as if it had to be eaten.

The hair grows about half an inch in a month, on an average; faster in summer than in winter.

The light hair comes from Germany. The black hair comes from Italy and the South of France, collected by a single hair merchant himself, who goes from fair to fair, where the peasant girls go expressly to sell their long, beautiful tresses; they stand together in a kind of semicircle, with the hair all combed out; with a single feel of the finger, and a smell, the merchant determines in an instant the value of it to him, and pays for it accordingly; each fleece is hastily tied in a knot or hoop, thrown in the basket. A common fleece brings in merchandise what cost the dealer ten or fifteen cents, but which there, is worth perhaps half a dollar. But now and then a very superior article has been known to bring twenty-five dollars an ounce for some special purpose or person, who wanted it of a particular tint and glossiness and length; this would be equal to some two hundred dollars for a fleece.

Railways break up hair fairs, because they carry with them progress, improvement, cultivation, refinement, and self-appreciation. It is only among the most ignorant, petty, and debased communities, that the hair can be purchased. Brittany and Normandy, "my Normandy," furnish the largest supplies, nearly twenty thousand pounds apiece every year. Belgium sends sixteen thousand pounds of hair to market every year.

Three heads yield a pound of hair on an average in Italy; in Belgium it requires six.

The coarsest hair comes from Auvergne, the finest from Belgium, the blackest and longest from Italy. The most beautiful hair in the world and the prettiest is from Bretagne or Brittany, a French province.

GRAY HAIRS

sometimes come prematurely by inheritance, some great trouble, or the large use of water which has lime in it; this is easily determined by taking half a glass of the water and blowing into it through a rye straw, or other tube; in proportion as it is limy it turns to a milky white, by the carbonic acid of the breath uniting with the lime, and making it solid. Lime water also makes the hair harsh and dry and brittle; these things can be obviated, remedied, or prevented by using only rain or distilled water, either for drinking purposes or in tea and coffee. If lime is the cause, the color may be restored sometimes by washing the hair well every morning, and by mixing half a pint of bay rum, half a pint of the best brandy, and one pint and a half of the best sweet oil; this mixture must be kept in a bottle well stopped, and must be thoroughly shaken before using. A patient perseverance in the use of this preparation frequently gives a very gratifying result. There is a

TURKISH HAIR-DYE

of considerable value. Take finely pulverized galls, make into a little paste, with sweet oil, roast this in an iron pan until no vapor rises; add water to the residue, until another paste is formed; heat this also until it is dry; make this into a powder

and keep it dry in a bottle, well stopped; when it is wanted to
be used, take a little of it between the thumb and fingers, and
rub the hair or head with it; or it may be put into the palm
of the hand and rubbed well into the hair every day once or
twice; in a few days the hair becomes of a glossy black, is
soft and pliant, and retains its color for a considerable time.
When the hair becomes suddenly gray, it is most generally from
great mental shocks; we all have felt the effect of it, to a greater
or less extent, about the heart, hence the instinctive carrying the
hand to the left side of the breast; and it is the office of the
heart to throw the blood to the most distant parts of the body;
but this it fails to do, to a proper extent; hence the hair suffers
for want of its proper amount and quality of blood, hence it is
clear that the sudden change of the color of the hair is owing to
the unnatural action of the heart. A lady who had a remarkable quantity of jet-black hair was called to endure a very great
change for the worse in her pecuniary circumstances; on the
very next morning her hair was of a lily white. On the journey from Varennes to Paris, the hair of Marie Antoinette
turned white.

As the Duchess of Luxemburgh was escaping during the
French Revolution, she was caught, put in prison, and the next
morning her hair was white.

It is related that an attempt was made to test the courage of
a Spanish officer who had a great reputation for bravery. He
was waked up at midnight out of a deep sleep, and informed
that by order of the Viceroy he was to be executed in fifteen
minutes. He said he was prepared to die, but was innocent of
the charge; when told that it was a joke, he laid his hand upon
his heart, instinctively, as if there was something there which
influenced his whole nature and was irrepressible, and only said,
" You have done me an evil service." In the morning his hair
was as white as snow.

The grief and mortification in consequence of the disasters
at Magenta and Malegnano turned the hair of Generals Hurn
and Benedek perfectly white in a few days.

Dr. D. Parry, Staff Surgeon at Aldershott, England, writes
that on the 19th of February, 1858, a sepoy of the Bengal army
was taken prisoner; I saw him stripped naked and surrounded
by soldiers; he trembled violently; despair and horror most in-

tense were depicted on his countenance; he seemed almost stupefied with fear, and under my observation his hair, from being a glossy jet black, became gray on every portion of his head within half an hour; the sergeant, whose prisoner he was, exclaimed, "He is turning gray." It is supposed that under the influence of fear or any great mental shock, the fluids of the hair retire to the interior, as under the same circumstances the blood of the surface retires to the interior of the body, to the heart, and its place in the hair is supplied with air bubbles which are colorless, and which remain there, becoming a permanency.

DRESSING THE HAIR

indicates the character of the wearer, especially in ladies, for it gives infinite scope for cultivating and exercising the taste; it affords a wide field for studying the adaptations of things. There is as much in the dressing of the hair as in the dress of the body; and few there are who understand either, who have by instinct the valuable secret of arranging all, so that the whole person shall be improved, "set off" to the best advantage.

A great bunch of hair on either side of a little, thin face, makes that face a caricature, makes it thinner and more tiny than before; not much better would it be for a dumpy person to wear enormous quantities of hair on the back of the head; and yet these are the very persons who affect the largest possible waterfalls, making them dumpier, more dwarfish than before.

A lady with a low forehead may brush her hair backward from the face, but that is no reason why another with a very high and broad forehead should do the same thing.

Round and broad faces are set off with drooping curls; but they make a long and flat cheek look more gaunt and skinny.

By studying the fitness of things, a curl has many a time caught a husband as whiskers have won a wife, and so it will be while the world stands.

A SINGLE HAIR

once held a sword; and frail though it is, it has power over mind and memory more enduring than its own ability to resist physical decay, for long after the body and its clothing have wasted away to their original dust, the hair vies with the bones in a protracted existence; the coffin and the solid plate are gone, but the hair is still there, the solitary remnant of one who lived an age ago.

A LOOK OF HAIR.

How carefully treasured! What a flood of loving memories crowd around the heart as we gaze upon it; how it carries us back to the loved and lost, a part of whom it once was, the only thing unchanged that they left on earth; for a moment it seems as if the departed were almost present; for a brief instant we can almost look into the eye or hear the voice; the expression of the countenance, the smile on the lip—how they all flit across memory's waste, and tell of happier days departed, fully authorizing the apostrophe of the poet:

> " How often has this lovely curl
> Been bound with flowers and decked with pearl;
> How oft round snowy fingers twined,
> How often fluttered in the wind !
> Aye, 'tis a thing to love and bless,
> This little sweetly shining tress.
> The one by whom this gem was given
> Seems to my heart a thing of heaven.
> An angel dream—a gentle dove
> Sent forth from out the ark of love;
> A vision come from Paradise
> To bless and gladden mortal eyes."

THE VOICE.

SOUND is a series of air-waves, extending and widening as in the water when a pebble is thrown into it. Musical sounds travel farther than others by one half. A strong, healthy man can " fill " a room measuring seventy-five feet each way ; if he sings, he can fill a room half as large again.

There may be a hum of voices in a room, and a fife playing at the same time ; you may not be able to hear the fife in the room, the hum drowns it; this hum will travel a hundred yards perhaps ; but far beyond that you can hear the fife with great distinctness. At the same time, as between speaking in a monotonous or sing-song tone, and a distinct enunciation with an appreciable interval between each word and syllable, there can be no comparison as to the greater ease in understanding the latter, although the volume of sound in the former is much greater. Many a public speaker is pleasurably understood with much less power expended in vocalization, while another, with stentorian lungs, fails to convey his ideas to the hearer, the difference being in the manner of enunciation.

Monotonous speakers are heard painfully, because the sounding of one word runs into another, and the attention is kept on the stretch all the time to catch the intervals, which it is necessary to do in order to comprehend the idea. A certain method of avoiding this great and unfortunate mistake is for the speaker himself so to pronounce each word that his own ear can easily measure a distinct interval, not only between each word, but between every syllable. If a public speaker will pay the proper attention, he will discover that there exists a certain instinct within him, which will enable him to feel whether his voice fills the room and reaches the whole audience.

A blind man was once sent to an office to deliver a message. On returning, he reported that on opening the door he found no person there. On being asked how he knew it, he replied that the rebound of the voice, its force and character, were different in an empty room and one more or less full. There is a ring in an empty room; if full, the voice falls more like a thug or muffled sound.

A man may cast a pebble fifty yards, and fifty other men of equal strength and skill could each cast it fifty yards; but no one of the fifty can throw that pebble farther than fifty yards. So five hundred voices, although very loud within the sphere of one voice, will not be heard farther than one voice of the five hundred. Thus a man may be singing in a crowd where the general hum prevents him hearing himself, yet he will be heard at a distance far beyond that which the hum reaches, because a musical note travels farther than one of prose.

To speak without an effort of mind or voice or person, the whole consciousness must be absorbed in the subject itself. Then only can a man speak with Nature's eloquence. He must for the instant feel that his subject is overwhelmingly real, overwhelmingly important; hence it is that all the " arts " of oratory, such as studied gestures, attitudes, attention to the modes of breathing, and efforts to speak so as not to exhaust the lungs fully, are so much wastes of physical power, as well as moral force, because just that much attention is taken from the subject, and deprives it of its life. The oratory of the heart, which is effective the world over, whether in assemblies civilized or savage, cultivated or all untutored, is that which comes from a man whose consciousness makes him feel that material and immortal destinies hang upon his utterances.

CLEAN FEET.

THE majority of people pay little attention to the cleanliness of the feet, and yet any square inch of the sole of the foot demands cleanliness, perfect cleanliness, more than any square foot of surface of the body, as far as health is concerned, because the "pores" are much larger there than anywhere else; so large indeed that they may be called "sluices" for carrying away the impurities of the system. Hence the bottom of the feet should be well washed and well rubbed every day.

PIES, PASTRIES, AND PUDDINGS

are as healthful and more nutritious than pork steaks, roast pig, or boiled ham; and yet there will not be perhaps two readers in ten who will assent to the statement. But when Old Christmas is coming, and the tables of the country will be loaded with this "forbidden fruit," it would be a great misfortune to let so many good things be neglected; but there is no danger of that, which proves that the reader practically admits the truth of the "monstrous statement" of the opening sentence, so contrary to preconceived opinion, that "pies, pastries, and puddings are as healthful and more nutritious than pork steaks, roast pig, or boiled ham." Nine readers in .ten will regard this statement with almost contemptuous surprise. But as the year is closing in, when these things will abound in every household, let us look into the thing, with a view to eat, drink, and be merry during the grand holiday time.

Every man of science knows that there is twice as much nourishment, meaning thereby power to give warmth and strength, in a pound of sponge-cake, gingerbread, or plum-pudding, as in a pound of roast beef, for more than half the beef is water. To be specific, two-thirds of the best roast beef is water, and one-third nutriment at most, while puddings and "sweet cakes" of every description contain more than two-thirds nutriment, and have less than one-third water; hence a man will live longer on five pounds of sweet cake, than on five pounds of roast beef. Sweet cakes, pound-cakes, and the like are bread sweetened, with trifling additions, as to weight, of eggs and butter; but the flour alone out of which the cake is made, which when baked is called "bread," has all the elements of nutrition, and man can live on bread alone. But neither the eggs, nor the sugar, nor the butter, nor the milk, which added to the flour complete the ingredients of pound-cakes, are unhealthful nor innutritious; hence it is difficult to conclude that if each of half a dozen of ingredients which make up an article of food are healthful, all combined are unhealthful, especially as, if eaten singly at one meal, they would all be mixed together in the stomach, where it will be found that in the course of two or three hours after an ordinary meal, the contents of the stomach, if the owner of it is in vigorous health, are to all appearance identical in color, consistency, and general appearance. The same general principles hold good as to pies and puddings. A pie is stewed fruit added to a little bread and butter; the butter being mixed with the flour before baking, making pastry, cannot by the mixture make the combination unhealthy; it will scarcely be asserted that bread and butter outside of the stomach can become unhealthy when put inside well mixed, as they are in chewing. The same things hold good as to the prince of puddings—

"PLUM-PUDDINGS."

The plums, the flour, the butter, and the several other ingredients are healthful to eat individually; and why not collectively is difficult to comprehend.

The universal error as to the unhealthful nature of pies, puddings, and pastries, taking it for granted that they are well made and properly cooked, has arisen from the simple fact that being eaten after we have made a full meal of other things, the stomach is oppressed by them, and, if the process is repeated, becomes eventually dyspeptic; that is, has not power to work up the food, because it has been "worked to death" already. It would be quite as philosophical to say that if a man has become very tired by ploughing all day, and then by chopping wood he had " worked himself out," it was very unhealthy to chop wood.

It has frequently occurred to observant persons that having made a good meal, the unexpected appearance of a toothsome pie, or splendid pudding, or irresistible cake, instantaneously and miraculously changed their sentiments. A moment before they thought, felt, and believed that they had eaten enough ; and now they believe no such thing, and forthwith eat as much in bulk as they had already taken, with the result very often that they are

" AS SICK AS DEATH."

Whether death is ever sick or not, is another question; but the meaning is, they feel as if they were almost sick enough to die. The legitimate conclusion is that pies, pastries, and puddings are as healthful as roast beef or boiled tongue, if properly prepared, and eaten judiciously as to time, quantity, and quality. There are multitudes of dyspeptic persons in the common walks of life and on our farms who very rarely can afford to indulge in pies, pastries, and puddings, showing that they have become dyspeptic by eating bread and meat and vegetables at improper times, in improper quantities, or after improper preparation.

The healthy method of taking pies, pastries, puddings, and other forms of dessert is,

First. As a luncheon, take a moderate amount, and nothing else.

Second. Leave room for them at dinner-time, by eating half as much dinner as you would have done had you known there was to be no dessert.

Third. Take your dessert at the beginning of dinner; and if any man eats too much dinner after that, he will be the greatest curiosity in existence.

THERMOMETERS AND BAROMETERS.

THERE ought to be a barometer in every family, and a thermometer in every chamber, that every child may be taught their uses, which, if properly explained, and with sufficient clearness, will become a fund of amusement, and interesting and intelligent observation for a lifetime.

The barometer measures the heaviness of the atmosphere; the heavier it is, the farther up does it press the mercury, for the column of mercury in the barometer exactly balances a like column of air extending to the top of the atmosphere. The lighter the air, the lower the barometer, the heavier are we relatively to the air, and the more lifeless and depressed are we apt to feel. At places near the sea-level the mercury in the barometer averages about 30 inches high, sometimes rising there to 31 inches, sometimes falling there to 28 inches. The higher above the sea the barometer is, the lower the mercury in it.

It is a comfortable thing to get up in the morning when we have a pleasant visit or excursion in contemplation, to know that it will not rain that day; and many a time it will save a best dress or best bonnet to be told by the silent friend that it will certainly rain before night. But to be thus informed, the height of the mercury should be marked at night, and there is a convenient arrangement for that purpose; if, on rising in the morning, the mercury has fallen an inch, it will certainly be followed by rain or storm before night; if, on the other hand, it has risen largely, it will clear away in a few hours, although it is raining at the instant.

The uses of the thermometer are to indicate the temperature of our chambers, and to warn us beforehand of the state of the out-door air, that we may adapt our clothing to that day's climate.

The Duke of Wellington's nose was his thermometer, and it was about the longest and biggest we ever saw; he never failed to hoist the window and put his head outside the first thing every morning, " sniff " the air, then give his servant directions what clothing to lay out for him that day. Many a life has been lost by not being dressed warm enough on going out for the day, in consequence of a great change in the weather during the night; for it requires a day or two for the cold "to get into the house." On the other hand, if it suddenly changes to a much greater warmth during the night, thirty or forty degrees warmer, and we go out with the clothing of the previous day, we are oppressed, and change to a lighter dress, and a bad cold is taken. It is never safe to change to a lighter dress, after having dressed in the morning; if we want to "leave off" clothing, let that be at the first dressing, and at no other time. This observance alone will prevent much sickness during a lifetime.

In summer time, if we sit in a room of sixty-eight degrees, the system will be certainly and quickly chilled; but in mid-winter a room of sixty-eight degrees will feel almost "suffocating," especially if entered soon after a brisk, out-door walk. Ordinarily a church feels comfortably warm in winter, if the thermometer stands at sixty-five in the centre of the building, and about five feet from the floor.

COAL FIRES.

SERIOUS inconvenience to health is sometimes occasioned by tardiness in kindling a coal fire; passengers in railroad cars have often undergone incalculable sufferings from this cause.

Before coal kindles it must be heated through and through, made hot enough to blister the fingers in an instant, although still black. It is easy to see that a small bit of coal will get thus heated sooner than a larger one; hence the smaller the coal, the sooner will it ignite.

Coal must be kindled with wood. This wood will give out a certain amount of heat, and no more; and as a given amount of heat is necessary to kindle the coal, the more wood, and the less coal, and the smaller the pieces, the sooner and more certainly will the fire be lighted.

In the face of these facts, persons are frequently seen in rail-cars, when the fire in the stove is low, to put on a large amount of coal, the result being that the more coal put on, the more the fire will not burn, because the small amount of heat is distributed over a large amount of coal, all of which is heated some, but

22

none of it heated enough for ignition. The more a coal fire is stirred, if a little low, the more certain it is to go out.

The best way to replenish a coal fire is to put on a small amount of coal while it is burning well; and after this is thoroughly kindled, and has been red for a short time, add a little more coal. In this way a fire may be kept burning a whole day in a grate without using the poker once; and good housekeepers know that every time a poker is used, the ashes fly in every direction, and valuable time is expended in brushing them up. If a poker must be used, the time to do it is when fresh coal has been thoroughly kindled, for then there is no danger of its going out.

If a coal fire is burning too much, either cover it with some of the ashes which have fallen through the grate; this makes the mass more compact, and diminishes the draught; or if it is desirable to put the fire out altogether, as when going to bed, press the coal down from the top with a shovel or blunt-edged poker.

It has been the custom to use the largest-sized coal for the furnace; this requires a great waste of wood in kindling, besides much time is lost in firing up in the morning, the very time when most heat is wanted, and wanted quickly. It will take less coal, and give incomparably more comfort, to feed a furnace with coal, the largest piece of which is not larger than a hen's egg, only taking care to put on a little coal every hour. Observation and close-calculating economy has shown this to all our river boats, tugs, and steamers.

As a well-warmed house and a brightly burning fire in the grate add greatly to the comfort, and life, and enjoyability of winter calls, these items about coal fires are seasonable. The most beautiful, the cheeriest, and the most healthful open fire known is that which is furnished by Dixon's low-down grates.

RICE.

BOILED rice is among the most nutritious of all foods, and is the most easily digested, and, being cheap in all countries, it is the principal food of more than half of the human family, and is especially suitable for cold weather; for one pound of it gives as much warmth to the body as four pounds of roast beef, and it is digested in about one-fourth the time, that is, in one hour; but it does not give one-quarter the power to work which roast beef gives. It is more universally used among the Chinese than any other nation, and is on that account, perhaps, prepared most philosophically by them, as thus: " take a clean stew-pan with a close-fitting top, then take a clean piece of white muslin, large enough to cover over the top of the pan, and hang down inside nearly to but not in contact with the bottom. Into the sack so formed place the rice, pour over two cupfuls of water, and put on the top of the stew-pan, so as to hold up the muslin bag inside, and fit tight all around. Place the pan over a slow fire, and the steam generated from the water will cook the rice. Each grain, it is stated, will come out of the boiler as dry and as distinct as if just taken from the hull. More water may be poured into the pan, if necessary, but only sufficient to keep up the steam till the rice is cooked. The pan must not be heated so hot as to cause the steam to blow off the lid."

It ought to be extensively known that ordinary boiled rice, eaten with boiled milk, is one of the best remedies known for any form of loose bowels. Its efficacy is increased if it is browned like coffee, and then boiled and eaten at intervals of four hours, taking no other food or liquid whatever; its curative virtue is intensified if no milk is taken with it, and the patient will keep quiet in a warm bed; then it becomes an almost infallible remedy.

COMPLAINING.

While those who are never well should have our warmest sympathies, very different is it with that innumerable host of chronic growlers who are pouring into our afflicted ears the interminable tale of their sorrows, the whole of which are imaginary, are from mere habit, or are from their own making.

Some persons, after having been sick a short time, are very liable to fall into the habit of complaining, which becomes so inveterate that they unconsciously begin to detail symptoms which long before had ceased to have an existence.

For that unfortunate class who are forever looking out for symptoms, and seem to feel a real gratification to have something to growl about, and will shake their heads into a headache, or poke their sides in search of a "hurt" if they have none, there is no hope; they are clean gone daft. But let the reader take a hint on the subject; except in your own family, no one cares a straw about your complaints, and, for the sake of getting rid of your rigmarole in the shortest time possible, will thrust a piece of advice under your nose which cured somebody a great deal worse than you are, and of course it will cure you; and, having fixed you off, they are then for business.

If you have nothing better than a complaint to make of yourself, hadn't you better go on the principle, "If you haven't anything good to say, say nothing"?

What good can it do for you to be talking about your imperfections? If you are speaking to a real friend, it only saddens him to think that you are suffering, and the more so as he is helpless to aid you. There is some sense in a man's speaking of his actual virtues, or what he has done for the good of others; but to be telling Tom, Dick, and Harry, the instant you lay your eyes on them, that you have a sore toe, or a boil on your body, or the "rheumatiz" in your joints, or a hole in the spine of your back, man alive, be ashamed of yourself, and from this day forth, if a friend asks you "How do you do?" say, "Pretty well, I thank you," and then talk about something else. In this way you will at least get rid of trying a thousand and one things which have cured a man "no worse than you," or "a great deal better than you," don't know which.

TOOTH-PICKS.

Some one has said, "one tooth-pick is worth a bushel of tooth-brushes." The people must get into the habit of weighing every practical statement in reference to the health and well-being of our bodies, or they will be led by specious statements, or striking comparisons, or popular names, to many hurtful habits, practices, and observances. Every dentist knows that the more a tooth-pick is used, the more the yielding gum is pressed upward; and the larger the space becomes between the teeth next the gum, the larger will be the pieces of food that will lodge there, and the greater the necessity of the use of the tooth-pick for the remainder of life, and to some extent the solid tooth itself may wear away.

If the tooth is hollow, it ought to be extracted or filled with gold at the very earliest moment possible, so as to prevent decay and a noisome breath.

To be under the necessity of spending five or ten or more minutes after each meal in picking the teeth is a great and useless waste of time, and is essentially a loafing and indecent practice, unless done in one's own private room. On the other hand, the intelligent dentist knows that the judicious use of a toothbrush immediately after each meal, twisting it up and down sideways, so that each bristle becomes a soft tooth-pick, and gently dislodges particles of food, while at the same time it hardens the gum, makes it more firm, causes it to grow more fully into any crevices, and fills them up more perfectly. Whether by pick or brush the same important end is sought, to keep the teeth clean, because it is the only means of preserving them, and the want of it the certain means of their speedy destruction in almost every case.

THE NEW ANODYNE.

THE medical world is delighted with the discovery of a new medicine, and the newspapers abound with advertisements, setting forth the peculiar advantages of each preparation, every man claiming that his own is the best. It is called

CHLORAL HYDRATE.

The object of taking this medicine is to promote sleep, and thus far, when administered pure and in a proper manner, it has advantages above all others known hitherto, whether in the form of Opium, Morphine, Laudanum, or Paregoric.

This Chloral Hydrate is in white crystals; almost every liquid dissolves it; hence it is largely advertised in the shape of syrups, anodynes, and various fluid mixtures. When it is dissolved in any fluid, it begins to lose its peculiar power within an hour; hence it should be mixed and used on the spot. Therefore, if employed at all, each person should purchase it in its white crystal form direct from the apothecary, and mix it himself; then only can he get all its advantages, and know what and how much he is taking; all preparations of Chloral Hydrate other than in white crystal form are gross impositions on the public.

There can be no doubt of its advantageous use under the physician's care for a few times; but any one who takes it on his own responsibility, especially if used night after night for promoting sleep, acts most unwisely, for it has not been in use long enough to allow proper observations to be made as to its safety. There are several medicines which can be taken a few times without any apparent ill result; but if their employment is continued, the most ineradicable and deathly consequences follow. A man may drink water brought into the house by a faulty lead pipe, and notice no inconvenience; he may repeat that drinking for days and weeks, and be apparently as well as ever; but continuing to use it for months, the most incurable poisoning follows, and in multitudes of cases fatal, after months and years of torment.

All anodynes act more or less directly on the brain, the most delicate and dangerous part of the whole body to be tampered with, and Chloral may have its far-reaching tendencies there to impair and to destroy. Sleep, healthful, delicious, and invigorating, comes only from the exhaustion to a certain point of that store of strength with which we leave our chambers in the morning, which "store of strength" is the result of rest to body and brain. This store of strength comes up, accumulates as naturally as the water accumulates in a well which has been left almost dry from excessive use; the water rises higher and higher, simply from the well being let alone. So bodily strength rises up, as it were, during a state of repose, while asleep at night, and does this more favorably if left alone to its own natural actions. The best and only healthful anodyne in the world, the most unobjectionable sleep-producer, is sturdy, honest out-door labor; for the Bible has said it: "The sleep of a laboring man is sweet."

WINTER SHOES.

In the sloshy weather of winter, when the roads and streets are covered with mud or half-melted snow, India-rubber shoes are a perfect protection; but to wear them longer than an hour or two, especially if the person is not in continuous exercise, has the certain effect to make the feet cold and clammy, thus preparing the system for colds, croups, and inflammation of the lungs.

Workmen and business men must be on their feet more or less all day; and to have the feet dry and warm is essential to health and comfort, and even to life itself.

The soles of shoes can be made impervious to dampness if they alone are soaked for twenty-four hours in kerosene oil, and are then allowed to dry thoroughly. Let the sole be deep enough in the oil to cover the top of it, so that the oil may sink in among the stitches, and fill in the seams of the sole and upper leather; then the upper leather may be polished with blacking, but it could not be made to shine as well if soaked in oil, nor is it desirable to have the upper leather impervious, for then it would be no better than India rubber.

All persons should have cork soles in their shoes, the cork being covered on the side next the foot with Canton flannel; but it would be well to take them out every night, and place them where they will be well aired and dried. Another benefit of cork soles is, they save about ninety per cent. of darning. Nine shoemakers out of ten fail to rasp off the pegs and nails on the inside of the sole, the result being in many cases that holes are worn in the stockings in twenty-four hours after their first wearing. But even if the wooden pegs are ever so well rasped, or the iron pegs clinched, still wood and iron are harder than leather, have no yield, and wear holes in the best stockings in a short time; and as a large portion of the time of our industrious wives at the close of the week, especially on Saturday nights, is spent in darning stockings, these suggestions are worth consideration.

CHILL AND FEVER

is the all-pervading blight within fifty miles of New York City, causing multitudes who go to the country for health to return in the fall of the year saturated with disease, which the slightest indiscretion or exposure develops into some troublesome fever or mysterious form of sickness. Chill and fever, intermittents, and the old-fashioned name of

FEVER AND AGUE,

are one and the same disease, arising from the one cause of low, damp lands or stagnant water, whether in the shape of mill-ponds, lakes, sluggish streams, or pools of water here and there in the beds of half-dried creeks and rivulets. Many neighborhoods are the hot-beds of disease in summer, because the ponds are not filled up or the lowlands drained. If standing water is drained in warm weather, it exaggerates the sickness a thousand-fold, because the slimy bottom is exposed to the hot sun, and the deadly miasm is generated in incredible quantities and of concentrated virulence.

The time for draining ponds or other forms of stagnant water is midwinter. Then fill up or plough and cultivate in early spring, keeping all the drains free. To show what intelligence and public spirit will do through a single individual, it may be stated that a gentleman living near New York, observing that there was a great deal of sickness near his country place every autumn, quietly purchased all the ponds in his neighborhood, to the great astonishment and wonderment of everybody. He subsequently drained them, and, when the bottoms were dry, ploughed them deeply, thoroughly, and well; then sowed his seed. The fall gave a crop which surprised "everybody;" such a yield had never been heard of in all that section of country; and September, 1871, when Staten Island, New Haven, Poughkeepsie, and other places were overrun with chill and fever to an unremembered extent, the village of West Farms is not known to have had a single case. In many parts of our country intelligent enterprise can prevent disease, produce unheard-of crops, and add one hundred per cent. to the value of adjoining lands. Fever and ague is said to be cured by dissolving a heaping tea-spoon of common salt in half a glass of water, and drinking it on rising, three mornings in succession. It would not be wise to call this ridiculous, until thoroughly tried. An old negro once said that he knew a tree, the bark of which would cure chill and fever; the people tried it, and, finding that it never failed in that country, gave the man a large amount of money to show the tree; from this bark quinine is now made.

If common table salt can cure fever and ague, it may be added to the increasing list of "Food Cures," for salt is on all our tables. Still it would be better to have no fever and ague, by draining all ponds within five miles of the locality where it prevails, in the winter; then either fill them up or plough the bottoms and cultivate them, thus obtaining a large amount of healthful food from spots which caused disease and death to make their ravages through whole neighborhoods.

TOMATOES AS FOOD.

It is known that the essence of the tomato made into a pill acts upon the liver, and to that extent must counteract biliousness and all forms of fever.

The free use of figs is known to multitudes to obviate constipation in a great many cases; every intelligent druggist knows that a tablespoon of white mustard-seed, swallowed without chewing, is useful in the same direction, has been used for that purpose for a century, and for that reason is kept in every good drug-store for sale. The seeds pass from the body unchanged, but are supposed "to act" on the bowels mechanically. The seeds of the delightful tomato act in the same manner; hence the fruit, while it is palatable to the taste, and nutritious to the body, has a health-promoting effect on the liver and the whole digestive system.

MAKING COFFEE.

Make a bag of felt or heavy woollen flannel long enough to reach from the top to the bottom of the coffee-pot, with a wire attached to keep the bag upright; put the fresh-ground coffee in the bag, pour on boiling water, and it is at once fit for use; the water takes the strength out of the coffee and passes through the flannel clear with all its aroma.

Americans persist in boiling the coffee, thus driving away its most delicious quality.

The French put the ground coffee in a tin cup with perforated bottoms, pour on boiling water, and then give it time to drain through; but if the liquid is then boiled, its most essential and distinctive quality is evaporated and lost, although not to as great an extent as in the most unphilosophical American method

HEARTY SUPPERS.

It requires about five hours for the stomach to work up an ordinary meal and pass it out of itself, when it falls into a state of repose. Hence, if a man eats three times a day, his stomach must work fifteen hours out of the twenty-four. But the multitude of mechanics who are wildly clamorous for only "eight hours a day," are the very ones who, while they are angered at being required by others to work more than eight hours a day, do not hesitate to impose on their stomachs fifteen hours' work; nearly double. After a night's sleep, we wake up with a certain amount of bodily vigor, which is faithfully portioned out to every muscle of the system, and every set of muscles, each its rightful share; the stomach among others. When the external body gets weary after a long day's work, the stomach bears its share of the fatigue; but if when the body is weary with the day's toil, we put it to bed, giving the stomach meanwhile a five hours' task, which must be performed, we impose upon the very best friend we have, the one that gives us one of the largest amounts of earthly enjoyments; and if this over-taxing is con tinued, it must certainly wear out prematurely, as the body itself will, if it is overworked every day. And if persons eat between meals, then the stomach has no rest from breakfast in the morning, until one, two, three, or four o'clock next day; hence it is that so many persons have dyspepsia, the stomach is worked so much and so constantly, that it becomes too weak to work at all. It is to be hoped that every intelligent parent will press these things on the attention of their children as a matter of conscience, because dyspepsia, like consumption, has its foundations laid, in a large majority of cases, during the "teens" of life.

THE LIVER.

AFTER food is eaten, it is made into blood, and sent direct to the liver to be filtered; the office of the liver being to withdraw from the blood all that is waste, impure, and imperfect; this filtered blood is then sent to the lungs through the heart, to be prepared still more perfectly for imparting health, and strength, and warmth, and life to the whole body. Hence, if the liver does not do its work, it is said not to " act," to be " torpid," to be " lazy," to be " asleep ; " and the man soon becomes " bilious," the blood becomes so impure, so heavy, so thick, that the whole body becomes heavy, the head aches, the mind is depressed, there is no life, no animation, no appetite. This waste and impure matter which is withdrawn from the blood is called the " bile," is collected together in a little receptacle holding a few table-spoons, called the

GALL BLADDER.

The almost universal " symptom " or sign that the liver is not doing its work properly, is an aversion to food, accompanied with a kind of sickish feeling ; the very thought of eating is almost enough to cause vomiting. The point in all such cases is first to carry out Nature's instinct by eating nothing whatever until the appetite becomes voracious, keeping abundantly warm all the time. If persons are in a hurry to get well, then exercise in the open air from sunrise to sunset; exercise moderately, steadily, in something which is agreeable, and, better still, profit·able.

The advantage of this method of causing the liver to work is that each additional use of the remedy, if promptly applied the very hour the liver is noticed to be " out of order," will make the cure surer, easier, quicker, safer, every time.

Exercise makes the liver " work," because in exercise all the muscles of the body are put in motion, and this motion is communicated to the machinery within. The exercise should be out of doors, because out-door air is purest, goes pure into the lungs, but comes out so impure that if rebreathed without any admixture of pure air, we should " faint " on the spot. The air going out being so freighted with the impurities of the blood, it in a sense lightens the burden of the liver, helps to unclog its machinery, and it starts off to work itself with almost the instinct that an animal rises from the earth when pressed down to it with an over-weight, the moment that weight is lightened. But there is a still more speedy method of making the liver " work."

This important organ, the largest manufactory of the body, is at the lower edge of the ribs on the right side, extending nearly from the right hip over towards and near the navel. In one sense it is like a sponge, which, if pressed upon, parts with the liquid which it contains ; or like a bladder with an open mouth, pressure " squeezes " out its contents. Then with the ball of the hand, at the body end of the thumb, press in towards the liver and downward, beginning at the right hip and coming round to the centre of the body over the stomach ; press firmly, aiding the pressure with the other hand if you choose ; do this eight or ten minutes night and morning ; this may be called " kneading the liver," and is an excellent substitute for medicine. To persons who are troubled a great deal with biliousness, this is a very efficient means of remedying the trouble.

A more speedy method still of making the liver work is to take medicines which are known to " act " on the liver, but this becomes more properly the province of the physician to advise, with this warning to all who prefer taking medicine : each successive dose must be larger, in order to accomplish the same object, while the intervals become shorter, until after a while the man is all the time taking medicine, and is all the time sick ; hence the unmedicinal means of keeping the liver at work are safest and best, because they offer no violence to the system, and become more and more efficient at each repetition. But some-

times life can be saved only by giving relief within a few minutes; this is done by giving an

EMETIC,

the operation of which is to give a heave; this brings the stomach
and other muscles up against the liver, making a kind of
pressure, as with the ball of the hand mentioned a while ago, but
more efficiently; in fact, so much so, that the gall bladder sends
its contents toward the stomach, causing by its presence there
such deathly sickness that out they come through the mouth as
" bitter as gall," literally. But as this heaving and straining has
sometimes ruptured a blood-vessel, causing a bleeding to death,
the reader is advised never to take an emetic on his own responsibility to make the liver work promptly, but rather consult a
physician, or use the milder means previously named.

PRIVIES.

" WATER-CLOSETS," " Necessaries," or by what other name they
may be called, were known by the ancient Romans as the " Temples of Cloacina;" she being the goddess of purity. A gentleman living in beautiful Tennessee, whenever he has a new
guest, takes an early occasion to show him around his premises:
the parlor, the library, the bath-room, his own apartment while a
guest, and last, not least, the privy or water-closet, which is
among the most faultlessly tidy portions of his establishment.
His neighbors say of him sometimes he is " queer in some
things." Pity is it that there are not a million to one like him.
There is delicacy, wisdom, and healthfulness in the idea. How
furtively has the reader, many a time, on going to a strange
place, looked around for a servant, and with averted eyes and
whispering tone made inquiry as to this point; and then again
how much afraid of encountering the opposite sex in going or
returning, to say nothing of a most disagreeable apprehension of
intrusion or interruption.

On farms and on all country places, it should not fail to be arranged to have what is necessary, in connection with the stable;

for among other reasons a gentleman is naturally supposed to have an interest in horses, and they could saunter around in that direction, those who saw them supposing they were going to look at the noblest of animals, while the man himself persuades his own mind that any one seeing him would suppose he was visiting the stable to take a look at its arrangements and occupants; so subtle a being is man.

Constipation and piles are brought on in innumerable cases by deferring the calls of nature for the above or other causes, and standard medical works give detailed cases where persons by delays have induced inflammation of the bladder, dying in three or four days. Every mother should consider it a duty to impress upon the minds of children, beginning at the age of three or four years, the danger of delaying the calls of nature, and the influence it has in impairing the health, and in bringing on life-long ailments.

Almost all our common ailments are attended with costiveness, and as the bowels become free again, recovery takes place. If a mother were to draw the attention of a sick child to this fact that when the bowels began to act, the health improved, and that when sick, the bowels had failed to act that day and perhaps the day before, it would make a practical and a radical impression on the child's mind, with life-long benefits.

NOSE DRENCHING.

Some individuals are in the habit of drawing water through the nose into the mouth with an indefinite idea about its being advantageous in reference to catarrhal affections. The more this is done the greater craving there will be for its repetition, because cold water of fifty or sixty degrees applied to a surface whose natural temperature is near one hundred, inevitably chills it; the reaction of that chill is fever and inflammation, thus drying up a surface which Nature intended should be always moist.

If warm water is used, the results are not so harmful, but warm water is harsh and hard in comparison with Nature's lubricant, which is the mildest and softest possible. The internal passages and surfaces were intended to be always in a state of lubrication; if water is habitually used, it being harsh in comparison, the system learns to rely upon these artificial moistenings, and the surfaces must be dry for a greater part of the time, as it is impossible to be sniffing water up the nose every half-hour in the twenty-four, the result being a feeling of want of something whenever the parts are not sufficiently moist. All know what clots of hard substances are blown from the nose at times; these are loosened by the natural lubricants poured out under them, and pushing them off from the surface as fast as is needed, keeping the nasal passages clean and clear of obstructions, and admitting a full supply of air at each breath: certainly these are important considerations; every one has felt what a delightful sense of relief there is the moment after a large clot has been discharged from the nose.

If these considerations are not sufficient to induce the abandonment of the unnatural and hurtful habit, let it be remembered that the water sniffed through the nose into the mouth carries with it whatever of the natural secretion of the nose happens to be there. Our whole nature revolts at the idea of taking into the mouth what has been discharged from the nose, and yet the sniffers do this in effect.

Very many persons are in the habit of closing the mouth and making a forcible suction of air through the nose into the mouth, the effect of which is to carry the contents of the nose into the mouth, and then spitting it out or swallowing it, instead of discharging it through the nose into the pocket-handkerchief. The habit is so common, and so utterly disgusting, that one would think that it was only necessary to draw attention to it to secure its universal abandonment.

SICK AND POOR.

MANY a man who has not a dollar ahead thinks it a great calamity that he has not the means to enable him to get well, while every physician knows that in multitudes of cases the only obstacle to health in the case of the rich is that they are not obliged to work. There is many a "fair ladie," the occupant of a splendid mansion on Fifth avenue, who, rustling in costliest silks, taking her daily drives in her splendid equipage, walking on velvet carpets, and receiving in her saloons the culture and grace and elegance of the city, is at the same time a martyr to maladies all unsuspected by admiring outsiders: yet thin, and frail, and pallid she exists rather than lives; life is a burden rather than a blessing; all that she lacks to put the rose on her cheek, and make existence a happiness, is the necessity of scrubbing floors at a dollar a day, or washing clothes at fifty cents a dozen, to purchase meat and bread enough to keep body and soul together. Hence it is infinitely easier for a poor man to get well than a rich one. The poor man can turn his hand to anything; the unfortunate rich, knows nothing; he can't split a rail, or drive a wedge, or draw a cart, or curry a horse, for if he tried the last, he would be so awkward the poor brute would think it was some animal gouging out his ribs, and would incontinently kick his brains out, if indeed there were any there. Hence it many times happens that the fortune of the poor is their poverty. A poor clergyman on consulting a physician, after having taken all the medicine he could get within ten miles, and getting worse fast, was advised to go to work. Some time after, in relating the improvement of his health and the means employed, he writes, "I am making collections for a company and selling farm implements for the most part, stopping on a farm now and then, and working for my board." He was told that he was a fortunate man; that boarding around gave him a wholesome variety of food; and that collecting bills and selling agricultural implements was an honorable and useful employment; that it kept him exercising a great deal in the open air, and was an admirable means of cultivating the powers of persuasive oratory; that bartering in a country store was the foundation of Patrick Henry's immortality, as it gave him opportunities of meeting the sophistries of the common people, of overcoming their prejudices, and observing what kind of arguments reached common minds; and he who can persuade money out of the pocket of a dilatory debtor, and can make a miser buy what he don't want, will soon be skilful enough to move the masses as Patrick Henry did, and win souls for his hire, besides curing himself of dyspepsia, hobgoblins, and other maladies. Many invalids and a great variety of ailments could be certainly, permanently, and happily cured, if the unfortunate sufferer only had the moral courage to engage in some out-door employment, requiring but moderate activity, even if it yielded only money enough to pay expenses; but mind, in proportion as the yield was greater, the sooner will the patient get well, for money-making is a medicine more efficient than the most potent pill of the apothe cary.

HOW TO SLEEP WELL.

THERE can be no healthful sleep except that which follows the sleepiness resulting from the voluntary and involuntary action of the muscles of the human body. Weston, the great walker, falls into a sound, deep sleep almost as soon as he is put to bed, at the appointed time for rest. This is the sleep from voluntary muscular exercise. A person in good health sits around the house all day; an invalid may all day sit, and lounge, and lie down from morning until night, without sleeping; and both the healthy man and the invalid, in the course of the evening, will become sleepy, and fall into sound repose, the result of the weariness which involuntary motion brings about; for the various organs of the body, the heart, the liver, the stomach, the eyelids, work steadily every day. The intestines are as ceaseless in their motion as the waves of the ocean; as these latter are always dashing towards the shore, so is the great visceral machinery working, working, working, pushing the wastes of the body downwards and outwards from the first breath of existence to the last gasp of life.

There is not a movement of the system, voluntary or involuntary, external or internal, which does not require power to cause it. When that power is to a certain extent exhausted, instinct brings on the sensation of sleepiness, which is the result of exhausted power intended by nature to secure that cessation from active action which gives time for recuperation, very much as a man who runs for a while stops and rests, so as to get strength to run again.

We get up in the morning with a certain amount of reserve or accumulated strength; in the course of the day that strength becomes expended to the point necessary for the commencement of a new supply, which supply comes from rest, the rest of sleep.

23

Opium, narcotics, all forms of anodynes, cause sleep artificially, by compelling rest. A horse may be tied so that he cannot move; he is compelled to be at rest; it is not the rest of tiredness, hence is unnatural. Anodynes in a sense, tie a man down; they take away his power of motion, they compel a rest, but it is not the rest which is a result of used-up strength, hence it is an artificial rest, causing artificial sleep, not natural; and sleep which is not natural cannot be healthful; hence the truth of the first utterance of the chapter: healthful sleep comes from the expenditure of the strength of the body in various forms of exercise.

SLEEPLESSNESS AND INSANITY.

There are more insane persons in the United States than in any other part of the world, by fifty per cent. " I can't sleep " is a complaint becoming every day more familiar to the city physician, and sleeplessness always precedes the ordinary forms of insanity; on the other hand, an improvement in the ability to sleep is a certain indication of coming restoration to reason. Hence the want of ability to sleep well, soundly, and connectedly should always meet with prompt attention, to prevent its becoming a habit, a second nature. The speediest method of doing this is to break up the present associations, whatever may be the sacrifice; get some different employment, something more active or stirring. The next best thing is a long journey on horseback, with a good companion; a journey which has an end in view, the selection or location of lands for investment; camping out for months together as far as is practicable from human habitations, relying for provisions wholly on what can be caught or hunted. Visiting new and strange countries is another method of breaking up the treadmill sameness of some kinds of business. The great point for those who cannot sleep satisfactorily is to be a large portion of the time in the open air, and to be occupied in a way to bring into activity other muscles and other mental operations; and in proportion as they are of pleasurable and absorbing interest, so much the happier will be the good effect, and the more speedy will be the return to that " balmy sleep," the very thought of which, as enjoyed in youth, is a happiness. Neither money nor medicine can purchase healthful sleep; it can only be procured in all its deliciousness by large out-door activities or homely toil.

"REST FOR CONSUMPTIVES."

One of the most beautiful of the many magnificent charities of liberal New York, the largest-hearted city of the world, is an institution, a year old, called "The House of Rest for Consumptives," where those who have no money can find a comfortable home, if there is any vacancy. To be doomed to certain death, to know that it is an inevitable event, to occur only after weary weeks and months of insupportable, wasting cough, and restless nights, and not a pillow for the head, nor a cover for the body, nor a single penny for medicine, nor a morsel of food, has scarcely its equal for the terrible; and yet there are loving, thoughtful, and humane hearts in New York who have had a care for such, whose names we are glad to record in the following statement. Reader, if you have a single dollar to spare, send it on right away, and the angel of goodness will make a note of it to be forwarded up to heaven.

The first anniversary of the founding of the House of Rest for Consumptives was held in 1872, at the House, at Tremont, N. Y. About 150 persons were present, among whom were Bishops Potter and Littlejohn. The annual report was read by the President, Mr. Henry J. Cammann. Through the agency of Miss Bogle, the lady now in charge, the present Board of Trustees was organized in October, 1871. A building, with about one and a half acres of ground, was obtained at Tremont, and on the 1st of November the House was opened for the admission of patients. The Institution was supported by voluntary contributions from surrounding churches, and many of the articles of furniture were thus received. During the past year, about $10,000 have been expended; 38 patients (21 men, 17 women) have been admitted; 14 have been dismissed, most of them much benefited; 12 have died, and 12 are now in the care of the House.

ASTHMA

is an incurable disease by human agencies. An attack can be modified or shortened, and this is all that the thousand and one vaunted remedies for the "cure" of asthma can do; they alleviate or remove for the time, nothing more. Sometimes the disease lies dormant for months or years, only to reappear in some change of life, or some more terrible form of human affliction. In some cases it disappears in childhood, to show itself again after forty years. Children sometimes "outgrow" it. If it disappears at the "change of life," it may not be heard of again, but that life will seldom reach threescore and ten.

It is very certain that persons troubled with asthma may be exempt from it for a succession of years, and even for life, by removing to a different atmosphere or a different climate; hence, instead of losing time in the attempt to "cure" asthma, or of being satisfied with shortening or curing merely an attack of it, it would be a wiser course to change localities or climates. Standard medical works give interesting cases in which exemption more or less permanent is secured by moving from the city to the country, from a level to a hilly locality, from the seaside to inland, from Maine to Florida, from Cape Cod to California, and the reverse of all these; that is, an entire change of air does sometimes exempt from asthmatic attacks.

When such changes are impracticable from any cause, the next best thing is not to have asthma at all. It is exceedingly inconvenient to be blowing like a porpoise, to feel as if fifty thousand feather pillows were piled upon your face, to have the sensation that you would certainly die if you stopped breathing long enough to say "Yes" or "No;" and yet such are the sensations during an attack of asthma. And what is worse, these worse than inquisitorial tortures usually come on towards daylight, the very time when sleep is most delicious; you are obliged to sit up in bed, and with your head leaning forward on your drawn-up knees, you feel, until the longed-for daylight comes, and sometimes for hours later, as if every breath would be your last, and mortal agony is depicted in every lineament of the face.

But there is, as the poet says, "comfort in brooks and stones, in everything." Asthmatics never die; they can whistle at consumption, and bronchitis, and all such tough customers; that is, asthmatics generally live to old age, unless this form of the disease disappears; asthma itself is antagonistic of consumption. In consumption you can't get air enough in to support life, because there are not lungs enough to receive it; in asthma you can't get the air out, hence, remaining in, it gets warmer, and distends the lungs by its increasing rarefaction, and thus develops them.

Asthma is almost always the result of a bad cold attacking an asthmatic constitution. This cold forms phlegm in the branches of the windpipe,—a tough, sticky phlegm, which adheres to the insides of these hollow branches of the windpipe; and as the air goes into these branches with more force than it comes out, it has the effect to carry the phlegm before it, downwards, in the shape of a plug, into a narrowing orifice, and so to speak, the cork is driven in tighter and tighter by every breath that is drawn. But it is with asthma as in other diseases; when they reach their worst, that is, their " crisis," they begin to get better. It is not necessary to say how, just here, but the suggestion is repeated, that it would save a great deal of suffering and trouble if persons would only not have asthma; and all that one has to do is simply to never take a cold; and certainly a man need not take a cold once in a year or five or ten years. All that he has to do is to dress abundantly warm to avoid getting chilled, and to cool off slowly after being overheated; that is, after being warmer than is natural. Such is the true philosophy of common asthma.

WARMING COUNTRY HOUSES.

ONE of the most important items in the preservation of the general health is being comfortably warm all the time, for then we should never take cold. There should be a room in every farmer's family which should be kept at a temperature not under sixty-five degrees Fahrenheit from daylight until bedtime, all winter, by stove or furnace heat; stove heat is better, because it will bring up the heat more quickly. When the farmer comes in from his work he is generally overheated and tired, both conditions making him greatly more susceptible of taking cold; or if, on the other hand, he is very cold from having been riding or engaged in something which has not involved activity enough to keep him adequately warm, a well-heated room is exceedingly grateful, and gradually raises the temperature of the surface of the body to its natural condition.

Large stoves consume less fuel in proportion than small ones, and give out more heat, hence are more economical.

It is a common error in the country to have too small stoves, so as to economize space, and under the mistaken notion that they consume less fuel in proportion. A circular stove, six feet high and about two in diameter, lined with fire-brick two feet high, will keep a large room more equably warm, and maintain a purer atmosphere, with a very much less amount of fuel, than our common stoves. Stoves of this shape, made of porcelain, are used in Germany and Russia, where wood is grown for fuel; and from personal observation we think that about half the amount of wood is consumed, giving a greater, better, and more comfortable heat than we have here. In farmers' houses an immense amount of heat is used in warming all out-doors. The longer a flue is, the stronger the draft; all flues should be built from the ground, thus securing a good draft, and also saving millions of property every year from being burned.

Two sitting rooms on the same floor and one or two chambers above may be adequately warmed by one stove, thus: Let the stove stand in one room and let a pipe of good size be sent through the partition into the adjoining room, where it should expand into a large drum; from this drum the ordinary pipe should extend through the floor into the chamber above, with a drum there if needed. Only a moderate amount of heat is needed in a chamber; but that moderate amount is needed in winter time. There is no advantage in going to bed in a cold room, nor in sleeping in a cold room, nor in getting up and dressing in a cold room; persons may survive it, many have lost health by it; to have the chill taken off the air on going to bed, and when dressing, is comfortable and healthful. A room under forty-five degrees is a cold room for a sleeping apartment, and sleeping in an atmosphere in-doors lower than that is always hurtful, is always positively pernicious, for the simple reason, that such a temperature causes the carbonic-acid gas of a sleeping apartment to condense and settle in the lower part of the room, where it is breathed into the lungs, with all its pernicious results. Sleeping in a room cooler than above named is especially dangerous to feeble and aged or invalid persons, as it tends to cause inflammation of the lungs. Persons may sleep out of doors with impunity when the temperature is many degrees lower;

that is because the out-door air is pure, is full of life, full of oxygen, without any admixture of in-door poisons, hence gives a vigor of circulation which keeps the whole body warmed to its natural point, resisting cold and all diseased conditions.

DRUNKENNESS A DISEASE.

UNDER this view of the case it is said that more than half the persons who submit to the treatment are cured in the hands of Dr. Dodge, at the New York State Asylum for Inebriates, at Binghamton, and Dr. Parrish of Philadelphia. The method of treatment adopted by Dr. Dodge, a gentleman of wealth and culture and professional ability, is to remove the cause promptly and completely on entering the establishment, then to gain the coöperation and confidence of the patient. Such food is provided for each as is calculated to tempt the appetite and promote digestion, and thus bring back the power of a debilitated and outraged stomach; for it is a good digestion which gives strength of body as well as a vigorous and healthy working brain, which of itself is a great aid to strong resolutions not to touch, taste, or smell the abominable thing. To give varied occupation to the mind, and exercise to the body, with a motive, a great variety of amusements are inaugurated—as billiards, chess, backgammon, dominos, and out-door sports, with a well-appointed reading-room, and a variety of social gatherings, reunions, and conversations; then there are pianos, organs, violins, banjos, harps, and vocal music besides. When patients have been there long enough to acquire force of will sufficient to enable them to resist any ordinary temptation, they are allowed to range over field and wood, and employ themselves in cutting canes, making curious toys, and contriving devices for diversion and amusement. Everything done is of a nature calculated to elevate, refine, and ennoble.

This is the bright side. Drunkenness is a habit, an appetite cultivated to the extent of becoming inappeasable, like a natural passion, one which will not be satisfied without an indulgence, to return again forever, like the sense of hunger for food, or thirst for water; like the passions of our nature. Now and then a man may have such an extraordinary force of will as to overpower the passion, just as some men have force of will enough to resist eating until they die. But such powers of will are not found oftener than once in a thousand. The only safety from a ruinous life, a disgraced name, and a beastly death, is the systematic, habitual avoidance of spirituous liquors in all their forms, from cider and lager beer to wine, brandy, and absinthe; for the use of the mildest beverage now and then, in courtesy to friend or hostess, is but the first step to a ruined fortune, and name, and body, and soul; and to avoid these first steps to death, so disgraceful and inevitable, is to make home the pleasantest place in the world for children, so as to keep them out of the city street, and away from the country grocery, the circus, the theatre, and railroad station. Train the children early to the conviction that they must do something for a living; teach them that to earn money honestly is a first virtue, and next to that, saving it; any child practising these once, is saved for all time.

Whether drunkenness is a disease or an inappeasable appetite, the unfortunate individual ought to have our sympathy, and all the aid which can be given to save from the ruin which threatens. The Asylum at Binghamton is under the direction of Dr. Dodge, the founder of the Washingtonian Home, at Boston, Mass.; it is literally a home, and not a prison with bolts and bars. There is only one restriction—that upon liquor; its use must be promptly, wholly, and forever abandoned; in all other respects, there is as much liberty to go and return, to eat, drink, sleep, dress, hunt, fish, and recreate, as a guest would have in the house of a friend. The inmates pay for everything they get, and are as perfectly independent as if they were at an Astor House or a Fifth Avenue. There are libraries and reading-rooms, with newspapers, magazines, and periodicals from all parts of the country; and the associations are as cultivated, scholarly, and mannerly as can be found on board a first-class steamship for the Continent. An ex-patient states that the rules governing the inmates are of the mildest sort. Most excellent attention is given to the sick, and a great variety of rational amusements are provided.

Dr. Parrish, of Philadelphia, presides over another "home," and for his intelligent, self-sacrificing efforts, for years together, to perfect a reform intended to save some of the best hearts and the greatest intellects of the country, he, with those who are engaged in a like humane work, merits and receives the admiration and respect of all good men.

Applicants who are able, pay their own expenses; and often arrangements are made to accommodate those who have no means. In view of all the dreadful calamities which befall a man, sooner or later, who becomes enslaved by drink, let every parent begin early to inspire the minds of children, girls as well as boys, with a terror of the despotism of alcohol; and let it be woven in the framework of their minds from day to day, that there is only one way of safety, and that is, never, under any conceivable circumstances, whether of sickness or of pain, to swallow a drop of the accursed thing. Alcohol for the sick is never a necessity; in no case whatever is it more than an inferior substitute or makeshift for something that is much better.

"The most confirmed drunkard cured by a remedy which can be given without the knowledge of the patient" is announced in the daily papers. Should this be true, it will be a great blessing.

There is no family in the land who has not or may not have a personal interest in this admirably managed institution. A letter addressed to Carrol Hyde, Secretary, Binghamton, N. Y., will secure a report, which is full of interest. The object of this institution is to break up the habit of drinking liquor. Some of the statistics are suggestive. The number treated during 1871 was 315. Thirty per cent. of the inmates paid twenty dollars a week; twenty-five per cent. fifteen dollars; twenty per cent. could not pay anything; showing that more than one-half of the inebriates are from the wealthier classes.

One-fifth were discharged unimproved, meaning hopeless, utterly hopeless of reform; a terrible lesson to those who ever taste or touch the "flowing bowl."

One-fifth had a collegiate education; two-fifths had an academical education; all had been to school.

Two-thirds were of a lively, cheerful disposition; of the temperaments, nervous, sanguine, bilious, each had a third. Two-thirds were whiskey-drinkers; a fourth wine and brandy; fifteen used opium.

One-third had intemperate ancestors. Two-thirds drank habitually before meals. One-fourth from trouble or pecuniary embarrassment.

One-half were constant drinkers; one-third had sprees now and then. One-half were married; one-third bachelors. The oldest, sixty-three; the youngest, nineteen.

One-third were from the city. Nearly one-half were merchants and merchants' clerks. One in twelve had no occupation. The chaplain reports that the inebriate is physically, mentally, and morally deteriorated; that he loses self-control, and that if left to himself to reform, he is, nine cases in ten, lost! because in the popular estimation there is little hope of his reformation; consequently all business confidence is withdrawn from him; he sees it; next he begins to be regarded with pity and contempt, and becomes conscious of his position; he loses all self-respect, becomes an outcast, and generally falls away into the darkness of a dishonored grave.

There were two clergymen, six physicians, and twenty-five lawyers. We visited Binghamton in August, 1871, purposely to become acquainted with the workings of the institution; but unfortunately there was no official in the house higher than the man who was sweeping the floor; but he did it well, and took a polite pleasure in showing and telling all he could; his views of inebriate management were thoughtful and philosophical. Little did he know the inexpressible sorrow a single sentence of his shot across our heart, when he said in answer to a question propounded in reference to an only son of one of our oldest, and best, and most cultivated and happy households, " Beyond remedy." Young, high-born, and heir to large estates, "beyond remedy." The institution is " beautiful for situation," commanding one of the loveliest views in the land. The rooms are large and airy. There are various pastimes, games, libraries, reading-rooms, music, regular public worship under the judicious conduct of Rev. Samuel W. Bush, Chaplain, whose report is worthy of circulation in every household.

A very sad report comes from the Inebriates' Home at Fort Hamilton, New York, that nearly one-half were women! Of seventy-two married, forty-five were separated from their partners because of intemperance. Two-thirds of the whole number of inmates were separated from their partners because of their intemperance. Four-fifths were whiskey drinkers; one-third hereditary drinkers. Beer-drinking Germans had not a single representative, nor had a single case of delirium tremens ever occurred in the institution as a result of drinking beer or other fermented liquors.

The reformed inebriate from Binghamton rejoices in the fact that instead of placing the bottle on the table to every visitor which was almost universal less than fifty years ago, "It is no longer deemed obligatory to provide strong drink at christenings and funerals; that it is possible in New York city to have a wedding reception without wine and brandy; that some noble ladies have the courage on New Year's Day to place nothing stronger than tea and coffee before their callers." He closes by saying, "And last of all, and best of all, there exists an organized army of temperance men, who are determined to prohibit by law the sale of strong drink." This last sentence shows the sentiment of an educated man, who has been through the fire, that the most efficient engine for the prevention of intemperance is that which makes it most impossible to obtain anything to get drunk on. Prevention costs less than punishment and remedy. The philosophy, the theory, the practice of this whole subject of the banishment of intemperance as a national and social vice, is contained in half a dozen words of Holy Writ,

TOUCH NOT, TASTE NOT, HANDLE NOT.

Drunkenness is unfortunately so prevalent, even creeping in among the wives and daughters of the land, that there is scarcely a family into which this book may come which will not have a special and personal interest in the details above given. A sudden fit of drunkenness may be cured.

If a man is almost dead drunk, or has just taken a large amount of liquor which would kill him if allowed to remain in the stomach, raise the head, loosen the clothing, and give an emetic of a large tablespoonful of ground mustard, and as much common salt, stirred quickly in half a glass or more of water; the more water the better.

VELOCITY.

	H.	Min.	Sec.
1 mile locomotive	1.	00	
1 mile running, Henry Perritt	1.	42¼	

	H. Min. Sec
1 mile pacing, Pocahontas	2. 17¾
1 mile trotting, Bonner's Dexter	2. 18¾
2 miles trotting, Flora Temple	4. 50½
4 miles running, Lexington	7. 19¾
3 miles trotting, Dutchman	7. 32¼
16 miles trotting, Prince	50. 00¾
20 miles trotting, Trustee	59. 35¼
100 miles trotting, Conqueror	8. 55. 00
100 miles, couple, Busk and Robin	10. 17. 22

	Miles.
Ocean steamers average per hour	11
River boats	20
Race-horse at the rate of	30
Bird	60
Hurricane	80
Sound	804
Earth round the sun	68,000
Light	690,000,000
Electricity	1,000,000,000

A telegram could go to the sun in five minutes. If a cannon ball were shot from the earth towards the sun, and on the instant of the flash a telegram was sent to that effect, the inhabitants of the sun would have two months to get ready for it, but it would be ten years before they would hear the explosion. All have seen that light travels faster than sound.

But it is not wholesome to be in a hurry. Locomotives have been reported to have moved a mile in a minute for short distances. But locomotives have often come to grief by such great rapidity. Multitudes in their haste to get rich are ruined every year. The men who do things maturely, slowly, deliberately, are the men who oftenest succeed in life. People who are habitually in a hurry generally have to do things twice over. The tortoise beat the hare at last. Slow men seldom knock their brains out against a post. Foot-races are injurious to health, as are all forms of competitive exercises; steady labor in the field is the best gymnasium in the world. Either labor or exercise carried to exhaustion, or prostration, or even to great tiredness, expressed by "fagged out," always does more harm than the previous exercise has done good. All running upstairs, running to catch up with a vehicle or ferry-boat, are extremely injurious to every age, and sex, and condition of life. It ought to be the most pressing necessity which should induce a person over fifty to run twenty yards. Those live longest who are deliberate, whose actions are measured, who never embark in any enterprise without " sleeping over it," and who perform all the everyday acts of life with calmness. Quakers are a proverbially calm, quiet people, and Quakers are a thrifty folk, the world over.

DOMESTIC SERVANTS

are human beings. This announcement may surprise some who read it, but it is true for all that. Half the housewives in the land, at the very least one-half of them, have forgotten this important truth, if, indeed, they ever knew it.

Domestic servants are full of human nature ; in fact, they are a great deal too full of it ; and the only remedy is to take out some, and replace it with grace ; that is, let mistresses, instead of heaping upon them all the epithets of the " catalogue," as Dame Partington would say, lift them to a higher plane of life, by considerate courtesies and humane forbearance. They are ignorant, and allowance should be made for it. They have feelings, and those feelings should be respected. They need encouragement ; they need a good example. Uniform civility and politeness to servants is a power over them. Servants, with all their want of learning and with all their disadvantages of birth and rearing, are quick and accurate observers of character ; and they fix in their own minds the moral status of the mistress, even a little quicker than the mistress forms a true estimate of their availability as aids in housekeeping ; and whatever they see which lowers their estimation of the mistress, diminishes their respect for her, and makes them less ambitious to please her and to secure her good-will.

If the mistress is passionate and impatient, if she is changeable, if she has no mind of her own, if she is double-faced, has one bearing towards visitors when present and another when they are gone, if petulant at the table, if unreasonable in her exactions, if inconsiderate in the amount of services required, if, in a measure, regardless of the personal comfort and welfare of those in the kitchen, every deficiency is measured, and the standard of respect lowered accordingly.

Scolding, loud talking, depreciating epithets, never made any servant better, always makes them more inefficient and unreliable; it is much better to appeal to their intelligence, their self-respect, seldom, if ever, to their religion; that is too sacred a thing to be brought into the daily affairs of common life.

Familiarity with servants is always a mistake; keep them at a respectful distance; let them be made to feel your superiority, not by mere assertion, but by your high bearing. Encouragement, courtesy, patience, consideration, and sympathy—these are the qualities which will seldom fail to make bad servants good, and good servants better, especially when the maid sees that the mistress knows how things ought to be done. Domestic rule should be one of love rather than of fear.

FAILURES IN BUSINESS.

What untold agonies wrench the heart of an honorable business man, as he sees himself approaching the maelstrom which is to ingulf the savings of a lifetime, and more than that, which leaves him a debtor to those who once trusted him, to say nothing of the enduring wretchedness of seeing his own loved ones living in self-denial and destitution, hopeless of any remedy from his hands! During 1870, three thousand five hundred men failed in business, owing to other persons one hundred millions of dollars.

To be old and poor, and have no home, is terrible beyond expression; but how many these failures have sent to a premature grave, and, worse, to a mad-house, and, worse still, to crime and bodily degradation, only the Judgment can disclose. What hopes have been blasted, what hearts wilted and withered away, no one may know. But a near question comes home to the reader: "Who knows but I may fail before another year? who knows but that I may be in an early grave, my wife in the mad-house, my son in the penitentiary, and my daughter on the street, as not remote results of such an event, and how may I certainly prevent it?"

Some men fail by trusting others, some by being trusted. The man has never yet been found who was willing to acknowledge that he failed because he had no more sense. It is always somebody else that broke him.

Solomon said, "He that hateth suretyship is sure." Wonder if he found that out by having indorsed somebody's note!

"THE MASTER"

would not trust Himself to man, because He knew what was in man, that the human heart was deceitful above all things, and desperately wicked.

The man who trusts, and the man who is trusted, aim at the same result; both hope to make money by the operation, and very often both lose. If all business was done on the basis of a "cash transaction," or, as John Randolph expressed it,

"PAY AS YOU GO,"

human suffering, and sorrow, and sickness, would be diminished by one-half, and human crime and human curse would largely disappear. Two short rules might serve to abate much of the mental misery and moral degradation of debt:

Never trust out more than you can afford to lose.

Never engage to pay more than you have money to pay already in your pocket, and the next minute pay it out.

If everybody were to observe these two simple rules, this world would be better and happier in a year than it has been since Eve found out that she wanted a better dress.

ACONITE

Is wolf's-bane or monk's-hood, from the shape of the tall, spike-like, dingy yellowish or purple blossom. The leaves and root are both medicinal—the leaves while green, the root only after the leaves have fallen. The leaves have a bitter, acrid taste, giving a tingling and numbness to lips, mouth, and throat, lasting some-times for hours. The root is sweetish at first, but leaving the sensation which the leaves do. Aconite is a species of Crowfoot, and is allied to the buttercup, with five petals, the highest arched with three or five pods. The ancients regarded it as a powerful poison. It was first used as a medicine in Germany in 1872. The blossoms give out an odor in summer, which causes sick-ness and fainting, and is even poisonous to children and sickly feeble people who go too near the plant. Fatal results have fol-lowed the taking of its root for horseradish. It is frequently used, both root and leaves, for causing sleep, perspiration, and urination. When applied outwardly, it relieves rheumatic and neuralgic pains. Take one scruple of extract of aconite, one ounce each of soap liniment and compound camphor liniment, rub it well into the part night and morning; or. pour some alcohol on the root and leaves, and rub in a teaspoonful two or three times a day.

For internal use, take from a quarter of a grain to two grains of the extract.

MENDING FINGERS,

Or toes or nose, or any other part of the body which has been cut, may be done successfully by taking the part cut off and press-ing it against the other portion attached to the body, so arranged that the pressure should be steady and continuous, hard enough to keep the parts in contact. We all know that in case of a gash in the flesh, if the parts are immediately pressed together and kept in contact, they will soon unite; so will solid bone, sometimes, only keep the parts in steady contact, and keep the air out by ap-propriate wrappings or bandages.

A Mr. B. had his left forefinger severed by a straw-cutter; he came down-stairs, leaving his finger behind him, but another gentleman went up for it, held it against the stump until the physician came, who secured it in its place, where it grew together; the joint, however, remained stiff.

The sharper the instrument the cleaner is the cut, and the more readily will it unite, especially if the bowels are regular, a fruit and coarse bread diet is adhered to, and no jar or jolt or other violence is offered to the wounded part.

-----∞-----

DIPHTHERIA

Is a Greek word, meaning a membrane which forms in the wind-pipe, as in croup, and arises from the same causes—wet and cold acting on a debilitated system, as if it were a typhoid type of croup; croup attended with too much debility to allow the system to rise without help.

Filth and over-eating, bad air, etc., seem to cause diphtheria, but that might be because these debilitate the system and make it more liable to bad colds from slight causes. It is a disease of the mucous membrane of the throat, like croup. There is a resemblance in several points between croup, diphtheria, and scarlet fever: they all attack the throat, all arise from wet and cold and debility of the system at the time, habitual or transient.

Croup generally comes on very slowly; it usually requires several days for it to come to its height; or it comes on suddenly, the child having been in seeming perfect health a few hours before. Scarlet fever is preceded by some derangement of the stomach and bowels always, although not always noticed. Diphtheria often comes on suddenly with nausea or vomiting or dizziness, palpitations, faintness, neuralgic pain in the legs; or sudden attacks of loose bowels, debilitating greatly; or difficult urination or menstruation, or some irregularity in it; there is chilliness, irritability, and then the throat begins to be inflamed.

There are three great distinguishing symptoms in diphtheria:—
Excessive debility.
Very foul breath. 24

Patches all about the mouth, tongue, inner cheeks, and throat, whitish, yellowish, ashy, varying; in severe cases these patches extend up into the nose, and downwards towards the lungs; in bad cases the glands of the parts swell, blood oozes from the internal mucous surfaces, often throwing out an acrid and extremely offensive fluid.

HOMŒOPATHIC TREATMENT

of diphtheria consists in attacking it promptly, in the earliest stages, with belladonna in mild cases; twelve globules in a tablespoonful of water, one teaspoonful every two hours until there is a change for the better. When there is not much fever, but great uneasiness and debility, with bad breath, take acidum muriaticum, three drops of the second decimal solution in one teaspoonful of water, every two hours, until there is a change for the better.

If the throat is swollen, of a deep red, and specks, and the saliva flows abundantly, take mercurius protiodatus. If no improvement in twelve hours, take kali bichromicum. If the surface patches continue to present themselves, and throat is getting painful, give acidum nitricum. If these symptoms remain stationary after twenty hours, give kali chloricum.

If there is great fever and headache, and violent pains in back and limbs, with weakness, administer phytolacca. If there is great debility from the first, give apis mellifica. When patches appear, and there is a scarlet redness in the throat, and there is burning or scalding urine, give cantharides.

If there is great restlessness after midnight, with prostration of strength, give arsenicum.

Sometimes the exudations of diphtheria tend downwards and the voice begins to alter; then give sodium. In desperate cases when blood oozes from the mucous membrane of the mouth, then give ammonium causticum, merc. iod., and kali bichromicum.

Glycerine applied with a camel's-hair brush seems to dissolve the false membrane; when this disappears, then the true membrane should be painted with acidum muriaticum, giving it internally also, if there is any tendency to a re-formation of the membrane.

The food should be strengthening, as eggs; beaten up with a little wine or brandy, milk and water with some sugar, strong beef-tea; if the strength seems to be failing give wine, champagne, in small quantities often repeated, or mix them with the milk and beef-tea.

management of diphtheria is to give a hot bath at the onset, to young and old, in the form of a whole bath or a sitz; if the latter, cover the patient with a thick dry blanket, and let an attendant put the hands under and flap the water against the chest and ribs with the hand, so as to aid in producing sweating; to this end keep on adding hot water until the object is attained, then the symptoms will begin to abate; then, as soon as the sitz-bath is over, go direct to a pack of cold water, with additional wet cloths over the chest and around the neck up to the chin. If the patient is chilly use hot-water compresses about breast and throat; if sleep comes on it is a favorable indication; let it continue four or five or six hours, it will strengthen the patient; if there is no sleep, continue the pack for an hour, unless the patient becomes weary or restless. The bath-room should be seventy degrees; but when packed let in cool air gradually, down to sixty or even lower. But when the pack is ended have the room up to seventy again; rub the whole body until quite dry, and then give a good rubbing with the naked hands; this, if properly done, leaves the skin in a soft, healthy condition. Then put wet bandages to the throat and chest so as to fit well, covering them with dry cloths. Put the patient to bed with a wet cap on the head, and hot bricks or water-bottles to the feet, for they must be kept warm. The room should be kept quiet, and not too light.

The great object aimed at in the water-cure treatment is to relieve the internal congestions, to bring the blood to the surface, and thus equalize the circulation; hence the after-treatment is to keep the feet warm by frequent and plentiful frictions, or apply warm or hot flannels, wet or dry. The dry are best, and the warm hard rubbings still better.

Remember that the essence of diphtheria is debility. The patient needs rest and quiet. Keep out company, court sleep; encourage, avoid all anxious questions on business matters, and by all means give an abundant supply of pure air, out-door air warmed.

Encourage the patient to drink boiled or rain water only; to eat nothing whatever, until all the symptoms have greatly abated, until the patient desires food, and then give such in a fluid form regularly at intervals of three or four hours, with little sugar or butter or fat. The hot water and steaming appliances above named dissolve the false membrane, causing a very copious expectoration, amounting to quarts in the course of twenty-four hours.

Relapses are of frequent occurrence from over-exercise; hence persons should remain in the house several days, undertaking no severe labor, no hurried or straining work.

The bowels should be moved daily with enemas.

Forty years ago Bretonneau of Tours gave his name to a disease which is now so familiar, so fearful, yet it was known in Egypt, and was described by Aretæus of Cappadocia. Hecker described it in Holland in 1337; Carnevale, at Naples in 1620; Dr. Douglas of Boston, Mass., in 1736, and Dr. Saml. Band, of New York, in 1771. It was epidemic in France in 1855, passed over to England in 1857, appeared in California, and in 1860 prevailed in the Eastern States. It is now believed that Washington, Josephine, and Stephanie, the beautiful Queen of Portugal, all died of diphtheria. The very first symptoms are a general feeling of discomfort, slight sore throat, and a swelling of the glands behind the jaws, with fever, headache, furred tongue, and some difficulty in swallowing. On examination, the jaws and throat are reddish or purple. Its real cause has not as yet been determined; it prevails in limited bounds as in a small town, a crowded school, a large family, several perishing in a short time, children being more liable than adults. It is known from scarlet fever or putrid sore throat by having no eruption on the outer skin, but a substitute in the whitish or gray or yellow patches about the tongue, fauces, and surrounding parts, and a brick-dust, flush, or strawberry-colored tongue.

In thrush and aphthæ the splotches are not so large and are more dull; there is, besides, not so much general disturbance. Thrush also begins in the mouth, not in the throat, and is very rare except in young children.

Diphtheria is known from croup in its severer form; croup does not spread, is not "catching," is not attended with such excessive debility, nor has it a fetor in the breath. In diphtheria the membrane is more conspicuous than the tonsils and upper part of the throat; in croup it is lower down, in the windpipe.

Diphtheria is more of a disease of the general system, a disease of debility, and needs building up from the start. Open the bowels with salts, a teaspoonful every hour until there is free action; then give to a child of four years five grains of the chlorate of potash every two hours, or for adults twenty drops of chloride of iron, or twenty drops of the sesquichloride of iron in two ounces of pure glycerine; dose, half a teaspoonful; to adults a grain or two of quinine, every two hours, aids to keep up the strength; or a drachm of permanganate of potash in a pint and a half of water—dose, one teaspoonful every hour. Only concentrated liquid food with brandy to it, beef-tea, milk and water, wine whey, or some kind of punch. Let ice melt in the mouth as much as is wanted; honey and muriatic acid, half and half painted on the membranes, or diluted in water, may be used as a gargle; if there is much heat in the throat, use ice-water or compresses of flannels wrung in boiling water, as in croup. Ice kept in the mouth for several hours seems to have cured a patient in France in twenty-four hours, when the whole inside of the mouth was covered with the membrane. Smoke tar, by dropping it on a coal in a tobacco pipe and swallow the smoke, making it come out of the nostrils. Gargling the throat with lemon-juice, every two hours daily, is highly beneficial in loosening the membrane.

LADIES' HAIR

Can be kept in perfect order and healthy condition by cleanliness of the scalp and hair by means of comb and brush, and pure soft water, that is, rain or snow or distilled water; the nearest to this last is water which has been boiled and allowed to cool. Nothing is equal to water in dressing the hair for purposes of cleanliness of the scalp; twice a month is sufficient, and if water is not oftener used, and no other thing—oil, pomatum, grease, or anything else ever named—was ever allowed to touch it, the hair would not fall out as it does; it would have enough of its natural oil to keep it sufficiently smooth, it would not soil everything it touched, the scalp would not be plastered with an almost impervious coating of grease, and dust, and perspiration, thus effectually preventing the air from coming to the roots of the hair, to impart to them its life-giving virtues, and also to convey away such gases and emanations as are calculated to rot the hair itself, poison the circulation which supplies the bulb of the hair with nourishment, thus allowing it to perish for want of nutriment, with the result of irremediable baldness, for the root is gone, and hair can never grow there again unless the upper skin is removed and a part of the scalp is taken from a healthy head and put in its place; in this way hair can be made to grow on the baldest pate; this surgical transplanting can be done just as an old tooth can be drawn from one jaw and a tooth of the same size taken from another person put in its place, and if done deftly by a dentist who understands his business it will become fixed as the original one, with the advantage that it will never ache. The scalp should be brushed plentifully with a hard brush, in the direction of the hair always, hard enough to redden the scalp a little; this is to remove dandruff and stimulate the blood to come to the surface to nourish the hair bulb and roots; this should be done by ladies night and morning, but never use so hard a brush, or bear so much on the scalp as to scratch or bruise or wound it in any way; then in dressing the hair use a soft brush, use it patiently, as is done in brushing a silk or fur hat; the fur after being crumpled with use will not lie even down at first, but will if the brushing is continued. The truth is, the human hair is like that of a horse, and every groom knows that the more freely and judiciously his horses are brushed, the more glossy and beautiful will be their coating.

Let ladies bear in mind that the use of oils on the hair is an utter absurdity, as much so as to oil a carriage horse before taking a drive to the Central Park.

CURLY HAIR.

The hair sometimes has a natural curl; then be particular to curl it always in that direction, and no other. If the hair is wet at any time, or damp with perspiration or the humidity of the atmosphere, curl it and let it lie in that state. This is a good plan in dressing the hair of girls, which should be kept cut short until thirteen years of age, and allowed to curl as much as it will; if on special occasions it is desired to keep the curls in place, nothing is equal to weak solution of isinglass.

Never twist or knot or strain the hair by plaiting it, or drawing it hard in any direction; it is just as injurious as it is to pull upon a tender plant: it loosens the root, and endangers the life of the hair. As it gets long it should, as before stated, be twisted in a very loose coil, to lie on the back of the neck, or allowed to fall down the back behind, with a loose ribbon around it, just below the ears, no tighter than will allow the hair to cover all the space between the ears, and as much of the shoulders as possible, as then there is no possible strain, and the air, with its life-giving influence, has the freest access to it; the great ruiners of the hair of ladies are grease and straining; the great preservators are soft water and good brushing.

Sometimes there is an unnatural dryness of the hair-scalp and harshness of the hair, arising from a flaccid atonic state of the scalp; then wash it twice a week with a solution of green tea, with as much alum or tannin in a cup as would lie on a dime.

The Eastern nations, China, Japan, and India, have long, black, glossy hair. They wash the whole hair and head in cold water, then rub in a handful of pea-flour (perhaps any other flour would do); this is well rubbed into the hair and scalp for a quarter of an hour, a little water being added from time to time until it becomes lathered all over; finely powdered borax will answer quite as good a purpose. After rubbing this lather into the scalp and about the roots well, wash it off with several rinsings of cold water, comb it out very slowly and tenderly, using a very coarse comb (horn is the best by all odds); then press a soft dry cloth on the hair to absorb the moisture, and keep at it until it seems to take up no more; then run the fingers through the hair to let the air get in among it, and also to add to the facilities for drying it. Next brush with a hard brush plentifully, then use the soft brush. The result will be that the hair will be clean, and will be in a condition of silken fineness, without having any oil or grease or impurity of any description. This method of treatment gives vigor to the hair and to its growth, and keeps it at its own natural color. Such a washing ought to be given to the whole hair and scalp of every class and age and sex and condition, every month.

But it should be remembered that "good" hair, beautiful hair, is by inheritance, but may be improved by careful and judicious handling

GLYCERINE HAIR-DRESSING.

Sometimes it may be desirable to have the hair handsomely dressed, as on a wedding occasion or reception. Oil and grease came into fashion simply because they keep moist longer than water, making a less frequent dressing necessary. But glycerine has become an article of commerce of late years, costs but little, and as it evaporates at a less temperature than most other liquids, it keeps the hair damp for a long time; and as it is so perfectly mild in its nature, not objectionable on account of color, quality, or odor, it is incomparable as a dressing for the hair—in fact, is next to soft water. Take four ounces of good, thick, pure glycerine, and mix it well with twelve ounces of soft rain, or distilled, or rose water; put it in a bottle, shake it well before using it, and keep it well stoppered in a cool, dry place. This makes a pint of material at a very small cost, and will last for months. It will keep for years.

No hair-dressing should ever be used which contains litharge or any other form of lead. It ruins the hair, injures the skin, and has brought on paralysis in a great many cases—in fact it is poisonous, whether used internally or externally.

BLACK HAIR-DYE,

which is not hurtful in any way, is made by getting the juice of the covering or hull of walnuts before they fall from the trees, while this covering is yet green; then put in enough of sweet-oil to make it thin enough. A little of it applied to the hair night and morning will make it black.

TEA WASH.

Take three ounces of black tea, pour on a gallon of boiling water, strain it so as to keep back all the leaves and tea dust, add three ounces of best glycerine, one quart of bay rum, and half an ounce of the tincture of cantharides. Let it remain two or three days, and rub a tablespoonful of it into the scalp twice a week, when the hair is too dry, or is disposed to fall out, or needs to be quickened in its growth. These are merits claimed for it, it is given with others, at the same time it should be borne in mind that the essential point in all cases is to keep the scalp clean and healthy, to keep every possible stain from the hair, and let as much air get into it as possible, down to the very roots, and between every hair.   The statement has been made that hair growing gray gradually, owes the change, when premature, to using water which has lime in it.   Wheat bread has as much lime in proportion ; the prevention and the remedy in such cases is the avoidance of everything made from grain of any description, to use no bread, but rice, sago, and tapioca in its place ; to drink no water unless it has been distilled, or rain or snow water, these being the products of nature's distillation.

LOSS OF HAIR,

when premature, as in the case of most of our daughters, is the result of negligence, bad treatment, or want of cleanliness of the scalp ; hence if, when the hair begins to fall out prematurely, proper means were adopted, it might be arrested, and the growth become strong again.   Put a tablespoonful of cologne water into a pint of common, pure water ; shake it well.   Brush the hair in the direction of its growth with a stiff brush until the scalp reddens, work one-fourth the mixture into the hair and scalp, and all down its roots with the ends of the fingers, for these can best rub it in ; then dry as before ; do this thrice a week.

SUPERFLUOUS HAIR

can always be got rid of permanently, infallibly, and safely in only one way ; pull one hair out by the root with a pair of pincers which will not cut it in two as soon as applied ; then take another hair ; if this is done leisurely, until five, ten, or fifteen are removed, then wait a few days until the irritation is passed away, and repeat the operation.   Depilatory powders, pastes, and other preparations will not only fail, but most of them do harm, and sometimes serious harm.   So much has been said about the hair, because it is the most beautiful natural ornament a man or woman possesses ; in addition, its uses cannot be safely or healthfully dispensed with ; it preserves the scalp from chills ; keeps the head at a healthful warmth, and is a most important protection against sudden changes of temperature. The hair of a woman is said to be her " glory," and certainly the world over it wins the admiration of the sterner sex ; and as for the man, it adds to the manliness of his appearance, and is essential to the highest physical beauty. Coal oil rubbed well twice a day upon a place on the scalp made bald by a sore, has been followed in a month or two by a plentiful, and even abundant crop of hair. Dandruff in many cases is removed very effectually by taking one drachm of carbolic acid, four ounces of glycerine, and two drachms of oil of bergamot, mix well, rub it thoroughly into the roots of the hair with the ends of the fingers, and in a few minutes wash freely with bay rum. Use it once a week for some time, and then once a month; it is an admirable means of keeping the scalp free from accumulation of dandruff, to see which on the collars and shoulders of gentlemen's coats and ladies' apparel excites in every beholder of cultivation and refinement most disagreeable suggestions; it is an index of being low bred, as unmistakable as a rim of black under the finger-nails; or rub into the scalp every morning, with the balls of the fingers, two tablespoons of the following: Put one ounce of flowers of sulphur in a quart bottle, nearly fill with water, shake it well and let it settle; use the fluid only.

The skin of the scalp is very tender, hence the brush used should not be very hard or harsh, but stiff enough to part the hair and reach down to the scalp so as to loosen the scurf; the hair of a lady should be thus brushed at least a quarter of an hour night and morning, and when the toilet is made in the middle of the day. This is not lost time; the exercise is good for the arms, tends to cleanliness and the prevention of headache; let the brush begin at the root of the hairs, and be continued to the extreme ends. In combing do the same thing, only as soon as the comb leaves the scalp hold the hair behind the comb in the hand, so as to be on no strain whatever between the hand and the scalp; this is to prevent all dragging on the roots of the hair, which is just as injurious to it as a similar process would be to a delicate plant. The best hair has been ruined by too fast or jerking use of the comb or brush.

The natural oil of the hair is sufficient usually; but if any ointment or oil or pomade is needed, there is nothing better than castor-oil and alcohol, named elsewhere.

A weak solution of isinglass is a good curling preparation, or a quarter of an ounce of Iceland moss, boil in a quart of water, and add some spirits to make it keep.

If the hair is oiled any day, it should be well rubbed with a dry flannel at night. The hair ought to be

SHAMPOOED

once a month. Put one teaspoonful of hartshorn in a pint of water, put the whole hair in it in such a way that it can undergo a washing operation with the fingers; this is to take out all the oil with the hartshorn; wash the whole well in tepid water, not failing to clip the extreme tips, which are likely to split, which will deaden the hair if let alone.

If the hair is short, as in girls, or boys, or men, a thorough washing of the whole scalp in cold water every morning would keep every hair clean, healthy, and oily; always being careful to wipe it dry; this is a great protection against headaches and colds and catarrhs.

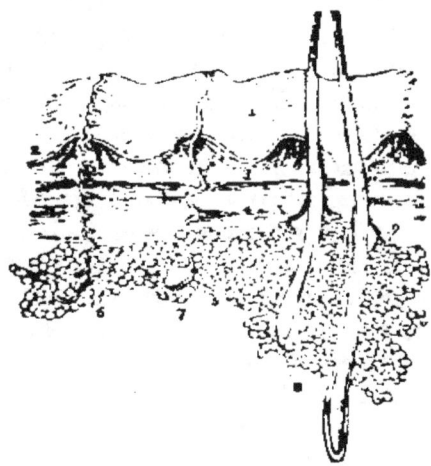

SKIN AND HAIR.

1 shows the outermost layer of the skin, called the epidermis or cuticle; it is this which, when rubbed or pressed with a shoe, forms corns by thickening. 2 is the second layer, called the rete mucosum. 3, the little mountainous ridges, are a collection of nerves, terminating in a cone, and give sensibility to the skin. 4 is the corium or deep layer of the skin, or the real true skin, varying in thickness in different parts of the body, from the fourth of a line to a line and a half, a line being the twelfth of an inch, thickest on the soles and palms, thinnest on the eyelids. 5 are the sweat-glands everywhere under the skin which supply the oil to the hair; these little glands send the oil upwards through little tubes as seen above. 6 and 7, a hair-gland; at 7 being larger and the tube straighter. 8 points to two hairs rising above the scalp. 9 shows two little ducts reaching from the glands and entering the side of each hair.

The hair is really of a horny material, like the finger-nails, and grows like them, being pushed out; the bulb of each hair is embedded in the true skin, reaching down to the fat-glands. It may be interesting to notice by the way that the silk dress is made of a kind of hair; so is the spider's web, only inconceivably smaller and finer than a human hair, for under a spider's body are six little knobs. When it wants to spin a web, it presses these knobs with one of its legs; from each knob one thousand threads come, these six thousand strands are twisted into one by the two hind legs of the spider, each leg having three claws each; and yet it takes a dozen strands of spider web to make one as thick as a hair—that is, the original spider's strand is seventy two thousand times finer than a hair from the human head.

THE PULSE.

Every intelligent person, every parent, should have some general idea of the nature and indications of the pulse; it beats with the heart and just as many times as the heart does, and very nearly at the same instant of time. The pulse is best felt at the wrist on the thumb side, or at the temple, or bend of the foot below the ankle, because it comes nearer the surface there, and the bone is immediately under it, compelling it to distend the artery in the direction of outside. The arteries have pulsations; hence if an artery is cut the blood comes out by pulses, by jerks and spirts. The veins have no pulsations; if they are cut the blood comes out in a steady stream not endangering life; but unless the bleeding of an artery is stopped at once, death follows in a few minutes; arterial blood is of a bright red; venous blood of a dark red. The pulse beats per minute in

Infancy	 110	Manhood..	70
Childhood	 90	Old age ..	60
Youth	 80		

A feverish pulse is quick in proportion as it is ten or fifteen above nature.

Inflammation is indicated by a quick hard pulse, as if a fine wire was vibrating under the fingers, while the natural pulse feels as if a soft yarn were under the fingers.

A thready pulse is barely felt; it is always fast, merely vibrates, is very weak; it is the pulse of the dying.

A jerking, quick, variable pulse indicates nervousness. A double pulse indicates typhoid symptoms, debility—always dangerous; it beats twice very close together, all of it making but one pulse, as if the heart was not working together in all its parts.

Palpitation of the heart should not, as a general thing, be regarded as an important symptom, as it is often emotional or nervous ; if it thumps or flutters, let it thump, but do you go at once and think about something else. An over-meal may cause it. Quietude of body and diversion of mind is the best remedy ; sometimes it is instantly arrested by drawing the fullest breath possible, retaining it as long as you can. Irregular pulse, one or two or three beats, then a stop or slower beats ; pay no attention to them, for almost always it means nothing, and if it did you can't help yourself.

Some persons have inherited a quicker pulse than usual, others a slower pulse. Every intelligent person owes it to himself, and parents owe it to their children, to ascertain the healthful pulse of each one, that should a physician be called he may take it into account whether it be slower or faster than natural.

There are a few general facts which should be known in reference to the action of the pulse. Midway between breakfast and dinner, or in the afternoon, are the best times to determine the natural rate, after having been at rest for a quarter of an hour or more, for a regular meal excites the pulse ten or fifteen beats, and hunger makes it languid.

The main point in all ordinary ailments is the rapidity, seventy beats in a minute being the average standard of health in middle life; all above that indicates that the heart is excited, and is exhausting the vital forces. The quicker any machine runs the faster it wears out ; so with the body ; in proportion as the heart is beating over seventy in a minute, fever is wasting the system.

The pulse of the consumptive is always fast, and the consumptive certainly dies. A pulse of seventy-five indicates fever ; if it is ninety or a hundred it is a very high fever.

If the pulse is simply fast, it is fever; if it is fast and hard, beats like the vibration of a hard string tightly drawn, it is inflammation, and there is danger always. The pulse is infallible as an index of inflammation in any part of the body; it is immaterial where it is, the wrist says it is in the body somewhere, and always alarms the physician. It would be really five dollars well laid out, if it had to be earned by sewing, for a mother to have the family physician to take her to a person who was suffering from any inflammatory disease, and teach her what an inflammatory pulse was; then she would be warned in time, or be saved from unnecessary alarm, according to the nature of the case.

There are, then, four kinds of pulses with which the intelligent reader should be at pains to acquaint himself:

First. The number of the healthy pulse per minute.

Second. The fast pulse, measuring the degree of fever.

Third. The fast, hard pulse, showing the degree of inflammation.

Fourth. The quick, indistinct, thready pulse, reaching at last to a hundred and thirty and over, or so fast that it cannot be counted; the pulse of death.

In all disease man begins to die at the extremities; the heart, which has been pumping from infancy, at the rate of a hundred thousand times a day, begins to grow weary of its labor, and works more feebly every hour; it can no longer send the living current to the tips of the toes and ends of the fingers; each successive beat sends it shorter and shorter of the mark, and carries less away from the heart, leaving it and the lungs more and more full, and finding that it does not carry out as much at each stroke, it endeavors to make it up by working more rapidly, but it is suffocating; each beat is now faster, but feebler than its predecessor, so feeble that it sends the living stream barely to the lungs, in limited quantities; they, too, receiving so little life, begin to pant for breath, faster, feebler, and still feebler, until the last breath, and then the last throb, and life's work is done, its task is ended now, all is literally "still as death."

THE TONGUE

Is, next to the pulse, the best index to the skilful physician of the condition of the body; because the skin of it is a continuation of that of the bowels and stomach, and its healthful condition measures that of the internal organs which we cannot see; for example, if the tongue is white, it indicates internal fever; if the tongue is coated thickly, so are the bowels and stomach; and there is no healthy appetite, if indeed there is any at all.

If the coat is yellow it shows that the blood is more yellow than it ought to be, for the coating is made out of the blood.

If the blood is yellow it shows that the bile is in it, which would not have been the case if the liver was doing its proper work, which is to withdraw the bile from the blood ; and when it ceases to do this it is said to be torpid, does not work, does not act, and means must be taken to make it act, or the man dies. It is purposely repeated here that there are four successful methods of making the liver work :

1. Nature will do it.
2. Hygienic means will do it.
3. Water will do it.
4. Medicine will do it.

Nature will cure a man as a pig cures himself—fortunate pigs, who never have any doctors' bills to pay, nor any "doctors' stuff" to swallow ! In truth, a pig is a practical doctor himself; he medicates by example ! When he is sick he rests, and keeps on resting until it is "kill or cure" with him ; and when he feels better, gets hungry, he gets up and goes to work in hunting up something to eat.

If the liver does not work, let it alone ; let it rest until it does feel like going to work, and then it will pretty certainly do so.

If the liver does not work, it is because it cannot work any more than the body can, unless it is unnaturally stimulated by some lash, physical or moral. Man constantly forces himself to work ; nerves himself up to his task, when really he knows that he ought to rest. Pigs don't do anything of the kind ; pigs have no notes in bank, they haven't any debts to pay.

HAPPY PIGS.

Hence when they get sick they can afford to rest. Ah ! what multitudes of mankind are there who literally can't afford to rest. There are a dozen men in New York any day of the year, who would be financially ruined by a "lost" day ; that is one of the penalties of doing business in all our large cities. Nothing in all the wide universe is as remorseless as debt. We gather around the dying couch ; how greedily do we run to the bedside at the slightest whisper or motion or look, to see if we can do some little something for him. What would we not give to be able to do the slightest service. How reverently do we watch and wait for the last intelligible word, to treasure it up for life long; for the last look, the last feeble pressure of the fingers, the last sigh, the last expiring breath; but

The clock strikes three, the note is not paid, and the fatal letters

" PROTESTED,"

are written all the same. But go back again; nature would generally cure man and beast alike if rest were given, when the liver would get up and go about its work "as if nothing had ever happened."

Hygienic measures will hasten the liver's resumption of its duties, as air, exercise, and kneading, which articles see.

Cold and warm water judiciously used according to the intelligent applications of it, after the hydropathic system; as will also the liver pills, or any other medicine acting on the same principles.

If the tongue is red, especially at the edges, there is internal inflammation, the redder the more dangerous, and the physician should be always sent for. Suppose all mothers knew this one point about the tongue, that bright red edges and tip meant dangerous inflammation, many little children would be saved from a premature grave.

If there are deep cracks in the tongue it means dyspepsia, although all dyspeptics do not have them.

A black tongue, not made black by something swallowed, and sometimes swollen, means death, as it proves that the bowels are mortifying.

A very dry tongue, a "parched" tongue, means high fever.

A natural tongue is about the color of the lips and is moist; away on the back part it is always more or less coated; in proportion as the coating is thick, and extends towards the tip, the man is sick.

If the tongue is coated and seems "glazed," the person is very sick, and as such a tongue roughens, he is getting better.

Sometimes the tongue looks very much coated on rising, but if after breakfast it is pretty much all removed, it proves that the system has been out of order, but is getting better.

A pale tongue means poor blood, no health.

A cold tongue is the collapsed state of cholera, and means death.

Red tongue is always seen in scarlet fever, and inflammatory conditions of the stomach and bowels.

Furred tongue is indigestion.

Brown or black, typhoid.

If protruded with difficulty it indicates low fever or apoplexy.

If always put at one side it indicates paralysis, apoplexy, or softening of the brain.

A tremulous tongue indicates indigestion, and often habitual drunkenness; the indigestion implicating the spinal marrow.

The tongue is too red all over, with little elevated points, in scarlet fever.

It is red and dry in inflammation of the brain, stomach, or bowels.

In typhoid fever there is often a red streak down the middle.

If the tongue turns pale in the progress of a fever, it means that death will follow.

A shrinking tongue indicates inflammation of the lungs and liver.

Swollen tongue is in nervous diseases and consumption.

BISMUTH

Was once supposed to be lead, but in 1520 Agricola discovered that it was a metal, white, pulverizable; it is this which forms pearl-white to paint the face, and is an ingredient in pewter. With nitric acid or aquafortis it forms subnitrate of bismuth, and in some forms of chronic diarrhœa and irritated state of the bowels it is used for a mechanical influence, sheathing their tender surfaces from injuries; it is astringent, absorbs foul gases in the intestines, hence is largely used in diarrhœa, dysentery, and various painful affections of the stomach. Very beneficial in the loose bowels of consumption and typhoid fever. Dose from five to thirty grains, or a quarter of a small teaspoonful three times a day. It is very heavy, and cannot be well taken in water; it tastes and looks like powdered chalk; it is easiest taken between layers of boiled rice or softened bread or mush or stirabout. It colors the discharges to blackness and makes them more consistent, showing that it is doing good.

25

ABRASION

Is the scraping off of the external skin. In ordinary cases, cover the part with cotton or soft rag, give it rest, protect it from friction and violence, keep it warm, and if the person is in good health it will be well in a few days, if the bowels act freely every twenty-four hours. At the same time the scratch of a pin is an abrasion and has many a time caused life-long sufferings, not unfrequently death itself, attributed by the common people to the poisonous character of the pin, when in reality it is the poisoned condition of the blood. A gentleman of wealth in stepping into his carriage one day, missed his footing, the fore part of the leg scraped against the sharp edge of the iron step, and took off the skin from the shinbone or fore part of the leg. As his constitution was impaired by long years of liquor drinking, there was very little vitality in his system, the wound would not heal, inflammation set in, and he died.

The London brewery draymen, as a class, get to drinking several quarts of porter or beer every day, and by the time they are forty years of age they seldom drink anything else, with the result that although they look large and stout and corpulent, there is no strength, no endurance, no stamina; their blood is impure, black, stagnant, full of poisonous ingredients, has no life-giving influences, no power of healing; hence when such persons have the " scratch of a pin " on the back of the hand, it does not perfectly heal for weeks and months and years, sometimes never; so with cuts and bruises on other parts of the body; the reason is, that the blood is so much inflamed by the spirituous, the alcoholic ingredients it contains, a poisonous quality is imparted to it, and instead of sending renovation and life to a wounded part, which it would if it were healthy blood, it sends poison and fire and death, especially when the wound is on any part of the body where there is but little flesh, as on the back of the hand or fore leg. But not only in scratches and abrasions, but in all cuts and bruises and wounds and contusions the chances of cure diminish in proportion as the person is in the habit of using ardent spirits, whether in the shape of manufactured whiskey, strong brandy, or beer or ale or porter or wine, and in such proportion is it necessary and imperative to follow with promptitude and fidelity the directions which follow for the treatment of an abrasion, which is literally a "shaving off."

But since the slightest abrasion may produce erysipelas, lockjaw, and death in any person not in vigorous health, it is safest in any case, however slight, to keep the part warm and protected, from violence, as just named.

If the abrasion covers a large surface, or is deep, especially in the old and young and feeble, from whatever cause, the additional precaution should be used to give the person and part quiet, to practise regular and abstemious eating, see under head of "eating;" soak and wash the feet well in warm water, so that the very large pores in the soles may be kept in vigorous and healthful action, so as to give free and speedy exit to any impurities which the blood may contain, as also to invite the blood there, and to that extent divert it from the abraded part, for this directly lessens the inflammation and heat and fever of the part. In addition the bowels should be made to act freely and fully at least once in twenty-four hours, either by the use of castor-oil or salts, which see, or mineral waters or enemas, which see. In more decided cases, or where there is tardiness of cure, it is better to take some liver medicines to hasten the purification of the blood and reduce its quantity.

If persons cannot remain in the house, or if in the house must work, two things are important: protection against friction, rubbings, and other violence; and from the cold air, which is said by the common people to "poison" it, which in reality is inflammation caused by the cold air, thus the parts become chilled, the reaction of chill is fever and inflammation. In ordinary cases use a spreading of soft clean cotton, with a bandage over it to keep it in its place, or cover it with a piece of gold-beater's skin, or oiled silk; these latter keep out the dust and keep in the warmth, and are less cumbersome.

As a better covering in some cases, as also more convenient in parts of the body where a bandage cannot be applied without being unsightly or cumbersome, as on the forehead, glycerine or collodion may be applied with a soft pencil. These same things are applicable in excoriations and chafings—scratches.

If a person knows that slight wounds or scratches heal rapidly in his case, then he need give only a general attention to these suggestions; on the other hand, if he knows that all sores and scratches and things of that nature heal very slowly in his case, he cannot be too prompt or particular in giving the above suggestions a judicious attention, in proportion as he has a dread of lockjaw or erysipelas.

Put four parts of the yolk of fresh eggs in a mortar, with five parts of glycerine, rub them most thoroughly together, and spread some over any broken or scalded or abraded surface; it is a kind of varnish, and most effectually excludes the air. If there is much pain, expose the part to the smoke of brown sugar on burning coals, or of burning leather.

FRUITS, BERRIES, AND MELONS

ABOUND most and in greatest perfection in those latitudes where their peculiar agencies on the system are most essential to the preservation of human health and life. Wherever miasmas prevail, there are most indispensably needed certain qualities, in whatever is adapted for the nutrition of the body, which can antagonize miasmatic influences. All know that bilious diseases abound in low, flat, moist, luxurious localities, as on river bottoms, along the banks of bayous, and on undrained prairies; and these are the very places whose neighborhoods produce uncounted millions of bushels, spontaneously and in their wild state, of almost every berry that can be named, which contains that peculiar acid, so efficient in its influences on the system as to keep it open, cool down its fevers, and enrich its blood.

The liver, in its agency in purifying the blood from many of its waste, useless, and poisonous constituents, is second only to the lungs; whatever of these one leaves, the other eliminates.

A man has bilious fever; from time immemorial, calomel, blue pills, or other forms of mercury have been considered the sheet-anchor of safety, and doubtless will be till time shall be no more. It is because calomel "acts on the liver," meaning thereby that in some unexplained way, either directly or indirectly, it causes that organ to do more of its appropriate work, which is to separate, to secern from the blood many of its impure qualities, while it is passing through it to other parts of the system. At times the liver is so full of blood, so congested, that in a sense it cannot " work it up," and there it accumulates, getting more and more impure, more and more full of bile, which, instead of being yellow, is as " black as tar " in its concentration. This was found to be the condition of Daniel Webster's liver after his death. He was of a bilious temperament, and his habits of life were such as, combined with the temperament, were well calculated to make him bilious. But suppose in this condition a " good dose of calomel " were given a man with ordinary vitality and strength of constitution, it would so "act on the liver," as commonly expressed, that in twelve hours after, the patient would feel himself another man, comparatively well. Chemical research has lately ascertained, demonstrably, that the acid of fruits, in their natural state, and thus eaten, has this self-same effect on the liver; "acts" on it; makes it go to work and separate the bile from the blood : and thus taking away the yellowness from the skin, the fever from the cheek, and the languor of disease from the eye; hence it is that in the summer and fall of the year persons who live mainly on fruits and berries and coarse breads, bread made of the whole products of the grain, are exempt from fevers, diarrhœas, and dysenteries, at the very time when whole households who eat meats and vegetables three times a day are wasting away with disease.

THE HOUR OF DEATH,

IN a natural way, comes to more persons in the neighborhood of five o'clock in the morning, than at any other of the twenty-four; the fewest about the hour of one in the afternoon.

In the early morning the world is still, the atmosphere heavy with the damps of the night, and the body debilitated, often with the long fast from supper-time, with nothing to rouse the spirits or the circulation.

At about one o'clock in the afternoon the air is most generally fully dried by the sun, has more life, more oxygen in it, hence is more purifying, more invigorating, while the bright daylight itself has an elevating, vitalizing tendency.

These facts should be borne in mind by those who are nurses to the sick, for by extra attentions of various kinds, the critical hour might pass, and if so, the patient is more liable to live over for another twenty-four hours.

It is said by observant physicians that each seventh year of life is critical; which means that every seventh year is liable to be fatal; but that if passed over with improved health, it gives a reasonably certain lease of another seven years; for example, the most of those who become consumptive do so about the age of twenty-one, a year sooner or later, but twenty-one is the period when the disease becomes decided in the greatest number of cases.

About forty-two, the six times seven, is by far the most critical time of life in women; if that is passed healthfully, they have a good chance of seeing threescore.

It will perhaps be found that a larger number of persons die within a year or two including sixty-three than at any other specified time between forty-nine and seventy; these things suggest that increased attention should be given to the health at these critical periods.

LIVING TOGETHER.

THE art of living together pleasurably is greatly promoted by the habitual exchange of the little courtesies of life; they are never unimportant, never unacceptable, are always grateful to the feelings, and are a constant well-spring of agreeable feelings in every household. Shall brothers and sisters be less careful of the feelings of one another than those of a stranger! And as between husband and wife, should there be less effort at gentleness of deportment, of suavity of manner, and courtesy of expression than is extended to outsiders, who have no special claims, and may never be seen again? Shame upon any member of any family who neglects those affectionate attentions, and those suavities of deportment toward the members of the household and even to the lowest servant, which cannot fail to elevate the giver, and draw from the receiver those willing and spontaneous reciprocities which make of family associations a little heaven below.

Fault-finding is an apple of discord in multitudes of families. There are some persons who, from ugliness of temper arising from bodily infirmity, or an inherent blight of nature, are forever finding fault, either with something said or done, or omitted to be said or done; if not in the family, then out of it. Somebody or something is always going wrong with them; in every remark they make there is vinegar and bitterness; their whole nature seems to be in a condition of chronic snarl; their objectives are of a most sweeping character; every person is a " liar," or " swindler,"or " scoundrel," even if their short-comings are of the slightest character. Such persons are demoralizers of the community in which they live; and of those with whom they reside they are a perpetual storm, a tornado, and a curse. This complaining, fault-finding trait does not assume these gigantic proportions of enormity at once, but always comes by slow degrees and long practice. Let the reader fear falling into this great condemnation, let him be afraid of it, and resolve never to find fault with anybody or anything, or characterize any one's conduct for omission or commisson, until he has " slept on it," thus giving the clearer judgment of a renovated brain an opportunity of more dispassionate exercise.

Let every person of intelligence, refinement, and culture bear in mind that in " living together " with others pleasantly, happily, it is of essential importance to practise the virtues of uniform gentleness, deference, and courtesy, remembering that one of the most cardinal points in the promotion of domestic enjoyment, and of family happiness, is to cultivate self-sacrifice; for it is this which cherishes love in the heart of the giver, and kindles it in those for whom the self-sacrifice is made; or, to frame the principle into a phrase which all can comprehend, remember, and apply, that is the noblest heart in any household which gives to the others the first choice, and leaves to others the best places and the best things.

LONGEVITY.

The following table shows that men have attained a good old age, and there is no necessary reason why these might not be the average ages of men and women in our time :—

Dryden,	70	Loewenhoeck,	91
Petrarch,	70	Cato,	91
David, King	70	Hans Sloane,	93
Linnæus,	71	Whiston,	95
Locke,	73	Michael Angelo,	96
La Fontaine,	74	Titian,	95
Rev. Dr. Wardlaw,	74	Isocrates,	98
Handel,	75	Elisha,	100
Reaumur,	75	Hervelius,	100
Galileo,	78	Fontenelle,	100
Swift,	78	Zeno,	100
Roger Bacon,	78	Terentia,	103
Corneille,	78	Stender,	103
Marmontel,	79	Helen Gray,	105
Solon,	80	Georgias,	107
Thucydides,	80	Thomas Garrick,	108
Anacreon,	80	Democritus,	109
Juvenal,	80	Joseph,	110
Kant,	80	Joshua,	110
Pindar,	80	A. Serush,	111
Young,	80	Mittelstedt,	112
Willard,	80	H. Thauper,	112
Sophocles,	80	R. Glen,	115
Plato,	81	Moses,	120
Buffon,	81	Prastus, King of Poland,	120
Goethe,	83	Sarah,	127
Dr. Chas. Caldwell,	83	Ishmael,	137
Claude	83	Effingham,	144
West,	83	Countess of Desmond,	145
Franklin,	84	Drakenberg,	146
Metastasio,	84	Jacob,	147
Herschel,	84	Thomas Parr,	153
Madison, Pres.,	85	Thomas Damme,	154
Newton,	85	Epimenides,	157
Voltaire,	85	Henry Jenkins,	169
Halley,	86	John Rovin,	172
Simeon,	90	Abraham,	175
Fabius,	90	Isaac,	180
Eli,	98	Peter Torten,	185
Protagoras,	90	Monga of Kentigen,	186
Livia,	90		

CANCER

RARELY attacks persons under forty-five years of age. Women are more subject to it than men. It most often attacks the female breast, next the lips, the tongue, the stomach, and the neck of the womb, sometimes the gum. Its growth is exceedingly slow in the beginning, but proceeds with great rapidity in its later stages. In the breast it comes with a hard, knotty, uneven feel ; this it may maintain for many years, but as it is nearer development, sharp, lancinating pains strike across it, or from it, as rays from a star. They are as instantaneous as the stroke of the lightning. In process of time the skin is puckered at the hardened part and begins to assume a leaden hue, and then begins to discharge a thin fluid substance which irritates and even excoriates the surrounding parts. The base of the sore is hard, at the same time it spreads, seeming to eat its way along, wider and deeper, throwing out more and more the fetid matter, so exceedingly offensive, and so different from anything else, that it can never be forgotten.

When it appears on the lips, or where the skin is thin, it is in the form of a hard pimple or lump, which soon becomes an eating, running, noisome sore.

It is well to know that cancers are sometimes developed by causes which, had they never been put in operation by the person, would never have led to so deplorable a result. For example, there is a little sore on the lips, it begins to heal, is almost healed, and the scab is picked off, instead of being allowed to drop off. That picking irritates, causes a little tearing away from the tender, new-formed skin, and often there is a little bleeding. A new sore is made which must go through its regular process of healing, to be picked at and picked off ; by this thwarting of Nature she seems to get discouraged, the power of healing is lost ; that is cancer, and cancer is death.

It is also developed in the breast in early life thus : girls get to know generally that some undefinable thing is going to happen to them before the first change of life comes on, and instead of being proud of it, as a boy is of his first pair of suspenders, or of his first coat-tail, the general feeling is one of shame or shyness, leading them to conceal, having had no proper instructions from mothers. Hence when the bosom begins to develop they not only do not let out the dress, but draw it more closely; this arrests the fluids in the glands; they are reabsorbed or congested, the glands harden, and there is the lump which forty years later is the seat of the fearful cancer.

Pregnant women generally, at the first time, prefer to conceal the coming event; they do not care to have it known that the first processes are manifesting themselves which are to end in motherhood; at other times the symmetry of form, for appearance' sake, leads them to tightening the bosom; not infrequently vanity induces it in persons of middle life, the effect being to arrest the natural flow of the various fluids, with a resulting hard lump. Hence the uniform injunction of the best medical men in the world, that as soon as gestation is known to have been inaugurated, all the clothing should hang from the shoulders until after confinement.

Lumps are formed in the breasts by injudicious handling in the nursery; the milk is not drawn with that regularity and completeness which is essential to the healthy condition of the part, it dries up, and there is the foundation of the lump again.

The same result takes place if the child is weaned too suddenly. Turn to the article "Weaning."

Unlucky blows on the bosom are frequent cause of cancer in the breast. Mothers should teach these things to girls before they are twelve years old, beginning with the fact that the beginnings of womanhood are things to be proud of.

Cancer is a disease of the blood; hence to cut one out leaves the taint behind, to sprout up with more vigor elsewhere, and often in more places than one, and in more critical places; always hastening the sad result. The only thing to be done for cancer safely, as far as is yet known, is to keep up the general health in every way possible. A condition essential above all others is a free and full action of the bowels every day, and so much the better if brought about by the use of fruits, berries, coarse breads, and vegetables as a diet, with cleanliness, pure air, and outdoor exercises.

But it must be remembered that there is a spurious cancer; it seems to be a real one, but it is not. These, having been cured by various means, have given rise to a great number of cancer cures, some of which are here given, that any sufferer may try them, inasmuch as in any given case it may not be a real cancer.

Some of these "lumps" have been gotten rid of thus: take pounded ice and salt, half and half, put it into a silk bag, so as to make a little pad large enough to cover the lump; lay it on the part, with some pressure, twice a day, long enough to freeze the part so much as to make the skin very white. Cut the skin crosswise, the knife not to enter the tumor. Then insert a preparation made of equal parts of chloride of zinc, carbolic acid, and tannin, to remain five hours, when it becomes very painful, and must be removed. Cover with a mild poultice, and within a week the parts slough out; the theory being that the ice and salt freeze the cancerous part down to the very roots, and the other application loosens and destroys utterly, by reaching to the utmost end of every fibre of every root; whereas if it had been cut out, the knife might not have been extended far enough, and left a fibre outside, to spring up into a new cancer.

An old Spanish woman had the reputation of curing cancers by making a salve of the yolk of an egg; mix with it as much salt as it will take up. Spread a portion of it on linen or other material, and lay it over the spot. This plaster must be renewed night and morning, until a cure is effected; the bowels being made to act freely every day.

Salt has been claimed as a cure for consumption. The statistics of this country show that where consumption prevails the people suffer most from cancerous affections. Medical men of ability have long contended that they were essentially the same disease, acting on different tissues with different manifestations, yet originating in the same depravity of blood. These things put together give color to the idea that a most plentiful use of salt would cure both cancer and consumption, the two most incurable, hitherto, of all human maladies. A case is given where a man, apparently in the advanced stages of consumption, seemed to have had such an overpowering appetite for salt meats and salt, that he would put a tablespoon or two in each vest pocket every morning; pinch by pinch it would be diminished, and by night it was all gone. He recovered. But it may not have been consumption, any more than the old woman's cases were real cancer.

Dr. Fell, an American physician in London, has a reputation for curing cancer. He places a sticking-plaster over the cancer, having cut a hole in it large enough to receive the cancer and a rim of healthy skin besides; then a piece of muslin is cut of the size of the opening. This is plastered with the following mixture : equal parts of chloride of zinc, blood-root, and common flour ; to remain twenty-four hours, when the cancer will appear to be a piece of burned leather, and the circular rim of skin outside of it is white and parboiled, as if by hot steam. The chief ingredient is the zinc, the three being made into a paste with any convenient material, or water.

As this article will be read by women with great interest, very many of them cherishing an apprehension of it, further statements will be made of its nature as far as ascertained. Cutting out a cancer which seemed to be a true one, has been followed by permanent recovery. Some cancers dry away by spontaneous degeneration, as consumption is sometimes spontaneously cured. Cancer is inherited, but also is a result of constitutional causes. Bilious persons, those of a bilious temperament, of a dark skin, are liable to cancer, especially if their habits are sedentary, if the bowels are habitually torpid, and the passages are usually hard, or in little hard lumps or balls.

Persons of the bilious temperament are liable to depression of spirits unless they lead active, energetic, exciting lives, and nothing tends more to originate and develop cancer than a desponding habit.

Rokitansky, the most eminent medical writer of the time, gives the following as the order of attack of cancer, the first being least frequent, the last-named locality being most common :—

Throat,	Brain,	Rectum,
Tongue,	Skin,	Stomach,
Ovary,	Bones,	Breast,
Testicle,	Liver,	Uterus.
Eye,	Glands, lymph.	

In proof that consumption and cancer go together, it is found that both diseases are more frequent near the sea, diminishing as we go westward.

Also both diseases are more frequent north, and diminish in frequency as we go southward. This statement must be modified from the consideration that the census returns and mortuary reports are more exact north and east. The rate of deaths from consumption is as follows :

Going West is in	per cent.	Going from West to South	per cent.
Massachusetts	25	Michigan	16
New York	20	Indiana	14
Ohio	16	Kentucky	14
Indiana	14	Tennessee	12
Illinois	11	Alabama	6
Missouri	9		
Kansas	8		
Colorado	8		
Utah	6		
California	14		

The above statements confirm the fact that the sea and lake shore localities favor consumption; the raw damp atmosphere and chilly winds give colds, and drive the blood from the skin inwards upon the lungs; these same conditions tend to develop cancer by their impairing effect on the general health. Practical use can be made of the following

Table, showing the percentage of deaths from consumption, as compared with the total number of deaths from all causes, in each State and Territory:

Alabama	6	Missouri	9
Arkansas	5	Montana	9
California	14	Nebraska	9
Colorado	8	New Hampshire	25
Connecticut	20	New Jersey	20
Dakota	12	New Mexico	8
Delaware	26	New York	20
District of Columbia	20	North Carolina	8
Florida	6	Ohio	16
Georgia	5	Oregon	12
Illinois	11	Pennsylvania	16
Indiana	14	Rhode Island	25
Iowa	12	South Carolina	5
Kansas	8	Tennessee	12
Kentucky	14	Texas	5
Louisiana	8	Utah	6
Maine	25	Vermont	25
Maryland	16	Virginia	12
Massachusetts	25	Washington Territory	16
Michigan	16	West Virginia	16
Minnesota	14	Wisconsin	14
Mississippi	6		

. Michigan surrounded by lakes, Delaware on the Atlantic, are the most deadly from lung diseases. Minnesota, next to Michigan, notwithstanding the contrary reputation given it, is the grave yard of consumptives. Consumptives, it would seem, should go away from the northern sea-shores and lake situation, and retire to inland places, protected from bleak cutting winds; the same remarks are applicable to cancer. But after all, both cancer and consumption can be indefinitely postponed, as to fatal results, by keeping up a high state of general health.

Some cancer salves are made with great precision; for example, green wood-sorrel juice, poured on a pewter plate and allowed to evaporate in the sun, its oxalic acid combines with the lead in the pewter, and forms a compound which has efficiency in curing some sores.

The cundurango plant obtained from Ecuador has obtained a great notoriety from the fact that a high official has certified that a relative, a lady, was cured of what seemed to be cancer, by taking this remedy internally as a tea, or infusion. It may not have been a real cancer; besides, there is a spurious cundurango. Between these two statements a cancerous person might take the remedy hopefully, as prepared in New York by men who import the plant. Boil the best Turkey figs in new milk; as soon as they are quite soft, split one open and apply it as hot as can be borne to the cancerous sore; change this poultice night and morning and at noon, first washing the part well with the milk from the boiling; night and morning drink half a pint of the same fig-boiled milk.

SUNSTROKE,

MORE properly "Heat-stroke," because it takes place in cloudy days and under any circumstances of exposure to great heat in a debilitated condition of the body, when obliged to walk or work, whether that condition results from overwork, from a weakly frame, or from intemperate habits; for it is found that in numerous cases the persons attacked have used intoxicating drinks more or less freely. Still, the direct rays of the sun hasten or aggravate an attack; hence a large green leaf worn in the hat, or a moist light muslin or silk handkerchief, very certainly prevents sunstroke. The great heat and the small amount of oxygen in the air breathed, seem to cause a chemical change in the condition of the blood, or overheat the body.

Symptoms. The person falls suddenly, unconscious, as in a common fainting fit, but the head is very hot; so, instantaneously take the patient to the shade, keep off the crowd, and pour a continuous stream of cold water on the head, crossways, in every direction, so as not to fall on one spot.

Sunstroke seldom occurs on farms, or in country villages, but in cities mostly. In New York, during the summer of 1868, eight hundred cases occurred; and during July of 1872 there were several hundred deaths. Horses also perished with something similar.

If the patient is restless a quarter of a grain of morphia injected under the skin seems to have restored some persons; but in all cases let the person be placed in a sitting position and have cold water poured on the head, or a cushion made of equal parts of salt and pounded ice; give an injection as soon as possible, and rub spirits of hartshorn on the upper lip; if the salts are held too close to the nose and the patient is insensible, great injury may be done to the nerves of smell. Mustard plasters may be applied to the spine and stomach alternately.

Some are quiet, insensible; others restless, furious, or depressed; as the breathing becomes more noisy the case is increasingly desperate.

If the skin is cool, it is not sunstroke; it is always dry and hot in this case, and the heat sometimes increases after death, and the body begins to decay at once, while the heart seems as dry and hard almost as a piece of wood.

If you find a person on the pavement insensible lay your hand on the skin of his bosom, and if it is cool lay him down horizontally in the nearest shady place; if the skin is dry and hot keep his head up as if sitting in a chair, dash on cold water by the bucketful; if you can strip off his clothing the better, or take him to a pump and pump the water over him continuously until he is perfectly sensible and the skin is of a natural temperature; but a substitute is a cushion of ice and salt on his head, if it can be had; if not, have several folds of cotton or linen and keep them wet with cold water, for it is the brain which suffers most from the great heat; pouring water is best. The Egyptians pour salt water over the head and ears.

SUMMER-COMPLAINT

Is a too frequent action of the bowels of teething children. Every mother ought to know what is the healthful frequency and appearance of the bowel discharges; then she can be on her guard against the approach of disease. At first it is better that the infant should have three or four passages every twenty-four hours, yellowish and of the consistence of thin mustard,. without any sour or fetid smell; no white curdy matter, no lumps, no pain, no wind; in a few weeks the color is darker and the consistence greater; they should never be less than two daily, the first year. If during any day there has been but one passage since daylight, give before bedtime a teaspoonful of castor-oil in a tablespoonful of warm milk, and repeat next morning and noon and night, until two passages are secured for each twenty-four hours; this simple precaution would prevent much infantile sickness, and save many a little darling's life,—during teething it is of infinite importance, for summer-complaint is almost always preceded by costiveness, to prevent which use the following: one ounce of castor-oil, two drachms of calcined magnesia, three drachms of loaf sugar, two drops of oil of anise, mix it well, and give one teaspoonful thrice a day, or often enough during teething to keep up two actions of the bowels every twenty-four hours; or one or two teaspoonfuls of manna in a little warm milk. But castor-oil is the best stand-by, and it is better to learn its uses, and rely wholly on it. In ordinary cases of loose bowels of infants feed more entirely on boiled milk, with sago, tapioca, or boiled rice. If there is wind and griping, and the infant takes hold of the breast eagerly, and yet it is not satisfied, and is pale and thin, the milk or food is not suitable, and the only remedy is healthy milk.

If, after nursing, the milk is thrown up unchanged, and the infant is disposed to play, it has had too much; feed it less often, and at regular hours, on no account between; this will generally overcome looseness of bowels, especially if the diet is made to consist of the articles of food named.

Sometimes teething children with irritated gums and looseness have been cured in an almost marvellous manner by being allowed to chew a piece of the rind of boiled ham, to which some of the fat adheres; give a large piece, so that it cannot be swallowed; and safer still to run a strong thread through it and tie the other end to the child's wrist; this will certainly cure in very many cases; sometimes the little sufferer is so greedy for it as not to allow its being taken away.

The chief signs of summer-complaint in children are vomiting and diarrhœa; the discharges from the bowels are usually colorless, thin, greenish, without odor, with shreds of mucus coming away without effort, or squirted out; sometimes there is pain and griping and straining; there is a whining, plaintive cry, restlessness, a drawing up and stretching out of the limbs, with languor, emaciation; the discharges look like the washings of meat; and stupor or convulsions follow.

Homœopathy relies on aconite when there is fever and thirst; arsenicum, if there is great weakness; ipecac, if the stools seem fermented; chamomilla, if there is colic or griping; veratrum, if great purging and vomiting; secale, if face is pale and eyes sunken; mercurius, if stools are slimy and bloody; croton tiglium, if stools come with a gush; belladonna, if face is flushed; sulphur, if stools are white and watery; opium and china in desperate cases. Give the mildest food—milk diluted, oatmeal gruel. Keep the whole body warm, the feet and hands particularly.

Hydropathy gives cool water injections; abdominal compresses when there is fever and heat; if the evacuations are bloody give cold-water injections, as often as the discharges occur; give pure cold water to drink; if the case is protracted, give tepid sitz-baths, and spend a good deal of the time in rubbing the whole back with the hands, eating mainly rice, mush, sago, with a little sugar or boiled milk.

Allopaths prefer calomel and magnesia, or calomel and chalk. Two grains of calomel, twenty grains of bicarbonate of soda, twelve grains of ginger powder—make into ten doses, and give one dose three times a day, or a quarter of a liver-pill night and morning, until the discharges thicken and are not oftener than two or three times a day, eating boiled rice, sago, or tapioca.

In many cases, the loose bowels of infants and children are corrected by eating ice-cream—taking nothing else for nutriment or drink but a little boiled rice, it acts by cooling that inflammatory condition which causes the looseness, as lumps of ice swallowed often cure dysentery in adults.

26

FIRE ESCAPE.

IF you wake up and find the room on fire or full of smoke, fall on your face and crawl towards the door or window, for the smoke is least dense on the floor and the flame less severe.

If you have to pass through smoke and flame, as in carrying a person out, throw a silk handkerchief over your head to fall down over the face; if none at hand, use muslin or linen, or tear part of a sheet or pillow-case off. If neither can be dampened, do not use them. If there is a

CHIMNEY ON FIRE

throw some brimstone on the coals, or throw on a peck of salt; or close every door and window, dip a sheet or blanket or carpet in water and hold it close over the fireplace.

Many persons are burned up for want of presence of mind, most likely to happen if waked suddenly out of a sound sleep. Horses are thus so confused sometimes that they cannot be induced to come out of the burning stable; but many times it can be done if the bridle and saddle are put on them; this diverts their minds and gives them a chance to think, and they leave the stable as a kind of habit.

It is the same sometimes with a balky horse. Put some salt to his nose, or a handful of mud, or tie a string tightly around his ear, anything to divert his mind, and he moves on. So with a stupid man in a fire: divert the mind from the sense of excessive danger, and thus give him a chance to have his wits about him.

The first thing in a fire in house or on boat or shipboard, is to stand still, say nothing, and think a minute; time immensely valuable will be saved by it. Cast your eye around and take in the situation. Don't go with the crowd, necessarily. Never jump from a window or ship until the very last moment. If you find you have to go through flame or smoke, get if possible a blanket or carpet, or any woollen thing, and wrap it around you; if you can wet them, the better. Instead of jumping from any height, make a rope of sheets and blankets, or old trousers, or anything else; draw the bedstead to the window, tie one end to the post, the other around your body under your arms; then take hold at a part near the bed-post, and let yourself down, provided you have ascertained certainly that there is no chance to go down-stairs. But don't go up-stairs, unless there are houses adjoining; for then your leap would be from a higher point.

If the clothing takes fire lie down instantly; for flames always would go upward, and would burn your face and would be breathed into the throat and lungs. The instinct is always to run, which makes a draught and increases the flame. Lie down then on the instant and roll over and over; or, better, take the corner of the carpet firmly in your hands and roll over, bringing the carpet with you; or blanket or overcoat, or any woollen thing, for then it would not catch on fire very easily.

BAD BREATH

SOMETIMES results from disordered gums and teeth, which ought to be attended to by a dentist; but almost always the cause is in a bad digestion, constipation, or other form of disease which corrupts the blood. The better the health, the less offensive the breath is. But it must be remembered that no breath is pure coming out of the lungs, because the air goes into them pure and fresh; it is the oxygen in it which gives it its purity and freshness; but when it gets into the lungs all that oxygen remains there, has been absorbed into the blood, and its place is taken by the waste and impure particles of the body, the carbonic acid gas, which has no life or freshness in it. Hence, every one's breath is more or less offensive, but that of some is so much so that it is observed almost as soon as they enter the room, or come within several feet of you. Some are conscious of this, and endeavor to rectify it by using various drops and drugs; but it is only a seeming correction; for the bad breath is there, with the addition of the overpowering drug, making the air doubly less pure. Take two ounces each of catechu or other gum, white sugar and orris root, made into a paste, with peppermint or other perfume, and carry a bit of it in the mouth. This is good for a specific occasion. The better plan is to eradicate the trouble, not cover it over, by making efforts to secure a higher state of general health.

BILIOUSNESS

MEANS that the bile, which in reality is the waste of the system, the washings out of its used and useless particles, has not been separated from the blood, and remains in it, keeps it dark, thick, impure, poisonous, and unfit to carry on the life processes; this blood, being thick and heavy, is sluggish, does not pass along the blood-vessels freely, but clogs them, dams them up, becomes impacted in them, congested; this congestion making itself felt most in those parts of the system which have been weakened, either by accident, disease, or hereditarily.

It is the business of the liver to withdraw from the blood those useless particles, which, being mixed together, make what is called bile; these particles are naturally conveyed from the liver into the gall-bladder, out of which it passes, drop by drop, into the top or beginning of the bowels, near the point where the food passes from the stomach into this same top of the bowels, and is especially active after meals. It is a strikingly beautiful exhibition of the economy of nature, that this bile, which is perfectly useless to the body, is waste matter, is made to have a purgative effect on the bowels, stimulates them to pass from them the refuse of food which contains no nutriment. The Creator could as easily have added another apparatus to the machinery of man which would have had a specific effect, the same effect as the bile has; but that would have made the machine more complicated; and He preferred to make nothingness useful; He preferred to order the adapttinos so that a useless thing should do a useful work, a work absolutely necessary to the well-being and safety of the body; for we all know that if the bowels cease to act, we certainly die; this is of a piece with the divine operation in the moral world; worthless men, wicked men, are made use of to forward his great purposes, as clearly expressed in the Holy Record, " making the wrath of man to praise Him."

The effect of this presence of bile in the blood, of this congestion, compaction, is to clog up the whole machinery of the body, like a clock that is so dirty it scarcely runs at all; the limbs don't work, and the man feels indisposed to do anything; the brain does not work, and the bilious man can't think to advantage; his head is heavy, his eyes are dull, there is no life, no animation, no appetite ; and instead, a universal feeling of discomfort ; the feet are cold, the head aches, the bowels costive; in short, the whole mental, moral, and physical nature is in a state of demoralization. Now for the remedy :—

First, cut off the supply of blood, for there is too much in the body already, and as the blood is made out of the food eaten, if nothing is eaten for a day or two half the work is done, and eventually the whole, by continuing to eat but little, thrice a day for a short time, until the symptoms have disappeared. This is the doctors' method.

Another is, stimulate the liver; make it work, by taking such things as are known to " act " on the liver; we don't know why they should act on the liver, or how, but we know they do do it. One thing acts on the brain, as whiskey; another acts on the stomach, as tartar emetic ; a third acts on the bowels, as a dose of salts ; so there are medicines which " act on the liver ;" this is the quickest way, and the laziest way, and the least self-denying way of getting rid of biliousness ; but it is not the best way ; it is the worst way. So no information will be given here as to what medicines would best act on the liver ; for then, when a man became bilious, he would take a dose of physic, and in a short time he would be all the time dosing. Besides, after a while all remedies begin to lose their legitimate effect, and either become useless in any quantity, or must be taken in large quantities, so large sometimes as to become poisonous and fatal.

There are, however, two things which we can take for biliousness, and either of them will cure in all curable cases ; but they won't be taken ; hence no harm will result from imparting information.

Blood, like many other liquids, is thinned by being warmed ; hence warm up the blood. Nature teaches this, for bilious persons are very chilly. One way is to

TAKE A SWEAT,

a good old-fashioned sweat, by getting into bed with hot bricks to the feet, and bottles of hot water under the arms, and a quart or two of hot catnip tea, or any other kind of tea, although hot water will do quite as much good, only it is not so pleasant to take ; ginger tea, red pepper tea, all have their virtues, but the most virtue is in the heat of the fluid swallowed ; then have yourself tucked in all around in a feather bed, so as to have the sweat roll out of you in great big wholesome drops for an hour or two ; repeat this daily until well ; eating in the mean while bread, fruit, soups with bread crust in them ; this treatment not only renders the blood more fluid, so that it will circulate more easily, but it diminishes the bulk of the blood, the weight of it, for the sweat comes out of the blood, being its more watery particles. But after a "sweat" the person should cool off slowly, gradually, in the course of an hour.

But there is another plan and a better : " take exercise." The best is steady work in the open air, as in ploughing, chopping wood, splitting rails, threshing grain, etc., but if you are so unfortunate as to have nothing to do, no useful work to perform, row a boat, or take a steady walk of an hour or two's duration ; a walk with a pleasurable result at the end of it ; a walk involving such physical activity as to cause a gentle and general perspiration, and such mental or moral energy as to cause self-forgetfulness, and an entire absorption in the thing in hand. This interested, pleasurable exercise not only does all the good of the sweating operation, but has an additional power in diminishing the quantity of the blood, in working the waste particles out of the system, by that friction of the multitude of muscles which are employed in walking. If, in addition to the exercise of walking, there are brought into requisition various bendings and twistings of the body, all these have the effect to stimulate the liver, by pressing upon it, like pressing water out of a sponge ; because it is a large, soft body, weighing several pounds, at the left side, above the lower edge of the ribs.

Hence it is that persons, even of the bilious temperament, who are on their feet for a great part of daylight, stooping down, straightening up, pushing, pulling, and lifting, are seldom troubled with "biliousness," unless they take cold. There are many ladies in New York who keep off biliousness, or get rid of it when an accidental cold brings it on, or close confinement to the house for several days, by taking an active walk of an hour or more every day, in marketing, shopping, calling upon friends, or making visits of charity and good-will to the sick and suffering and unfortunate. Who does not see the wonderful wisdom and beneficence of the great Creator of us all, who punishes to save, who brings blessings out of cursing? for in that He said, "In the sweat of thy face shalt thou eat bread," He so arranged it that the very labor which man was destined to perform, would by the very sweatings keep the human system in a healthy condition, making labor a pleasure and a means of glorious good health.

A bilious condition of the system, known by one or more of the following symptoms, can always be removed, if possible by any means, by taking one of the liver pills, according to the directions. If one does not accomplish the object, take another at the interval of a week or ten days, and a most triumphant result will be the general reward. Improvement is to be measured by the return of the appetite and a clean tongue, which see. The symptoms of biliousness are costiveness, headache, bad morning taste, variable and poor appetite, cold feet, chilliness, and depression.

RESTORING FADED WRITING.

In case a doctor's prescription should become illegible, dip a feather in tincture of galls, or a solution of ferrocyanide of potassium, slightly acidulated with hydrochloric acid; apply either of these washes as nearly as possible to the ink lines, and thus prevent the spreading of the ink.

DIGESTIBILITY OF FOOD

in the order of the easiest of each class :—

EASIEST.	LESS EASY.	HARDEST.
Ale,	Porter,	Champagne,
Claret,	Coffee,	Chocolate,
Sherry,	Cocoa,	Pickles,
Black Tea,	Cooked Fruits,	Peas and Beans,
Toast Water,	Rhubarb Plant,	Mushrooms,
Sweet Apples,	Marmalade,	Carrots, Parsnips,
Peaches,	Jelly,	Cucumbers, Onions,

EASIEST.	LESS EASY.	HARDEST.
Strawberries,	Farina,	Pineapples, Cherries,
Grapes,	Bread,	Pears, Plums, Nuts,
Oranges,	Raspberries,	Custard,
Cauliflower,	Currants,	Pastry, Cakes,
French Beans,	Sour Apples,	Toast and Butter,
Sea Kale,	Apricots,	Muffins,
Asparagus,	Celery,	Fresh Bread,
Arrow Root,	Lettuce,	Cheese,
Sago,	Artichokes,	Hard-boiled Eggs,
Tapioca,	Spinach,	Melted Butter,
Rice,	Cabbage,	Oil,
Stale Bread,	Turnips,	Mussels,
Roasted Oysters.	Beets,	Shrimps,
Fresh Fish,	Potatoes,	Crabs,
Sole,	Oysters	Lobster,
Flounder,	Trout,	Salt Fish,
Haddock,	Pike,	Halibut,
Turbot,	Cod,	Herring,
Milk,	Turtle,	Salmon
Mutton Broth,	Butter,	Eels,
Beef Tea,	Eggs,	Mackerel,
Grouse,	Soups,	Hashes,
Pheasant,	Snipes,	Sausage,
Partridge,	Woodchuck,	Salt Meat,
Turkey,	Wild Water-fowl,	Brain,
Chicken,	Duck,	Heart,
Sweet Bread,	Young Pigeon,	Liver,
Hare,	Rabbit,	Goose,
Venison,	Lamb,	Veal,
Mutton.	Beef.	Pork.

The preceding table is approximate to the truth as a general rule, but now and then one article is easily digested by one person and very hard to digest in the stomach of another.

The practical use to be made of the table is to read it thus:

Ale is easier of digestion than porter, and porter is easier than champagne.

Mutton is easier of digestion than beef, and beef easier than pork. Roast mutton, for example, is digested in about three hours and a half; roast beef in four, and roast pork in five or more hours.

Each table presents a certain variety of food; the first is more easily digested than the second.

The first article of each class is the easiest of digestion; each following one less easy, until the last, which is the most difficult in that column; thus, sweet apples in the first column are digested within two hours, and so is rice; mutton requires nearly double the time.

When it is said that an article is digested easily, it is meant that the juices of the stomach soonest dissolve it, soonest melt it up, pass it out, fit to be made into good blood as soon as it gets into the heart, and thence passes into the lungs; and here the subject which most naturally presents itself for consideration is

DYSPEPSIA,

which means literally "hard to digest." Some prefer the name of "indigestion," but that is not literally true, for it means no digestion at all or without digestion, cannot be digested, which is not the idea to be conveyed; for an article may be taken into the stomach which could not be digested in three hours, but it might be in four or five; but if it ought to have been digested in three and was not until five, thus requiring two hours extra work of the stomach, it was "hard" to digest, but was not indigestible, hence the Greek word dyspepsia is more truthful than the Latin name indigestion. Dyspepsia in the United States is a national disease; it almost seems that every third person is more or less troubled with dyspepsia; it is a rare disease, comparatively, in England and on the Continent; it arises from improper eating in one of three ways:

Eating too fast.

Eating too often.

Eating too much.

Medicine cannot cure dyspepsia; it can only be remedied by adapting the food to the strength of the stomach, by which is meant the solvent powers of that liquid which accumulates in the stomach for the purpose of dissolving the food preparatory to its being converted into blood. The idea is better comprehended by comparing a dyspeptic stomach to a faithful maidservant who is just recovering from a long sickness; she is willing to work and anxious to please you. If you give her, in her weak state, a small amount of work to do, she will do it, and will do it well; if you give her a great deal to do, she will try to do it all, and in the effort may go through it, but none of it is well done. The dyspeptic stomach will digest a small amount of food well, and make good blood out of it; but if a large amount is taken into it, it is dissolved, but not perfectly dissolved; it makes blood, but not good blood; and it, going to the heart, and being there mixed with the other blood of the body, is not only not pure blood itself, but renders impure and imperfect the whole mass of blood in the system; hence it is that as the blood goes to every part of the body, being bad, unnatural, it is capable of causing unnatural feelings in any and every pin-point in the human frame; hence dyspeptics sometimes truthfully express themselves as being miserable all over, although, as a general rule, the misery congregates itself at one point, most generally at the stomach at first; but as the blood becomes more and more disordered it begins to affect the nerves; and since the nerves go everywhere, and are fed by the blood, the blood being its natural aliment, they become disordered and complain. The nerves are in pairs generally, in corresponding sides. Sometimes they complain on one side, then change to another; when there is a pain at one spot, there may be one on the other side of the body at a corresponding spot, alternating. Sometimes these pains spread upwards from the stomach, and develop themselves on the sides, about the ribs and chest, causing persons to apprehend approaching consumption. The experienced physician always feels relieved when persons having cough, or some throat trouble, begin to complain of pains in the sides of the chest, under the ribs on either side or both sides, or any pains whatever which are changing, especially to corresponding places on the other side of the body. Such pains are neuralgic, depend upon a bad condition of the blood, arising from imperfect digestion, from

DYSPEPSIA,

and so far from such pains threatening consumption, they are proof that the stomach is the ailing part, being actually a protection against consumption; these very pains in the chest and side are favorable, for being neuralgic and of dyspeptic origin, they tend to draw away disease from the lungs, and in that direction are a positive benefit.

It was not meant to say that errors in eating were the only causes of dyspepsia; there is a nervous dyspepsia, or dyspeptic symptoms arising from a disordered condition of the nervous sometimes become dyspeptic for the want of sufficient food, from want of nourishment; not a few have dieted themselves into dyspepsia, for knowing that eating too much has given dyspepsia, they thought that safety consisted in eating the smallest amount possible, forgetting that all strength to every part of the body comes from the food eaten, and if the stomach itself is not nourished, it will get so weak after a while as not to be able to digest anything, and the man dies; persons who have been starved on wrecks at sea, get in eight or ten days to have such weak stomachs, that they cannot take more than a teaspoonful at a time of the very lightest food; of all others, a dyspeptic needs nourishing food; starvation will kill him.

Sometimes persons are made dyspeptic by too close mental application; they sit down to study immediately after a hearty meal; do this daily, habitually, for weeks and months together, with the result that the nervous energy which ought to go to the stomach to aid in digesting the food is forced to the brain, to be expended there, with the inevitable result that the food is not well worked up, the strength of it is not withdrawn, the body every day becomes weaker, the stomach has its own share of weakness, and there is the

STUDENTS' DYSPEPSIA.

Debility of the stomach, inability to convert the food into healthful nourishment, is the essence of dyspepsia; the stomach juices, whose office it is to dissolve the food, are either deficient in strength or quantity; in either case the effect is the same.

Vinegar is more allied to the gastric juice in its nature than any other liquid known; but if diluted with water or any other liquid, it is less strong, less fit for its appropriate purposes; hence dyspeptic persons should take little or no liquids at meals.

If the stomach is too weak to digest much food, then it follows that the dyspeptic should eat but little at a time.

If the stomach is weak, a little work wearies it; hence it must have rest; hence dyspeptics should not eat often, there should be a considerable interval between meals, except in peculiar cases; but as it is known that it requires about five hours to digest an ordinary meal, and to pass it out of the stomach, it follows that a dyspeptic should not eat at shorter intervals than five hours in the daytime or three times in twenty-four hours, especially as it has been noticed by the naked eye, through a hole in the stomach, by Dr. Beaumont, that if more food was eaten in an hour or two after a regular meal, the stomach, in a sense, ceased to digest what was there before, until the last food taken in was brought to the condition of what was there before, thus continuing the work of the stomach that much longer.

The finer food is divided before swallowing, the more speedily is it dissolved; as the smaller bits of ice are, the more rapidly do they disappear; they, like the food, being dissolved from without inwards; hence food should be chewed well or cut up in bits as small as a pea; to chew it well requires time, hence the dyspeptic and those who wish to avoid dyspepsia should chew very slowly, and take good care of their teeth.

THE STOMACH.

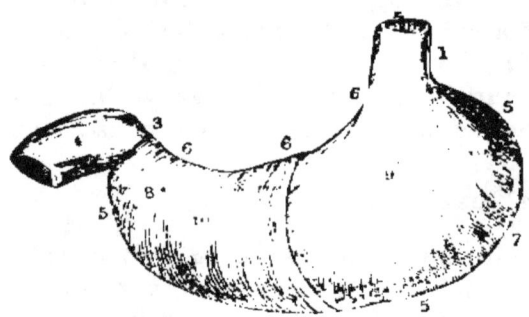

1, Entrance to the stomach, called the cardiac orifice because near the heart; at this point the food enters the stomach from the œsophagus, popularly understood as the throat. 3 is the pyloric orifice, or gate, which opens to let the food pass out of the stomach after it has been sufficiently digested. There seems, with our present knowledge, to be a human rationality in the action of this curious part of the body; if the food is not in a proper state to be passed this gate does not open, and the particle is sent back to go another and another round; but after a while, if it still presents itself, it is allowed to pass along, although wholly unsoftened, as much as to say, "It is of no use to keep you in here any longer; pass on." This is why hard substances, pieces of coin and other things, are voided; at other times undigested articles of food have been vomited after having remained in the stomach ten or fifteen hours.

4 Is the first part of the intestines called the duodenum, meaning twelve, the Romans giving it that name because it was about twelve finger-breadths long; then comes the "cæcum," meaning blind or closed at one end, like the bottom of a bag;

next the colon, which is the longest intestine, ending in the rectum, at the bottom of the body, the exit of which is called the anus, which is kept closed by muscular bands acting very much like the string of a reticule, to keep the contents in until the time comes for passing them outwards. This operation is called by physicians "defecation," a word which ought to come in common use, as it would displace the names of water-closet, privy, necessary, with two or three other words to be attached to them before the full meaning is expressed. The stomach lies across the body in a horizontal position. It will be seen that if a person lies on his right side, for example, in going to sleep, the contents of the stomach pass out of it as water passes out of a bottle when turned upside down; if on the left side, then it has to be lifted as a bucket is lifted out of a well, requiring more stomach power. While, therefore, it is better to go to sleep lying on the right side, it is not advisable to lie down on that side always or all night; better let instinct take care of the position after having gone to sleep.

It will be seen by the cut that the stomach has several muscles to work in various directions, the object of which is to keep the food in motion all the time, as we keep anything in motion with a spoon in a glass when we wish it to be dissolved. If you attempt to wink your eye more rapidly than usual it gets tired out in a minute. This shows that it requires strength to wink the eye, and so to move any other muscle of the body. This strength comes from the nerves. If the body is tired or weak there is very little nervous power for it or any part of it; hence, if persons eat when they are very tired, there is but little strength in the nerves which move the muscles of the stomach, hence the food is not digested.

Hence, also, as stated before, if all the nervous power goes to the brain of a student soon after he has eaten, the muscles of the stomach lack their proper supply of nervous power, and the food is not digested.

For the same reason it is very imprudent, especially for feeble persons, to eat when very tired, because the muscles of the stomach are weak in proportion to the other parts of the body. Persons have been thrown into convulsions by eating when greatly debilitated.

Working people and others, on returning from a ride or an excursion, often enter the house very ravenous and very tired; they can scarcely wait until the food has been placed on the table. Hence it is a good plan to take a bowl of hot soup at the beginning of dinner, the heat stimulates the stomach to action, while the small amount of nutriment in it requires but little stomach-power. If much tired and the meal must be eaten, a person will be greatly revived by prefacing it with a cup of hot tea, and will be otherwise benefited thereby. This tea will be absorbed rapidly without diluting the gastric juice, but, if solid food is taken, any liquid causes a hurtful dilution.

HOW MUCH TO EAT,

is a question proposed by every dyspeptic with a great deal of interest, because, if he eats much of anything it causes discomfort; that discomfort is proof that it is not digested. At the same time his appetite may be ravenous, he feels as if he could never eat enough, and even after he has eaten he soon gets hungry. The reason is, that but little nutriment is extracted from what is eaten. There is not power to withdraw it. Instinct really seems to think in this case; thinks that the body wants more food when it really wants more nutriment; there is food enough in the stomach already, but it is not extracted in consequence of want of stomach-power. Thus it is that all dyspeptics eat many times too much. It is the quantity which injures more than the quality; although in the cure of dyspepsia attention must be paid to quality, two things being requisite: easiness of digestion and nutritiousness; not a concentrated nutritiousness, there must be bulk as well as nourishment.

No medicine has cured dyspepsia, nor ever can. No physician can ever cure a dyspeptic, he must cure himself.

No one man who has had dyspepsia and is now well, can cure any other man who has dyspepsia by teaching him how he recovered, for no one man is a safe guide for any other; because the symptoms, the constitutions, and the surrounding circumstances of any two dyspeptics are never the same; each man must be a rule for himself, must observe for himself, and act accordingly.

All must eat regularly three times a day, nothing between meals, and very slowly, of well-divided food, not in a tired condition of body, not concentrated food, nor poor, unnourishing food; these points have already been discussed, with some general principles as to quality and quantity. As dyspeptics are babies and have very little common-sense about eating, they must be encouraged and helped along, especially as to their great weak point, eating too much. The first step is to diminish the variety of the food at any one meal; not that there is unhealthiness in variety, for, as elsewhere stated, half a pound of food made up of a dozen different articles would be as easily digested as half a pound made up of only three kinds, equally digestible; the point is, that variety tempts the appetite, and it is tempted too much already; the dyspeptic always wants to eat more than is good for him. A man who sits down to a dinner of bread and butter, roast beef and boiled potatoes, will eat until he is satisfied, until he feels that he wants no more; but the weight of it will be perhaps a third less than if, in addition, he had tomatoes and cauliflower and egg plant and delicious pastry, ending with fruits and ice-cream or champagne. Hence it is abundantly easier to avoid excess in eating, to have only three items of food on the table at any one meal. The quantity must be determined by systematic experiment and observation. You eat so much to-day; if there is the slightest unpleasant sensation in any part of the body, any sensation which uniformly follows a meal, unpleasantly attracting attention, then you have eaten too much; at the next corresponding meal diminish the amount a sixth, and keep on diminishing the amount, bravely, determinedly, until no discomfort is observed; then you are half cured, because you have only to persist in taking this amount for a few days, when you will find that you not only can take a little more, but that you are not as hungry all the time as you used to be, and that you are a little stronger and have more cheerful spirits. This is the only rational foundation for the cure of dyspepsia. It will meet every case and will cure every curable case, other things being equal.

The cure will be greatly facilitated and expedited by attending to several other things.

First. Strict personal cleanliness.

Second. Several hours should be spent every day in out-door activities, interesting, agreeable, profitable.

Third. Regular hours of sleep and plenty of it.

Fourth. Be busy, if anything a little pushed all the time; this gives no leisure for desponding thoughts and depressing influences, prevents the mind from dwelling on contemptible trifles, and senseless exaggerations of the many disagreeable things which come up, more or less, every day.

Fifth. Take special pains to cultivate a lively, cheerful, generous, and lofty frame of mind. This will be a most wonderful help towards a speedy cure.

AVOIDABLE THINGS.

Avoid cold feet.

Avoid costive bowels.

Avoid cooling off too soon, after all forms of exercise.

Avoid fatigue; always stop before you are much tired.

Avoid chilliness.

Avoid all tonics, stimulants, spirits, bitters, tobacco, or any other excitant.

Avoid eating before the time comes, merely to quiet the craving or gnawing or goneness.

Avoid fats, sugars, sweet milk, eggs, and coffee; you may favor yourself greatly by selecting your food. It might be well to begin on the "Special Fruit Diet," elsewhere spoken of. At all events you are safe in beginning with roasted beef or mutton, lean; cracked wheat, or wheaten grits, or Graham bread, and good butter, with all you can eat of berries, cherries, currants, melons, grapes, and peaches and apples, after breakfast and dinner, as dessert, taking them in their natural, raw, ripe, perfect state; if not in the season, take them stewed or baked, but not preserved.

It was not intended in this article to detail any curious cases or to waste space in long disquisitions, but to present simply the main features of the disease as presented in ninety-nine cases in a hundred, so as to reach the masses of the people. If compelled to state the certain cure of dyspepsia in three rules, they would be:—

Eat regularly thrice a day.

Eat just as much as will not be followed by any discomfort.

Spend from five to ten hours every day in interested and profitable out-door activities.

The almost universal cause of dyspepsia is error in eating; the almost universal symptom is an unpleasant reminder that there is a stomach; the almost universal principle of cure is never to eat so much at any regular meal, of not less than five hours' interval, as will attract the attention unpleasantly to any portion of the body. No method of cure ever succeeded which did not involve this principle, and when regarded, this alone will permanently cure any curable case, without one atom of medicine of any kind, and the cure will be expedited in proportion as the time from after breakfast to sundown is expended in profitable, agreeable, and absorbing out-door activities.

ADIPOCIRE.

WHEN great numbers of human or animal bodies are buried together under certain circumstances, or exposed to the action of water, the flesh forms into a kind of soapy or gelatinous substance.

ADIPOSE TISSUE is that formation under the skin that holds the fatty portion of the system, composed of very small cells collected together at points which are filled with oil.

ADVENTITIOUS is a membrane or other thing which may form, and is not natural; the tough substance which forms on the lining of the windpipe in croup, and which grows thicker and thicker if not removed, is an adventitious product.

PAPER SHIRT COLLARS

ARE glazed with a material containing white-lead. The perspiration of the skin dissolves the mixture; the warmth opens the pores of the skin, and the poison is absorbed, carried into the blood and thence to the nerves, causing paralysis, which will soonest manifest itself in that part of the system which is most debilitated. If a collar or cuff or any other article of dress made of paper is burnt, the ashes will be found on cooling to show particles of lead. It is this same glazing, made of acetate of lead, which is used on visiting cards; there is a sweetish taste to it—hence sometimes called sugar of lead. Young children, attracted by the sweetness, have eaten them and have been poisoned. Drink warm milk until free vomiting has been induced, or eat the white of eggs.
27

A HANDSOME FACE

Is an attainable possession, for it is the mind that makes it, and keeps it handsome till threescore and after. It is mental activity, it is a busy life in stirring scenes, in heavy responsibilities, constantly calling out all the latent fires; these are they which give a fire to the eye, a firmness to the lip, and a clear, sharp outline to the features of the face; on the other hand, those who are born handsome soon grow dull and flat and flabby, and jejune in face and form and mind and heart, when they give themselves up to idleness and inactivity and animal indulgences. To get handsome and remain handsome, be busy in the execution of high resolves.

THE PLAGUES AND PESTILENCES

Of centuries ago were nothing more than miasmatic poisons, precisely such as in our own times cause every variety of epidemics, from fever and ague, diarrhœa, dysentery, and the dengue, up to yellow fever and Asiatic cholera; more destructive in some years than others, and sometimes not appearing for long years together, simply for the want of the proper combinations of heat and cold, rain and drought, in relation to decaying vegetation. When the yellow fever first appeared in Charleston, South Carolina, in the year 1700 it was called the plague; so again in 1703 it was called the plague; this not appearing for just a quarter of a century, it was then spoken of as

YELLOW FEVER.

For future reference and information the following statistics of its visits to Charleston are given:

1703.—The same disease occurred, with similar results, and was still called "the plague."

1728.—Twenty-five years elapsed, during which no mention is made of epidemic sickness, when the disease of 1700 and 1703 appeared, and was called yellow fever.

1732.—It began in May and continued until October.   During its severest period eight to twelve died daily.   The population of the city was then about 10,000.

1739.—It appeared, but not violently ; also, in 1745 and 1748, with some severity ; but the deaths cannot be ascertained.

1753 and 1755.—A few sporadic cases appeared, after which, until 1792—some writers say 1794—a new series of epidemics commenced, appearing in 1795, 1796, 1797, and 1799, when 239 died ; 1800, 184 deaths ; 1802, 96 deaths ; 1804, 148 deaths ; 1807, 162 deaths.   The population of the city at these periods was about 20,000.

The fever passed then over the ten succeeding years.

1817.—There were 270 deaths, of whom a great many were children.

1819.—There were 176 deaths of yellow fever.

1820.—A few sporadic cases.

1824.—231 died of yellow fever, and this year it reached Sullivan's Island, causing many deaths.

1727, 62 deaths ; 1828, 26 deaths ; 1830, 31 deaths.

1834, 49 deaths ; 1835, 24 deaths.

1838.—The year of the great fire ; the fever was destructive, causing the death of 353 persons.   Population, 30,000.

1839.—133 deaths—the fever epidemic.   From this date, for ten years, the city maintained a high state of health.

1849.—A sickness prevailed, strikingly similar to that existing in 1872.   The weather was followed by heavy rain.   The beginning and progress of the disease, the gradual change into a very " mild type of yellow," or a " broken bone," or a " bilious attack," were like those of 1872.   The fever began 1st August, and ended 1st October ; 123 died.   During its progress there was very little alarm, and no panic.

1852.—An epidemic prevailed ; 280 died.

1854.—Was a severe year ; 624 died.

1856.—There were 206 deaths.

1858.—The most distressing sickness ever known here prevailed, when 680 died.   Population, 45,000.

1864.—There was some sickness.

It will be noted that there was no yellow fever in Charleston from 1739 to 1792, a period of over half a century.

One point cannot possibly be placed before an intelligent mind without securing the most fixed attention, that whenever the moist surfaces of the bottoms of ponds and summer streams are presented to a hot summer's sun for days in succession, epidemics will inevitably follow, to be destructive of life. in proportion to the heat of the weather and the extent of the muddy bottoms. Sometimes an area of a few square yards has sent death into whole households. If such bottoms were filled a foot or two in depth with water no harm would result; it is the muddy bottom which does the mischief—the little shallow lakes in the depressions of dried-up creeks.

THE ITCH-INSECT,

Sarcoptes Scabiei (*Acarus Scabiei* of Linnæus), burrows in the human skin, and thus causes the common itch. The itch-insect, cheese-mite, and other mites, and cattle-ticks, belong to the same group of animals with spiders and scorpions. Many of these breathe by tracheæ or air-tubes in their bodies; hence the impression that if the skin is kept well greased, even with lard or sweet oil, these little breathing-tubes of theirs are closed up, they die of suffocation, and the itch is cured.

LONGINGS, FRIGHTS, SHOCKS,

are not supposed by the most eminent men in medicine to be capable of giving marks or blemishes to the child. The great Dr. Hunter, who had no equal in his century, noted down two thousand cases of childbirth. He asked each of these two thousand women, as soon as the child was delivered,

Had you any longing?

Had you any shocks?

He put every answer down in his note-book; and among those two thousand cases he did not have a single instance where a mother who had a shock or a longing had given a mark or blemish to her child. He did find marks and blemishes where the mother did not remember to have had a shock or longing.

POISONOUS BED-CHAMBERS.

PLASTERED walls, uncarpeted floors, and uncurtained windows, and a large open fire-place are the healthiest places to sleep in, as they afford the least shelter for dampness, dust, insects, mould, and poisonous emanation from fabrics made of unhealthful material or ingredients.

Another source of ill health in sleeping apartments is the exclusion of sunshine. In old countries and in Rome to this day apartments facing the south command double prices over northern rooms.

A son of one of our wealthy citizens was sent West some years ago, to settle on a farm. It bordered on a prairie; the largest and most commodious room in the house was on its north side, an upper room with wide windows, making it a delightfully cool summer room. But the young man's health began to decline, compelling him eventually to come home. The physician saw at once that there must have been a slowly acting cause, for the inroads were very insidious and their manifestations not very distinct, comparatively speaking; all, however, looking to an impairment of the lungs, indicated by a trifling "heck" insufferable in its tantalizing frequency; but patient questioning brought out at length the remark that whenever he went to his wardrobe, the clothing appeared to be mouldy, showing the want of the healthful, drying sunshine. He died of consumption.

A third and more frequent and fatal cause of unhealthful chambers is a vitiated air, made so by the room being kept too much closed against incoming pure air, while that already there, being breathed and rebreathed, is more and more contaminated at each act of respiration.

Dr. Nichols, in his "Fireside Science," well says that the crowded, ill-ventilated school-room is often the place where, early in life, rebreathed air commences its deadly work. Not one school-room in a hundred in this country is a fit place in which to confine children six or eight hours of the day. The little ones are herded together in a promiscuous crowd: those of tender years and those more advanced, the feeble and the strong, the sickly and the well, are all subjected to the same hours of study, the same school discipline, and all breathe the same deleterious air. The hardy and the strong may be able to resist the influence of the poison; the weak and tender ones grow pale and haggard, and, struggling on through their school-days, live perhaps to the age of puberty, and then drop into the consumptive's grave. Will parents never awake to the enormity of this evil?

Small, ill-ventilated sleeping-rooms, in which rebreathed air is ever present, are nurseries of consumption. These are not found alone in cities and large towns, or among the poor and lowly. Well-to-do farmers' daughters and sons in the country—those who live among the mountains of the New England States, where God's pure air is wholly undefiled—are often victims of consumption. How is this explained? Look into their bedrooms; examine into their daily habits of life; and the cause is made plain. Old-fashioned fireplaces are boarded up; rubber window strips and stoves have found their way into the most retired nooks and corners of the land; and the imprisoned mountain air in country dwellings is heated to a high point, and breathed over and over during the days and nights of the long winter months. It is certainly true that girls in the country take less exercise in the open air than those residing in cities. They appear to be more *afraid* of pure cold air than city girls. Consumption is not less rare among females in the country than in cities, in the present age. It was not so formerly. The declarations of grandmothers and old physicians go to show that, fifty years ago, consumption was hardly known in the rural districts. The winds whistled through the dwellings then, and the fire blazed and roared upon the hearth. Half the time, in the cold winters, "the backs of the inmates were freezing, while the front parts of the persons were roasting;" and yet there was less rheumatism than now, and no consumption. It is the want of an habitual breathing of pure air, night and day, which is so surely undermining the constitutions of multitudes. The first step towards removing the evil should be in the direction of sleeping in large rooms, in single beds, with open fireplaces, and either wide swinging doors or window sashes arranged to admit outdoor air.

TREATMENT OF TAPE-WORM.

TAKE about forty grammes of gourd seed, or 620 grains, an even ounce and a-half is near enough, peel them, and make into a paste, add thirty grammes each of honey and castor oil, an ounce each is enough, or one tablespoon each; mix these with the seed;

mix well, take it at one dose in a glass of milk. Two hours later take one or two tablespoons each of castor oil and honey, enough to make it operate well on the bowels ; eat nothing until the operation, and then eat moderately, at not less than five hours apart for a day or two. Nothing whatever should be eaten for twelve hours before the gourd seed are taken. Pumpkin-seed tea, strong, a pint of it, fasting for at least twelve hours, and in ten hours more take two tablespoonfuls of castor oil.

SPIRITS OF TURPENTINE

half an ounce, which is a tablespoonful, with two tablespoonfuls of castor oil, take it all at one dose, not having eaten anything for at least twelve hours, and in ten hours two tablespoons of castor oil ; this generally brings it all away.

PINK ROOT

and senna, each half an ounce, half a drachm of jalap, one drachm of bitartrate of potash, let the whole stand for an hour in boiling water ; give one tablespoon every three hours until the worm is expelled, not having eaten anything for twelve hours.

A leisure way of removing tape-worm is to bruise a pound of pumpkin or gourd seed, having taken off the skin, pour on a quart of boiling water, stir it well, and drink half a pint of it every morning before breakfast until a cure has been effected ; if not, take a dose at bedtime also, all the time eating moderately, being out of doors several hours every day, keeping the feet warm, and avoiding chilliness.

The ethereal extract of filix often fails ; in such cases, one or two grains of the oxide of copper, combined with three or four grains of aloes, two or three times a day, brings away masses of mucus loaded with pieces of the worm, and sometimes the whole worm itself. No mischief has ever resulted from taking this remedy.

Oil of turpentine, in doses of one or two tablespoons at a time, will generally bring the worm away. The Egyptians treat it by administering twenty or thirty drops of petroleum, fasting, two or three times a day. The oil of male fern, from one to four teaspoonfuls, fasting, three or four times a day, has been effective.

In Abyssinia, kousso, the flower of the Brayera anthelmintica, half an ounce, mixed with water, before each meal is certain to remove the worm or kill it. Kameela is also a cure; botanists call it Rottlera tinctoria. All medicines for the removal of tape-worm should be given on an empty stomach, thus compelling the worm to take it also, or to imbibe it through its skin.

ANOTHER REMEDY.

Six grains of jalap.
Six grains of extract of colocynth.
Four grains of podophyllin.
Make into nine pills. For one whole day eat nothing but meal gruel, half a pint every four hours. The next morning take three of the pills on an empty stomach, and repeat every three hours, eating nothing that day but a pint of meal gruel before bedtime. Next morning take one ounce, that is two tablespoonfuls, of turpentine, and at noon one or two tablespoons of castor oil. This will very certainly bring the worm away. If not wholly successful, wait a week and repeat the course. The general treatment of tape-worm by homœopathy is to give aconite first, three globules in water, until fever abates, then cina in twelve hours. In twenty-four hours after this last give filix mas, which is mother tincture. Give this in large doses, followed by doses of castor oil or oil of turpentine. One drop of mother tincture in a teaspoonful of water, night and morning.

THE ARMY ITCH,

As it is persistently called, not because it is confined to the army, nor only got by going into the army, but because it is so common among soldiers who have not the means of attending to it promptly. It never gets well of itself, but always gets worse, because of the opportunity, by not being disturbed, which the insect has of multiplying into millions. Infection very certainly follows if a person who has this itch is touched, or clothing handled, or the same bed or berth is slept in; hence the amazing rapidity with which it spreads when it once gets among large companies of men. Sometimes it is so long neglected that the whole blood of a man becomes poisoned, his whole constitution is impaired. This must be rectified in addition to getting clear of the insect itself. To this end dissolve four grains of arseniate of soda in four ounces or eight tablespoons of syrup of sarsaparilla. Dose: one teaspoonful on getting up in the morning and on going to bed at night. In addition, take once a week one dose of purgative pills at bedtime, not taking the other mixture that night nor until the next night.

In addition make an ointment of four drachms of Burgundy pitch, one drachm each of Venetian turpentine, red-lead, and red precipitate, and twelve ounces of fresh butter; the first three articles named should be mixed together and reduced to the finest powder; put the other two in a vessel and melt them slowly, stirring in the powder until all are most thoroughly mixed together, then place it on ice or in a vessel of cold water; stir it until it cools to the consistency of an ointment, a small portion of which must be rubbed into the skin affected, night and morning. The underclothing should be changed at least twice a week. Once a week the whole body should be washed with soap and warm water. The diet should consist of cold bread and butter at meal times, with a cup of hot drink, using coarse bread and fruits and berries; at dinner may take some lean meat and a vegetable, but no other article of food than those mentioned, and then only at meal times. In bad cases, time and patience will be necessary, but a cure permanent and satisfactory is certain if the instructions given are followed and the preparations named are made with care and of good materials.

The sovereign homœopathic remedy for itch is six globules of sulphur in a tablespoonful of water, night and morning, not having eaten anything in four hours; do this for ten days, omit a week, then go on as before, continuing thus until cured, using sulphur as a lotion or ointment externally, at the same time. A lotion is made by adding six drops of the saturated alcoholic tincture of sulphur to two tablespoonfuls of water, and apply night and morning with a soft rag.

If cases have been of long standing take a good hot bath daily and a good scrubbing with a coarse cloth dipped in strong soapsuds, with the following diet, employed when it is desired to adopt an

ERADICATIVE TREATMENT.

Diet.—Which should be nourishing, light, and easy of digestion, taken regularly in moderate quantities; equal proportions of animal food with vegetables—roast beef and mutton are much preferred, soft-boiled eggs, stale home-made bread; only one beverage, universally safe, water. Stimulants and ferments are to be strictly avoided.

Air.—Dry, cool, in elevated situations, no bleak winds, as little time in-doors, as much out as possible, never, however, to a fatiguing extent. Exercise should be free and unrestrained, particularly avoiding any check to the perspiration; never remain still or uncovered for a moment while out of doors. If weather prevents, then exercise in-doors in any and every way calculated to circulate the blood, enliven the spirits, and engage pleasurable attention.

Water.—Take a cool bath every day; if not practicable, give the whole body a good scrubbing every morning with a coarse cloth dipped in cold water. Let this be done vigorously and rapidly, within five minutes.

Cleanliness.—The most perfect, perpetual, and universal, extending to person, to clothing, to bed, to chamber, to home, to premises, to everything. To a homœopathist filth in every form is an abomination not to be tolerated a moment. It is the low, the vulgar, the ill-bred, who have filthy habits, which keep them degraded.

Habits regular—in everything regular as a clock, if possible—in eating, drinking, sleeping, exercise, recreation, work. Method should be infused into everything. From this it will be seen that in the three " pathies,"

Allopathy,

Homœopathy,

Hydropathy, the same general hygienic principles are advocated.

STIMULANTS IN SICKNESS.

THAT there may be no doubt left on the mind in reference to the injurious effects of alcohol in disease, referred to in another part of this book, an official report is here given, published as long ago as 1865, in the *British Medical Journal*:—

Some remarkable statistics regarding the employment of stimulants, and the mortality in the London Hospital during some years past, appear in the last volume of the *Reports* of that hospital. In 1862, the number of in-patients was 4,519, and the general mortality 7.6 per cent. The quantity of stimulants consumed was 1,281 gallons of wine, 162 gallons of brandy, 38 gallons of gin, and 1,100 ounces of cinchonine.

In 1864, the number of patients was 4,619, and the general mortality 10.5 per cent.; the stimulants consumed by these being 1,558 gallons of wine, 359 gallons of brandy, and 77 gallons of gin. But as a set-off, if it may so be called, 760 more leeches were employed during this year than the average for the five preceding years, viz. 3,840. However, here we have a great increase in the amount of stimulants consumed, and also a great increase in the mortality of 1864 as compared with that of 1862. We state the facts, let it be understood, without in any way pretending to connect them as cause and effect.

Other statistics Dr. Frazer gives us under this head:—" From 1854 to 1858 the annual average quantity of wine employed by each physician was 12,803 ounces;" each physician having an annual average of 391 patients under treatment. The annual average mortality was 11.87 per cent. But from 1860 to 1864, the annual average quantity of wine employed by each physician was nearly quadrupled, being 48,136 ounces; his annual average number of patients was 413; and the annual average mortality was 12.65 per cent.

From 1854 to 1858, each surgeon employed annually 38,016 ounces of wine; his annual number of patients was 1,036; and the annual average mortality 4.48 per cent.

From 1860 to 1864 (five years) each surgeon employed an annual average of 142,951 ounces of wine (nearly four times more than in the previous years); the annual number of patients under him was 1,065; and the annual average mortality 6.65 per cent.

Hence we have, in the practice of both physicians and surgeons, a distinct increase of mortality coincident with great increase in consumption of stimulants.

Dr. Fraser also tells us (referring to a former paper of his) that in 1851 there were 4,051 in-patients in the London Hospital;

that in 1857 there were 3,935 in-patients; and that the mortality was greater in 1857 as 8 to 6.5 per cent., although £962 more were spent in 1857 than in 1851 for articles of luxury.

It is curious to note that the only comment which Dr. Fraser makes on the above remarkable statistics is this:—

" It is evident that a steady rise in the employment of stimulants . . . is still going on; and whatever be the cause, we may rest assured that the practice is imperative and needful; for it would be a monstrous assumption that a whole staff could be blindly following an objectless routine."

Not a single word of comment does Dr. Fraser bestow on the constant fact of the coincident increase of the mortality !

The summary of these statistics stands thus:—

From 1854 to 1858 each physician employed 12,800 ounces of wine annually; the deaths being 11.87 per cent. From 1860 to 1865 he employed 48,136 ounces; the deaths being 12.65 per cent.

During 1854 to 1858 each surgeon employed annually 38,016 ounces of wine; the deaths being 4.48 per cent. During 1860 to 1864 he employed annually 142,951 ounces; the deaths being 6.65 per cent.

In 1862 the general mortality of the hospital was 7.6 per cent.; the consumption of stimulants being 1,281 gallons of wine, 162 of brandy, and 38 of gin.

In 1864 the mortality was 10.5 per cent.; the quantity of stimulants consumed being 1,558 gallons of wine, 359 of brandy, and 77 of gin.

To these statements nothing need be added.

ABSORPTION

Is to draw up, to suck up, as a sponge sucks up water, or as a lump of sugar or salt draws up into itself any liquid with which it comes in contact. Applied to the human body, it means that process by which various things may be introduced into the blood, as water through the skin, or as the poison of a viper is drawn up into the circulation from the point bitten.

Sometimes when persons could not swallow, nutriment seems to have been conveyed by means of passing soup or other nutrient materials into the bowels by injection.

ABSTINENCE

Is usually applied to a voluntary restraining one's self from taking food, as in ordinary fasting as a religious observance, or compulsory as in shipwreck, or from fanaticism. The course to be pursued in all cases is the same; the stomach is weak in proportion to other parts of the body, and almost as incapable of action; hence give but a very little food at a time, and at short intervals, proportioned to the duration of the abstinence, if over three or four days. If there is sickness at stomach give five drops of morphia and ten drops of camphor water in a tablespoon of water; then give two or three tablespoons of soup or milk, thickened with bread, every half hour, for two or three times, and then every hour, and if no discomfort is experienced the feeding may be more liberal, but at longer intervals; if these articles are not hot a sip or two of hot tea is a great relief; it warms the body within and wakes up the circulation.

Sometimes persons become fanatical, believing that all eat too much; that the less is eaten the better, and carrying this out in practice, the stomach becomes so debilitated that it cannot work at all, even if food is given it at the last hour, and the person dies as certainly as if compulsorily starved.

MEASLES

Is a disease of childhood, but occasionally attacks grown persons. The older a person is who has an attack of measles, the more likely is he to suffer permanent ill effects. Many have consumption in its most incurable form, from an attack of measles after childhood, they not having come out well, or having "struck in," to use a common expression, that is, disappeared suddenly, which is often occasioned by draughts of air, chilliness, or loose bowels, whether by medicine or by other causes.

This is a disease which runs its course, and seldom attacks a person more than once. The sooner children have it the better, for there is less suffering and less danger of troublesome "sequelæ," as physicians term it, meaning, less ill effects are left on the constitution.

After having really taken the measles, it is ten or fifteen days before the disease manifests itself by a depression of spirits, fever, running at the nose as if a cold had been taken; there is a slight cough, and red and watery eyes. The rash appears on the fourth day on the face, spreading all over the body, not so bright as in scarlet fever; on the seventh day it begins to fade, with fading fever, and the scaling off of the skin.

If the disease is not properly attended to it is followed by various maladies, as sore eyes, diphtheria, bronchitis, and consumption; the chief things to be attended to are to keep the bowels acting not more than once a day, either by enemas or a teaspoonful or two of salts or castor oil night and morning; take more or less, so as to have but one movement in the twenty-four hours. Take thrice a day some cracked wheat or boiled rice, with fruits, berries, bread and butter, sago, tapioca; keep comfortably warm; never by any possibility allow a feeling of chilliness, nor a draught of air; the room ought to be well ventilated; the most favorable circumstances for measles are a cool, well-ventilated room and to keep warm in bed; for a chill or draught will strike the measles in, with liability to all the bad results named.

If the phlegm is tight, shown by a cough, or tightness in the chest, take a teaspoonful of syrup of ipecac or some compound syrup of squills, not enough to vomit, but merely to loosen the phlegm; but it is better to do without these things, as they tend to take away the appetite and make tonics necessary during the convalescence.

Great harm results in numberless cases from impatience to get out of doors; after the rash has disappeared it is better to avoid leaving the house for at least a week.

Measles is a contagious disease; nothing is gained by trying to avoid it, for the sooner it takes place the better and safer for the patient.

Flax-seed tea is good to allay the cough. The feet and hands may be bathed two or three times a day if they burn. Tepid water applied to the body once or twice a day cools it off. Drink tea plentifully while in bed to promote perspiration, but avoid cooling off afterwards too soon, or it will strike in the measles. Sometimes lemonade makes a cooling and pleasant drink. Take no cold drinks whatever.

Measles present the appearance of a patchy redness of a circular form, and the pimples made by the internal and external application of the skin have a feeling of a number of little hard points. Scarlet fever is also red, but it has a smooth feel in the skin, and the redness is suffused like a blush.

When the rash is fully out, the skin is as red as a raspberry.

If the eruption strikes in, recall the rash at once by a hot mustard bath; keep the feet warm by all means when in bed, with bottles of hot water under the arms, until the rash reappears, drinking hot teas meanwhile, so as, if possible, to bring on perspiration. If the breaking out delays, keep warm in bed and give good doses of hive syrup, and drink warm teas abundantly, and keep the bowels open. If at any time there is a fixed pain in the chest following measles, keep it away by mustard plasters, applied and reapplied, with such other things as are done in pneumonia.

There is a disease called

FALSE MEASLES,

something between common measles and scarlet fever, it is to be treated on the same general principles.

Saffron tea was given by our grandmothers to " bring out " the measles, and if it was followed by an increased redness it was considered favorable; it was truly a good sign, but it was not the saffron principle; it was the heat in the liquid, which, throwing the blood to the surface, carried with it its impurities through the pores of the skin.

Late discoveries seem to point to the fact that measles and scarlet fever are the product of the same living insect, or at least that insect is present in both maladies, as if they were one and the same (which article see).

In all cases keep the patient quiet, composed; avoid the excitement of company, and keep the feet and body warm all the time; this is of great importance, so as to prevent striking in.

The homœopathic practice is to give aconite and pulsatilla, which, separate or together, are considered infallible. Ipecac is given when there is oppressed breathing before the eruption appears; euphrasia, when there is severe headache; coffee, when there is a dry cough, or hep. sulph. Nux vomica is given to dark-complexioned persons when there is a dry cough. If the eruption is inclined to go in, give bryonia at once; pulsatilla, if there is looseness of bowels. If the brain is affected, give belladonna or stramonium. If the lungs seem to be affected, give phosphorus or sulphur. The diet should be as in other eruptive diseases.

SCARLET FEVER.

Is a blushy or brick-dust redness of the skin, with a smooth feel to the fingers. In about five days after exposure—for it is a contagious disease—the appetite fails, with pains in the limbs, sore throat, often very sore; this is the dangerous part; the redness appears on the face and neck, and in ten or twelve hours it is all over the body; there is some swelling and great heat, reaching to 106° Fahrenheit. The skin burns, and sometimes feels sore. There is a strawberry look to the tongue, little points coming up through its coating. The pulse is very high, intense thirst, constipation, vomiting, headache, and stupor in bad cases; there is an abatement the fifth day of the attack, and by the ninth it is pretty well over; the skin begins to clear, sometimes quite large pieces peel off. If there is great depression, some chilliness, stupor, with a livid appearance of the rash, as if it was going in, there is great danger.

In scarlet fever the rash comes out on the second day; in measles, the fourth. In scarlet fever there is sore throat, none in measles.

In scarlet fever the patient seems to have no cold, but does have symptoms of it in measles.

Scarlet fever has a brighter red, and is diffused; in measles the redness is in patches.

As dangerous as scarlet fever is, no treatment is needed in mild cases; the same course is to be pursued as in measles, but in addition, if there is not free urination, drink freely of flax-seed tea or lemonade; if the throat is much inflamed, swallow little lumps of ice all the time until relieved.

Gargle the throat with red pepper, vinegar, and water.

If there is bad breath, make a mixture of equal parts of muriatic acid and honey, dilute it so as to be used as a gargle, or twenty grains of sulphate of zinc in an ounce of water as a gargle.

The great points to be labored for in scarlet fever are:

First. Keep the bowels free by a free use of fruits, berries, and cracked wheat.

Second. Keep out the rash by the prevention of chilliness and looseness of bowels.

Third. Keep down thirst and fever by acid drinks, lemonade, buttermilk, etc.

Fourth. Keep the room cool and well ventilated.

Fifth. If there is a tendency to debility, add some meat, poultry, and soups, with bread crust, to the diet.

Sixth. In great heat of the skin, sponge it freely and often with tepid water.

Homœopathy gives belladonna as soon as any dryness or burning is noticed in the mouth and throat, and there is a desire to drink, but no ability. Give mercurius in six hours after the second dose of belladonna; and six hours later, arsenicum, if there is great prostration and the ulcers emit an offensive odor. If arsenicum does not restore reaction, then give nux vomica. If inflammation, give aconite, followed by belladonna, if the pulse falls and fever abates. If the skin burns and there is drowsiness and stupor, give opium. If convulsions are present and are not relieved by opium, give zincum. If the eruption is intense, give sulphur.

A favorite treatment of scarlet fever in England is to immerse the patient in a warm bath in the early stage of the disease, and this is repeated frequently, or as often as the strength of the patient will allow. The first effect is to produce a soothing and refreshing feeling in the patient, to be followed soon by such an

28

eruption on the surface, of so vivid a color, and in such amount as would astonish those who have never witnessed it. Thus one of the greatest dangers of this fearful disease—the suppression of the eruption—is escaped.

The appetite generally returns after the first or second bath, and the strength of the patient is kept up by nutritious food. The bath prevents the dissemination of the disease, by removing the excreta from the skin as soon as it is deposited. This treatment promotes cuticular desquamation. The body should be gently dried by soft linen cloths after the bath.

By this procedure the various secretions are deprived of their noxious properties, and the irritation of internal organs is quickly relieved, thus dissipating infection. Another benefit is, that a very serious case is soon reduced to a mild one, and the patient recovers in less than half the usual time.

An eminent London practitioner claims that in fifteen years' practice, the adoption of this treatment has not failed to cure scarlet fever in a single instance.

AMMONIA

WAS first made from the soot of burning camel's dung near the Temple of Ammon or Jupiter Ammon, whose representation was in the form of a ram, strong smelling; it consists of three parts hydrogen and one part nitrogen. It is found in largest quantities for commercial purposes in a liquid product of coal in the process of obtaining the gas from it for illuminating purposes; by mixing carbonic acid with this liquid, ammonia is produced; this liquid boils, becomes gaseous at thirty-eight degrees, and freezes, becomes solid, at seventy-five; hence if not corked well it evaporates, leaving nothing but a scentless water, or if in a solid form, disappears entirely.

AMMONIA

in a solid form is called smelling-salts; if liquid, it is hartshorn, because if the horn of a hart or deer is reduced to fine shavings and soaked in warm water and distilled, it produces an impure kind of ammonia; this ammonia is composed of nitrogen and hydrogen. Aqua ammonia is the watery preparation, and tincture of ammonia is an alcoholic solution, and is called spirits of hartshorn. Hartshorn is often applied to the nostrils of persons in an insensible condition, "to bring them to." It should be applied with care, if applied at all, as it has caused violent and even fatal inflammations of the breathing organs. If a person has his senses, there is no danger in breathing it, because if too strong for him he instinctively withdraws from it.

If taken by mistake, it acts as a corrosive poison to the throat and stomach, when vinegar or lemon-juice should be swallowed instantly, as the latter is an acid, the former an alkali, and they antagonize each other like cold and hot water mixed.

A half-pint bottle of aqua ammonia, and also of the spirits of hartshorn, should be kept in every household, well stoppered with a tight cork or ground-glass stopper. Aqua ammonia, eight or ten drops in a tablespoon or two of water, often relieves belchings, eructations, wind in the bowels, heart-burn, sometimes called acidity of stomach; all these meaning indigestion, that is, the food in the stomach, whatever it may be, is not digested, is not acted upon naturally by the juices of the stomach, for either they are not strong enough, or the quantity of food is too great for them; so the food sours, ferments, rots, and being sour, the ammonia, being the very opposite of sour, causes it to disappear, arrests the fermentation.

About ten drops of this aqua ammonia in a pint of warm water, about every five days, greatly revives and invigorates house-plants and flowers. All rain-water contains ammonia; and it is that ingredient which so freshens and revives them, the ammonia acting as a nutriment or food.

All observant farmers know that the deeper and longer the snows of winter, the richer will be the crops of summer. This is because snow is frozen rain, and has all its ammonia; guano, the richest manure of the world, is thus rich because of the great quantity of ammonia it contains; and this, too, is the reason why barnyard manure enriches the soil upon which it is spread.

The substance which causes the poisonous effects following the bites of insects, serpents, and animals is acid; hartshorn is the strongest alkali, hence an instantaneous cure of these bites is often effected by dipping a soft rag in hartshorn and applying it to the spot, constantly renewing it. This spirits of hartshorn acts beneficially in another way : it evaporates rapidly, hence carries off the heat, the inflammation of the part, cools it, and thus gives grateful and instant relief. Persons whose monthly turns are difficult or painful, have had a grateful relief afforded them by sitting over a chamber in which has been placed half a table-spoon of spirits of hartshorn. Sometimes the pain disappears in a minute, not returning until the next time, when it is as efficient as at first. Those who have ill-smelling feet, or have odors aris-ing from their persons, often antagonize it completely by wash-ing their feet and their armpits with a mixture of a tablespoon of spirits of hartshorn in half a pint of warm water, a tablespoon of the mixture to each foot, especially between the toes, and a table-spoon under each arm every night. If used in the morning, it may impart a disagreeable odor to the clothing during the day. A tablespoon of spirits of hartshorn to a pint of warm water makes the best

HAIR WASH

in the world, because the alkali of the hartshorn unites with the grease or oil on the scalp ; the hair is naturally oily, and makes a soap which, if rubbed into the roots of the hair, cleans the scalp perfectly, uncovers every pore obstructed by dandruff and dust; and nothing known so much promotes the health of the hair and its healthy growth as the cleanliness of the scalp, and nothing can do any good to the hair, towards promoting its growth or res-toration, except in proportion as it cleans the scalp, and in addi-tion stimulates the circulation of the blood about the roots of each hair; this the hartshorn does. We know it does so by its reddening the skin if it is rubbed briskly upon it. This reddening means that there is an increased flow of blood to the part; and what it does on the skin of the body it will do on the skin of the head. Rinse the hair well with cold water afterwards. Hartshorn water makes a very cleanly wash for the whole body, by uncovering every pore of the oily matter mixed with dust which clogs it, and gives a delightful feeling of coolness and freshness of a summer's day, when the whole atmosphere is hot and sultry and lifeless.

WASHING PAINT

is best done by dipping a soft flannel in a mixture of one table-spoon of spirits or water of hartshorn in a quart of warm water; simply wash off the wood work—no scrubbing is necessary; if the mixture is strong enough of hartshorn, it takes off all grease-marks easily.

If you want to remove grease-spots from any delicate fabric which will not bear washing with soap, dip a piece of white blot-ting-paper in strong spirits of hartshorn, lay it over the spot, and iron it lightly.

If you want to

WASH LACES

nicely, put twelve drops of spirits of hartshorn in warm soapsuds.

TO CLEAN SILVER,

nothing is better, easier, or more convenient than a wash made of two teaspoonfuls of spirits of hartshorn in a quart of hot soap-suds; put the articles in the water, and use any kind of old nail or tooth brush.

HAIR BRUSHES

are easily cleaned in the same mixture, rinsing them in cold water afterwards, and putting them out to dry in the open air or hot sun.

It is an excellent thing, also, to wash off finger-marks from gilt frames, and other places—a few drops of hartshorn on a moist rag; rub it quickly and lightly.

Sometimes blue and black fabrics are stained red by strong acids having fallen on them; hartshorn will remove these red stains.

FADED WRITINGS.

Dampen a piece of soft white paper, lay it on the faded writing, press it down closely; put a tablespoon of spirits of hartshorn in a tin vessel, with a candle or lamp under it; hold the soft damp paper over it, so as to receive the fumes of the hartshorn; if the writing is not exhibited on the soft paper plain enough, dampen it again, and repeat the whole process until it is plain enough. Sometimes a physician's prescription may become faded by water or other fluid, and it may be a matter of life and death to have it renewed or made legible. It adds greatly to the comfort and convenience of human life in many ways, and at various times, to know all the uses to which what we have at hand may be applied. Hence the statement of several uses of hartshorn, which have no immediate connection with health or medicine; and the same course will be pursued in reference to other articles possessing a medicinal effect, but which may be applied to other and important purposes.

BRONCHITIS

Is a cold settling on the branches of the windpipe, which are called bronchia, hence the name; the word "itis" being added, which means "inflammation," whenever it ends a word. Bronchitis is acute or chronic: acute, when it lasts a few days or weeks; chronic, when it lasts for years or a lifetime. The acute form comes with a chill, then fever; the eyes and nose water, there is a binding, a cord-like feeling across the breast, more distinct when there is an attempt to draw a long breath. There is a harsh, dry cough, which fails to loosen the phlegm which plugs up the bronchial tubes and keeps the air from passing in and out freely, hence the shortness of breath and the tightness. Go to bed; have hot bricks or bottles to the feet; put a mustard plaster, a large one, all over the chest; take a liver pill or four purgative pills; keep warm in bed, get into a perspiration, and you will be relieved in half an hour, the more decidedly so when the pill begins to take hold, in about two hours; when it operates, you will feel like a new man, if you don't renew your cold or check the perspiration suddenly. Do not be in a hurry to get out of doors; live for a few days on bread and butter, and fruits or berries at each meal; nothing else but a little lean meat for dinner added.

CHRONIC BRONCHITIS.

The principal feature is a hard, dry cough, mainly in the morning on getting up and stirring around in dressing, with spells of same kind of cough during the day; seldom troubled with cough during the night, because the body is kept warm in bed. After coughing a while the phlegm begins to loosen, and the cough subsides. Some do all their coughing in the morning, and, for the remainder of the day, are pretty well. The morning cough is so violent in some persons, lasting for an hour or more, that a looker-on would think they were in the last stages of consumption, and yet, twenty years later, they are still coughing. It is wholly different in its nature from consumption; it seldom ends in consumption. As a general rule, not much can be done for it in the way of cure; it can be kept down, can be modified very much by a fruit and coarse bread diet, dressing warm all the time, keeping the feet comfortable, avoid taking colds, and having the bowels to act very freely and fully every day, by any and every means. A chill, a cold, even a slight one, biliousness and costiveness, always aggravate the ailment, hence they should be constantly guarded against. The chest should be well protected, especially from November to June, by wearing a buckskin jacket during the daytime over the flannel shirt. It should come half-way down the arms. The whole neck and scalp of a man, and arms and armpits, should be well washed in cold water every morning throughout the year, keeping the feet always warm, so as to draw the excess of blood from the lungs. Great injury is done by following the advice of ignorant persons to take various preparations, keeping the stomach gorged with medicines, interfering with digestion, debilitating the body, most of them aggravating the malady in the future by affording temporary relief. Every medicine in the world sold for a cough does an injury in bronchitis, because it contains opium.

It may be convenient or necessary sometimes to aid in loosening the phlegm; in such cases take as little medicine as possible, and that the least bulky. Avoid cough remedies with sweets in them; they soon cloy the stomach and impair the digestion. Coxe's hive syrup, called the compound syrup of squills, is always more or less efficient in loosening the phlegm; about half a teaspoonful at a time, more or less, so as not to induce gagging or vomiting. Anything which has a nauseating effect brings relief. Perhaps the simplest and least objectionable remedy is

TINCTURE OF IPECAC.

Put a teaspoonful of powdered ipecac root in a vial, pour upon it two tablespoonfuls of any kind of spirits, shake it well daily for several days; it can be used in ten minutes after the first shaking; let it settle, and take from ten to twenty or more drops on a lump of loaf sugar, or in a little water, or as it is; take enough to cause some nausea. None of these nauseants should be taken within two hours after eating a meal, for they may cause vomiting.

This tincture of ipecac should be kept well stoppered; it is the safest, simplest, and best remedy ever known for a troublesome, dry, hacking cough of any kind; it has no after ill-effects, is of little bulk, can be carried in the vest-pocket, and may be always relied upon to loosen phlegm, if there is any phlegm to loosen, and anything can loosen it. In the author's book on bronchitis and kindred diseases, the nature of the ailment, and how to distinguish it certainly from consumption, is more fully stated.

Let it be remembered that keeping chronic bronchitis under control, and eradicating it from the system, is greatly expedited under any form of treatment in proportion to the greater number of hours spent in out-door activities, with abundant bodily warmth all the time, with fruit and coarse bread diet, lean meat, and one vegetable once a day, and a full, free action of the bowels every twenty-four hours. This course cures of itself often.

A disagreeable remedy, yet one of the best known to control morning cough, to loosen it, and to prevent a good deal of distress in aggravated chronic bronchitis, is thus prepared:

One thousand grains of gum ammoniac, an exudation from a tree growing in Persia and Hindostan; one hundred grains of sulphate of copper, known as blue vitriol; and twenty-four ounces of water, which is a pint and a half, or forty-eight tablespoonfuls. A dose is one drachm, or one teaspoonful, containing half a grain of sulphate of copper and five grains of the gum. Take one teaspoon or more on first getting up in the morning, about an hour before breakfast, so as to cause free vomiting. The relief is such, that persons troubled greatly with night and morning cough, have voluntarily taken it at bed-time, not having eaten or drank anything within five hours. The author merely states the facts coming under his own observation, leaving the reader who is troubled with a

BRONCHIAL COUGH

which is really distressing, to decide for himself whether he will try the experiment on himself or not.

Under the daily use of this seemingly disagreeable remedy, the author has known his patients to begin to gain flesh within a week, to improve the appetite, to invigorate the digestion, and to increase in flesh and strength, and to recover from coughs which seemed to indicate that the person was in the advanced stages of consumption. It is worthy of a fair, persistent trial.

PORES OF THE SKIN.

IF all the skin of a man was stretched out against the side of a house, it would cover about thirty square feet; this skin is filled with pores or openings, through which the perspiration is constantly escaping, carrying with it several ounces of waste, useless, and poisonous matter every day, depositing it outside the body. There are about twenty-five hundred pores in each square inch, or five millions in all; they are of different sizes, the largest are in the soles of the feet. This shows how important it is for the skin of the body to be kept scrupulously clean, so as to give the freest exit to those particles, which if retained only poison the blood. In fever all the pores are closed, and there is no health, no appetite, no comfort.

More especially ought the feet to be kept clean, the soles of the feet; the pores there are almost sluices; the soles should be kept as clean as the face, should be dipped in water every morning for an instant, and then wiped smartly, rapidly, and hard. If they are not thus wiped, the foul matters which they would have carried outside the body are reabsorbed, and thus are a double source of poisoning the blood; and yet very many people do not wash their feet oftener than once a week. It is a very great mistake.

If these little pores were joined end and end, they would make a tube twenty-five miles long.

It is said that in China men will sometimes replaster a small sleeping-room for nothing, feeling themselves paid by scraping from the walls, as manure, the dried breath of the sleepers in the course of years. Through the five million pores in the skin of an ordinary adult, there passes out in common life about one pint of liquid matter, of which one ounce is a solid substance, made up of waste, useless, and poisonous particles, which if kept in the system a few hours would cause death; hence the wisdom of keeping these pores open by cleaning off from the skin every particle of dust and dirt and oil. But in addition to this pint of liquid and ounce of more solid matter, there is a large amount of carbonic acid gas escaping from these pores, a gas so deadly that one full breath of it would fell a man to the earth as instantaneously as would a thunderbolt; no wonder, then, that personal cleanliness is such an important element in the preservation of health. Cover up every one of these five million pores, death would follow within five hours. By all means let every reader have so much respect for himself as to make it a point to keep the whole surface of the body strictly clean, not merely the face and the hands, but the soles of the feet, under the arms, in the groin, behind the knees, as well as the general surface, for purity of mind comes with purity of body, as well as personal elevation; for the world over, dirt degrades the mind, corrupts the morals, and destroys the body. The proverb taken from the Hebrew Talmud is true: "cleanliness into godliness;" meaning thereby, that cleanliness leads into a godly state, naturally.

The feet of some persons have such an odor, that it scents a room when they enter it. Ill-smelling feet is inherited or constitutional with some, in others it is acquired, but in both cases it may be overcome by washing the feet every morning or evening, wiping them well, and then rub over them a little of the mixture made by adding a teaspoonful of spirits of hartshorn to half a pint of water.

INTERESTED EXERCISE.

A VERY great obstacle to the improvement of the health, as well as maintaining it, is found in the failure to take that daily amount of out-door exercise which is absolutely essential to those who are most of the time in-doors, including wives and daughters, and those men in towns and cities who have no special occupation, or who are recovering from sickness.

Exercise, to be highly beneficial, should be of a character which interests the mind—which is more or less exciting, and agreeably calls out both the physical and mental activities. An objectless walk does very little good, nor is a listless ride in a carriage calculated to benefit any one. This principle ought to be taken into consideration. Exercise is advised as a means of promoting the health. There are multitudes of cases where medicine is utterly unavailing; where the system is brought to that condition when it must be let alone, to recuperate by its own natural' powers; in many such cases judicious exercise is invaluable, but to be effectual there must be a motive ahead, something sufficiently absorbing to bear the mind away from the consciousness of bodily ill.

Persons are often without a motive to go outside the door, because they do not know what might be seen in an hour's walk or ride. To give a case in point of which advantage may well be taken by any New Yorker whose eye may chance to fall on this page, or by any person in the country who may have occasion to come to the city: starting out some sunny morning from any point between the Battery and Harlem River, there are routes to be taken for almost every day in the year, even by an old New Yorker, which might be found full of novelty, interest, and instruction, especially with a cheery companion or a guest in the family, to say nothing of the health-giving influences which would be necessarily experienced.

Suppose it is a summer morning; have an early breakfast; be ready to leave your door at 6 o'clock; enter a South Ferry stage, which will take you to a Staten Island boat, giving you an hour's ride down the bay, and bringing you in sight of the ocean, to breathe the salt sea air in all its freshness. Stop at Vanderbilt's Landing, take the cars for the interior of the Island, and in a run of a dozen miles there will be found a variety of scenery, of forest and garden, of hill and plain, of cabins and country-seats, which will be perfectly charming in its contrast with the unvarying brick and mortar of the city. Order a dinner at any of the good stopping-places found in every direction, with fruits, native and tropical, berries and melons and ice-cream, in all their abundance and lusciousness ; then, an hour's saunter through the woods and by the sea, returning by cars to the boat, thence up the bay in the cool of the day, a while before sundown, steaming through whole fleets of ships and barges and floating hotels, those mammoth constructions, which will house and feed a thousand people ; some going out, some coming in ; the departing expecting no return for months or years ; those coming home after long absences in foreign lands, so full of joyous expectation of seeing familiar faces and friends and kindred waiting on the shore to give them a glad welcome ; with sights and associations like these, to fill the mind and wake up its activities, you seek your home, tired it may be, but the delicious sleep which will follow, the renovation of the blood which has been occasioned, and the waked-up appetite for the next day, with all the accompanying feelings of wellness and vigor, what a pity is it, that there are literally thousands in New York City, who, until this reading, have never imagined such a trip for a dollar was possible.

Or take an early breakfast and boat up the Hudson to Cornwall Landing, to arrive at noon ; make your way to the "Mountain House," with an appetite which you have not had in a year ; take a leisure walk after dinner to the brow of the Storm King, and see a panorama before you which travelled men and women declare is not surpassed in beauty and magnificence in all their journeyings in the world ; that Switzerland has nothing equal to it ; where the air is as pure as that from the poles, and the breezes as sweet as those which come from Araby the blest. Remain over night, to gaze upon the scene at sunset, by moonlight, and in the early morning, and impressions of loveliness will be left on the mind which time will not efface. Returning to New York next day, there will be renovation, a "making over" of body and mind, perfectly delightful to think of. Just think of it : a trip to the bay of Naples, or what is more beautiful ; and a trip to Switzerland, or what surpasses, to be had in a day from New York !

For another day take the Central Park. A few cents will

carry you to its gates by the Eighth, Sixth, or Fourth avenue cars, starting from near the Astor House. At one of these gates will be found vehicles in waiting, which, for a quarter of a dollar, will carry you through winding ways and gardens of flowers, by lake and waterfall, along terraces and through tunnels, for miles and miles together, and will, in an hour or two, set you down in safety at the place you started from. But a better plan would be to take a leisure walk of half a day, if you please, which will give you an opportunity of seeing places far more beautiful than a ride will afford ; and when you have been delighted with the graceful swans of the lakes, have sat and contemplated in summer for hours on the shores of the lake, have been floated in gondolas over the smooth bosom of the sparkling water, and have ordered a dinner at the Casino which would tempt a king, then visit the Menagerie, to

See the monkeys dance.

And instruct yourself as to the habits of those bears and lions of which you read in ancient days,

Who so delight
To growl and fight.

Then do not fail to visit the Museum of Natural History, where you will see the most instructive and interesting exhibition in all departments to be found anywhere on this continent—enough itself for a whole day's delight. At the Arsenal, near by, are to be seen the elephant, the rhinoceros, the seal, the alligator, and foxes and wolves and birds and fishes so beautiful and full of life as they skim along on the bosom of the liquid lake. Besides these, you wander through the long halls one after another, and up stairs and down with their magnificent variety of minerals and insects, so delicate, so rare, so beautiful and so numerous, collected by various hands, from clown to emperor, getting new views, and wider and more comprehensive, of the universe of things than you ever had before.

Another day, drop yourself down at the corner of Broadway and Tenth street, where Brady's Gallery, free to all, displays its unrivalled beauties in photographic art, and gaze by the hour in wonder and delight at the life-like presentations of the men of our time, of accomplished women, of distinguished singers, of nameless girls in all their coyishness and childhood and infancy, so sweet, so pure, carrying you back in delighted reminiscence to other and earlier days of your own, departed now, never to return.

Then pass across the street to that magnificent structure with its more wonderful containings, of the costliest fabrics of all climes and countries, with their crowds of busy admirers and the thousand deferential and courteous attendants, ready at a word and without a murmur to make their rich displays, so tempting to purse and pride and prudence. Taking nothing with you but the boast, if you are not a New Yorker, that you have been to

STEWART'S STORE.

You cross a street in the rear, and one block to your right, brings you face to face with a world's wonder of Christian beneficence, the

BIBLE HOUSE,

covering a whole square of ground, looming up toward the sky in seven or eight stories, in the lowest of which you may chance to see unwieldy wagons delivering their tons of paper, which forthwith begin to rise through story after story, and when it reaches the topmost height it begins to descend stair by stair, until it comes to earth again; but with the change, it went up a bald blank sheet, now it is the

BLESSED BIBLE,

in cheap or costly form, from a few cents to fifty dollars a volume, to be sent away to the ends of the earth to "show to men benighted" the way to immortality and eternal life, where the toils of the present are ended, its sorrows and its tears all cease, forever and forever. And just across one street there stands a stately pile of dark-brown stone. Seventy years agone a poor little boy, working for twenty-five dollars a year, was wishing one day he had some books to read; he wished too that he could go to school; he wished other little boys could go to school, and read books too. "I would like to give them books, and teachers to show how to use them. Wouldn't I be glad one of these days to do it." He worked on for that poor pitiful sum of twenty-five dollars a year, never faltering, never idle; after ten years he was "better off;" after twenty he had money ahead; in half a century he said to a man, with a whole armful of drawings stretched out on the broad table, "Here are six hundred thousand dollars; build that house; let there be rooms in it where 'poor little boys like me,'" and he went back fifty years in his mind, thinking for the instant that there had been no change in him, "can have books to read and teachers to teach, all for nothing; and away down under the earth, away from all noise and bustle and confusion, let there be an assembly room to hold two thousand people, who can hear lectures, and listen to music, and have sermons preached to them about the great future, and towards the top another spacious apartment, light and cheerful and airy, with newspapers from all parts of the world, and pictorials and magazines and useful books, to be visited by any of woman born, for all time, black or white, old or young, male or female, to remain an hour, or all day, from year's end to year's end, to be cool and quiet in summer; in winter cozy and warm, with brilliant lights to read the tiniest print, until away on in the night, when it is time for bed. And then there must be other rooms for painting and for design, and for instruction in all arts and sciences, all for nothing for 'poor little boys like me.'" And when you have gone up and down and through, and looked at it all, and thought it all over, carried away with admiration at what has been done by

PETER COOPER,

turn it all over in your mind, and decide for yourself what you can do, what you ought to do for poor little boys and girls in your neighborhood to help them to help themselves to be something in the world, while they are in it, and to be above the angels afterwards.

Now you can go one block back to Lafayette Place, a short street parallel with Broadway, and not a hundred yards from it. If it is not earlier than ten o'clock in the morning, nor later than sundown, you can enter an imposing structure built by the munificence of a poor little Dutch boy, with a

PACK ON HIS BACK,

a pack of "wild varmint" skins, to be sold to somebody. A purchaser came who was glad to give his money for them; the little boy knew where he could get more, and he set his traps for them and got others to set traps for them, until there was a line of traps across the Continent to the great Pacific Sea, ending at Astoria, in Oregon; and dollars came tumbling in until they amounted to many millions, and out of these was built the

ASTOR LIBRARY,

with its scores of thousands of the rarest and best and costliest books in the world. You can go there and read any of them all day, from ten till sunset, any day in the year and all days in the year, or you can copy them or study over them and make other books out of them without let or hindrance. Everything so clean and nice and comfortable and cozy, and so respectable too and quiet; a perfect elysium to one who has time and leisure and taste to avail himself of treasures so unspeakable in value.

If you are not tired, go two blocks westward to Second avenue, and you will be near Eleventh street, where is the building of the Historical Society. It is not open to everybody, yet a ticket of admission can be had for the asking from any of the members, but as you may not receive one, you can go to the *Tribune* office, or that of the New York *Express*, or the *Observer*, founded, like the telegraph by a

MORSE.

With such a ticket, the doors will wide open swing, and entering, you will see what you never expected to see before. You can handle as well as see some of the very bricks which Moses' people made, or so near like them, you couldn't tell which was which, with a collection of interesting antiquities gathered in a lifetime's wanderings through Egypt and the Holy Land, by that plain little old man, Mr. Abbott himself, a poor boy once, and who, when he was living, was very enthusiastic in his descriptions to the author of the wonderful things which he was then exhibiting on Broadway. But he is dead now, and has left his wonderful treasures to delight all comers' eyes for the ages afterwards; the mummies and the men; the beasts and the birds; the seals and the signets; the gems and the jewels, which glistened and glittered on the breasts and fingers of the Pharaohs of near four thousand years ago. And there, too, are the marbles from Nineveh, the very building stones upon which Jonah gazed ; the pavements on which he trod, and the curiously sculptured figures by fingers which plied the ready tool a thousand years before Rome was.

You are tired now. Go another day to the Mercantile Library, near Broadway and Eighth Street, with its hundred thousand well-thumbed volumes, the product of busy brains, great and small, living and dead ; then a leisure walk along Broadway, northward, brings you to the Academy of Design, into which you can enter for a small fee, and gaze with wonder and delight upon those creations of the pencil, which the men and women of taste in all ages so love to contemplate and study and admire. And just across the street, above Putnam's handsome book store, the same Putnam who was a friend of

WASHINGTON IRVING,

making by his foresight, his energy, and his enterprise uncounted dollars for the great writer, so loving and so loved. Well, in the upper rooms of that splendid building, the

ASSOCIATION HALL,

will be found, and persons to explain to you its origin, its workings and its accomplishments ; how that, a very few years ago, some thoughtful young men noticed that boys coming from the country to the city to make their fortunes, with high resolves, and honorable aims sometimes, often made their ruin instead, by falling into the hands of bad men, who, seeing their ignorance of city ways, led them into evil paths and places, out of which they came—lost ! and that others coming and not finding employment, became discouraged, their money spent, no acquaintance, no friend, nothing to eat, no place to sleep, and forced to adopt any plan to save dear life ; plans, too often, leading to degradation and crime. Others there were who would get sick, and, without care or food or medicine, would lie down and die ; some mother's son, without a mother's tender watching, she herself all unknowing what was going on in the great city where that son was ; gone there to try and do something to keep her now, and to be able in after years to give her a home of comfort and quiet and peace in her old age ; but that same son was dying now, to be buried by stranger hands in a pauper's grave ; things like these were happening all through the

29

months and years, had been so happening for a century; and these young men—how pleasant it would be to record their names!—resolved that they would get other young men of like mind to join with them and devise a plan by which, whenever a young man or youth or boy was noticed to be a stranger, his acquaintance should be made, his confidence should be gained; he should be invited to church on Sundays, and be helped to find a "situation," and when obtained, some one would have an eye on him, would visit him now and then, and prompt him to vigilance in his duty, to fidelity to his employers, to rectitude in himself; warning him against dangerous places, to keep away from the restaurant, from the corner grocery, from the engine house, from the theatre, and the dancing saloon; to visit him when sick, to help him to money if his funds failed in emergencies. Then they bethought themselves of having a cheerful, warm, tidy, well-lighted room, where, when night came, and the business places were all shut, especially the long nights of winter, instead of sitting for hours in their lonely rooms at their boarding-houses they could sit down and read the papers and keep themselves informed of what was going on in the city, of who wanted such help as they could afford, at better wages, and kindred things; then, there were magazines to read, and books to study, with pleasant conversable acquaintances between times. And the thing went on, and went on, rising and widening, until it required a building to accommodate all who came, and successfully carry out all that was wanted; a building which would cost a hundred and fifty thousand dollars to erect; and then young men took a paper and wrote down their names for so much, and got others to write down their names for so much; and some of them, having rich fathers, got them to put down their names for so much, and when they came to "foot it up," they had money enough to buy the ground and contract for the building, and this is the hall of the Young Men's Christian Association of New York City, the city's honor, the honor of the State, of the nation, of civilization. With your heart all swelling with human sympathy at the contemplation of deeds so disinterested as these, so honorable to humanity, cross two blocks westward, which brings you abreast of the far-famed Fifth Avenue Hotel, and going along that magnificent street at your easiest convenience, for hurry is never healthful, and on, and on, and on, you pass the palatial mansions of the rich, costing, some of them, with their contents, nearly a quarter of a million of dollars. Yes, just think of it, living in a house, costing, with its furniture, a hundred thousand dollars, two hundred thousand dollars, their owners some of them poor boys less than forty years ago, and when you have passed several hundred such mansions, and several churches, Catholic and Protestant, at half a million each, stop at number six hundred and eighty-one, where you will take a comfortable seat to rest your body, while the mind and the heart will be delighted at the contemplation of the splendid paintings in the

METROPOLITAN ART MUSEUM,

provided you had taken the precaution, when you were at the Association Hall in 23d Street, to ask Mr. Putnam for a ticket of admission to these treasures of the easel. Then, make yourself happy for as long a time as you desire to remain. These details have been made at length, to show New Yorkers, and those who may come to New York, how they may have motives to a kind of exercise in quite a number of conditions of the human body, which fail to be benefited by any other human instrumentalities; —exercise which brings into requisition the whole man, body, mind, heart, so renovating, so recreating to the body, so elevating and so enlarging to the mind; waking up the activities of brain and muscle and moral sentiments.

If persons get tired of these home sights they can live them over again in taking to them their callers and guests and friends who come from a distance; for next best to enjoying a thing for one's self is putting a friend in the way of its appreciation, under our own guidance.

There is, it is true, not a New York everywhere, but there is no locality which has not its beauties, its places of interest; none that has not, at no great distance, something that is strange enough to excite inquiry or study, or amusement for one's self and then for one's friends, all inviting to muscular activities in the open air, with motives powerful enough to wake up, to amuse, to interest; and this is the kind of exercise which, if persevered in, if habitually taken day after day, when not actually raining, would save many an in-door, sedentary person from a life-long invalidism; and would keep in enjoyable health others, who, without these exercises, daily exercises in the open air, of a few hours, are destined themselves to become invalids, and thus crowd their later years with endless complaints of bodily discomforts, of mental disquietudes; to blight the life, to blunt the heart, to dwarf the mind, and make of human existence a failure; to be counted nothing, at the great day of reckoning, but

"WOOD, HAY, STUBBLE."

HEALTHFUL WALKING.

THE easiest way to walk erectly is to have the chin a little above a horizontal line, as if looking at the top of a man's hat or of a house in the distance, then an erect walk can be easily maintained without an effort.

If the shoulders are thrown back and the chest thrown forward, such a mental and physical effort is required that it becomes wearisome to maintain the position for five minutes, or it is forgotten, and there is both a feeling and an appearance of awkwardness as to make it altogether uncomfortable. But if the head is thrown up, and the arms carried behind, as in the cut, a naturally erect and easy gait would soon be acquired, having the effect to throw out and develop the chest, making way for the reception of a larger amount of pure, fresh air into the lungs at every breath, to say nothing of the greater manliness of look and independence of gait, which of themselves give a presence which at once commands attention and respect; but to see a person approach you, stooping, shoulders thrown forward, with bowed head, gives an idea of cringing and supplication, inspiring at once a pity and contempt, while the influence which such a carriage of body has on the health is pernicious, only pernicious, and that

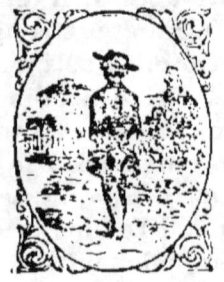

continually. Walking briskly, with an exciting object or pleasurable interest ahead, is the most healthful of all forms of exercise except that of encouragingly remunerative, steady labor in the open air; and yet multitudes in the city, whose health urgently requires exercise, seldom walk when they can ride, if the distance is a mile or more. It is worse in the country, especially with the well-to-do; a horse or carriage must be brought to the door, even if less distances have to be passed. Under the conditions first named walking is a bliss; it gives animation to the mind, it vivifies the circulation, it paints the cheek and sparkles the eye, and wakes up the whole being, physical, mental, and moral. We know a family of children in this city who, from the age of seven, had to walk nearly two miles to school, winter and summer; whether sleet, or storm, or rain, or burning sun, they made it an ambition never to stay away from school on account of the weather, and never to be "late;" and one of them was heard to boast that in seven years it had never been necessary to give an "excuse" for being one minute behind the time, even although in winter it was necessary to dress by gaslight. They did not average two days' sickness in a year, and later they thought nothing of walking twelve miles at a time in the Swiss mountains. Sometimes they would be caught in drenching rains, and wet to the skin; on such occasions they made it a point to do one thing, —let it rain,—and trudged on more vigorously until every thread was dry before they reached home.

There is no unmedicinal remedy known to men, of more value in the prevention of

CONSTIPATION

than a few miles' joyous walking; let one follow it up a week—a walk of two or three miles in the forenoon, and as much in the afternoon— and except in rare cases, when a longer continuance may be made, the result will be triumphant; and yet nine persons out of ten would rather give a dollar a bottle for some nauseous drops or poisonous pills, than take the trouble to put in practice the natural remedy of walking.　Nor is there an anodyne among all the drugs in the world, which is the hundredth part so efficacious in securing refreshing, healthful, delicious

GLORIOUS SLEEP,

as a judicious walk.　To be judicious it should not be continued so long as to make the person feel fagged out; this can be prevented by turning back when there is only a little tiredness; then after resting awhile on a sofa or bed, without closing the eyes, repeat the process, until in the course of the day several hours have been spent in the open air.　Then after a light, early supper of a piece of bread and butter and a cup of tea, spend several hours in pleasant conversation or in games and amusements, not retiring before ten o'clock, going to bed with warm feet, not sleeping any after five in the morning, yet not leaving the bed until you feel like it, and not sleeping a single moment in the daytime; and if in less than one week you cannot sleep deliciously for several hours unbrokenly, there is something the matter with the brain, and you are a candidate for the asylum, unless you take prompt and able medical advice.

No drug or drop or pill or potion can by any possibility give refreshing, invigorating, healthful sleep; they all, without exception, aggravate the

SLEEPLESSNESS;

and it is greatly to be deplored that such multitudes, especially in cities, are constantly resorting to the drug stores for something to make them sleep,—even young men and women.

Nervous people are specially inclined to take something to make them sleep, with the effect to keep them nervous, and prevent refreshing sleep year after year, thus embittering their own and the lives of those in the same household.　In all such cases there is an excess of nervous energy, and that too of an unhealthful character; there is too much steam aboard; the remedy is to work it off in pedestrian excursions.

In walking, as in all other vigorous forms of exercise, the object fails to be accomplished, sickness is induced, and not unfrequently life itself is lost, for the want of taking a common-sense precaution to cool off slowly after the exercise, before a good fire in winter, in a warm room of seventy-five degrees in summer, with every window and door shut, no garment removed, even hat or glove for five minutes; then shawl or overcoat by degrees, so as to cool off very slowly in the course of half an hour. It is no exaggeration to say that thousands of lives are sacrificed every year from failing to

COOL OFF SLOWLY

after the exercise has been taken. It is not so much going out of doors and being out of doors that gives people coughs, colds, and consumption, as the getting of these things after coming into the house, by cooling off too quickly.

PHYSIOGNOMY OF WALKING.

Observing people move slowly, their heads move alternately from side to side, while they occasionally stop and turn round.

Careful persons lift their feet high and place them down flat and firm. Sometimes they stoop down, pick up some little obstruction and place it quietly by the side of the way.

Calculating persons generally walk with their hands in their pockets, and their heads slightly inclined.

Modest persons generally step softly, for fear of being observed.

Timid persons often step off from a sidewalk, on meeting another; and always go around a stone instead of stepping over it.

Wide-awake persons " toe out," and have a long swing to their arms, while their hands shake about miscellaneously.

Careless persons are forever stubbing their toes.

Lazy persons scrape about loosely with their heels, and are first on one side of the walk, and then on the other.

Very strong-minded persons have their toes directly in front of them, and have a kind of a stamp movement.

Unstable persons walk fast and slow by turns.

One-idea persons and very selfish ones toe in.

Cross persons are not apt to hit their knees together.

Fun-loving persons have a kind of halting movement.

Good-natured persons snap their thumb and finger every few

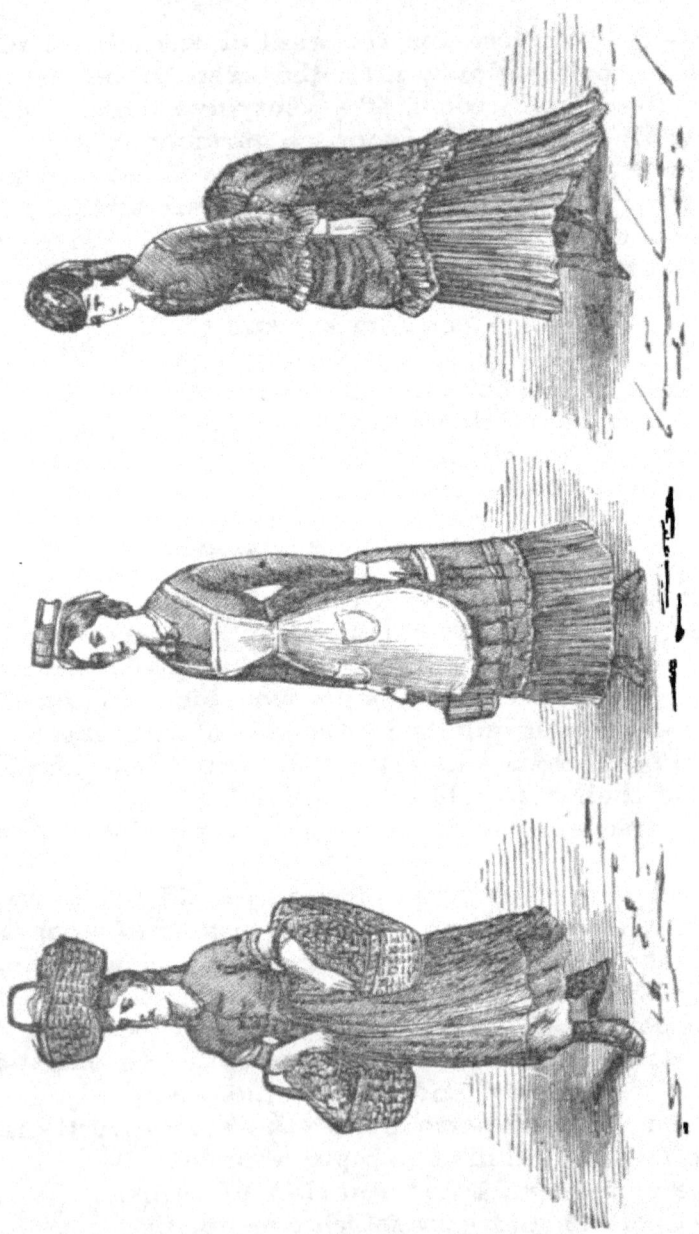

steps.   Persons having a long stride, show directness, firmness,
courage, and persistence.   Such men force their way up to success.
Persons walking with a kind of throwing the head back-

ward, as if each touch of the heel on the ground jarred the head, are hasty, weak-minded, want firmness, and can always be bought.

Cautious people, reliable people, take short steps and slow.

Men who take long, quick steps, with a kind of lifting up of the body at each step, are fearless and honest, and expect to win success by their own unaided forces.

Lighting on the heel means anticipation of obstacles, and a determination of purpose and a firmness of will which nothing can daunt.

Stepping on the toes with a quickness and easy spring indicates activity, vitality, and confidence.

A fashion of wearing high-heeled shoes was adopted by the ladies in 1871; by throwing the body forward, an attitude is required, as seen in the cut, which makes an erect position in walking impossible; too much weight is thrown on the toes, causing backache and spinal deformity and corns, but the discomfort of such a fashion will soon rectify itself. The handsomest, most graceful, and best shaped women in the world were the mulatto girls of New Orleans, before the war. In performing domestic errands they carried the most of their burdens on their heads; the author has seen them, year after year, carrying large baskets of fruit and clothing, and dry-goods packages on their heads through the crowded streets, with their hands at their sides, or gracefully deposited in their little apron pockets, or if the load was heavy, their arms were akimbo, it being rarely necessary to carry either hand to the head; there was an instinct for balancing the head-load which was amazing.

A hint is here given which is of incalculable importance in cases of spinal deformity: nothing will correct it sooner than to carry a weight on the head for half an hour at a time, several times a day, the very weight compelling the person instinctively to assume a position as nearly perpendicular as possible. The intelligent physician who chances to read this, or a parent who observes in any child a tendency to a crooked position while sitting in a chair, can readily turn the hint to an important practical account.

The mode of exercise shown by the girl with a book on her head and weights in her hands is, perhaps, more effectual, and will sooner give a graceful carriage than dumb-bells or any amount of calisthenic exercise; the same may be said of the basket-girl.

SITTING POSITION.

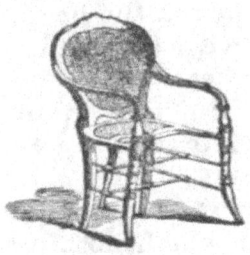
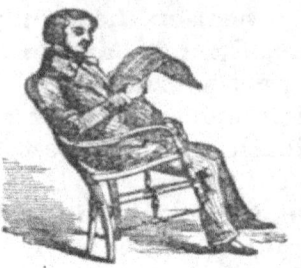
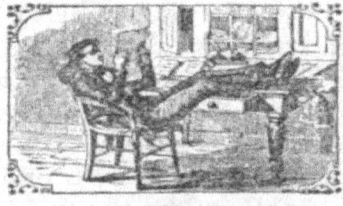
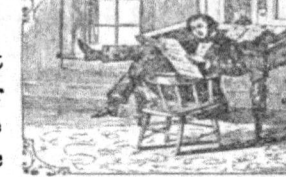

The first chair on the left has a seat eight inches deep, compelling the sitter to an erect position, by throwing the lower portion of the spine against the

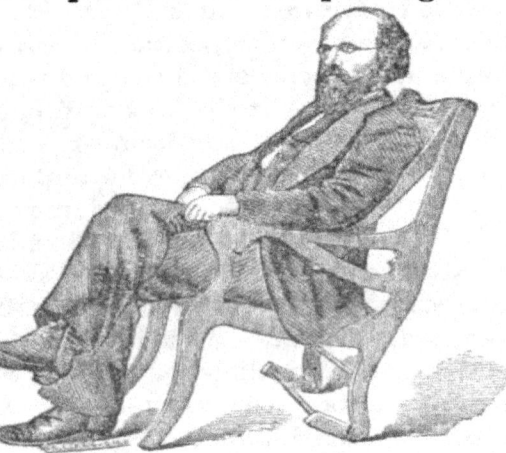

back of the chair; the next cut shows a fifth leg, preventing the tilting back too far. The man with his feet on the table, and the one below him with the legs hanging over the arm of a chair show a very common position of gentlemen when alone. Charles O'Hara, of Hillsborough, Ohio, having given the public several valuable agricultural inventions, has devised the best chair for the weary and feeble, as its back adapts itself to the spine of the sitter, whether in the position of ordinary conversation, or at the writing-desk; it affords a grateful support to the small of the back to all who sit much.

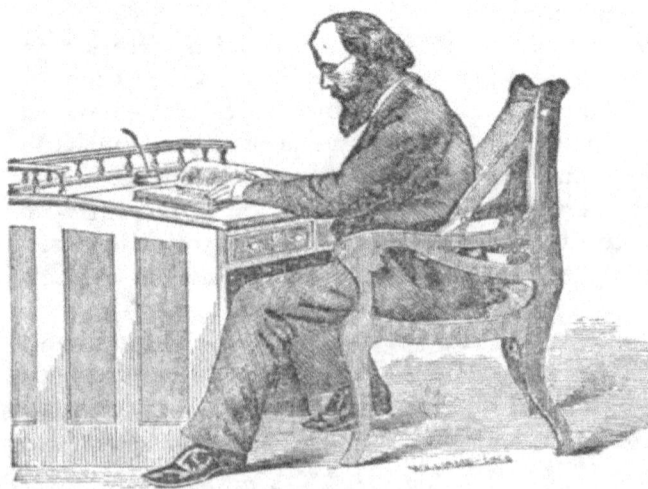

The cut, showing the legs over the arm of the chair, is not an uncommon position, the other person above

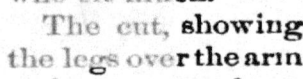

this cut, is more nearly in a horizontal position, and the heart has less labor in sending the blood to the extremities than if he were sitting bolt upright. Besides, the blood in the veins, in this position, is aided in getting back to the heart from the feet by gravity; hence a tired man in that position will get rested sooner than if he were sitting erect. The point is this, that a frequent change of position in reading, or in any sedentary employment, is better than "sitting up straight," and that, if very tired, the nearer we can get to a horizontal position, the sooner will we feel rested.

ANÆMIA

is literally "without blood," and means that the blood is poor, thin, watery, hence the pale face and wan appearance; there is no animation, no life. This condition is brought on by frequent bleedings from any part of the body, severe sickness, long protracted disease, bad food, insufficient eating. It is often found in young girls; even the lips are pale sometimes, also the tongue. There is a general debility, feeble pulse, nervousness, and palpitation of the heart, attended generally with cold feet, costiveness, bad taste in the mouth of mornings, and very irregular appetite, with changing pains to any and all portions of the body. Such persons take cold very easily, are subject to chills from slight causes, have no stamina, no vitality, with the result very generally that they die early or soon fall into a consumptive condition.

In all such cases prompt means should be taken to build up the general health, and these should be persevered in for weeks and many months, if necessary, for, to give up because there seems to be but little change, because the progress towards health seems slow, is to abandon the person to a premature death.

The first thing to be done is to regulate the eating to thrice a day, nothing whatever between meals. For supper take a cup or two of hot drink, with some cold bread and butter, or bread crust broken into tea.

Any drink at meals should be warm, with cold bread and butter, and a piece of fresh meat of any kind for breakfast, and nothing else. Dinner same, adding one vegetable and nothing else, no dessert unless ripe, raw fruit or berries or grapes.

Great pains should be taken to keep the feet warm. (See "Cold Feet.") If one plan does not do, after a systematic, persevering effort, try another, remembering that until the feet become warm and remain so habitually, there is no real approach towards health. Cold feet show that the blood does not properly circulate through the system, and when that is the case there is no health, there is always disease, which can be removed in one way only—vigorous and healthful circulation of the blood.   Another essential requisite is a daily action of the bowels.   To that end take a dose of liver pills once a month, and between times use castor oil or salts in the manner named in the article under the head of Liver Pill.   But there is a far better way—walk or work in the open air during the forenoon and also during the afternoon, beginning with one hour at a time, increasing ten minutes every day, until an amount of time is spent in this way which will secure not only a regular action of the bowels, but will get up a good appetite and a vigorous digestion.   This plan will seldom fail if persevered in ; if it fails, all others will fail.   The point is to ride on horseback, or walk, or work in the open air enough every day to get really hungry.   If spirits or liquors are taken in these frequent forms of disease, the result is to quicken the pulse and thus wear out the strength more rapidly, without adding any ingredient to the blood to increase it in quality or quantity.   Ale and beer and porter sometimes seem to increase the flesh, but never by any means add to the real strength of the body, much less to improve the blood.   Various preparations of iron are given in these bloodless, pale-faced conditions of the system, but there is only one safe, healthful, certain, and natural method of adding iron to the blood, and that is to supply it through a vigorous digestion of substantial meat and bread; these will give all the iron which the blood requires.   Warm feet, regular bowels, a good appetite—these are all important, they are essentials, they will cure, if cure is possible, if several hours are given to exertive exercise in the open air, every day, rain or shine.

ACACIA

MEANS sharp, as it is the sharp spines in certain trees and shrubs, from these a gum exudes, called gum arabic, useful in some forms of irritation, such as tickling in the throat, or inflamed condition of the bowels.   Powdered gum arabic has been known

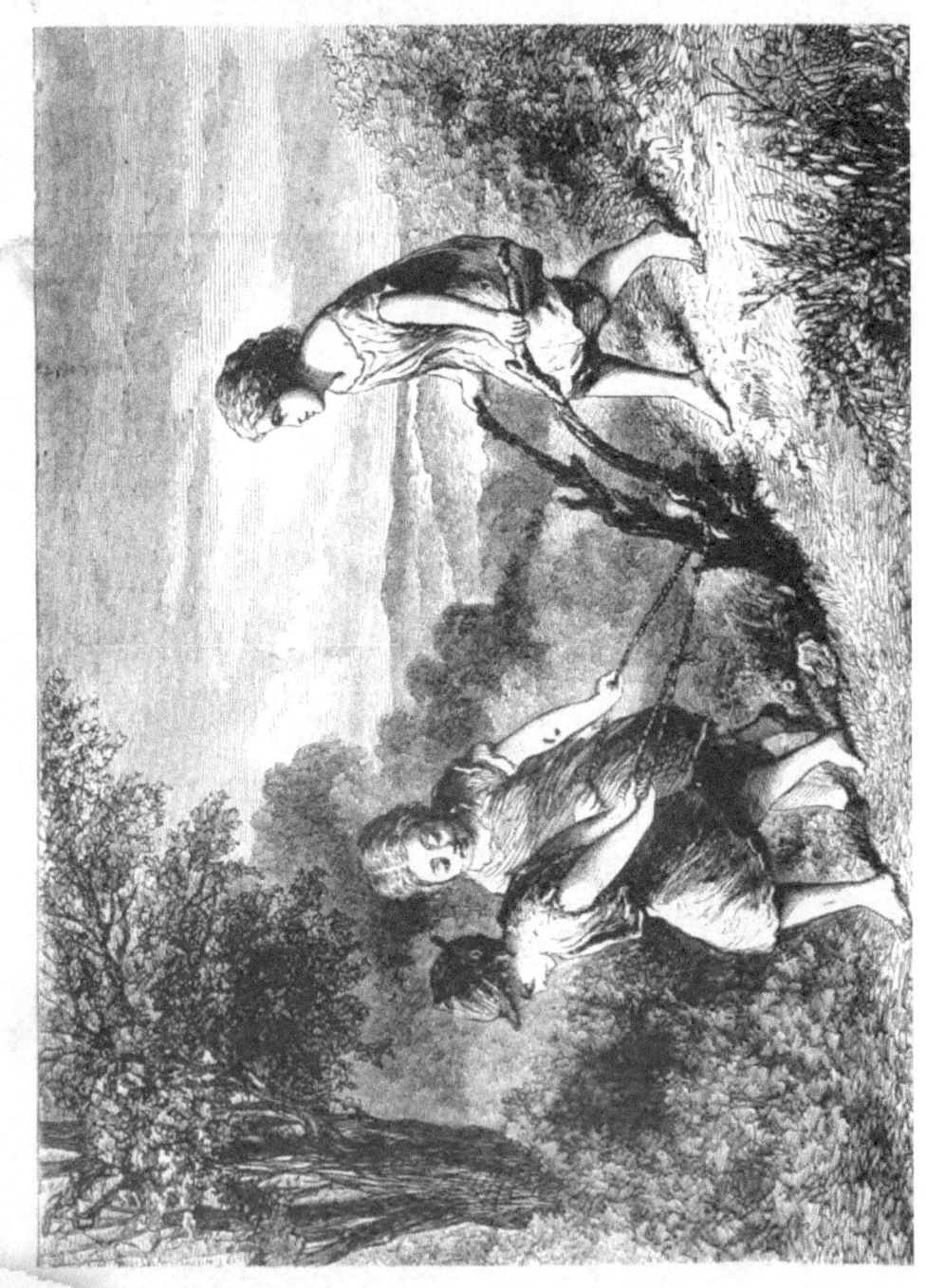

to stop certain bleedings when other things failed, by simply sprinkling or dredging it over the parts.

ACHILLIS TENDO,

THE great muscle; the calf of the leg narrows off until it becomes a band attached to the heel, enabling us to lift the foot and heel; sometimes from jars, or strains, or jumping from heights it is torn in part from its place, and causes intense suffering. The great point—as in all other strains or sprains, for they all mean that the tendon has been dragged or torn—is to keep the part cool, either by applying leeches to draw up the blood, or, which is better, let a stream of cold water fall on the part until the pain has subsided; the water carries off the extra heat of the inflammation, it cools the part, in addition to this the essential of cure is absolute rest until the parts are perfectly restored, regrown to the spot from which the tendon was more or less dragged. Many persons protract the cure of sprains for months and even years, by getting resprained, by use of the part when it was only partially healed. (See Strains and Sprains.) To facilitate and hasten the cure, eat moderately and regularly, and keep the bowels free and feet warm.

PRIMITIVE PLOUGHING.

THE most available form of exercise to the masses of men is ploughing, and it is a most perfect form as a means of restoring health; because

First. It keeps the person out of doors.

Second. The exercise is moderate and continuous.

Third. It can be left off at any time, as there is no hurry.

Fourth. It need not exhaust the strength, and there is no occasion for hurry.

Fifth. The hours of exercise and the time of its duration can be arranged to meet the wants of each case.

Sixth. It can be always made useful and remunerative enough to encourage and to keep the mind away from the ailments of the body. Under these conditions, for men there is no form of exercise which combines with it so many advantages, and is infinitely preferable to going to sea or on long journeys abroad and to the South, where other invalids congregate, and where pale faces and distressed countenances are met at every turn, and the sound of the sepulchral cough is heard at every street corner, or rings like the knell of death through hall and corridor, and hut and hovel, wherever the feet are turned. The iron ploughshare is of modern invention; in primitive times wood was used, and is met to this day in eastern countries. The cut illustrates the kind of plough which it may be supposed Cain and Abel used when they were boys, just outside of Paradise.

WHAT SHALL I DO?

Is often the anxious inquiry of persons who really do not require any medicine to restore them to health, needing only a reasonable amount of out-door exercise. It is the inquiry of many who are in that desperate condition which cannot be improved by medicine, for medicine has lost its power; it is the inquiry of that other large class whose only hope of restoration to health and happiness is in spending a large portion of every day in the open air. As has been before insisted upon, work and exercise, especially in the open air, tend to improve the health, but their beneficial effects are greatly intensified if the work is encouragingly remunerative, or is deeply interesting. The mass of mankind are too poor to be able to "keep up," if they are not earning something every day; but to be earning nothing, and to be on expenses besides, must necessarily have a most depressing effect on the mind, and always retards improvement. The city physician is often called on to aid in putting the sick in the way of recovery. But there are multitudes who do not know how to do anything well enough to earn wages; yet it would seem that almost any one could rent or purchase a single acre of land near a railroad station which was within an hour or two of some large city. It may therefore be profitable to know what may be done with an acre of land, which will give moderate exercise and yield a revenue worth working for. The Florida yield is about the same; in California seventy orange-trees will grow on one acre, each yielding fifteen hundred oranges, or a hundred and five thousand oranges, which, at a cent apiece, is a thousand and fifty dollars.

In Los Angeles, one tree seventeen years old yielded twenty-eight hundred oranges. If from the seed, a tree will grow in a dozen years, yielding two thousand oranges at from $15 to $55 per thousand; sixty trees to an acre would yield a handsome profit; one orchard of nine acres yielding its owner eight thousand dollars a year.

An old man of eighty-six years, who wanted something to do, writes, I planted an acre with corn, beans, peas, and other vegetables and tended the whole myself, having only my hand and hoe, yielding four bushels of beans, twenty-four of corn, thirty of potatoes, besides a good supply of sweet corn, cucumbers, squashes, cabbages, beets, onions, parsnips, carrots, strawberries, raspberries, gooseberries, currants, tomatoes, and grapes. Fifty apple-trees to an acre, at a thousand apples to each—and some yield four thousand—would be a profitable care. The Ramie plant is a kind of nettle with such a silken fibre, that it is not impossible that it will one day be as valuable as cotton. It is propagated from the root. One planting will last three or four years. California yields two crops in a year. In April, 1872, the product of one acre yielded in England three hundred and fifty dollars.

The cultivation of the ground has many important advantages; it compels you to be out of doors every day, this involves exercise and the breathing of a pure air; it is steady work, no need of hurry or fatigue, and leisure exercise is worth more than all others. You can work and rest as suits the strength of the body, and there is a quiet and repose about it which admirably adapts it to building up the health and strength of both body and mind; exercise without end or aim, except as a means of health, is a doleful penance at best. Half a year's amusement might be derived from

CULTIVATING FLOWERS.

The very sight of what is beautiful tends to purify the heart and elevate the character; while the cultivation of flowers directly promotes physical well-being. The following list of flowering plants affords a succession of bloom throughout the season, and will be regarded with interest by every intelligent reader in the beautiful May. In this connection may be premised a striking exemplification of the instinct of plants, by the naturalist Hoare, who placed a bone in the strong, dry clay of a vine border. The vine sent out a leading or tap-root, directly through the clay; the main root threw out fibres, but when it reached the bone it entirely covered it by degrees with the most delicate and minute fibres like lace, each one sucking at a pore in the bone, like a litter of pigs at their dam, as she lies down on the sunny side of the farm-yard. On this luscious morsel of a marrow-bone would the vine continue to feed as long as any nutriment remained to be extracted. What wonderful analogies there are running through the various forms of animal and vegetable creation, to stimulate curiosity, to gratify research, and, finally, to lead our contemplations from nature, in a feeling of reverence "up to nature's God."

As to the vine spoken of by Hoare, it is worthy of remark that the root went no further than the bone, which it seemed to have literally smelt out, as would a hungry dog, in passing.

FLOWERING SHRUBS.

Pink Mezereon.
Dwarf double-flowering Almond.
Double Purple Tree Peony.
Chinese White Magnolia. (*Conspicua.*)
Soulange's Magnolia.
Sweet-scented Magnolia. (*M. glauca.*)
White Fringe Tree.
Garland Deutzia. (*D. Scabra.*)
Broad-leaved Laburnum.
Rose Acacia.
Tartarian Tree-Honeysuckle, red and white.
Double White Hawthorn.
Double Pink Hawthorn.
Fragrant Clethra.
Oak-leaved Hydrangea.
Venetian Sumac or Purple Fringe.
Buffalo Berry (male and female).
Siberian Lilac.
The Althea or Hibiscus Syriacus.
Colutea Arborescens.
Chinese double-flowering Apple.
Deutzia Gracilis.
All the Spireas.
Snowball (common though beautiful).
Dwarf Dogwood.
Pyrus Japonica.

Euonymus (burning bush).
Forsythia.
Philadelphus (Mock Orange).
Symphora.
Wiegeila Roses.

PERENNIAL PLANTS.

Dicentra Spectabilis.
Plumbago.
White and Pink Phlox.

[There are from twenty to thirty common Phloxes, many of them dwarf, of beautiful colors, and much admired.]

Companulas.
Chrysanthemums (summer and fall).
Double Hollyhocks.
Pæonias (white and red).
Iris (pale blue, very fragrant).
Sweet William.
Valeriana.
Persian Lilac.

CLIMBING SHRUBS AND VINES.

Some of the finest and best climbing shrubs are the following:—

Large flowering Trumpet Creeper.
Queen of the Prairie Rose.

Chinese Glacine (Wistaria).
Double Purple Clematis.
Clematis Flamula, Florida and Siboldii.
Monthly Fragrant Honeysuckle.
Chinese Twining Honeysuckle.
Yellow Trumpet Honeysuckle.
Scarlet Trumpet Honeysuckle.
Japan Evergreen Honeysuckle.
Chinese Bignonia.
Virginia Creeper.
Periwinkle (as a creeper for shady places).

CLIMBING ROSES.

Queen of the Prairies.
White Multiflora.
Laura Davoust (half-hardy).
Baltimore Belle.

TRAILING ROSES.

Fellenberg.
Glory of Rosamond.

Monstrosa.
Baron Prevost.
Noisette Superba.
La Reine.

MONTHLY ROSES.

Hermosa, pink.
Cels, blush and pink.
Devoniensis, creamy white.
Archduchess, pure white.
Giant of Battles, crimson.
Louis Philippe, red.
Souvenir, blush.
Luxemborg, buff.
Queen of Lombardy, deep rose.
Saffrana, yellow buff.
Daily, light pink.
Prince Albert.
Garibaldi.
Triomphe d'Exposition.
Monthly Cabbage.

THE MICROSCOPE,

DISCOVERED by Janssen, in 1619, meaning the " looking at small things," is a contrivance which enlarges an object to many times its natural size, thus enabling the eye to see what otherwise could not be noticed.   One of these useful little instruments, magnifying to the extent of a thousand diameters, that is, making a thing look a thousand times larger than it really is, may be obtained for two or three dollars, and be a source of amusement, instruction, and wonder to a whole family gathered around the fire of a winter's night, affording a varied and most lively entertainment to a whole household, especially the little ones, filling the mind with wonder and admiration of the wisdom and power of Him who " hath done all things well."

The family which makes the fireside attractive is the family in which sons and daughters grow up loving and loved, saved from the contaminations of the street, and from the corrupting influences of bad associations after nightfall ; for that is the time when the young are most readily tempted to go astray, as if the darkness covered their wrong-doings from human view.

30

The evening is the best time to use a microscope, as with a lamp, or gas, or candle, the light can be better directed to the exact spot where it is wanted. It is a delightful thing, before a winter's fire, to have the little ones gather around, with inquiring looks and wondering eyes and brightening countenances, so full of joyous expectancy; and then how easy to lead the mind upward, in loving admiration of Him who made all things, from an insect's eye, or a snowflake, to the sun in his glory!

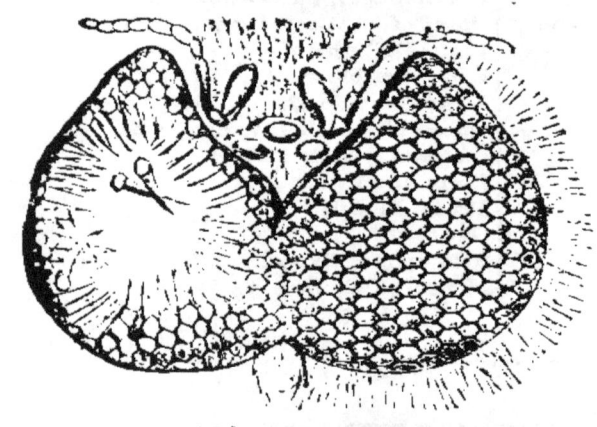

ANT'S EYE MAGNIFIED.

The accompanying cut represents the eye of an ant. It does not move around, or from side to side, nor even turn its little head to advise it of coming danger. The eye is firmly fixed, and no more moves than the nose or ears; but in each eye there are multitudes of eye-balls, which face every possible direction, and every image which comes within their scope is perfectly portrayed and seen, whether it be a particle of dust brushed from a feather, to a man or a mountain.

By this magical instrument, when of great power, insects of various sizes may be seen in the hollow of a grain of sand. Every hair of the head is found to be hollow, and covered with scales, like those of a fish; indeed, these can be felt by drawing one between the finger and thumb-nail the wrong way, for, in one direction, with the scales, the hair is smooth. Our very bodies are covered with scales, a hundred of which can be covered by a single grain of sand from the sea. Look at a butterfly's wing and its beautiful hues. Every bright spot is made of uncounted little feathers, while the mould on a crust of bread looks like a luxuriant forest. The smallest mite will take a hundred steps in a second. Every leaf is fed upon by millions of miniature cattle, while a drop of stagnant water has uncounted monsters wriggling in it with the freedom of a whale at sea. But it is well to know that running streams and deep wells contain none of these; they are too cold for their life, and the dashing of the waves and the dancing of the waters over pebbly beds are too boisterous for their frail frames.

THE BEAUTIFUL SNOW!

so pearly white, so soft and feathery, and to us appearing to be of one universal sameness, when seen under the microscope, as freshly fallen from the sky, is composed of many flakes, yet every flake is different from every other. Of the myriads which fall of a winter's night, no two have yet been found to be alike, except in one amazing point: there is not one which by any chance has a jagged edge, all have a wonderful evenness and regularity. Every single flake is composed of perfect crystals, and of the most beautiful and varied forms imaginable, as seen in the following cut.

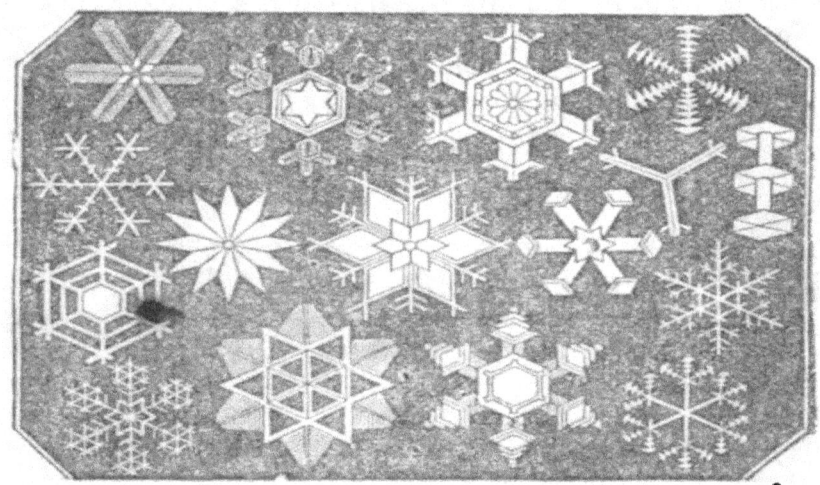

SNOWFLAKES, MAGNIFIED.

In examining the sting of a bee, the point *a* is arrow-shaped, formed like the barb of a fish-hook, easy to enter, but the drawing of it out tears the flesh, and aids in the hurting; but at the same instant through the sting, which is hollow, the poison from the little sacs, *b*, *b*, *c*, is injected, and constitutes the

VENOM OF THE BITE.

On the same principle are formed the bill of the mosquito, and in part the fang of the rattlesnake, which is hollow; and the sac of poison being at the bottom of it, is pressed, and the poison makes its way into the wound which the fang made, there to rankle and rage and destroy.

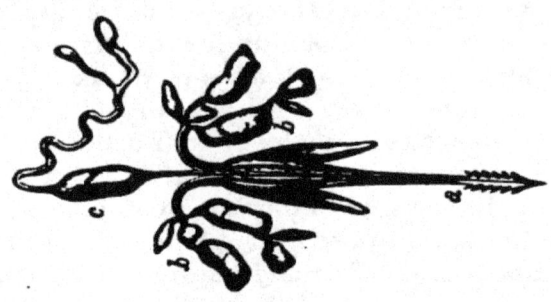

STING OF A BEE.

In the foot of a fly the microscope shows a single hair as large as the foot itself, with the marvellous little pads, or soles, which enable it to cling to the ceiling, with its head downwards, all unconscious of its doing anything wonderful. The end of the bee's

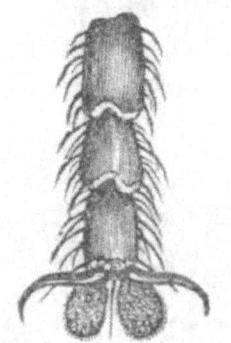

FLY'S LEG AND FOOT.

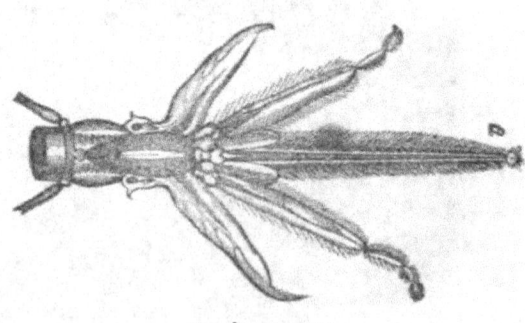

BEE'S TONGUE.

tongue is seen at *a*. It is through this that the substance is drawn up from the flowers, which is made into honey and wax, the other parts seeming to be used in steadying the little worker's body while exploring the flowers.

The uses to be made of the microscope in the detection of disease, or in the investigation of diseased conditions of the system, have not yet been determined, as microscopy is still in its infancy. Suffice it to say, that insects, cells, and all forms of vegetable and animal life are found everywhere, in the body and out of it, in the corners of the eye, in the ear, the nose, in fact, almost everywhere in the

HOUSE WE LIVE IN,

a worm for almost every mechanism of the system, making it a pasture-field on which to graze, to flourish, and to thrive.

Of late it has become quite a common thing to examine the discharges connected with various forms of disease; and each one, thus far, seems to have abounded in a specific form of life, either vegetable or animal, forms of amazing fecundity, paralleled only in the process of fermentation, as in the making of a loaf of bread. One kind of life cell has been found in the discharges of

CHOLERA,

which begins to rise in the air the instant of leaving the body, and is thus drawn into the lungs, and swallowed into the stomach, giving the disease to others, to work the wise behests of the Infinite One, or else to be

THE SCAVENGER

of creation, to remove from human sight all that can offend, as the maggot eats up the carrion, then dies, and passes itself into the impalpable dust.

Briers and thorns were sent into the garden and the grain-field and the orchard, to compel man to make his bread by the sweat of his face, and thus earn for himself also an immeasurable happiness,—the happiness of a hearty appetite, a vigorous digestion, delicious sleep, and

GLORIOUS GOOD HEALTH!

We do not yet know but that even the infinitesimal insect which multiplies into a million in a minute to propagate disease, if it finds dirt to propagate it in, was intended to be the thorn of the animal world, to compel man, the master, to such watchfulness and industries as would banish from his person, his chamber, his dwelling, his garden, his fields, and his pastures, every possible thing which could harbor a disease-producing worm, or which by any possibility could afford filth enough for it to feed upon for a minute.

THE BLUE-BOTTLE FLY

deposits eggs in ulcers and sores, and at the various outlets of the human body, flesh-wounds, etc., and these eggs are developed into worms in a few hours. By cleanliness and care such a result will be avoided.

COURAGE LUMPS,

named under the impression that they result from grossness of body, or are connected with the transformation period from youth to manhood. They are often a disfigurement, as well as a source of mortification. Either let them alone, or when ripe, yellow at the top or centre, put a thumb-nail on either side, press inwards and upwards, and a whitish, cheesy, thread-like worm comes away.

MEASLES AND SCARLET FEVER

have associated with their appearance a living germ, as also the common

ITCH.

But whether they cause disease or were intended to prevent it, one point is clear, that it is man's duty, in either case, to prevent the filth which feeds them, or to remove them with the filth in which they appear, and thus be perfectly clean in his person, in his habitation, and in all his surroundings, that there be no unseemly object anywhere in sight, it being a condition of health of body and purity of mind and heart that the man himself should be pure and clean as the precedent of his being good, and made fit for angelic associations.

It is worth having the itch, to enjoy the bliss of scratching; there is nothing like it: why? You feel as if you could dig your nails an inch deep into the flesh. If, however, you get tired of scratching, take grease, and you will soon be well. The books tell us that the common itch is occasioned by the bite of a living thing, so small that it takes a hundred microscopes to see one of them. But the peculiarity of these little insects is, that they are full of noses. A man has only one nose; and if you plug it up with putty, he will die in five minutes, if you can only induce

him to keep his mouth shut ; if he don't, putty it, too. So as to
the itch insect, you have only to putty him up ; if, however, you
are in a hurry to get well, keep the itching parts covered with
sweet oil, and every one of them will be smothered to death.

THE HAND

Is not only the great helper of man, his defence as well as his
support and protector, but it is his ornament and the index of his
position in society. A hard hand is the sign of an honest worker,
of one who had rather toil for a scanty living than steal for the
privilege of idleness. A soft hand shows that its owner is of
gentle birth, at least is not the slave of labor ; while the
soiled hand proves that its owner is uncultivated, unrefined.
To soften the hands, mild white soaps should be used, because
they are not strong of alkali, which makes the skin harsh, but
they are the purest, the freest from all foreign substances. The
old Windsor soap is the worst for the hands ; for its native ingredients of pulverized bone sometimes wound and poison the skin,
especially of the face. After each washing, some glycerine
should be rubbed into the skin, worked into it by the wringing of
the hands, especially on the back of them. This keeps the skin soft ;
the softening is greatly expedited if, the last thing at night, they
are well washed with white soap and warm water, then rinsed in
cold water until the skin is thoroughly divested of all the soap ;
then wipe with a soft cotton cloth ; next, just before retiring into
bed, put a quarter or half of a teaspoonful of sweet oil into the
palm of one hand, lay the other palm on it, rub them back and
forth and then wring the hands like a washing operation, so as to
convey the oil into every pin-point of the surface of the skin ; put
on a pair of old gloves—kid is the best. Repeat this operation
every night until the object is accomplished. For the cure of
chapped hands and cracked fingers it is the simplest, speediest,
cheapest, and most effective ever known hitherto. If it is desired
to whiten the hands in addition to softening them, you have only
to wear gloves all day as well as all night.

If the hands are stained with ink, or fruit, or other things, hold
them in a bowl of water into which five grains of oxalic acid has

been put. Stir it well, keep the hands in for five minutes, then wash them well in an abundant supply of cold water; or put ten drops of oil of vitriol in a pint of water, in a china or earthen bowl, a teaspoon level-full of saleratus, and stir and soak the hands in it five minutes, and then wipe dry, not using soap for half a day afterwards, as it returns the stain.

The hands are made harsh and sore in winter by frequent washings with soap and water, especially if the soap is not thoroughly rinsed off, or when the person is around the fire a great deal and has to handle cold metal, as iron cooking-utensils; this may be antagonized to a considerable extent by sleeping with greased hands in gloves, and wearing these as much as possible in the daytime. Even twenty-four hours of such wearing makes a striking difference in the comfort of their feeling.

It is an excellent plan, under all circumstances, to give the hands a good washing every night, before going to bed, using soap and water. In very cold weather, it is better to wash the hands but once a day, if the fingers are at all inclined to get sore or crack; or after each washing, rub into them a few drops of glycerine or sweet oil—no preparation in existence answers so good a purpose as the former article, to prevent and to cure chapping; or have finely-powered starch always at hand, and after each washing, on putting the hands in any liquid, wipe them, and rub some of this starch-powder well into every part of the hands and fingers. It at once cools and soothes and softens the hands, and gives immediate relief to their smarting; or, to melted tallow add some powdered camphor, with a few drops of oil of almonds, and let it cool. There are various preparations for this purpose, but glycerine is so easily had, and is so mild and otherwise unobjectionable, that it is not necessary to add to the list. When the hands have been blistered by sweeping the floor, or in any other way, let some melted tallow fall into cold water, gather it, then mix it with any kind of spirit or alcohol, and rub it well into the blistered parts; it is a most admirable relief and cure for blistered feet, if rubbed well into the soles.

The hands may be softened, whitened, and otherwise beautified, by mixing four parts of the yellow of an egg and five parts of glycerine, and rubbing them well together in a mortar with a pestle. Rub it well into the hands after each washing. It will keep for years, and is an admirable preparation for all bruises of the skin.

The paste of sweet almonds is very good to soften the hands and arms, it makes the skin elastic; and, where hardened by labor, the incrustations are soon removed.

Sometimes persons have a very ugly soreness in the hands in cold weather; the remedy is, to keep them warm all the time, indoors as well as out, and use the glycerine and egg preparation freely. If there is any smarting with the soreness, use the starch-powder. If the hands are cold, and otherwise uncomfortable, when you get into the house dip them in tepid water. This is much better than holding them to a hot fire, stove, or register.

Many stains of the hands and skin are promptly removed by keeping on hand a preparation made by putting a table-spoonful of salt of lemons or tartaric acid into ten table-spoons of water; rub it well into the stained part; or, if time presses, take the powder of the articles above named and rub it well into the parts after washing them, moistening a little with water.

FINGER-NAILS

should be trimmed once a week with toilet scissors. The use of a penknife makes one shiver to see. They should not be trimmed to the quick; there should be a rim left of five or six hairs' thickness. It is better to have the outer edges of the nail a little longer, otherwise the skin may grow up and spread over the nail, or become sore. The nails grow faster in warm weather than in cold; they grow by pushing outwards, and are renewed, grow out their whole length about every four or five months, and, in doing so, they sometimes drag the skin at their roots along with the nail, stretch it more and more until it snaps, making nail-tags, which sometimes are very uncomfortable, become sore and. much inflamed; this can be prevented by taking a soft towel every time the hands are washed, and push back the skin while it is yet soft, or it may be done with the finger or thumb nail; do it gently and slowly, and do not push it too far; if, by neglect, it has been dragged forward and the thumb-nail is not strong enough, take an ivory paper-cutter, or next best is a piece of money; by all means avoid the use of a knife about the finger-nails; some persons are seen continually scraping the ends of the finger-nails with a penknife, some have a little file, but neither leaves the edge of the nail anything like as smooth as the use of sharp toilet scissors and a day or two's wear. To remove the gatherings under the finger-nails with the sharp point of a penknife is a barbarism; it makes the nail grow thicker and less delicate, and often wounds the tender skin under, leaving painful inflammations. It is still more injurious to scrape the nails with a penknife at the junction of skin and nail—it causes those ugly white splotches which are so often seen on the nails, and prevents that even and regular appearance of the skin at those points which adds so much to the delicacy of the fingers.

The indecent habit of biting the finger-nails need only to be alluded to to prevent any one from repeating it, as it is really eating the dirt which collects under them. If at any time children get into the habit, make them dip into wormwood tea, several times a day, the ends of their fingers—a very good plan also for preventing nursing children from sucking their thumbs. The best means of keeping the finger ends delicately clean is the frequent use of soap and water; if, on occasion, these are not to be had, by no means use a knife or any metallic point. Employ a piece of sharpened stick or wood, but soap and water are best.

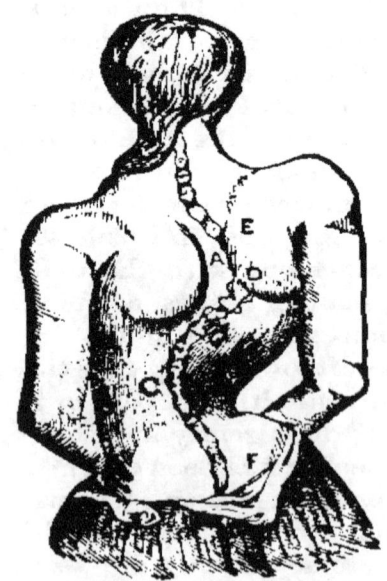

CURVATURE OF THE SPINE.

Induced by an erroneous sitting posture, as sideways, or one shoulder lower than the other. The scrofulous are most liable to it.

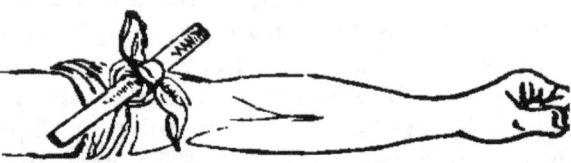

THE TIE TO STOP A BLEEDING ARTERY

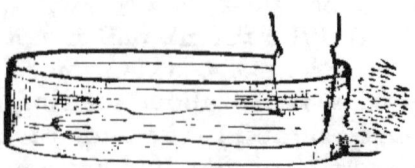

THE HAND OR ARM BATH.

PARENTS AND CHILDREN.

It is a very rare thing to find a parent turning against a child, except in old age, connected with a mild form of insanity; but it is far too common to find animosities in the minds of children, excited generally by trifling circumstances, arising from misapprehension or hasty judgments, and cherished for weeks and months and years, settling finally into a kind of impatient hatred or contempt. At other times these animosities have arisen from the innate ugliness of disposition of the child; so groundless, so unreasonable in its character, as to merit the pity rather than the resentment of a third person.

One of the most beautiful of all moral exhibitions on this planet is a whole family of parents, sons, and daughters living together in affectionate unity; where nothing is ever seen by any chance but kindness, courtesy, deference, and self-abnegation; a habitual preference in favor of the others—that kind of preference which lovers show, where the pleasure is in proportion to the self-denial; where it is no effort, and where there is not an instant's delay in yielding the best places and the best things, or in doing a service which can in the least aid another.

And when it is considered how short a time any family can remain together under the same roof, how rare a thing, indeed, that death has not already made a gap, and how he may make one any day, when it will be too late forever to atone for any wrong done, for any hurting of the feelings, especially under a misapprehension; any wounding unnecessarily of a loving mother's heart, or father's, or brother, or sister's, a wounding which, when they are dead and gone, like a Parthian arrow, flies backward, poisonous and rankling, never to be extracted, except by the great doctor—death! Well would it be for the happiness of many a heart to make it a study from this hour—the habitual study—how to live in the family so as never to be the cause of a heart-burning; how best to avoid the planting of those remorses which are thick this very hour all over the world, expressing themselves thus: " O! what would I not give to have them back one single minute, to let them know the bitterness of my repentance!"

FRENZY.

"'Are you ready for me! have you got the money?' and he went on heaping on me the most bitter taunts and opprobrious epithets; while speaking he drew a handful of papers from his pockets, saying: 'I got you into your office, and now I'll get you out.' I cannot tell how long these threats and invectives lasted. At first I kept interposing, trying to pacify him. But I could not stop him. Soon, my own temper was up. I forgot everything but the sting of his words. I was excited to the highest degree of passion; and in my fury I seized a small stick of wood and dealt him an instantaneous blow, with all the force that passion could give it. I did not know or think or care where or how hard I should strike, nor what would be the effect. He fell instantly dead! I then cut up his body, hid a portion of it, and burned the remainder in a furnace." This was the confession of a highly educated man, just before he suffered the ignominious penalty of murder; the murder of the best friend he had on earth! It was done in an ecstasy of passion, in a "phrensy," from a Greek word *phren*, which means the mind; or a state of the brain in which the mind is excited to a pitch which places it beyond all human control; it is a momentary madness. The lesson sought to be impressed by this narration is the danger of cherishing any mental excitement; and the consequent duty of studying how, in all possible ways, to keep the mental faculties in a uniformly calm, quiet, and deliberate condition. In the incident above, it was proven that half an hour before, the murderer had closed a philosophic lecture; and as he stepped from the rostrum into his own room was met, as above detailed, by a rich, remorseless creditor. In a very few minutes the calm philosopher was transformed into an ungovernable fury, by the utterance of a dozen taunting words; and had no more control over himself than an infant over an already sped thunderbolt. Cases are given in standard medical works, where the mental excitement has reached such an intensity, that the individual has fallen dead on the instant; even greater calamities are recorded; the loss of the mind forever, and the hapless victim has raved and raged in impotency behind the bars of a maniac's cell for the remainder of a long life; a fate surely worse than death! Sometimes the mind has gone out in eternal night with a fearful screech, combining the yell of the savage with the expressions of a demoniac.

Lesser degrees of mental excitement have found vent in words and manner so expressive, as to excite an uncontrollable horror in the minds of some of the hearers, and wilted the hearts of others, to bud and bloom no more. A single word uttered by a child to a parent, in a moment of excitement; of a parent to a child; of a husband to a wife, has many a time, before now, quenched every spark of human emotion and of human love, and a hate has sprung from the ashes, as virulent as the deadly upas, only to go out in the night of the grave. Human happiness, and life itself, then, often depends on a failure to control the mental emotion. An effort to practise such a control should be early made; the earlier the better. And let it be particularly remembered, that the most effectual practical manner of doing this is to cultivate a habit of speaking in a low, slow, deliberate tone of voice, under all circumstances; but whenever the circumstances are exciting, speak not a syllable until the thought, embodied in words, stands out plainly before the mind, " My God and Father is here," and then speak accordingly. The reason of this lies in the curious fact, that the mind has a faculty of being persuaded to believe what the lips express, although every word is a falsehood; for in the excited condition, that which is called imagination runs riot, and makes the merest presumption appear for a moment to be an actual fact. This is an every-day occurrence in domestic life, where an excited husband or wife begins to talk of a supposed insult, or deviation of a servant; and the more they talk the greater appears the aggravation. Reader, keep ever before you the fear of " frenzy," for in an unguarded hour, within any dozen minutes, it may lead you to utter a word against a heart that loves you, whose wound no tears can ever wash away; may lead you to commit an act which will send you to the gallows or a mad-house !

One of the surest and most infallible safeguards known to mortal man against life-long remorses, against the most withering mortifications, and in multitudes of cases against a fatal blow or stab or shot is within the reach, within the compass of every intelligent human being. In every excited conversation with friends, strangers, or kindred, wherever there is the slightest indication of impatience or anger, that very instant

KEEP YOUR MOUTH SHUT.

As you value your own self-respect, keep your mouth shut, closely, resolutely. As you value the Divine assertion, "that for every idle word that men shall speak, they shall give account thereof in the day of judgment," keep your mouth shut. As you value your life, your soul, your earthly happiness, say not a word, not one single syllable, and it will be a savior to you; besides, it will be so keen a mortification to the others, that it will never be forgotten. In a physical sense, keep your mouth shut habitually; it compels you to draw deeper inspirations through the nose, reaching down to the very bottom of the lungs, thus creating an increased development which adds to the chances of a longer life, and gives a more erect gait, a more manly carriage. In going into a colder air, keep the mouth shut, thus sending all the air to the lungs through the head, warming it before it gets there, thus preventing many a chill and bad cold.

VERATRUM VIRIDE

Is American hellebore, or poke-root. It has emetic qualities, increases the secretions, and has a powerful influence over the nervous system, indicated by faintness, somnolency, vertigo, headache, dimness of vision, and enlarged pupils. It will reduce the pulse thirty or forty strokes in a minute, when given in large doses. It is good for gouty, rheumatic, and neuralgic affections. An emetic dose is five or six grains of the powdered root, or one or two teaspoonfuls of the tincture made by six ounces of the fresh root in a pint of whiskey, brandy, or alcohol. It is an excellent remedy in all febrile and inflammatory affections.

Eight ounces of the dried root, soaked in eight ounces of alcohol for two or three weeks, gives a strong tincture; eight drops, repeated every three hours, with an additional drop at each dose, reduces the pulse very rapidly, especially in heart affections. If too much is taken by mistake, drink largely of whiskey or brandy.

FEEBLE INFANTS.

SOMETIMES infants are born with the smallest possible amount of life; the first thing is to keep them warm, wrap them well in flannel and hold each foot in a large, warm hand; next feed them; when they cannot swallow from any cause, or at any age, put a tube into the mouth, far back on the tongue, then lay the head on the left thigh of the feeder, the body being in a horizontal position, press the infant's cheeks, this naturally opens the lips some, put in a spoon half full of breast or other milk, as far back on the tongue as you can, and toss up the handle quickly; wait a while and the milk will gradually run down the throat without actual swallowing; do this at intervals of five minutes, several times, until the milk does not disappear from the mouth; repeat this feeding every three hours, night and day; in three or four days it will begin to suck, but in the intervals offer the breast, for although hungry, it may be too weak to cry.

STRYCHNINE,

OR Nux Vomica, is obtained from the nut of the strychnos tree of Ceylon, bearing rich orange-colored berries as large as a pippin-apple, containing flat round seeds near an inch in diameter, covered with silken ash-colored hair; this nut is of such a deadly poison that the natives give it the name of dog-killer. A nut contains about twenty grains, and is gradually learned to be eaten like opium, and with similar results; one nut generally lasts a week. It must be taken just before or just after having eaten, otherwise convulsions will follow. Strychnine, as we see it, is a whitish crystal, and is freely used by physicians, in small quantities, in nervous affections chiefly. If too much is taken death may ensue in a few minutes; hence drink warm milk and water instantly, a teacupful every two minutes until very free vomiting, then take in water twenty grains of bromide of potash.

FOMENTATIONS.

Put three or four folds of flannel in a basin, pour on boiling water ; when soaked, lay the flannel on the end of a towel, double the towel over and wring out the water, without burning the hands ; then lay this hot flannel over the part to be fomented, and a dry flannel overreaching the edges of the hot flannel ; draw over the bed-clothing, and in five minutes renew the application, with another flannel ready as soon as the first is withdrawn ; this may be repeated three or four times, not oftener, as a fomentation should not remain longer than fifteen or twenty minutes, thus debilitating instead of relaxing. Fomentations are pleasant reliefs in a variety of ailments, especially over the abdomen and chest, in hysteric attacks, suffocations, nervous and dyspeptic headaches, painful menstruation, sudden stoppage of the monthlies, asthmatic fits, convulsions, neuralgias, in great constipation, or difficulty of urination, nausea, vomiting, bilious or cramp colic. The fomentations should generally be large, covering the whole chest or abdomen in the severer forms of the above ailments, always remembering that, when the pains are sharp and severe, and the skin hot and pulse high, or other indications of decided inflammation, cold compresses are more appropriate, and hot fomentations are injurious.

LONGEVITY OF MARRIAGE.

The most carefully compiled statistics in the world, perhaps, are those of France, Belgium, and Holland. The latest figures show that

Married men from 25 to 30 years,   6 in 1,000 die annually.
Bachelors   "   25 to 30   "   10 in 1,000   "
Married   "   30 to 35   "   7 in 1,000   "
Bachelors   "   30 to 35   "   18 in 1,000   "
Married   "   35 to 40   "   7 in 1,000   "
Bachelors   "   35 to 40   "   13 in 1,000   "

Thus clearly showing that from 30 to 35 nearly three times as many bachelors die as married men.

Married women from 30 to 35 years, 9 die out of 1,000
Unmarried " " 30 to 35 " 11 " 1,000
Married " " 50 to 55 " 16 " 1,000
Unmarried " " 50 to 55 " 26 " 1,000

But let it be remembered that girls who marry before twenty-one are more likely to die than those who do not marry, by nearly double; that is, seven unmarried girls die out of every thousand, while twelve married die yearly from the same number. Girls should not marry until twenty-one; young men should wait until twenty-five.

DISINFECTANTS

ARE materials which take out of the air or clothing particles which, if breathed, would do injury to the human system; these particles are antagonized or destroyed. The only perfect disinfectant is

CLEANLINESS,

so that there shall be no impurity in the air or filth in the clothing, or that which is about us. The old-time method of destroying the foul odor of a sick-room was to burn tar, or sprinkle sugar on burning coals. This antagonized nothing, it only overpowered the other odor, and both were in the room instead of one. The cheapest and most convenient material for taking away the smell of privies, sinks, and the like, is a pound of copperas, called sulphate of iron, dissolved in a gallon of water; or,

One pound of chloride of lime in a gallon of water, and thrown down or sprinkled over noisome places; or,

Half a pound of chloride of lime to a pint of water.

For bed-pans or water-closets, one ounce of chlorinated soda to a quart of water; or,

Fifteen grains of the crude permanganate of potassa to a quart of water; or,

31

Take of carbolic acid, pure or impure, one ounce to a gallon of water.

Clothing had better be burned, or if not, boiled three or four hours vigorously, or exposed to a dry heat of 250° Fahrenheit.

Rooms can be ventilated by sprinkling chloride of lime in the fireplace or set in plates around, or one part of carbolic acid in a hundred parts of water, and sprinkled freely about; or,

Dissolve one pound of litharge in seven pounds of nitric acid and two gallons of water.

Powdered charcoal and fresh lime, half and half, make a most excellent absorbent.

Filth heaps covered with fresh earth lose their noisomeness immediately. Powdered charcoal absorbs an immense amount of ill odor.

The only true disinfectant is that which not only removes ill odors, but prevents the development of others, by arresting decomposition or fermentation. Sulphate of iron, for example, decomposes ammonia carbonate and sulpho-hydrate. Perchloride of iron precipitates albuminoid matters. Lime disinfects organic matters. Permanganate of potassa decomposes sulphuretted hydrogen, found in rotten eggs, rising from gutters, and blackening door-plates and knobs; it destroys all organic matters, and acts on all fixed compounds of that class. Chlorate of potash disengages the chlorine of cesspools, forming new compounds. Chloride of lime parts with its chlorine, and decomposes most foul odors by combining with their constituents and forming new compounds. Carbolic acid has the power to prevent miasms, and to that extent will arrest the progress of all epidemics depending on miasm—to which the reader should turn; and it may be well regarded as the best, most perfect, and cheapest disinfectant known, it being the same essentially as creasote, and the smoke which preserves our hams from decay.

MOTHER AND INFANT.

Of every two children born into the world, one dies before ten years have passed away.

Of every three children born, one dies before five years.

Of every five children born, one dies within a year.

With intelligent care, instead of half of all the children who come into the world alive dying within ten years, four-fifths of them ought to live, and would live. That so many die is owing to the fact, in part, that mothers do not know soon enough that anything is the matter with their children until the time is past for them to be saved; but they can know, they ought to know; and it is proposed here to show the mother how to know promptly that her child is not well, and to determine at once what part of the body suffers or is threatened.

If an infant is well its tongue is white, its eyes bright, its flesh plump and full, and its skin soft and cool; the breathing is regular and easy and natural; when awake it is lively, cheerful, always disposed to laugh; always pleased to be played with; and when asleep it rests quietly, the countenance is composed, and conveys an expression of happy enjoyment.

SIGNS OF DISEASE.

1. If the brow is contracted, there is pain in the head; if the head is hot, and turned restlessly from side to side, and the eyes stare, or there is a glare in them, there is inflammation, and

WATER ON THE BRAIN

is threatened. Relief must be promptly had, or the child is doomed. Put cold compresses or ice-pads on the head, and keep them there; compel the feet to keep warm, give a warm sitz-bath, and keep at these until the symptoms have abated, and the child sleeps quietly, or is disposed to feed or play.

2. If the lips are apart, with a kind of gritting, there is pain in the belly, and most certainly it has been fed too much or too often.

3. If the nostrils are drawn upwards and there is quick breathing, there is pain in the chest: something is the matter with the lungs.

4. If there is a squinting in the eye, or bluish tint about the lips, and a kind of rotating movement of the eyeballs, convulsions will soon follow; there is indigestion; and a warm bath with ice-pad on the head, and an enema or a warm-water emetic must be resorted to.

5. If the eyes are unusually dull, or there is an unnatural quickness, with a pearly look of the whites, brain-disease is approaching; give an enema or a dose of castor-oil, and feed with regularity.

6. If a child usually sprightly, holding itself up straight, is noticed to drop the head and seem languid or sleepy, or if it usually goes about from chair to chair, or is disposed to climb, but suddenly shows no disposition to do anything but lie down on the floor, there is something wrong in the stomach or bowels.

7. If there is crying and the legs are drawn up, there is indigestion, and the bowels are disordered.

8. In health a child seldom carries the hands above the mouth; if that is observed repeatedly, there is something wrong in the head; the feet are cold, and they must be kept warm; if the bowels have not acted within ten hours, give an enema or a teaspoon of castor-oil every hour until there is an action.

9. A healthy child, especially if not over two years old, is often carrying the hand to the mouth; but if it stops at the throat, croup is most likely to be forming; notice instantly if the feet or hands are cold, and turn to that article.

10. In the first months of infancy, if the little one is well, it nurses, plays awhile, and then falls into a gentle, easy, good sleep; if it does not, if it is restless, especially if it starts up in its sleep, or wakes and whines, there is disturbance in the brain, and it should be seen to that the bowels are regular, feet warm, and food given at proper intervals and of a suitable quality.

11. The first passages of an infant are dark-colored, called

THE MECONIUM:

to bring this away is essential; if this is not done, the child will suffer. But the first milk secreted, called

THE COLUSTRUM,

acts as a purgative and carries the meconium before it; but if it does not come away oil must be given; sometimes warm water will answer; and in first confinements no milk appears sometimes for several days, hence any uneasiness of the first-born for the first few days may be caused by costiveness.

12. In health, young children go to sleep at once, and sleep quietly and soundly; if they are not well they do not lie down willingly at the regular hour for sleep, nor do they fall to sleep at once, nor do they sleep continuously; there are frequent turnings and changings and wakings or startings up, often in alarm—then the bowels or head are out of order.

18. The dejections of a healthy child are yellowish and thicker than thick syrup, and are of uniform appearance, from three to four times a day; less than two is costiveness. It should be rectified with an enema or castor-oil. More than three or four, and as thin as milk, and light-colored, show diarrhœa, and are rapidly debilitating; keep the belly warm, especially the feet and hands; do not feed at oftener than five hours' interval, and let the food be boiled rice, sago, tapioca, exclusively, with a little boiled milk, until there is a reduction in frequency, and greater consistency is manifested. If the stools are curdy or green or smell badly, or come out with considerable force, there is disease, to be treated as just named.

14. Crying: young children never cry if all is well; if an infant cries, it is in suffering; each mother should notice the different cries of her child, for they mean different things; a cry from hunger is very different from a cry from hurt. A sticking pin causes a quick, instantaneous cry; a string or fastening which is too tight causes a fret at first, gradually increasing as the blood accumulates. The hunger cry does not come on suddenly, for the little thing begins to turn its head or face about, or makes motions with the tongue or lips; if it cannot find the breast it begins to make a noise, gets more and more impatient, and finally breaks out into a fierce, mad cry. The wisdom of the mother, then, should be called into requisition in deciding what cries mean, but in all cases attend to them; in a young infant it often means that a change of position is needed, or that it is too warm or too cold. A good plan always is, when a child is fretful, notice at once if the feet and hands are warm. If children are regularly fed as advised elsewhere, they will never cry for hunger, unless their food is not sufficiently nourishing. A tearless cry means pain or suffering. When tears are abundant it is the cry of anger or ugliness, and should always be disregarded; very young children will soon find out as to such crying, "It's no use knocking at *that* door any more."

A moaning cry always indicates suffering, and should never be neglected.

Breathing in a healthy child is regular, slow, easy, and full: in proportion as it is different in any case there is disease. If the breathing is loud or labored or quick or fitful, there is something wrong about the throat or lungs.

15. **Cough** of any kind, from the slightest heck to a deep or suppressed hoarseness, should always command immediate attention from its uniform connection with croup, which almost always comes on in the evening, seldom all at once: generally for several days previous there have been slight symptoms of a cold, increasing every day, but an occasional cough; the face a little flushed, a little more excitability than common; fitful temper, now a laugh, then a fret: it may be measles or it may be croup; notice the feet at once, and if there is any dampness in the clothing; inquire particularly about the exposures of the day preceding; the questions to the nurse cannot be too minute or searching: require specific, decided answers. Usually an attack of croup comes on after the child has been asleep a while, and is likely to wake with a cough, different from an ordinary one: it has a ring or whistle or wheezing with it, a dry cough, no loosening of phlegm is present. This first cough may not wake the child, but do not leave it for an instant; and if the second cough occurs, especially if the hand is carried to the throat, it is croup: act accordingly.

But let it be deeply impressed on the mother's mind that if the child is kept comfortably warm for every second of its existence, especially the hands and feet: if it is fed at stated hours only, and has regular and abundant sleep, three-fourths of all the diseases of infancy and childhood would be swept from existence.

ERUPTIONS.

The very instant a mother observes the skin of the child changed in appearance, even if it be for the space of a quarter of an inch, there is meaning in it: the child is not well: there is bad blood, and Nature is endeavoring to cast the poison out of the system. One thing should never be done,—put nothing on the eruption stronger than sweet oil or pure water; give the child an enema or a dose of cas-tor-oil, then let it have a warm bath, with a wet cloth or cap on the head, then adhere to regular feeding; keep the whole body, the feet, and the hands abundantly warm, so as to keep the erup-tion out until it very gradually fades away. The sudden striking in of an eruption is a serious warning, and instant measures should be used to bring it back, either by a warm bath or by get-ting the little patient into a healthy perspiration.

If the eruption be a swelling, especially if there is heat, apply cold compresses.

That the intelligent mother may be more deeply impressed with the advantages which watchfulness and care and timely precau-tion have on the lives of infants and children—infancy reaching to two years, and childhood to eight;—it is only necessary to state that during the last century, of every twenty-four infants born in the poor-houses of London, twenty-three died the first year. When the attention of the public authorities was drawn to the subject more care was given to the little ones; they were fed regularly, dressed warmly, and provided with well-ventilated rooms to sleep in, with the result that immediately only one in six died instead of twenty-three out of twenty-four, showing clearly that a hundred children died every month unnecessarily from avoidable causes; not only so, many infants are destroyed every year, even now, by intelligent mothers, from injudicious interference with Nature's operations, and very often in the direction of tampering with various eruptions and sores, endeavoring to heal them up when they are Nature's efforts to save the child. All those sores which break out about the head and ears during the whole teeth-ing of infancy are of this character; they should never be dried up, never washed with anything else than the purest, softest rain or snow water, generally cold; then apply cold water dressings, poultices, or compresses for a great part of the time; meanwhile keep the whole skin of the body perfectly clean, washed well with water, or put in a bath twice a day, rubbed well with the hands during and after the bath; keep the bowels acting twice a day; give several hours' outdoor airing, two or three in the morning and one or two in the afternoon, with regular feeding, not oftener than four times in the twenty-four hours—three would be still better. The same treatment is specially applicable to the multitude of skin-diseases to which infancy and childhood are subject, such as tetter, scald head, ring-worm, plica polonica, where the hair becomes glued together by the exudation from the scalp, and many others; taking care that in all scalp-diseases the hair should be kept cut very short all the time; remembering, too, that all poultices other than pure water keep the parts more filthy, and retard recovery, and that all washes in the nature of astringents, even although as simple as alum water, oak bark, and common tea, tend directly to cause water on the brain, or some other internal ailment quite as fatal.

FOOD CURE.

DIABETES has been cured in its early stages, and the symptoms greatly modified in incurable cases by the patient subsisting altogether on skimmed milk, all the cream carefully removed,—eating nothing, drinking nothing but three or four quarts of this skimmed sweet milk every day, taking a pint or two every four hours; the sugar begins to disappear from the urine within a week, but it should be persevered in for a full month, then for two weeks curdle it with rennet; then take lean meats, vegetables, and coarse bread.

Persons getting well can eat potatoes when they relish nothing else. They should always be cooked with the skin on, because the real nourishment—that which makes flesh—is found in the eighth of an inch, including this outer skin; but strange to say, this part is usually peeled off and thrown away. They should be baked, boiled, or steamed. Wash the potatoes in cold water as quickly as possible, put them in an iron saucepan, two-thirds full of potatoes, with no water, cover very tightly with a lid, place it over a hot fire; three-fourths of the potato is water, hence steam, which is hotter than boiling water, cooks them more rapidly; take them out as quick as possible when done, wrap them up in a cloth, or cover them over and they are ready to be eaten, with an almost floury mellowness. Or the potatoes can be cut in thin slices and then treated in the same way; experience will soon teach how long a time is required to cook them in either case.

SMALL-POX.

To set at rest the two questions—Does vaccination prevent small-pox ? Does vaccination introduce other diseases into the system ? it is only necessary to note a few facts and figures. In the kingdom of Bavaria every soldier was required to be revaccinated on entering the army for a period of fourteen years; during that whole time there was not a single case of small-pox, nor a single death.

Of fifty thousand soldiers revaccinated in the Prussian army, about one-third "took," showing that vaccination was a preventive, at least in two-thirds of the cases, for twenty years.

The chief English vaccinators, Drs. Mason, Stevens, Jenner, and West, vaccinated one hundred and nineteen thousand persons, old and young, without noting a single case where another disease was introduced into the system by vaccination.

The proper method of vaccination, taking it for granted that the vaccine matter is good, is to introduce it at four different points on the arm.

An attack of small-pox has been known to cure insanity; in all cases it leaves the system less liable to all attacks of other forms of disease.

If a person who has the small-pox is kept in a perfectly dark room during the whole time, allowing the light of but a single candle, there will be no pitting on the face; there never is under the hair, as it keeps the scalp always in darkness; then, also, there is but little pain, slight itching, and scarcely any smell at all; or varnish the eruption, as soon as it appears, with collodion, and then cover with a layer of fine wool or cotton; this adheres to the collodion; then brush the whole with a solution of gum-arabic, occasionally reapplying this gum, as the cotton may be disposed to rise at the edges; or, after painting the face with gun-cotton, sprinkle it over with the dust of pipe-clay, and repeat it thrice a a day, as the pustules break; this dust seems to absorb the matter which spreads the disease, and removes the itching and burning.

NERVOUS PROSTRATION,

Or debility, arises from three causes : worldly anxiety, over brain work, family troubles.

By the first is meant the constant strain on the brain in devising plans to " get along," to " keep up."   In cities particularly it must be dreadful.

By the second is meant excessive effort in the management of one's business, under circumstances of heavy responsibility.

In the third are included the loss of children, or what is a thousand times worse than death, their dishonor, their getting into bad habits, idleness, drunkenness, gambling, and crime ; these are the things which break a father's heart and send so many mothers to the mad-house.

Among these family troubles are those which come in the relationship of man and wife ; no one but a physician can form a proper estimate of these troubles, their depth, their frequency, and the little causes which lead thereto.   A good many men are meanly jealous.   It is the petty foible of the weak-minded.

In a woman it is a weakness, very often a misapprehension, but for all that it is a terrible trial to the heart.

Another source of trouble is a want of sympathy between man and wife.   The remedy for this is to take a greater interest in each other's department ; endeavor to save each other trouble ; do all you can for one another, to help each other along.   The wife ought not to be so concerned about being able to dress well as to be all oblivious of the means which the husband has to use to secure the money for the same ; nor ought the husband to see his wife worried by the servants and the children, and take no more interest in rectifying matters than if he were a member of another family. If a husband soils his clothing unnecessarily, his wife being his washer-woman ; if he stalks through the house without wiping his feet at the door, making ugly marks which it may require half an hour's work to remove ; if he causes meals to be delayed, or comes in long after they are over, not caring how much trouble he may occasion to prepare one anew ; if he permits his wife to get up and make a fire by which to cook breakfast, instead of getting up himself, allowing her to rest in bed until it is burning enough to cook by; if he brings in visitors and friends, inopportunely, and without notice, especially on wash-days; if he has the vulgarity to be always grumbling, finding fault with everything, pleased with nothing, as if he were perfection itself, never praising, never commending; no wonder that a woman who was once regarded as but little less than an angel should have her nervous system racked and ruined.

On the other hand, and it is not infrequent, that a woman is never satisfied with any exertions her husband can make to get along, but is always upbraiding him for not doing better; for not making money faster; for not being more of a gentleman; why don't you dress like so and so; then there is another large class of women as cold as icicles, who never meet fire with fire, always indifferent, always tardy, always log-like, or forever ready to interpose excuses and planting obstacles and making objections, and this, too, from sheer perverseness and not from injury experienced, —these are the things which drive men mad, which drive them to the club house, the drinking saloon, the corner grocery, and to the house of her whose "steps take hold on hell," and then when the die is cast, these same women wake up, as if they were as innocent as babes unborn, as if they had never done a harmful thing in the whole course of their lives.

Another frequent cause of utter nervous prostration in multitudes of cases is the inconsiderateness of married women absenting themselves from their homes for a week, or month, or a year at a time, leaving their husbands while they are enjoying themselves. Two examples will convey the author's meaning. A lady had been married six years, and had three beautiful children; she had often said that there was nothing within her husband's means which he would not willingly do to gratify her. She had her own beautiful home; carriages and horses were at her command. She thought she had too much family care, and proposed a housekeeper; it increased expenses, but the husband yielded; she made her own selection, that of an active, tidy, pushing, self-asserting young woman. The wife then thought that she would like to make a visit West. She did so, enjoyed herself very much, so much so indeed that from time to time she made excuses for staying a little longer, and at the end of eleven months returned home, soon became jealous, assumed an air of injured innocence, applied for a divorce, obtained it, and in three months her former husband was married. Twenty years have passed away, and she remains a broken-hearted woman.

Not long ago a lady in the very prime of life obtained her husband's permission to make a distant journey to remain a year. On her return she saw enough to overthrow her reason, and now spends her time in a private asylum with an allowance of five thousand dollars a year. The woman who leaves her family for a month defies fate; it ought never to be done for even a short week, unless there is an absolute necessity for it. Three men out of four are unwilling to be cheated; if they are, they feel themselves at liberty to make it up in some other way. They admit that in ordinary circumstances it is not right, but in their case there is a peculiarity, and is admissible. David wanted Uriah's wife; he did not think it right to order the husband's head to be taken off, but he persuaded himself that it was "all on the square" to put him in front of the battle where it was pretty certain he would fall by the hand of the enemy, and human nature is as subtle now as in David's day.

But as to the cure of nervous prostration, medicine in any and all of its forms may well be considered a miserable failure in comparison to proper hygienic measures, hence neither will allopathy or homœopathy be called to our aid.

In all these things the mind has gotten into a rut, and must be lifted out of it; other parts of the brain must be brought into requisition, and thus give those rest which have been at work too much, almost enough to disorganize them. In addition, the whole body must be forced into the large exercise of muscular activities, and as near as possible, compulsory; activities which must be engaged in every day, rain or shine; the best are those which compel journeying through strange countries, over untrodden deserts, intractable mountains, dangerous forests, where must be encountered the sierra, the ravine, the chasm, the precipice, the cañon, the untrodden prairies, the unnavigated river, and all along to be fed by chance, every now and then not fed at all; or as a hand before the mast on a sail-vessel by Magellan or the Cape of Good Hope. If none of these are available, then food and medicine and water must be brought into requisition. In all cases keep clean; breathe all the time a pure air, maintain a full, free action of the bowels every day. Be out on horseback, or walking or boating every available hour between breakfast and sundown, so as to compel the nervous energies to get out of the body through the muscles instead of the brain, thus giving it rest. If you have not strength to sit on a horse, have some one behind you to hold you up; if you can't ride fifty yards without great fatigue, ride ten, twenty to-day and twenty-five to-morrow, and so on, but ride, and remain in bed until you get rested, if it requires twenty hours out of the twenty-four every day, sending more of the nervous energy out through the muscles every day, less through the brain, meanwhile using a fruit diet, except that at dinner lean meats may be freely used, and if not too weak, a cool hip-bath every day; if very weak or chilly take a tepid bath, less and less warm until a bracing cold one can be taken, remembering all the time :—

The body must be nourished. The bowels must be kept free. The brain must be rested. The nervous power must be sent out through the muscles. The old business, the old occupation must be totally abandoned for the present. And sleep must be courted and indulged in to the fullest extent that the body will take, but not to be promoted by any drug yet known to man ; let it come from weariness ; for tiredness is the only safe anodyne.

———∞———

BRIGHT'S DISEASE

Was formerly called Albuminuria, because the albumen of the blood escaped through the kidneys; now called Bright's disease because a London physician of that name was the first to publish a more satisfactory account of the nature of the malady in 1827. It appears in two forms, acute and chronic; easily cured if promptly attended to when it first appears ; always fatal when it is allowed to go on so long as to become fixed or chronic ; hence it is of the utmost importance to know its first symptoms ; it occurs most generally from forty-five to sixty-five years of age ; one-third more common in men than in women. After exposure to wet and cold on a drunken fit, or an attack of scarlet fever, the skin becomes dry and cold, with headache, nausea, vomiting, pain in the back and limbs, and some difficulty in breathing. The urine is small in quantity, frequent, heavy and dark, because there is so much blood in it; the kidneys being so much congested in the small blood-vessels that the blood oozes through as well as the watery portion, as explained in the article on congestion. If the deposit is noticed through a microscope there will be seen blood-corpuscles, little tubes of albumen, and masses of fibrin. Within three weeks recovery or death takes place usually; some cases linger for months in the chronic form. Death generally results from dropsy, or some form of inflammation. About two-thirds of the acute cases recover. The most approved treatment by allopathy is cupping the loins over the kidneys to relieve the congestion, application of blankets dipped in boiling water and wrung out; free purging every day, and a nutritious liquid diet.

In the chronic form, which comes on very slowly in the course of months and years, there is a gradual loss of strength; the face is pale and puffy, some shortness of breath, and a frequent disposition to urinate.

But instead of showing these symptoms by degrees it sometimes comes on very suddenly in the form of a convulsion, amaurosis, difficult breathing, or violent inflammation in some one part of the body; then follow the symptoms named in the acute form, then getting better, to come on again with greater violence, at intervals of weeks, months, and years.

About one-third die from the blood being poisoned in consequence of the urine not being taken from it by the kidneys, as many almost die from general dropsy.

It was said that colds and wet and dampness and drunkenness bring on the disease. Drunken persons are very liable to just such exposures, going to sleep on the damp ground or grass. The kidneys are imbedded with fat, as may be seen in the butcher's shop, as if Nature intended them to be well protected from colds, as also from jars and wounds and bruises. All who wear a stout material of woollen flannel next the body habitually do much towards preventing Bright's disease.

Life and health are maintained by two processes: one of these is taking into the body from the external world materials which will sustain life; the other consists in casting out of the body that which, if allowed to remain, will destroy it. It is computed that almost as large a portion of the wastes of the system are carried out of it through the kidneys as by dejection through the rectum. The blood of the body passes through the kidneys,

whose province it is to withdraw from it certain waste principles, which, combined, are called urea, and are floated out of the
body by the urine. Bright's disease is a disease of the kidneys
in which they fail to unload the blood of those particles which it
ought to do, and at the same time allows a way of escape of certain other particles which ought to remain in the body, to be used
for purposes of health. The urea not being taken from the blood,
poisons it and affects the nervous system immediately, causing
convulsions, stupor, epilepsy, and death. These symptoms, in
connection with scarlet and puerperal attacks, are the result of
urine poisoning. If, therefore, the urea is not taken from the
blood, there is not so much discharged from the bladder; hence an
infallible result is a scanty discharge of urine, and that is a symptom never absent in Bright's disease; that is, a habitually small
discharge, for temporarily a person who perspires a great deal, all
healthy persons in warm weather send a large part of the water
out of the body through the skin, has less to be passed by the
bladder.

The usual amount of urine passed from a healthy person every
twenty-four hours is from fifty to seventy-five tablespoonfuls, that
is, from twenty-five to thirty-five ounces, or on an average about
two pints or pounds; if then there is not half that much for a
week or more, prompt attention should be given to it. In fact,
free, copious urination is a sign of good health; it "carries" off
internal fever, and keeps the blood pure. Hence medicines are
given to "act on the kidneys," that is, to prompt urination, as buttermilk, flaxseed tea. Water-melons are famous in that direction; when out of season, their seeds are made a tea of for the
same purpose. The common lemon has such a striking effect in
that direction, that it is used to cure dropsies, a case of which, in
an aggravated form, was successfully treated by taking one lemon
a day, one-third of it at three different times for three days; then
a whole lemon was taken morning, noon, and night, and in three
days more two were taken at a time, morning, noon, and
night, until eighteen were taken every day; then diminish the
number by one a day. At the end of the seventh day the urine
increased in quantity and kept on increasing until the dropsy was
perfectly cured. The same remedy might cure Bright's disease
in its forming stages, when the urine was observed to be scant
in quantity for a week or more, with the first symptoms of the
malady already described.

In the very first stages of Bright's disease, that of beginning congestion, there is too much urine, increased by the exudation of the serous portions of the blood, as before stated ; next, blood is exuded ; then there is disorganization of the structure of the kidneys, and death is inevitable. From all these statements the philosophy of treatment and cure is to begin promptly and give a liver pill, to be repeated every week; between these give some salts, so as to have two actions of the bowels every day ; take freely such remedies as act on the kidneys and promote urination, keep warm woollen pads or wet compresses to the small of the back, reaching to the shoulder-blades, and the special fruit diet ; all hope being in the prompt treatment of the first symptoms. Hydropathy and homœopathy treat this disease on the general principle of reducing inflammation and relieving congestion ; the latter is accomplished by hydropathists in the use of a loosening diet, compresses and fomentations and a general building up of the health. Homœopathy reduces inflammation of that important organ by aconite, cantharides, and hepar sulphur. If very painful, belladonna ; colchicum, if there is nausea and red urine, aided by abstaining from all forms of spirits, and cultivating quietude of body.

SHAVING.

ONE of the most disgusting face diseases, as well as tedious of cure, is often communicated to gentlemen by being shaved in a barber's shop with a razor which has just been used on the face of a man who had the malady. It ought to be a very urgent necessity which should induce us to go into a strange shop for a shave ; better go unshaven for a year than to run the risk of a disease which it sometimes takes a year to cure. The cause of the malady is a vegetable product which sprouts up by millions around the root of each particular hair, causing a filthy yellow matter, which scabs and scales, and seems to renew itself indefinitely long. This vegetable growth multiplies itself, and scatters its seeds by millions in a very short time. But there is an infallible preventive, costing nothing, yet the reader won't use it, not one in a hundred, simply from a reckless perversity, peculiar to the animal man. If the razor is dipped in hot water, carefully wiped, and dipped in hot water again, the contagion is impossible, because the hot water scalds the life out of the seed, as it would out of a grain of wheat, or any other farm product.

RULES FOR SHAVING.

Lather the face well, rub it into the skin and lather again; the soap takes the oil out of each hair and leaves it stiff and brittle. Then sharpen your razor and lather again.

Move the razor over the face in a sloping or mowing direction, not at right angles with the hairs; it thus mows or saws them off.

Do not tighten the skin with the hand, only as much as you can do so with the unaided muscles of the face, then you are not so likely to cut into the skin.

Let the razor lie as flat on the skin as possible; you may not shave as closely, but then you will very rarely cut the skin; the higher the back of the razor is above the skin the more likely are you to wound the face.

He is the most independent man who habituates himself to shave with cold water.

As soon as you have finished shaving strop your razor on the coarser side, because the razor then is warm and soft and sharpens sooner. Next wipe the razor well with soft buckskin, and then strike it flat on the pants or an ottoman, which will cover it with dust to absorb any possible dampness which may be left.

Wash the part shaved in cold water, flap it up against the face with the hands, not only to wash off all the soap, but to cool the skin, which has been irritated and inflamed by the sharp edge of the razor.

When you go to shave again, first lather your face as above, then wipe the dust from the razor carefully, strop it on the coarser side; for its being cold the edge is rougher than when put away, and these rough points are worn off; then use the smoothest side of the strop, do not bear hard; that rounds off the edge, as the leather rises immediately behind it before it gets away.

Draw the razor from heel to point and as diagonally as possible, for then a larger amount of razor surface touches the strop before you get to the end of it than if the razor is drawn more nearly at right angles across the strop.

32

It will require a longer time to sharpen the razor by pressing lightly, but it will be a smoother shave.

The last thing before shaving draw the razor a number of times from heel to point on the ball of the thumb, that is, the palm of the hand between the root of the thumb and wrist; this warms it and makes the edge a great deal keener.

Too much stropping will give a wire edge and a rough shave; in that case, draw the razor across the end of the thumb nail; if the edge is wiry there will be a feeling of roughness or filing or sawing.

COLD CREAM.

ONE ounce each of spermaceti and white wax, with a quarter of a pint of oil of almonds, mix and pour into a mortar which has been warmed by dipping into hot water, add while stirring four ounces of rose-water until it is cold, then let it stand in a convenient glass or glazed vessel. A pomade preparation consists of a hard, fresh hog's lard never salted, and well washed in cold water three times; in the fourth fresh water let it soak in a cool place for twenty-four hours; wash it once more; pour off the water and beat into it as much of the best rose-water as it will absorb during the beating. This is very useful to have in the family all the time as an ointment for sores, cuts, burns, bruises, irritated surfaces, chapped hands and lips. This is useful to keep on hand all the time; persons who have to be out in the cold a great deal should apply this freely to all sores, cuts, or scratches; it prevents inflammation.

PAIN EXTRACTOR, to be kept ready for use in every family, there is perhaps nothing of the kind equal to it. One ounce each of spirits of hartshorn, laudanum, and origanum; stir these into half a pound of mutton tallow, when it is nearly cooled. Rub it well into any painful part, and then spread some on a rag and apply it as a plaster; should be kept in a jar or pot well covered.

PHYSIOLOGY.

AT the top of the cut the convolutions of the brain are shown.

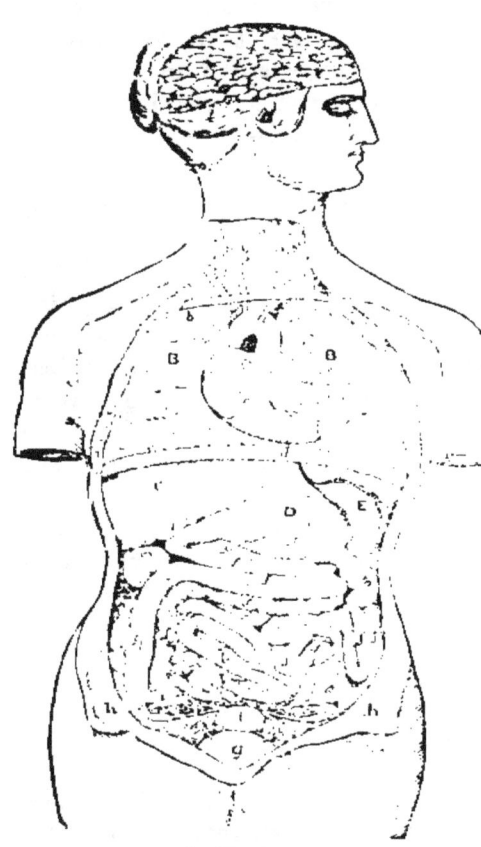

The windpipe is seen entering the lungs back of *a*, the aorta. The heart A is not exactly in the centre of the lungs, but a little to the left; if the lungs are fully distended it cannot be seen.

The bowels or intestines are seen in a number of convolutions; in health they are always in motion, more or less decided; if they move too much it is diarrhœa or cholera, hence one of the very best remedies in either case is a bandage of woollen flannel, over a foot broad, bound tightly around the abdomen, so compressing it that they have not room to move; this affords a delightful sensation of immediate relief, and a person who could not have walked half a dozen yards without stopping or resting, can walk half a mile with considerably less fatigue; besides the flannel imparts warmth.

As no sore can possibly heal if it is constantly picked, or is pressed apart every hour, so when a bowel is penetrated it rarely heals, for two reasons; either the part wounded instinctively rests on the instant, or the other portions are

A. The heart.
B B. The lungs.
C. Liver.
D. Stomach.
a. The aorta.
B. Lungs.
c. Windpipe.
d. Diaphragm.
f. The intestines.
g. Bladder.
h. Ligaments.
i. Uterus.
m. Kidneys.

in incessant motion, working their contents downwards, and when they come to the wounded part they escape into the abdomen, causing inevitably inflammation and death.   Hence the most important practical truth that if a sharp instrument enters the abdomen, or a bullet penetrates the bowels, the person more certainly dies than if the bullet entered the brain or the heart.   Unless a weapon or bullet divides a large blood-vessel, the person may live three or four days ; this fact is of immense importance at times, for while it shows that death must come, it gives time for the adjustment of various important matters.

If the intestines do not move enough they are said to be torpid, and constipation is an inevitable result.   This is a very common attendant of dyspepsia, and very remarkable cures have been sometimes effected by a regular, patient attention to kneading the bowels gently after each meal, that is, by pressing inwards and downwards with the ball of the hand for about five minutes, beginning at the lower edge of the ribs on one side and going round to the other side and backwards ; the intestines are thus made to move mechanically.   Others have been successful, remarkably so, by pelting the whole abdomen, to the extent before mentioned, with the balls of the fingers and thumb, spread out like a fan. Of course gentle means like these should be persisted in, but the cure is founded on philosophical principles and will seldom fail to compensate for the trouble taken.

LAXATIVES,

PURGATIVES, and cathartics are medicines which act on the bowels ; that is, being taken into the stomach they pass through the body and carry before them the contents of stomach and bowels, by causing more or less watery passages.   Purgatives so irritate the mucous membrane of the bowels as to cause them to push their contents onwards and downwards, as rhubarb.

Laxatives do not excite or irritate, they simply relax, and thus as it were open the gates of the system, and let the fluids pass out, as Epsom salts, an ounce at the time, dissolved in water, or a good tablespoonful ; a teaspoonful for a child. Unless there is urgency, it would be better to take half an ounce at night, and half in the morning on an empty stomach, the action would then be less violent, less weakening, and more protracted in its good effects, without leaving the bowels more costive than natural.

CASTOR-OIL

is another remedy for loosening the bowels. In full doses of two tablespoonfuls it goes through the body in a few hours; but in that case acts several times and largely, leaving considerable weakness and costiveness also, there being no action sometimes for several days.

If taken in small doses, night and morning, one, two, or three teaspoonfuls at a time, just enough to move the bowels once in twenty-four hours, it will be found to be the simplest, safest, and most unobjectionable remedy for constipation yet known. Each person can notice for himself how much it requires to act in his case once freely, keep it up for a few days until the system gets into the habit of acting; then first diminish each dose, then omit one dose, finally the other; but resume with returning costiveness. The great objection to its use is its taste, but pour the dose in the middle of any kind of fluid, put the rim of the vessel far back on the tongue, toss it up quickly and down it will slide, only do not draw the breath nor allow the oil to touch the lips; then it leaves no taste, only the taste of the vehicle. The castor bean grows in our gardens. The pressed seeds yield the oil. A good laxative in the form of a pill is made of forty grains of pulverized aloes, twenty grains of pulverized gum guaiacum, ten grains of pulverized gamboge, made into eighty-two pills with gum-arabic water; take two at bed-time, just enough to give one free action next morning; or,

Twenty grains each of aloes, rhubarb, and ipecac, made into thirty pills with gum water; take one or two, night and morning.

Perhaps one of the best pills ever devised for keeping up a moderate daily action of the bowels was formerly known as the

DINNER PILL,

first noticed in Paris in 1758. Take six drachms of the very best Socotrine aloes, two drachms each of mastic and red roses, made up with syrup of wormwood, made into pills of three grains each. They are also called and can be had at any good drug store; they were originally taken one at a time, about an hour before dinner, hence the name; take one or two at bedtime, just enough to act gently on the bowels next morning. But the reader should bear in mind, that the habitual use of any medicine to keep the bowels in a proper condition is always pernicious in the end; hence every means possible should be used to secure that result by natural agencies, such as coarse breads, fruits, and berries, aided by out-door activities. See "Medical Prescriptions," under the head of Laxatives.

POISON IVY VINE.

SOME persons are very liable to be poisoned by touching the leaves of this vine, or even coming near them; others are not affected at all; the skin of the face and hands itches, reddens, burns, swells, then watery blisters appear, break, and the skin peels off within a week. Bathe or wash the parts freely with sweet spirits of nitre, whether the skin is broken or not, or pour boiling water on a hard piece of lime-stone, called quick-lime, stir it, let it settle, and apply it to the parts with a brush or soft rag or sponge, night and morning until cured; or keep the parts well smeared with any kind of oil, but the first-named remedies are best. Keep the bowels acting very freely, three times in two days, with "special fruit diet." The same remedies are applied to other poisonous effects from plants. Or bathe the part thrice a day with sweet oil or common rum; if sores break, apply starch. Some wash with a decoction of witch-hazel bark, with the diet above.

The effects of the poison-oak or rhus toxicodendron are promptly controlled and removed by painting the eruption with the fluid extract of serpentaria, or Virginia snakeroot, night and morning, causing the bowels to act twice a day during the application, living altogether on coarse bread, rice, and fruits. Solutions of copperas, oxide of zinc, or lead-water are efficient, but are never safe without the free bowels and diet just named.

DISEASES
PECULIAR TO WOMEN,

WITH

SUBJECTS PERTAINING

TO THE

MARRIED RELATION.

DISEASES PECULIAR TO WOMEN.

TO PARENTS.

It is not profitable to children and youth to indulge in reading on subjects pertaining to the married relation, hence what is said in that connection is brought all together, and may be bound or secured with cloth or tape, in such a manner as to prevent the younger members of the family from having ready access thereto. Perhaps a better plan would be to keep the whole book under lock and key; parents making it a point from time to time to read such portions, with comments upon them, at such seasons and on such occasions, as might aid in impressing on the mind valuable practical lessons which may be applicable for a lifetime, attention to which might in very many cases prevent suffering and weary sickness, and premature death. A young man whose constitution was hopelessly broken by habits which naturally led to that end, but which he did not see, invoked curses on the memory of his father, in the author's hearing, for never having given him any instruction about guarding against disease or saying anything to him which was calculated to impress on his mind the immeasurable importance of taking care of the health.

A physician often hears the lament, coming with a sigh of agony from the bottom of the heart, "Oh! if mother had only told me a little about such things, I could so easily have avoided what I suffer." It is especially the duty of mothers to begin at the age of twelve years, with their daughters, to open up to their minds the coming change, to be looked for about fourteen, and sometimes a year or two or more earlier; it is safer to begin at twelve. They will hear at school hints about private diseases, especially such as are induced by bad practices, and when they see or feel anything unusual there is an instinctive prompting to conceal it, and to take measures in their own hands to remove indications, which very measures may have disastrous results upon the system, to last for a lifetime. A child, for example, observes a stain; the most natural resort is cold water; it is not effectual; more is used and more, until the parts are chilled, suppression takes place, liable to cause a variety of ill results.

About the same time also the breasts may begin to develop themselves; the same kind of shrinking is felt, means are taken to conceal it by a greater tightening of the dress at these parts, interfering with the circulation, arresting the flow of blood, hardening the glands, and laying the foundation for cancer in the breast; hence it is better at the age of twelve, in these latitudes, to begin to communicate by degrees such information as to these matters as may be serviceable under the circumstances. Make the communications in a casual way; do not make a mountain of it, let it be an incidental thing; not a long story at a time, and with no air of mystery, or secrecy, or in whisperings with closed doors; better to treat the whole subject as a matter-of-course affair, so as to have the child's mind at ease; this will enable it to give fuller attention to the subject and comprehend it more thoroughly than under other circumstances.

The same suggestion may be made to fathers in reference to their sons, who by instinct, without any teacher; or sooner, at the suggestions of vicious servants, or apprentices, or their own associates, fall into habits of procuring sexual gratifications, and about which some suggestions judiciously made would be a great advantage to the boy in various ways.

These things are spoken of in subsequent pages.

MATERNITY.

The noble Queen of England, with the intelligent coöperation of her lamented husband, reared a family of nine sons and daughters to maturity, without a single serious case of illness, by a firm and persistent attention to the ascertained laws of health and life in eating, sleeping, exercise, and manual labor, in accordance with the counsels of eminent medical men at court; and there is no necessary reason why other persons, contemplating parentage, should not secure a similar happy result. How this can be uniformly done, may be learned from the following pages.

LAW OF PERPETUATION.

" Whose seed is in itself," was the announcement of the great law of life by the wise and loving Father of All, before man was. " Like begets like," is a more modern and familiar expression of the same important practical fact. This law governs the perpetuation of every living thing, from the moss and lichen on the rocks, to the blade of the prairie, the flower of the field, the oak of the forest; from the invisible living things which float in ether, to insect and fish and animal and man. The truth is so generally recognized by savage as well as civilized nations, that it is acted upon in every part of the habitable globe in reference to the growth of our fields and the multiplication of our herds ; but in a direction infinitely more important, it is absolutely and everywhere disregarded.

Every farmer, even the most unintelligent, has mother-wit enough to endeavor to secure the very best " seed " wheat for his planting. The wild Arab who, upon his mettled courser, sweeps in kingly pride over the desert wastes of his country, spares no pains in improving by breed and culture the fleetness of his stock: while cultivated man, with science to direct and Christianity to urge to the execution, does nothing ; leaves to chance the impress of the physical, mental, and moral character of those who may be born to him ; and this, in face of the plainest mandate within the lids of the Bible, " Train up a child in the way he should go." Train him up for " length of days," for being useful to the highest intent, in his generation, and in such a way as will make it most certain that he shall secure a beatific existence beyond the boundary of time. The men and women who marry with a deliberate purpose like this, and will carry it out to the utmost of their ability, science guiding, and religious principle helping to execute, will be the forerunners of an evangel second only to that of him who came " crying in the wilderness ; " for the result will be simply this, that all who are born would grow up to be healthy, intelligent, and good.

Every parent can see for himself how wholly such ends as these have failed to enter his calculation and his deliberate plannings, except in part, at a time too late to accomplish the highest results.

THE LEPER.

The leprosy of the olden time was not only fearful in its rav ages upon the system, but the restrictions imposed on the unfortunate persons who were its victims, made it, if possible, a still more terrible calamity : to be an outcast from society ; to come in contact with no living soul ; to be shunned instinctively by all of humankind, and lest persons should approach unawares, to be compelled to give a loud warning to all coming near, " Keep away ! unclean, unclean ! " A disease for which there is no cure this side the grave ! The skin becomes dry and scaly ; the hair falls out ; the eyebrows and eyelashes drop off ; the nails of the fingers and toes are eaten away ; ugly excrescences and putrid sores deform the person. By imperceptible yet resistless advances, the miserable body, joint by joint, wastes away, yet not to be arrested by natural death, until the corrupted, disfigured mass has scarcely a relic to indicate that it had ever been human ! It requires no argument to prove that it would be a crime to perpetuate, to hand down to a child, such a horrible malady.

But here is a young man of wealthy parentage, of high social position, having a collegiate education and the means of an idle life. He soon finds the habitation of her whose " steps take hold on hell ; " every fibre of the system becomes diseased ; every drop of blood in the body rankles with an unquenchable fire of poison—a poison which no human remedy has ever succeeded in eradicating : irons heated to whiteness have failed and always will fail to burn out the canker, because it is in the blood ; splotches break out on the body, oftener on the face, sometimes eating away the nose ; as if Divinity intended to affix the mark of Cain, and to advertise all humankind to hold the victim in unutterable loathing. Medical skill sometimes patches up these men so far as to enable them to present an unsuspicious exterior, and by forced temperance and studied cleanliness of person and clothing, a semblance of health remains ; but only a semblance : the serpent poison still rankles within, only hidden enough to cause pardoning friends and kindred to sketch the whole history and character in the light sentence, " He *was* a fast young man." As much as to say, " It is a thing of the past ; it was among the

indiscretions of youth, but the effects have all been obliterated."
The assertion is a terrible untruth. A lifetime of purity and
temperance cannot wash away the taint, and every child born to
such a man will be born with a scrofulous constitution, to be for
a lifetime, with apparent intervals of reasonable health, afflicted;
with brain diseases in early childhood; inanition and wasting
away; predisposition to attacks of all prevalent diseases; to
slow and imperfect recoveries from the maladies of childhood,
followed by running sores from various parts of the body—from
the neck, in the shape of King's Evil; from the joints, giving
rise to white swellings, rickets, and St. Vitus' Dance; from the
ear, inducing life-long deafness; in later life a greater liability
to all diseases of the lungs, giving tubercles, the seeds of consumption; always being the foundation of various breakings out
on the body, of weak eyes, of slender bones, of frail constitutions, and of the dreadful cancer.

Now it is easy for a well-balanced mind to feel that it is a
crime in any man to perpetuate maladies like these. But the
principle is the same if lesser evils be entailed on the innocent
unborn. Hence the broad general truth cannot be denied, that
it is both a duty and a humanity on the part of all who contemplate parentage to make it a study how to avoid perpetuating disease, and how to secure to those who may be born to them the
highest possible advantages, physical, mental, and moral, not only
as a means of surrounding them with all the aids calculated to
insure enjoyment and usefulness here, but happiness in a blessed
hereafter.

GESTATION

means a "carrying," literally, and is synonymous with pregnancy, but is a more refined term. Catamenia is the better
name for the monthly turns, monthly sickness, menses, etc., conveying the idea of something which occurs monthly. If mothers
will accustom themselves and their daughters, as they grow up,
to employ the terms used by physicians, these being unknown to
most persons, it will be much easier to speak of them, as they
will appear less indelicate and less vulgar. If, after the catamenia have been occurring regularly, there should be a cessation,

without some more palpable cause, of shock or accident, or serious sickness or exposure to cold and wet, the wife may set it down as a fact that the foundation of a new existence has been laid, that

IMPREGNATION

has taken place, the duration of which is two hundred and eighty days, or forty weeks, sometimes sooner, sometimes later ; but in the great majority of cases of healthy women, that is the time, and is called "nine months." When that time will expire occasions thousands of conjectures and calculations, for the expectant mother wants to know the exact day as nearly as possible.

Impregnation or Conception takes place generally within ten days after being "unwell." Hence it is usual to count forty weeks from the day of the last cessation. Sometimes impregnation takes place just before the catamenia ; but the great general rule is that it occurs soon after, for then the woman is in a state of feeling and preparation and desire for the great generative act. Man is an animal, woman is purity ; he is always ready ; she seems to have the instinct of perpetuation only at the time the system is most susceptible of it, as if she lived to obey the Divine injunction, "multiply," rather than for purposes of passional indulgence.

Human inquisitiveness into the secret laws and operations of Nature has been carried to the extent of attempting to ascertain whether sex can be under the control of the human will. It is doubtful if the Almighty ever intended that the secret should be discovered, for it seems to be a necessity that the number of men and women should bear a certain proportion, that more males should be born than females, to answer the requisitions of war, and the accidents involving loss of life, which attend the more exposed occupations of men ; for many of them are perilous, as in working mines, and in sailor life. A law seems to prevail in animal existence, which in its application to the human race seems to show that if the impregnating act—which is generally denominated in these pages as the

" MARITAL RIGHT " OR " CONSUMMATION,"

being the thing which both husband and wife are entitled to, and which neither can refuse without invading the rights of the other, and which is consequently a great wrong, unless the demands are excessive, which subject is discussed elsewhere—if the marital right is performed within a day or two after the cessation of the catamenia, of the time of being unwell, the product will be a female; the longer it is delayed, the more probable is it that it will be a boy; usually no impregnation follows the marital act, when it is performed later than ten days after the catamenial cessation.

The first child usually comes two weeks earlier, in thirty-eight weeks instead of forty.

Another mode of counting is to calculate from the

QUICKENING,

which is the instant when the new being seems first to take up the life of motion; it stirs convulsively within the mother at the end of four months and a half from the date of impregnation. But a vigorous child moves sooner; then, again, the mother may be at the time so much engaged in important matters, that her mind will not take cognizance of the fact, but the quickening, in connection with the time of the catamenial cessation, serves to confirm the correctness of the " count." This quickening is not unlike the flutter of a bird or the involuntary twitching of a muscle, and occurs at the lower portion of the body or abdomen, just above the pubis; to some it feels like the motion of wind in the bowels.

The nearer approach of labor at the close of the nine months is the settling of the abdomen; the weight of the child seems to bear it downward; the parts seem more full, and there is increased mucous secretion, showing that the parts are relaxing preparatory to an easier delivery. At this time a chilly sensation, with nervousness, may pass through the frame, attended with an indefinable fear of impending evil, without any special reason for it. A more decided indication is a slight show of bloody mucus, before or after the pain, indicating a dilatation of the mouth of the uterus. If at the time there is a frequent desire for urination, or defecation, or both, this is kindly Nature's motherly preparation for greater safety in delivery, for the child passes out of the womb through the channel between the bladder and the rectum, and if these are both empty, it is easy to see how much more room there is for the exit of the child, and how much easier it is for the mother; if the bladder is full, there is danger of its rupture; hence, especially during the later weeks of gestation, the calls of nature, in both directions, should be promptly attended to. If nausea or vomiting occurs about this time, its effect is to relax the system still more, and to that extent insures an easy delivery. Synchronously, there is sometimes a nervous shiver or tremor, then comes the rupture and a flow of water; if there is no water, it is a

DRY BIRTH,

which is more lingering and less easy in other respects. Physical or mental shocks, from alarm or unwelcome news, may occasion a discharge of the waters several days, or in rare cases a week beforehand, but without materially unfavorable results.

FALSE ALARMS

are wandering and irregular pains; the real ones come at shortening intervals across the back, over the lower portion of the abdomen, or across the thigh; more frequent and more severe, until the last. About this time it is well to administer an enema slowly, of a quart or two of tepid water, not cold or cool even; this aids to unload the bowels more perfectly, with the advantage of its being less necessary to have an evacuation for several days after delivery. Constipation just before delivery may occasion false pains, and these may bring on the real ones. But after the thirty-eighth week or earlier, if there are indications of approaching birth, one full evacuation ought to be secured every day at the very least; better to have two, than to have less than one in every twenty-four hours It is always better, when these wandering pains occur, to take an enema; if it does not afford entire relief, and is likely to irritate or worry, add a teaspoonful of laudanum to a pint of water, and use half of it as an enema, or even less water, if the lower bowel or rectum has been just evacuated; the object being to allay the pain, which will be the more certain to be done, when the enema is retained. Sometimes, under such circumstances, an agreeable relief, comfortably soothing, is secured by sitting in a tub of water of ninety or a hundred degrees, or agreeably warm to the patient. If these things do not avail, it is because Nature wills the completion of her work. The patient should have on an easy dress, in which she can sit, or lie, or walk, with equal comfort, and that can be easily washed. Some impervious material should cover the bed or mattress, rubber or oiled silk; over this an old coverlid or comfortable, with folded sheets over that; then the ordinary sheet, and another at hand in case of need, with extra towels, handkerchiefs, and some sweet oil or lard; also a little soft blanket or flannel, a pair of scissors, and a soft string.

A few days before delivery, the uterus begins to contract, as if preparing itself for the important work before it, and by contraction diminishes, and begins to settle down in the abdomen. These contractions increase in frequency and strength. If they are not strong enough for delivery, they may be increased by friction over the back and bowels with the hand, or a damp cloth; a bandage around the abdomen, a little tightened from time to time, affords considerable aid. A great misfortune, however, if a physician is not present, is the disposition of the patient and ordinary midwives to become impatient, constantly attempting to do something in order to hurry up the delivery. The wise physician waits, and admits of no interference whatever, unless absolutely necessary; he does nothing in nine cases out of ten but to maintain the utmost composure and presence of mind; watchful, calm, and cool, and silent; only speaking now and then in confident, kindly, and encouraging tones, to sustain the strength and will power of the patient; he avoids equally unnecessary concealments and too confident assurances and unadvised predictions; he aims to maintain the highest and most implicit confidence of the patient, so as to enable her to lean upon him and look up to him in any emergency. He never speaks harshly or impatiently, but always in kind yet firm tones; now and then saying something to divert the mind to a foreign subject, so as to while away the time, and then it comes up to the case with more strength. Everything possible should be said and done calculated to compose and cheer, and inspire confidence in a safe delivery.

Great injury is often done by having too many persons in the room as assistants; each one thinks that something must be done, often they are in each other's way and are a positive hind-

33

rance ; the physician, the nurse, and the husband, each is equally indispensable, all necessary, and no more.

There should be always a good foot-board to the bedstead ; and better still, if a firm box were at hand, in case of need, to put against the foot-board, if the patient should be too high in bed ; this saves moving down ; a sheet also should be thrown around the posts at the foot, in such a way that it may be pulled upon, if necessary ; another at the head, as a brace to the arms and body, in bearing down.   If a side position is chosen on delivery, an attendant may support the patient's back, by pressing her own against it.   An extra pillow should always be on hand to place between the knees, to keep them apart if required.

Delivery sometimes comes so unexpectedly that the patient is entirely alone ; in that case, as soon as the head appears, if the cord which attaches the mother to the child physically is around the neck of the infant, lift it off over the head, let the air come to the face, and remove at once any obstructions of mucus or other thing, which may impede the breathing, from the nose and mouth ; lay the little stranger on its right side, a short distance from the mother ; if it does not breathe freely, sprinkle cold water on the face as long as it is a little purple.   When there is full breathing tie a soft string, moderately tight, around the umbilical cord, about two inches from the body, and another about an inch from that, and cut the cord between the two strings with a pair of sharp scissors—all this is to prevent any blood coming from the child or the mother ; the end next the child becomes the navel, that next the mother is called the " after-birth," and comes away at the next uterine contraction ; physicians term it the Placenta. If the contractions do not take place within a few minutes rub the hand gently over the bowels, grasp the ball-like protuberance with the hand, and give a little pressure ; and when the pain comes let the mother aid the expulsion by bearing down herself, and while the pains are continuing, not else, draw upon the cord gently and steadily, very much so.   Sometimes more blood comes away than is natural ; this is called

" FLOODING,"

and must be arrested by dipping cloths of several thicknesses in the coldest water, the colder the better, laying one over the abdomen; in two or three minutes replace it with another; if this does not arrest the flow of blood rub a flat piece of ice, as large as the hand, over the lower part of the bowels, and put a large piece up the vagina. Sometimes there is bleeding after the discharge of the placenta; this is

UTERINE HEMORRHAGE.

This bleeding may be external or internal, known in either case by the patient continuing weak and not promptly reviving after delivery; in that event do as before, change the cold cloths every minute, or lay a large flat piece of ice on the belly and keep ice all the time in the vagina; ice is best for all these purposes, because it does not wet the bedding; if there is no ice, and the wet cloths fail, pour water from a pitcher from the height of several feet, and if needed, give some stimulating drink, a glass of wine or a tablespoon of spirits in as much water, a teaspoonful or two at a time; or if much needed, drink it all down at once and repeat as often as necessary, until the patient begins to revive and the pulse comes fairly up.

As soon as the child and placenta have come away, the mother still on her back, knees bent upward, let her with her hands and feet help her body up a little so as to allow the soiled or damp cloths under to be removed; adjust the bandage around the abdomen tight enough to give it a comfortable support; it may be pinned or attached with tape strings. Next inject a pint of tepid water up the vagina to cleanse it thoroughly, put a cold wet compress over the parts and a dry napkin over this; but in case there has been no special bleeding use water at least milk warm. These injections should be used night and morning for several days and then omitted.

In first confinements the after pains are trifling, but these seem to become more and more decided after each birth; if they worry the patient apply hot fomentations to the abdomen or a tepid injection of half a teaspoonful of laudanum in half a pint of water, and retain it as long as possible. For a week after delivery the mother should eat thrice a day of gruel, mush, panada, fruits, toast and tea, and any kind of soup with the crust of bread broken into it; after that take at breakfast and dinner in addition eggs, fish, poultry, meats, etc., always eating regularly, nothing between meals, and lightly at supper; but at all times cut the food up very fine, fine as a pea, and chew it deliberately, and be careful that any vegetables used should be thoroughly cooked, known by their being very soft through and through before taken from the fire; this may be known by sticking the fork through them.

If the mother could be induced to begin ten days after confinement and continue, until the child is weaned, to use wheaten grits as a large part of her breakfast and as a substitute for bread, and at dinner and supper to use bread made of the whole grain of the wheat, the foundation would be laid for strong, healthy, durable teeth for the child, because the material which makes the teeth strong and supplies the enamel is in the bran, which is fed to animals; and if the child were required after weaning to make two meals of each day, breakfast and supper, mainly of this cracked wheat, the teeth would be still further improved in strength and durability, and thus materially add to the health and comfort of the body in after life, since good teeth are essential to the proper mastication, division, and digestion of food during the years of childhood and youth.

THE BREASTS,

after confinement, require special attention; for in about three days there is generally a feeling of chill, with more or less of headache and fever, which if very decided requires some attention; this is

MILK FEVER,

which may be greatly modified, if, as soon as the slightest chilliness is felt, bottles of hot water were put to the feet and under the arms. If fever comes on and is decided, bathe the hands in cool water, or sponge the body with water not cold enough to impart a shock, or invite back a chill; when perspiration follows fever, encourage it, but apply no liquid to the skin or any part of it; but after the perspiration has disappeared, if the body is sponged with alcohol and water, half and half, it is very grateful, if it is done quickly and not too much of the body exposed at one time.

If there is fulness or pain or heat in the breasts as the milk is appearing, have pieces of linen, four or five inches across, with as many thicknesses, at least four of these in a basin of cold water; apply one to each breast and cover with a larger piece of dry flannel, change every five minutes until fully relieved. The more decisive the symptoms are, the colder the water ought to be. If relief is not had, put flannels wrung out of boiling water to each breast every five minutes until relieved; repeat as often as necessary, and at the intervals apply warm compresses, renewing them before they become dry.

If there is any hardness remaining in any part of the breasts, patiently and gently rub such places with the warm, soft hand, or get an assistant to do it, half an hour at a time and several times during the day; by all means invite the flow of milk; if the child does not take away enough, use the pump or have it drawn by the nurse; these things are especially insisted upon as a certain means of preventing

"GATHERED BREASTS,"

which have been the occasion of incalculable suffering to young mothers; these abscesses are from allowing too much milk to accumulate in the breasts, and very rarely, if ever, from cold.

But if by any means there should be a gathering, the lancet should be used at the proper time; that is, when it comes to a head.

CHILD-BEARING.

THERE is scarce one woman in a thousand who does not have it in her power to have a safe and easy delivery, with little or no pain, especially if she has the coöperation of a generous and manly husband, and that, too, without the aid of any drug or medicine or vaunted anæsthetic.

Physical pain and danger were not involved in the primal decree in Paradise; for the perpetuation of the race, and not its destruction, was the very foundation of the plans of the Almighty. Nor was pain a necessary concomitant of child-bearing; it was "sorrow," taking the Scripture expression as it is; equivalent to trouble, physical and mental; the trouble of rearing children, the responsibilities, the anxieties inseparably attendant on the rearing of children, and that foreboding which is present during all the months of preparation for the important event of a child being brought into the world.

As it is, notwithstanding the neglect and gross ignorance of mothers as to the best means of preparing for delivery, notwithstanding all the disadvantages connected with the various conditions of human life and poverty, it may be safely said, that not over one woman in a thousand, taking the world over, dies in child-birth. The way of obedience to the commands of the Almighty cannot involve the loss of life of His creatures; it is disobedience that is death. "If ye love Me, keep My commandments," with the promise in return to be a Father and a Friend to all such; "a Friend who sticketh closer than a brother." This is the theory; the fact corresponds with the general testimony of mankind, that whole tribes and nations who live natural lives, nearly always in the open air, and their bodies unhampered by confining garments, have children safely, easily; so much so, indeed, that no confinement to the bed, or chamber, or house is necessary, even for a day. And in this very statement we have the general principles laid down for the

SAFE AND EASY CONFINEMENT

of every mother:

Abundant fresh air.

Temperance in eating plain food.

An easy mode of dressing; every garment perfectly loose from the shoulders downward, not a string, or button, or pin, or bandage below the top of the shoulders. It is proposed to examine these things in detail, and show their bearings.

Wandering tribes of barbarous and semi-barbarous people have safe and easy births, not delaying their journeyings a day, for four reasons: their plentiful exposure to the pure, out-door air; their being compelled to live on plain food, and even that not often over-abundant; to their large amount of exercise in the open air; and to the loose nature of their clothing. These things combined give a high state of general health. The exposure to the fresh, pure air not only purifies the blood, but im_____ ____ health and life, while the large amount of exercise _____ insures a vigorous digestion, and thereby secures that daily regularity of the bodily functions which is everywhere essential to good health, and these combined give a physical strength which is fully adequate to the emergency of bringing forth children easily and safely.

All these things can be secured in civilized life to a still higher extent, without the disadvantages of exposure, and acciuent, and scanty food, to say nothing of the dangers arising from storm and cold, and heating summer's suns, and the casualties of uncivilized life. Hence the real truth is, that the chances of easy birth in civilized life are greater than among the rude and uncultured, if we would only live up to the light we have; because we have comfortable homes, are sheltered from winds and rains and storms, from feverish heats, and the baleful night air with every required protection against changing weather and unseasonable seasons. In addition, we have the advantages of medicine, of surgical skill, in case there is necessity for their employment, besides the variety and suitableness of food to meet the varying wants of the system, and to satisfy its unnatural conditions. If accident occasions diarrhœa, we can at all times have quiet in a warm bed, with a dietary of boiled rice, which in nine cases out of ten is a prompt and radical cure, without which the system could easily fall into a state of irritation and debility, or convulsions, to endanger a miscarriage, which is ten times more injurious and fatal than child-birth.

If, on the other hand, by exposure to the weather, or accidental colds, the liver becomes torpid, and the bowels costive, or if from any other cause the system becomes disordered, and fever and want of appetite debilitate, at a time when all the strength possible is needed for an event which may take place at any hour, we can resort to the free use of the fruits of the orchard, and the luscious berries of the garden and the field, in their fresh or preserved state, and calculate on a speedy rectification of the untoward conditions—untoward, because if not corrected, and delivery comes on during a condition of obstinate constipation, confinement becomes an agony, even if a fatal rupture of the bladder or other equally grave injuries do not take place as a direct consequence of the constipation. And so with the easy rectification of other conditions, hurtful or dangerous, which observation and science have placed within our reach; besides the immeasurable advantages which the uncultivated can never command.

The one great essential for securing an easy and safe childbirth is vigorous general health; hence, the very moment it is known, or even suspected, that impregnation has taken place, by the failure of the return of the seasonable occurrence, the catamenia, it becomes the bounden duty of the individual to commence at once to inaugurate such a systematic and wise course of life as will be best calculated to give the highest possible state of general good health, that is, a good appetite and a vigorous digestion; for these will secure all else that is needed, and this can be done in almost all ordinary cases, can be done to a very great extent, even although the woman has been in bad health before, even although she may be in a decline, for this one overwhelming reason, and of which thankful and admiring note should be made, in justice and gratitude to the Infinite One who orders all things aright and mercifully: it is a fact and not an argument—a fact so universal that no intelligent mind familiar with the subject ever thinks for a single moment of calling in question, that the moment a woman becomes pregnant, the whole system begins to undergo a marvellous change; begins to arouse itself to the preparation for the work of Almighty decree, preparation for the production of another being, to appear in the image of the Maker of us all, in due time; this preparation is made under certain laws laid down by Omnipotence for the express purpose of bringing about a contemplated result. He commands to "multiply;" the command comes to every man and woman, that they shall do their part as far as they can; He does His according to laws fixed by Himself, and He does it in the very best way; that is, He has implanted an instinct in the system by which it becomes its nature, as soon as the foundation for another human being has been laid, to take upon itself a better and higher state of health. If there is dyspepsia, the dyspepsia begins to abate; if there are constitutional derangements, they begin to rectify themselves; and even in such extreme cases as consumption of the lungs strongly threatened, if a woman becomes pregnant the symptoms begin to disappear at once, and continue to improve during the whole course of pregnancy, and if properly managed they never reappear; or, if they do, it is not till child-bearing has ceased. And more, there are numerous cases recorded in standard medical works, where the lungs were in an actual state of decay; impregnation took place, the size of the abdomen increased, pressing up against the stomach, with the effect in breathing and otherwise to swell out the lungs in such a way as to cause the opposite sides of the cavity to meet and grow together, as the sides of a cut on the finger grow together if pressed in such a way as to keep in proximity; and as a deep gash on the arm will not grow together if the sides are not kept in contact, so in case of an excavation in the lungs it would remain so, unless the sides were brought together as above stated. To make this a little clearer, take three common bladders of India rubber, empty, hold them in a large glass tumbler; they do not fill it, there is space all around them and between them; blow in a little air through a quill, a little more, and a little more, and they will be seen to begin to touch each other at a greater number of points, and finally will press each other so closely that their sides meet, and no space is observed; the lungs are a multitude of little bladders, and are made to meet in the same way, by the space which they usually occupy being constantly diminished as they become more full and more distended; just as all know that when the stomach is very full there is more shortness of breath than usual, because it swells up against the lungs and gives them less room in which to have their full play; and so, in proportion as the child grows in the uterus, it presses upward, diminishing the room in which the lungs are to work. Thus it is that child-bearing sometimes cures consumption, the chances being greater the less time there is between the births. It is on this same principle that observant and capable physicians often see, that if a patient could be made pregnant, she could get well, even in so serious a disease as consumption itself.

There is another important operation going on in this connection, explaining how it is that a woman begins to be more healthy when she becomes pregnant. She then has to supply nutriment for two, instead of one; this nutriment being conveyed through the blood, hence more blood being needed, the appetite becomes more decided, and by a necessary arrangement in this connection, the digestion becomes more vigorous, by instinct, an instinct which the Almighty has implanted in order to insure the carrying out His designs of perpetuating the race; not allowing their success to depend upon the mere attention of the creature. Then again the surplus blood, for we all have a surplus in consequence of eating too much and exercising or working too little, goes to the support of the new being, thus relieving all those conditions of the system which have become unnatural in consequence of an over-supply of blood at particular parts of it, is a means of improved health throughout.

When those parts are thus kept relieved for months, of an overfulness of blood, they get at length into a habit of healthful action, and in many cases maintain that healthful action ever afterwards, and permanent health is thus restored to parts which, for a long time, had been in a diseased condition. For this and other legitimate reasons, the general truth is established that

SICKLY WOMEN SHOULD MARRY,

because in very many cases it is the surest means, as just explained, of regaining health. In this, Nature, as in many other cases of disease, accomplishes what art fails to do. In proportion to the chances of becoming pregnant, in ordinary cases, which are at least nine for and but one against, in such proportion is a woman likely to improve her health by marrying a strong, healthy man. But her chances for improved health are greater even if she does not become pregnant, in consequence of the complete revolution in all the habits of life, in going into another atmosphere, removal to another part of the country, changing from the prairie to the mountain, from the farm-house to the town, or their opposites; going into a new family, where the round of food and the modes of preparation are widely different; or in case of going to house-keeping, the excitements of mind, the activities of body, the bringing in of new activities, those ambitions and motives and moral qualities, which had been   lying dormant for long years; all these things involve radical changes, that " very change of air," which the physician has such frequent cause for recommend-ing, when all his special means of medicine and diet and exercise have signally failed to accomplish objects which, at one time, seemed within his easy grasp; changes general, radical, short, sharp, and decisive , which only marriage can command power of motive enough to bring about. Hence, a sickly maiden has not only in her favor the nine chances against one of pregnancy, but that multitude of other chances, which radical change of air and food and climate, and locality and company and association, and an entirely new set of motives and ambitions, imperatively bring about. And how many have their health improved by even a few weeks' changes!—as to a small part of these, let the universal habit of going to the country, to the sea-shore and abroad, every summer, testify; all these things together making it a reasonable probability, if not certainty, that a sickly single woman will have the health improved by marriage.

But, after all, this is a selfish motive for marriage. There is a more powerful one, a moral reason, which carries with it an overwhelming force. The command of no less than Divinity is

" MULTIPLY AND REPLENISH."

Marriage is the only means, and marriage is in our power; it is our duty to obey the command; to do what we can; that is all that is required of us; the rest belongs to the Omnipotent One, and He will carry it out or not, as seems best in His sight. The brave soldier obeys the orders of his superior officer implicitly, confidingly; he has nothing to do with consequences. The

NOBLE JACK TAR

has no other thought beyond obedience to the order from the quarter-deck, and shall a soldier of the cross, a child of Infinite Wisdom, hesitate to obey a plain, written command for fear this, that, or the other thing should happen?

The path of plain duty, of plain command, is the path of safety. When that command is given by the kind and wise Father of us all, we may reasonably look for a blessing to follow every step on that path, and as we have seen, the very first step taken in marriage is attended with improved health, thus encouraging us from the very outset. Suppose, then, in addition to taking measures for this pre-ordained improvement, we bring to bear all the knowledge and light we have to promote the general health, who can tell but what in any given case, by the coöperation of the creature with the Creator, in bringing about a desirable and laudable end, a miraculously favorable result will take place?

But we are bound still further. We bring upon ourselves our own sicknesses. A servant is not released from his duty to his master if he disables himself from performing that duty. If a man lives beyond his means, and thus becomes unable to pay a legal and honest debt, that does not relieve him of the obligation. Even if ill-health were an excuse for avoiding marriage, the duty presses to regain that health for the purpose of being able to marry, and thus fulfil the duty. Marriage, then, being a means of health, and health being necessary to the proper performance of any and all the duties of life; and, furthermore, marriage being legitimate, healthful, and honorable, it becomes a duty to all, whether sick or well; if well, they can perform the duty now; if not well, they should make a systematic effort to secure a better state of health, and then marry to complete the work.

It is not meant that those should marry who have any fatal disease, any malady which is ordinarily beyond cure, nor when in the last stages of any disease; but simply this: that if a person has not a good constitution, is not very vigorous, such one may marry as a means of health.

If in that worst form of disease, consumption, there is merely a tendency to it, marriage, as a means of health, is not forbidden, nor is it unwise. Many persons seem to think because they cannot find that any of their predecessors have died of consumption, that therefore it would be strange if they should have it; and are very prone to think that their symptoms are not those of consumption, while it is apparent at a very superficial survey of the case that it is present in the advanced stages.

The truth really is, that after making a great number of investigations, bearing directly on the point, the most eminent French physician in consumptive disease was compelled to acknowledge, against his former convictions, that consumption was not notably more frequent or more fatal in those who had consumptive parents, than among those who had no hereditary tendency to it; meaning, in other words, that very healthy persons were quite as liable to die of consumption as those who were weakly. And it is very readily and very satisfactorily accounted for. The weakly feel the necessity of taking care of themselves habitually; they know that they are very easily made sick; that even slight exposures make a lasting impression on the system for ill; hence, they are always on their guard. While the robust, feeling strong in their vigorous health, become possessed with the hallucination that nothing can hurt them ; they are contemptuous of exposure, with the result of falling victims to acute disease, and the distance between high health and the grave is measured by a very few days ; while the feeble, who seem as if a slight wind would blow them over, survive a score or two of years. And for the same reason, persons who are not very vigorous may marry and survive by many years those who are well and strong.

This is the reasoning on the case : hard facts confirm it—for it is indisputably true that more single women die between twenty and forty-five, than married. Two-thirds of the suicides among women are unmarried ; two-thirds of the inmates of lunatic asylums are single women ; showing in the most indisputable manner that marriage promotes health, that child-bearing is a means of health and longevity, and of exemption from the worst of fates—the mad-house. In the same direction it may be stated, with equal truth, that there is a multitude of human ailments peculiar to women which originate in celibacy ; the universally observed eccentricities of old maids are a direct result of their celibate condition, because the whole intent of their being is thwarted, and the whole set of purposes and functions of the womb, associated as it is with almost every other part of the system, is blasted ; the machinery arrested in its work, it is not possible that it should fail to shock the whole constitution, and to shake the entire fabric of a woman's being, which it indisputably does.

As marriage tends to the physical salvation of woman, it also improves the moral nature of man ; conserves it as well as his health ; very few men fail to improve in health within six months after marriage. A large majority of men in penitentiaries are under twenty-five at their first admission ; married men are more reliable in business ; the shrewd merchant will trust a married man when he would not think of trusting the same man if he were single, and had no family. The married man has a position, a stability in society which the bachelor never acquires. Voltaire said, with great truth : "The more married men, the fewer crimes. Marriage renders a man more virtuous and more wise. An unmarried man is but half of a perfect being, and it requires the other half to make things right ; hence, it cannot be expected that in this imperfect state he can keep the straight path of rectitude, any more than a boat with one oar can keep a direct course."

Marriage and child-bearing, then, are thus seen to be, beyond all dispute, a means of health and longer life to women, notwithstanding the drawbacks of nursing, and the pains and penalties and dangers of child-birth, arising from inexcusable ignorance, or a neglect, almost universal, to live in such a manner as would make delivery safe, easy, and painless to all. And if, with all this inattention, child-bearing promotes health and longer life, much more would it do so if, during the entire time of pregnancy, women would conscientiously live up to the laws and light which have been vouchsafed to them; these general laws are few, and are not difficult to be complied with on the part of any one who has a very moderate amount of intelligence and force of will. The first most important thing to be attended to as soon as impregnation has been surmised, is the

DRESS IN PREGNANCY.

Two things are indispensable—warmth and looseness.

There should be no binding on any one square inch of the whole body, but that which necessarily falls on the shoulders; every garment except the stockings should be suspended from them, whether worn day or night; it would be of incalculable advantage if women could be induced, at least during this interesting period, to have every garment, except the stockings, adjusted in a way that it would fit no tighter, nor bind more closely, and sit as loosely, as a morning wrapper; not even wearing garters; simply because the free flow of blood is arrested, and this disorders and deranges every part of the system, and corrupts every atom of blood in the body; for a free circulation is its health and its very life; stillness is a poison to the blood, just as stillness of the air we breathe in a room begins to vitiate every particle in that room on the instant. It is want of a free circulation of the blood which is the main feature of almost every ordinary disease, and to interfere with that circulation by anything which presses or binds in any part of the body below the shoulders is to invite to that body any and all diseases which are connected with bad blood. The ingenuity of each woman, when her head and heart are in it, will find out methods of adjusting dress which will meet the most important requisition of pregnancy. Next to looseness in dress, the most important item is

WARMTH OF DRESS.

Better be too warm than too cold. One sensation of chilliness pervades the whole frame in its evil influences ; but as some persons require more clothing than others, there is but one guiding principle ; let each one dress in such a way as to keep off a feeling of chilliness, to prevent the attention being unpleasantly drawn to any part of the body in that connection. Every one knows how the mind is led to the fact that the feet are cold ; it renders the whole person uncomfortable ; hence, direct special attention to that quality and quantity of dress which keeps every portion of the body comfortably warm ; this is the great overshadowing idea, be " comfortably warm " all the time ; but to secure this, and to avoid the danger of a chill, woollen materials should cover the body and limbs the year round, except at night, in bed ; the main reason for wearing woollen flannel is, that it helps, more than any other material, to regulate the heat of the system ; we cannot be always on our guard against draughts of air, against cooling off too rapidly ; and the wearing of flannel is a kind of self-operating arrangement ; it retains the heat of the body, absorbs it, and thus keeps a store of it on hand all the time ; silk and linen and muslin carry the heat away rapidly ; convey it off, take it from the body, and pass it directly away to the surrounding air ; woollen drawers should be worn on the lower limbs to protect them from cold and draughts, as well as the other portions of the body ; for the same reason, nothing should be worn to distend the lower part of the dress ; hoops, by doing that, open a wide door for cold air to come up and around the body, and keep it in a constant chill. As you value the health and life of the promised being, dress loosely, dress warmly, during the whole time of pregnancy, from the hour of conception to the moment of delivery ; it is of an importance in the direction of easy child-bearing, which ordinary words fail to express ; and scarcely less in value is

EATING DURING PREGNANCY.

Eat at three regular hours in the day, nothing whatever between, and at not shorter intervals than five hours, thus allowing the stomach full opportunity to pass from it what was last eaten, as also to give it some little time to rest; it is eating too often, and not allowing that rest, which makes half the dyspeptics in the land.

It is better to eat at morning, noon, and night; a great point gained would be to make supper, the last meal of the day, of a cup of warm milk and boiled rice, or oatmeal gruel, with a cup of hot milk and boiling water, half and half, with or without sweetening, or some oatmeal porridge; the object of such a supper being not to tempt the appetite. It is not likely that such a meal would lead to over-indulgence, and the stomach, not having much to do, would do its work well, would digest the meal most thoroughly, and would convert it into pure, nutritious, life-giving blood, without being overworked, or in any way distressed, with the result of allowing to that extent an opportunity of comfortable

SLEEP

for the rest, renovation, and recuperation of the whole being. A bad night's rest makes the ensuing day a day of discomfort, always; indisposing to the performance of ordinary duties, while the mind is discomposed, disquieted, unsettled, and the temper all awry; hence, to the extent that a moderate supper allows of good, refreshing sleep, it is of great importance.

It would be of incalculable advantage to the mother and to the new life, if, during the entire time of pregnancy, nothing whatever were drunk, except pure rain-water and very fresh, sweet milk; these things being drunk but at meal-times. Ordinary teas constringe, coffee has various injurious effects, while beer, ale, wine, and spirits in all their forms excite the circulation unnaturally, with the inevitable result of its sinking afterwards in the reaction, just that much lower than the natural standard, causing that derangement and inequality of circulation and condition which to that extent deranges the general working of the whole system; contributing not by any possibility one additional atom of strength to what was there before; for strength comes to the body only from the food eaten and healthfully digested.

Another important benefit of a plain and moderate supper is, that in less than a week, if it is persevered in, the appetite for

BREAKFAST

will be vigorous and strong, these being aids to a good digestion, with the advantage of having all the subsequent exercise of the day to expend its influences in converting the food into nourishing, invigorating blood, promising an enjoyable day. Too many know that when there is no appetite for breakfast, it is pretty sure to be followed by general discomfort, a want of bodily vigor and life, which take away all enjoyment, and instead of activity and exhilaration of spirits, there is a lassitude and indifference to what is passing around us which is as discomposing to others as it is uncomfortable to ourselves.

A good and sufficient breakfast can be made, in pregnancy, of tapioca, sago, boiled rice, lean meat, poultry, and a drink of boiled milk, and boiled rain or snow or distilled water, half and half, these having no minerals or metals in them; with a dessert of fruits and berries in their fresh, raw, ripe, perfect, natural state, making at least half the meal of these; it is better to omit all meats. If fruits cannot be obtained fresh, then use those which are dried and preserved. But use only one kind at a meal. Dinner may be made in the same way, adding any one vegetable most liked. If fruits and berries were used liberally, very liberally, at breakfast and dinner every day during pregnancy, at least one-half the meal made of them, they would have an opening, cooling, refreshing, and anti-feverish effect on the system, which would be of incalculable value. The acids of fruits and berries have a direct effect on the liver in stimulating it to its natural action of separating from the blood its waste matter and its bile, thus keeping the skin healthfully clear, removing from it those blotches of dirty yellow or brown which are often seen in pregnancy, and which are great disfigurements. Besides making the blood pure, sparkling, and bright, fruits operate directly on the bowels, keeping them open and free, which are inseparable from good health, as all persons of even limited observation know; preventing also a long catalogue of ailments which attend a confined condition of the system, as piles, diarrhœa, and dysentery.

THE DINNER

may consist of lean or young meat, or poultry, a single vegetable, boiled rice, oatmeal porridge, leaving off, when half done, to

34

complete it on some fruit. It is always best to take a cup of hot drink at each meal, and it would be much better if it should consist of half and half boiled milk and water, sweetened to make it palatable: it is the warmth to the body which a cup of good tea imparts, which does the good, more than the tea itself, although it has exhilarating qualities of its own, but not as much nourishment as sweetened milk and water.

It is a great aid to a temperate meal to confine one's self to three different kinds of food; it is variety which tempts to over-eat, and it is a constant temptation; one kind of meat, one kind of vegetable, one kind of substitute for bread, either rice, sago, or tapioca, and then one kind of fruit or berry as dessert. By discarding wheat bread and common well or spring water, a pliability is given to the bones of the parts, and a softness and yieldingness to those of the coming child, which aid most marvellously an easy confinement; the things allowed to be eaten are the natural products of the earth, and free from solid particles of lime and other hard substances, they all are very nutritious, and on them the pregnant woman will thrive and grow vigorous and strong for the important hour for which she is preparing.

In this connection, some narrations will be given, of which good use may be made by judicious persons, for they are very suggestive. A Londoner in eighteen hundred and forty-one, was apprehensive that his wife might not survive her next confinement, in consequence of the several preceding ones having been so exceedingly painful, even to all appearance endangering life. He started out on the conjecture that the more a pregnant woman lived on fruits and other food which contained little or no bone, earthy, or metallic materials, in such proportion would she have an easy delivery. His wife had two children in three years; during the last three months preceding both her confinements, her health seemed to decline, her strength failed, her veins were so much enlarged with stagnant blood, that it seemed necessary to bandage them to prevent bursting; she increased greatly in weight and bulk, so much so as to impede all her bodily motions and greatly interfered with exercise; at the end of seven months of her third pregnancy, she found herself in her previous conditions. She coöperated with her husband and began on the first week of the eighth month by eating an apple and an orange the first thing after waking up in the morning.

and the same at night; nothing whatever between, but light meals of fruits, rice and milk, or rain water; this at once cut off a great part of the supply of new blood; there was such an excess already, that the system was overburdened with it, and as by the natural processes of secretion and insensible perspiration the actual weight of the body decreases every twenty-four hours two pounds or more, this being from the blood, it is easy to see that the course pursued went directly to the root of the matter. On the fifth day, she took in addition to the apple and orange a whole lemon, with sugar, before breakfast, and at breakfast two or three roasted apples, besides a small amount of cold light bread and butter. During the forenoon, she took one or two oranges, and an apple; for dinner, a small quantity of fish, poultry, potatoes, greens, and apples in various forms, raw, roasted, or baked. In the middle of the afternoon, an apple, orange, or bunch of grapes were taken, and always a lemon, with sugar or molasses. For supper, apples or oranges, and rice or sago, boiled in milk; sometimes alternating apples with raisins or figs.

Two or three times a week she took a teaspoonful of the following preparation. The juice of two oranges, of one lemon, of half a pound of grapes, and a quarter of a pound of syrup. This course was kept up for a month and a half, with the result that the prominency of the veins was removed; all the swelling had disappeared from her legs and feet; her feelings of lightness and agility were such that she could run up stairs with greater ease than when in her usual health; her general condition was most unusually good. Up to the hour of her confinement she was free from bodily discomfort, and her breasts seemed to be in their natural condition, although in previous confinements they became sore, and remained so for weeks before and afterwards.

One evening, about two months after the treatment began, she was shaking a carpet in the back yard; an hour later there were indications of the important event; a medical man was sent for, and within four hours after the carpet-shaking, the child had been born and the physician had left, saying it was a safe confinement, and a more easy one than he generally met with; while the nurse declared that she had never witnessed a more easy labor. It was a boy; the bones seemed very pliable and soft, more like gristle, and he grew to be a strong, athletic man. The mother herself was up and about in three or four days, and could have been much sooner, if it had not been opposed by friends and neighbors, who adhered to the old prejudice of " nine days."

It is the testimony of others who have lived for the whole time of pregnancy regularly, and on moderate quantities of food which had but little earthy matter, that they had easy and almost painless confinements, with a rapid recovery ; plenty of milk, and healthy children.

Then it becomes a practical question of considerable interest, what are the kinds of food which have the least earthy and metallic substances? Bread is a daily necessity ; but wheat bread has more mineral matter than any other grain, hence wheat should be discarded in all its forms and preparations during the whole time of pregnancy. Water from ordinary rivers, wells, and springs contains a great degree of solid matter. It is known that in many localities, if a dead body is placed in the course of a running stream, it becomes a solid stone in a few years, with the features left at the time of burial. Any dead body may be petrified if a stream of cold limestone water falls upon it in such a way as to have the water run the whole length of the body. In the Mammoth Cave of Kentucky, in Weir's Cave in Virginia, in caves in the interior of the island of Cuba, visited by the writer, immense pillars of stone rise from the floor, and others like icicles hang from the ceiling. Sometimes the end of a stone icicle meets the top of a stone pillar and they become cemented together, one solid piece of stone ; this arises from the fact that in all these places the water is strongly impregnated with lime, and falling slowly in drops, it is evaporated, leaving the solid lime to adhere to what was there before. Stone in the bladder is formed in the same way in the interior of the body ; hence the bones themselves become more bony, for they are a preparation of lime ; therefore it clearly follows, that in order to make the bones of the foetus soft and yielding and compressible, the food of the mother which supplies the materials of growth to the child through the blood, should be such as has the least earthy or other hard substances in it : and for the same reason the water drank should be distilled or taken from the roof of houses as it falls from the clouds, for this is really distilled water, having been evaporated from the surface of the earth. The water which a man ordinarily drinks in thirty or forty years is computed to contain enough solid matter to make a statue of himself equal to his own size.

But it need not be considered a great hardship for a woman to be deprived entirely of bread and water during the whole term of her pregnancy; because, as for drink, healthy persons who spend most of their time in-doors are seldom thirsty, if they eat properly, and there is fluid enough in fruits and berries for all ordinary purposes. If thirsty, buttermilk is an admirably healthy drink. Still, rain-water and melted snow are admissible; a lemonade made of these could be drank every day to advantage by pregnant women, alternating with buttermilk; it is their acid constituents which are healthful. The farina and flour made of wheat contain a considerable amount of lime, a pound or more in a year's consumption. The pregnant woman should then seek to avoid as food and drink such articles as have solid matters in them, and in their stead use those which are known to contain little or none. Cheese, for example, made from the milk of the cow has one-twentieth part less of solid matter than wheat bread, while the fruits and berries have two hundred times less. But while wheat bread and water ought to be dispensed with during pregnancy, in order to give greater pliability and softness to the bones of the fœtus, there are many things which are not only not liable to the same objections, but are of a positive benefit in various directions, in the way of cooling the system, keeping it open, preventing fevers, and promoting a vigorous and healthful digestion, as the following list will show:

Apples,	Cherries,	Limes,
Apricots,	Cranberries,	Mangel Wurzel,
Artichokes,	Cucumbers,	Mallows,
Asparagus,	Dates,	Melons,
Beans,	Endives,	Mushrooms,
Beets,	Figs,	Nectarines,
Blackberries,	Fish,	Oats,
Broccoli,	Garlic,	Olives,
Cabbages,	Gooseberries,	Onions,
Carrots,	Grapes,	Oranges,
Cauliflower,	Leeks,	Parsley,
Celery,	Lemons,	Parsnips,
Cheese,	Lettuce,	Peaches,

Peas,	Raisins,	Savoy,
Pears,	Raspberries,	Strawberries,
Plums,	Rhubarb,	Tapioca,
Pomegranates,	Rice,	Turnips,
Poultry,	Rye,	Young Meats.
Radishes,	Sago,	

Any of the above articles can be eaten in moderation at regular meals, nothing whatever between ; only two or three at a time, with oatmeal porridge, rice, sago, or tapioca as a substitute for other forms of grain food or bread, but aiming all the time to make as large a part of each meal as possible of fruits, and berries, and lean meats, omitting altogether the whole list of spices, peppers, mustards, sauces, and whatever may come under the list of condiments, fats, grease, and sugars.

On the other hand, just as soon as the child is born, the food eaten in addition to fruits, berries, and lean meats, should consist very largely of those articles which help to make bone, the most prominent of all being that very bread which is said with great truth to be the

STAFF OF LIFE,

because, when made of the whole product of the wheat berry, it contains most of the elements of solid, substantial, nourishing food ; food which makes good flesh, firm bone, durable teeth. There is no science pertaining to human health and comfort and beauty which has made such large advances, so large, indeed, as to be almost wonderful, in the last forty years, as

DENTISTRY.

Earnest philosophical search in this branch has demonstrated that the teeth of the people are becoming more and more deteriorated with each successive generation ; they are so soft as to make them liable to injuries from such a variety of sources, that girls in their teens begin to lose their best teeth, and many persons at forty have false teeth, and some have not a natural tooth in their heads, all artificial. The cause has been traced largely, and as the very chief, in the increasing fanaticism of the people for

WHITE FLOUR,

not knowing that the whiter the flour is, the more worthless for all nutrient qualities. Flour can be made so white as to contain no more nutriment than the starch used to make a shirt collar stand up. For many years it has been a trick among the most wily millers, when they wanted to secure the first premiums for fine flour at State fairs, to take everything out of the flour but its starch; and they keep these "Premium" barrels in their mills, in this very city of New York, to show their customers what beautiful flour they can make, but they do not dare to sell it, because it would ruin their reputation; no one could make bread out of it; no intelligent baker would give a dollar a barrel for it, for baking purposes, because it would never rise; for there is no

GLUTEN

in it. This gluten is yellowish, but at the same time it is the element, and that alone, in the wheat grain, which contains any nourishment; it is the gluten of the wheat which makes light bread; it is the gluten which contains that which makes strong bones, durable teeth and firm flesh. This gluten is that part of the wheat grain which is found immediately under the outer coat, the part which is known as bran. But when the wheat is ground, containing bran, gluten, and all, so much of this gluten sticks to the little scales of bran which are sifted out of the flour as to materially diminish the value of the product for purposes of food and nutriment. Strict chemical analysis has shown that one-fifth of the actual nutriment of the wheat grain sticks to the bran, is lost for purposes of human food in the process of grinding and making into flour, and is fed to domestic animals; and as it is this which gives durability and beauty and strength to the teeth, and its absence is ruining the teeth of the rising generation, the most eminent dentists urgently recommend to all parents, who have the intelligence to appreciate these facts, to require their children from the age of four years to eat that bread only which is known as bran bread, which is made of the whole product of the grain, and thus save in the food of the child that very element which is absolutely essential to make durable teeth, strong bones, and well-developed muscles; and in order to make it more palpably clear to the masses, Dr. John Allen, styled the father of American dentistry, has collected numerous facts, showing how much solid matter is in bread made of the whole of the wheat grain, and how much of it is lost when the finest wheat-flour is used to make bread.

Liebig, the greatest chemist of the age, says, " nearly an entire half of the nutritive salts are wanting in flour," meaning thereby, that when we eat our finest, whitest, merchantable flour, one-half of its hard, its mineral portions, the parts which make bone and teeth, the lime and magnesia, are lost. This is the reason that our bread, our white bread, does not nourish us as much as it ought to do ; nearly one-half of the essence of the grain is irretrievably lost in our present method of grinding wheat into flour, lost to the bones, lost to the teeth, lost to the muscle, and lost to the brain ; hence, the immeasurable importance that nursing women should eat bread which is made of the whole wheat grain, as found in wheaten grits and Graham preparations.

These statements have been made at length for the express purpose of impressing on the minds of pregnant women the prime importance of not using wheat bread, and common spring or well water, during their pregnancy, if they wish to have a safe, easy, and speedy birth.

And for the same reason, this wheaten bread, made of the whole of the grain, should be eaten as much as possible from the day of delivery, not only as a means of strengthening themselves, but to develop the new-born child, to harden its bones, to give it firmness of muscle, and to lay the foundation for good, strong, durable teeth. It is impossible to conceive the full bearing on human health and happiness and prosperity in mind and morals and materiality, which a diet of the kind named during pregnancy, and of that advised after pregnancy, would have ; that after delivery being of fruits, berries, lean meats, and bread made of the whole wheat grain, not excluding now and then anything else that other people eat, in moderate quantities, and only at regular meals. The strongest of all human motives urge to adopt a course of this kind, personal health, comfort, and safety, the well-being of the fruit of the womb, its safety and health, and comfort during childhood, to say nothing of the advantages in after life of having a well-developed body, a strong, muscular frame, and that buoyancy of mind and heart which are inseparable from good health.   Surely the woman who is unwilling to submit to the course laid down, which really has no sacrifice in it, is not deserving the name of woman, wife, mother.

The subject is of sufficient importance to make it worth the while of the truly benevolent to have these statements printed in tract form, and scattered gratuitously to the four winds of heaven, until not a family in the land shall be without a copy.

If persons want to be aided in these modes of life, such assistance can be had by resorting to some of the best-conducted

WATER-CURES

in the land, where the modes of diet laid down are followed out, and where the guests have all these things spread before them on the table every day.   None of the bathings need be taken ; it is only necessary that they should enroll themselves as boarders, as at ordinary hotels.   To some extent this has been done ; women have been found who have had conscientious and intelligent views on this subject, and husbands of generous natures, and manly impulses, and hearts full of noble sympathies, and a pure love, who have heartily coöperated with their wives, and promptly and gladly aided them in carrying out their views; with the very uniform, almost unvarying, result of having their expectations most encouragingly realized.   Reports to this effect have come to the knowledge of the writer from individuals, and various publications, confirming in the strongest manner the general views that—

Such preparations can be made by women as to modes of life, eating, and dress, during pregnancy, as will insure, in all cases, deliveries more safe, more easy, more expeditious, than can possibly be had under the usual modes of living, and that—

Mothers may live on such a diet, and in such a manner while nursing their infants as will secure to those infants a certainty of survival of infancy, a healthfulness during childhood and youth, which under the ordinary mode of living during the nursing period are simply impossible.

Besides attention to loose dressing and a fruit diet during pregnancy, as means of insuring safe delivery, there are other things which have a favorable bearing in the same direction, all tending to secure and maintain a high state of general health.

OUT-DOOR AIR

is an absolute necessity to the pregnant woman; any kind of air, night or day, out-door air; but that is best which is dry and sunshiny. Three or four hours in the forenoon, two or three in the afternoon from the first of April until the first of December; but for the remainder of the year, two or three hours including one o'clock in the afternoon; for before that time in the morning, and after that at the close of the day, there is generally a dampness, a heaviness, and a rawness in the atmosphere, which had best be avoided unless the person is employed actively enough to keep off all feeling of chilliness.

The reader is urged to spare the writer the necessity of explaining and enforcing at length the value of out-door air in this connection. Let it be sufficient to appeal to your own observation of the actual facts. Go out any day as above, and see if there is not a joyousness in it, an exhilaration during the airing, a relish for the next meal afterwards, and a sleep the following night, either one of which would repay for the trouble taken. The truth is, every breath of out-door air is a benefit, for every breath takes away from the blood in the lungs an appreciable amount of its impurity, depositing in its place, literally, an equal amount of vigor and life, all of which goes directly to the life within, making it more healthful, making it more a life than it was before. Methinks a pregnant mother would begrudge every breath not drawn in the glorious out-of-doors sunshine. In this connection let the

MANLY HUSBAND

bring to bear the gallantry of his courting days, and be as ready as then to " take a walk," and talk over old times; talk of all the pleasant things and interesting things and encouraging things he can think of; and when he cannot go himself, arrange to have a substitute as near as possible, in obtaining some lively, cheerful, intelligent companion, one full of life and electricity, so that the time may be whiled away more pleasantly, the blood may have a more vigorous flow, and deeper draughts may be taken of the luscious air.

THE OCCUPATION

of the pregnant woman while in-doors is of considerable importance; all hard manual labor should be laid aside; everything
which is tedious or to be long continued; all work requiring
closeness of application should be dispensed with; everything
requiring haste or hurry or involving much responsibility;
everything should be kept from the mind calculated to worry;
all suspense, anxious anticipation, sudden announcements of
good or ill; in short, all that is possible should be done to promote tranquillity of mind, evenness of temper, and vivacity of
disposition. More is necessary; the husband and other members
of the family should aim in all they say or do to encourage, to
support, to strengthen. At the same time she should be busy,
but never to the extent of actual fatigue; better to be engaged
at one thing a little while, and before tiredness comes on, rest.
Exercise or work of any kind persisted in until the person is
fagged out, always does more harm than good; women are
peculiarly liable to errors of this kind; they often undertake
more than they are able to accomplish; they miscalculate their
strength; their ambition exceeds their capabilities; and their
anxiety to complete what they have begun frequently leads
them to continue in their work far beyond their ability; these
things in the pregnant woman are peculiarly injurious, and in
multitudes of cases cause miscarriages and premature births,
endangering, and not unfrequently causing the death of both
mother and child. At the same time exercise is a necessity, but
work is immeasurably superior to mere exercise; work which
interests the mind, which is agreeable, which meets the tastes
and inclinations and the ambitions; work which may be done or
not, as is agreeable; which can be abandoned any moment for
a day or week or month or more, or which may be committed to
others.

EXERCISE

is of such incalculable importance to every pregnant woman
during the whole time, to be kept up until she is admonished
that the hour has come, not only the exercise itself, but the kind
of exercise, and the manner of it, that the following narration

is made at length, with a view to give the fullest idea possible of the kind which will meet all the requisitions, with the assurance to every expectant mother who reads the statement, that the chances of an easy delivery will be very greatly increased by carrying out the general principles as far as practicable. All the facts came under the author's supervision; nothing is left for inference or stated on the information of others, and it covers the whole subject.

A lady occupied a beautiful home on the banks of the Hudson. She had been wishing for some time that she had a house in New York. Her husband purchased one in a very desirable locality in December, possession to be given on the first of May following. She was very greatly delighted; it seemed to her to be the realization of the dreams of many years. Being a lady of intelligence, of systematic habits and of forethought, she began at once to make the preparations necessary for a removal. Her whole being seemed to be absorbed in the work before her. She had been pregnant two months. She began to arrange matters in such a manner that moving should be attended with as little discomfort and loss and breakage as possible. She worked leisurely, everything was done with deliberation, done well, done thoroughly, running through several months. When the first of May arrived, everything was ready, every box was nailed, every trunk was locked, and these with every separate package were distinctly labelled; the whole thing was systematically done; so much so, that it is best illustrated by stating that the carpets were put in the conveyance last, because in going into a new house the carpets would be the first thing wanted, and they would be the first things to come to hand, as a matter of course. The whole removal and change was made without trouble, or annoyance, or breakage, or delay; safely deposited in the new home. Then began the work of arranging, and fitting, and fixing. Every room had to be furnished, every carpet laid, every painting hung, every curtain adjusted, to suit the circumstances of the case. Then there were the outside adornments; the grass-plot and the " borders," the vines and the bushes, the annuals and the perennials, all to be planted so as to meet certain desirable requisitions. One summer morning in August she was in the garden, and was called to the bedchamber; the family physician was sent for, her husband was reclining near her, holding her hand in his;

the doctor had barely taken his place at the bedside, a single strain, not two, a little wail, and the child was born; walking on the avenue to-day, in all the pride of womanly beauty and physical perfection, larger than either father or mother. This was the fourth birth. The third was widely different; it was tedious and painful, with a long and weary getting up; and such a tiny, puny child, that it was scarcely expected to survive the period of infancy. The nine months were spent in a boarding-house, with nothing to do but eat, and sleep, and dress, with all the discomforts and annoyances of that mischievous modern institution.

If nothing better can be done, walking is a substitute for interested occupations, and is better than nothing; this should be kept up until the day of confinement. The only direction to be given with safety in reference to the question, " How much am I to walk?" is that it should stop short of much fatigue; stop when a little tired, but continue it until there is a little tiredness. There may be circumstances which forbid walking; if so, it is a misfortune to be lamented; the exercise is necessary for all that. A man may be on the point of starving for want of something to eat; his not being able to get it does not make food less necessary. The idea is put in this light because there are now and then women of such little energy and force of character that they are glad of an excuse for not taking a walk.

The children of Israel increased their numbers with great rapidity under the task-masters of Egypt; it was not a whit abated when they had to hunt their own straw to make bricks; if anything, they were more prolific than before, and had more robust children.

The slave mothers of Virginia in the olden time brought an immense annual revenue to their masters in furnishing a supply to the more southern portions of the country, to work on cotton and sugar plantations. Steady work, plain nourishing food, these are the great requisitions for safe and easy confinements, for a rapid getting up, and for hale and hearty children. It would be an inexcusable oversight if nothing were said on the subject of influencing the moral character of the child as well as the physical, and yet that

MORAL CHARACTER

is moulded by the mother; whatever is her condition, during ges-

tation, as to the affections and passions and sentiments, will inevitably give color to the affections and passions and sentiments of
the child that is to be; and the more continuously the mother is
under the influence of these affections, passions, and sentiments,
the more deeply will they impinge themselves on the character of
the one yet to be born. So palpable is this, that the idea has
been advocated from the earliest ages, and among all nations, by
men of eminence and distinction. And yet during the present
times there does not seem to be any recognition of the important
fact; it appears to have been passed over as one of those indefinite and obscure things which are not deserving of special
attention, as being too much in the mist to be of any practical
value. It is hoped, however, that at no distant period in the future, men and women may begin to wake up to the fact that both
the physical condition, and mental and moral character of the
child, is shaped by the father and the mother, and that responsibility will be felt with increasing pressure in this direction. The
whole subject is commended to the thoughtful consideration of
cultivated minds, and to all those who endeavor to be guided in
the light of Christian principles and moral obligations. The following narration has come within the author's personal observation in its most important features, and is literally true.

Nearly a hundred years ago a young lady of education found
herself the orphaned daughter of a rich man. She married a
gentleman of good family, of a frank, liberal, and genial nature.
He lived freely, spent lavishly, and suddenly died, in the second
month of his wife's pregnancy. His affairs seemed to have been
left in a condition so complicated that his wife did not know
whether she was left destitute or not. Having all that pride
which naturally belonged to one who had been raised in wealth
and luxury, the thought of her changed condition, and the apprehension of some things which might be in store for her threw
her into a confirmed melancholy. Her dread of the future was
terrible. At times she wanted to hide herself away from human
view in the recesses of the forest. Under these mental and
moral conditions her daughter was born, but her forebodings
were never realized; she had an adequate income to the close of
life, and died at the age of seventy-five years, in circumstances of
unusual comfort. The daughter at a very early age would be
often missed, and when found would be sitting in some out-of-

the-way corner, crying most bitterly, and on being asked what was the matter, would exclaim in tones the most depressing possible, " we will have nothing to eat to-morrow." At other times she would run into the woods, climb trees, jump fences, wade into the water, bareheaded, barefooted, racing along the highway or through fields and orchards, her long black hair streaming in the wind, face sunburnt, and more like a young Indian than anything else ; if anything thwarted her, she would lie down in the road, stiffen herself, and remain there by the hour, yielding to no persuasion to move or change ; and through a life of sixty years, the one impending gloomy cloud hung over her, the undefinable fear of some future ill ; she could scarcely tell what, but which never came. Dying itself was so easy that, in reference to her fears of the last mortal agony, she said to a friend, " who would have thought it?" meaning thereby that death was so much easier than for a lifetime she had supposed it would be. It was a death without pain : life went out like the candle in its socket, like the embers on the hearth.

These narrations have been given at length, because they are known to be literally true, and because they shadow forth, in clear, shining characters, a great fact and a great lesson. The fact is, that the predominant states of mind during gestation mould the moral character of the offspring, give shape and tone and coloring to it, and not only to children, but to children's children. From the days of Hannah and Samuel it was so, and it may be set down as a law of nature, fixing, as it does, on the mother, to a large extent, the responsibility for the moral character of her children, thus presenting to her mind the highest possible motive, to live in such a way, physically and morally, during gestation, as to secure for her child a vigorous constitution, and a moral character which shall fit it for the highest duties of life and an immortality beyond.

Another object in the specifications is to impress upon the mind the

USELESSNESS AND HURTFULNESS

of anticipating evil; in both the cases named, the things feared not only never came to pass, but their very reverse took place— a reverse so signal, as to well merit a lasting impression on the mind of every reader; hence it follows that every gloomy thought, every foreboding, every hour of sadness and of shade was a clear loss to the sum of a life of sunshine, to say nothing of the fact that sad anticipations never by any possibility do any good; on the contrary, they are obstacles tending to bring about the very evils anticipated.

THE NEW-BORN CHILD,

being passed from the physician to the nurse, should be laid on its right side, a short distance from the mother, and covered over so as to be kept abundantly warm, care being taken to remove any obstructions from the mouth and nose; then, after a little resting, some rub a little oil all over the body, then gently wash with water not over ninety degrees, using Castile soap, with a soft sponge, rubbing a little hard to get from the skin that greasy, curd-like substance which covers it; special care must be taken to remove it from the eyelids, armpits, groins, behind the ears, as well as from all the creases and folds of the skin; a soft sponge will answer the purpose. In ten or twelve hours repeat this washing, so as to be sure to remove any remnants of the coating, for it is apt to get hard, and irritate the skin; after the sponging, wipe the whole surface dry with a soft cloth. Look at the navel-string before the physician has left, and if all right, double up an old soft rag of linen, five inches across, three or four thicknesses; cut a hole in the centre, large enough to allow the cord to be drawn through, fold the cloth over the cord, and secure it by a belly-band around the child of thin soft flannel, long enough to reach around the body, and about four inches broad; it is not really necessary, the original intent of it being to keep the compress at the navel in its place, the popular idea running into the absurdity of preventing protrusion of the bowels from the crying of the child. But such incalculable injury has been done to infants by making this girdle bind so tightly, that it is better to omit it altogether, and devise other means to keep the navel compress in its place. Grown persons have only to imagine the discomfort which they would experience, if they were bandaged tightly after or just before eating a hearty meal, as an infant is bandaged just before or after a nursing; it is a positive barbarism, and is enough to ruin the stomach of any infant subjected to such an infliction; 'and no doubt it has led to fretfulness and crying and severe pains, and a nervousness akin to convulsions in innumerable cases. No pin or button should ever be allowed about an infant; use strings, and

DRESS THE CHILD

very loosely, so that no motion of the body will be impeded; hence, no dress should extend beyond the feet, although it is almost universal to have the dress a foot or two longer, under the impression that it is necessary to keep the child warm. It is more necessary that it should have room to kick about its feet, and thus keep the blood in circulation, and generate the warmth from within; this is the only healthful warmth that ought to be retained by suitable covering to the feet and limbs, but by all means let these be free. Put no cap on the head, nor use a pin in any part of the clothing. The entire clothing should be changed twice a day at least, and always in such a way as not to endanger taking cold. Close all the doors and windows so as to avoid draughts of air, and the room should not be cooler in winter than seventy degrees.

If the breasts are at all hard, rub them gently and often with warm almond oil; let the rubbing be gentle and frequent. If the breasts are large, hard, painful, and red, cold-water compresses, renewed every half-hour, and a milk-and-bread poultice at night, especially if the bowels are kept a little lax, will remove the trouble in a day or two.

If, a few days after birth, any little tumor is seen on the scalp from any cause, rub it gently two or three times a day with spirits of wine or camphor; if it lasts ten days or longer, apply cloths steeped in lime-water or weak spirits every hour during the day, until it goes down.

If the child's head seems to be out of shape, let it alone, it will rectify itself; dangerous results have followed ignorant tamperings by nurses.

In difficult labor, the face and eyes of the child are at times discolored; let them alone; nature and the proper management of the child will bring it all right, as will also be done in reference to little scratches and wounds accidentally made.

If the child passes no water within twenty hours after birth, a warm bath will rectify it.

The child should be put to the breast within six hours after
35

birth. Do not delay it longer than ten hours. If necessary, give a teaspoonful or two at a time, a little barley-water, sweetened, or milk and water, or very thin gruel. It takes a baby just born a long time to carry into the stomach one teaspoonful, and the stomach at first will not hold more than two tablespoonfuls of liquid.

For the first week the infant should be nursed every two hours during the daytime; at three hours' interval from bedtime to sunrise; make it wait.

After one week, feed it every three hours during the daytime; then, at bedtime, once in the middle of the night, and then at daylight. This may be continued for six weeks or two months; then at intervals of five hours, from sunrise to ten o'clock at night, and no feeding during that interval. At three months old, the child should be habituated to take nothing from the time of its going to bed for the night until breakfast next morning. With this regularity of eating, a child may be allowed to take as much as it wants, whether nursed naturally or artificially.

It is impossible to convey to the mother's mind a full idea of the importance of this system of feeding children regularly, except that an infant should not be waked up to be fed, nor for that matter should any living being be waked up to eat, or to take medicine. If regular nursing were systematically followed out, it would materially influence the whole subsequent destiny of both mother and child. The child will not fret one quarter as much, nor will it interfere with the mother's sleep materially; thus saving her from exhaustion, and from a day of subsequent miserableness, as often as she is allowed to have all the sleep she can take at night.

It is the want of refreshing sleep at night which gives nursing women that draggled, exhausted appearance which is so common to them.

It is irregular feeding that kills half the children who die before they reach the age of three years, and which keeps so many households in a turmoil half the time, from the cries of colicky babies and sick nurslings.

It is the almost universal practice of mothers to put the infant to the breast the moment it begins to cry, supposing that it is crying because it is hungry, when nine times out of ten it cries because it has the colic, caused by wind on the stomach as a result of acidity or indigestion.

Nothing is more distressing to a young mother than the wail of an infant; a child's cry always pierces her heart; to hear that wail or cry for almost every hour of every day is a source of infinite worry; on the other hand, not to hear it, on an average, once a week, makes a difference wide as the poles asunder, in the amount of a mother's comfort; hence, she should bear in mind that nine-tenths of an infant's crying arises from a disordered stomach, arises from irregular feeding; and when she can infallibly remedy this by the simple expedient of regular feeding, it becomes a criminality to both child and mother, in fact, to every member of the family, servants, and all; for a sick infant interferes with the comfort of a whole household, in interfering with sleep, or imposing additional labor; to say nothing of the disquietude of mind throughout the house, for no human being can hear a child's cry without more or less sympathy or other annoyance. This exemption from crying procures an exemption from medicine, from taking those innumerable compounds of soothing-syrups which ignorance prompts to give, or which nurses are hired to advise.

All remedies given to quiet nursing children contain opium in some form or other, or some kind of anodyne, which never can be taken, by child or adult, a single time, without leaving its mark of injury. Half the cases of water on the brain, of

INFLAMMATION OF THE BRAIN,

in children, are the result of giving soothing-syrups, opiates, paregoric, laudanum, and similar drugs to

QUIET CHILDREN.

None of these things remove an ailment; by no possibility do they eradicate anything; they only smother, to eventually destroy, and they will inevitably destroy health, and life itself, if persevered in. One dose makes another more necessary. The use of these things this week makes them more indispensable the next; and thus it goes on, with increasing ill results, to leave life-long impressions for ill on the constitution, even when they

do not kill outright.   It should be borne in mind all the time
that when

THE BABY CRIES

it is because something hurts it.   If it is simply restless, fretful,
or uneasy, it is because there is bodily discomfort somewhere,
external or internal ; nine times out of ten it is external, in a
pin, or over-tight strings, or buttons, or some uneven thing in the
clothing or bed.   The first thing to be done is to lift the child
up, or change its position ; if still fretful, look for pins, or too
tight strings ; if still no relief, and it has had the regular feeding, it is very certain that the pain comes from within, and that
the stomach is the locality.   If so, relief is often had by rubbing
its little stomach with the mother's own hand, gently and patiently ; if more decided measures are needed, apply warm
flannels to the abdomen, or put it in a warm bath ; in some of
these ways relief will almost always be had in vomiting or
passing wind ; then at the next time for feeding give a little less.
    Suppose some quieting medicine had been given, this undi-
gested mass would have remained in the stomach, then passed
into the bowels, with the inevitable diarrhœa or convulsions ;
oftentimes laying the foundation for tedious summer complaints.
    But a very common practice is to give something to stop the
baby from crying ; then, when the diarrhœa follows, to give that
same thing to stop the diarrhœa, and so it does ; it becomes a
famous medicine : it keeps the infant from crying, it cures
diarrhœa, it is infallible in summer complaints ; but sooner or
later, or within a very few days, inflammation of the brain comes
on, and the child dies ; the mother does not note the connection ;
she does remember, however, how it kept the baby quiet, how it
stopped the diarrhœa, and how it promoted sleep ; and when the
next child is born, the same course is followed up with the same
results, blighting the mother's whole after life, for she never can
forget her first-born dead : its image rises up before her, ever
after to move to pity, or to tears, or to heartache.   It is literally
true that millions of little graves would be left unopened every
year, if nursing children were regularly fed with their mother's
milk on the principles detailed above.
    At the end of two years there is no reason why children should
not be limited to three meals a day, never by any chance allow-

ing anything between, unless, perhaps, a single apple, or orange, or banana, or a teacupful of berries in their ripe, raw, perfect, natural state, midway between meals; always, however, making the last meal of the day at the end of the second year of bread and butter and some warm drink, the most unobjectionable being a cup of milk and water, half and half, both having been boiled; now and then there may be substituted mush and milk, boiled rice and milk, or wheaten grits, or porridge; the point being one thing for supper, that one thing not meat; the object in being limited to one thing being, not that half a dozen things mixed up would not be quite as good, if the quantity was the same, not to tempt the appetite to take more than the system needs; if a child is at the table where but one thing is to eat, it will satisfy itself with that one thing, and will not eat too much, if it is plain food and is not a great rarity; but if there are several different articles, and the child is left to itself, it will eat as much in quantity of each as it would of one, the result being that it has been tempted by variety to eat three times as much as nature required, with inevitable ill results.   Then there is a

MORAL REASON

for placing children at the supper-table where only one thing is seen; they naturally want some of everything that is going, and if it is refused, their little feelings are hurt to an extent a parent does not dream of, especially if the parents partake of what is forbidden them.   For this reason it is greatly better that children should be seated at their own table for the last meal of the day, and when they are through, their hearts are light, their stomachs are full, and they are in a state of enviable joyousness, will play a little while, then go to bed, happy in heart and well in body, with the certain result of waking up to a good appetite for breakfast, having had a delicious sleep all through the night. If at breakfast and dinner children were confined to one drink and two or three different articles of food; that is, bread and meat and a vegetable, with one fruit or one kind of berry at any one dessert, they may be safely allowed to eat as much as they want.   But never, under any circumstances, compel a child to eat what it does not want; it is an unmixed and an unreasoning cruelty.   You may, if there is any good reason for it, require a child to eat what you wish it to eat, or eat nothing at all until the next meal; but to force it to eat should never be done.

But to return to the new-born infant: after its birth there remains a fluid in the stomach of a dark color, called

MECONIUM.

Nature generally causes this to be passed out of the stomach in her own way. The mother's milk, the first that comes, called the

COLUSTRUM,

seems to have a laxative effect by express design. If, however, this does not occur in five or six hours, take one teaspoonful of castor-oil and three of rose or rain-water; give one teaspoonful every four hours until relieved, mixing it well before each repetition; but it is better to try first a teaspoonful of whey, sweetened a little. Sometimes the same amount of sweetened water will answer the purpose.

It is necessary to go back to the birth of the child and its first dressing. Next in importance to proper feeding is the dress of the infant, bearing always in mind two things:

LOOSENESS AND WARMTH.

To keep the child abundantly warm from the hour of its birth doubles at once the chances of its life. An alarming number of infants die from exposure to cold, from the want of being kept comfortably warm every instant of existence. And as the weather is liable to great, frequent, and sudden changes, and as the warmth of a room is very apt to be neglected, the greatest safety is in abundant clothing, which for the first few months of life should be of flannel, very fine, very soft, and very clean. During the first weeks of infancy the dressing should be performed with great deliberation, tenderness, and care; no hurry, no roughness; everything should be as gently done as possible, and to this end the mother should do this as soon as convenient, for the child's sake, while the exercise and employment will do her good also. Everything done and said should be said and done most tenderly; no jerking, no loud words, no harsh tones, no impatient sounds or motions; the only words spoken should be words of cheerfulness, for there is no harshness there, and the new-born learns to note the difference in less than a week; by doing these things deliberately, tenderly, lovingly, cheerfully, you will encourage the little one to welcome the bathing and washing with a "crow" instead of a cry; with a glad flutter of the hands, instead of an angry kick of the feet. Let the mother note this.

WASHING AND DRESSING

should be performed at least night and morning. Wash the body well, and the parts liable to be soiled, after each evacuation. All the folds of the skin, neck, arms, armpits, and groins should be powdered well after each washing, and should not by any means be omitted. It would be a safe plan to arrange that the room should be at seventy degrees Fahrenheit at each dressing, and if this is done in the centre of the room, there is less danger from draughts of air. But sometimes from neglect of powdering there are ugly

EXCORIATIONS.

Wash these at least three times a day with two grains of sulphate of zinc dissolved in one ounce of rain or rose water, then dust with the following powder: Half a dram of oxide of zinc, one dram of powdered orris-root, and five drams of powdered starch, counting a large teaspoonful of each a dram; repeat this, dusting well after each use of the wash. If an ointment is preferred on any account, take three drams of spermaceti ointment, and one dram of carbonate of zinc ointment. In many cases any common pain-killer ointment will answer every purpose; spread this on lint, or very soft cloth or linen, and lay it on the parts; the cure will be facilitated by giving a tepid bath two or three times a week.

CLEANLINESS

needs no commendation, nor to be urged on any intelligent mother. But it will save a great deal of trouble if the mother will teach the child to hold out from urinating and defecations. This can be done, and the little one will soon learn to give notice, and even to submit to some uneasiness until the mother pays attention to it; but of course not an instant should be lost when the notice is given, and the mother should make it her study to show her approbation of such notice; make of it a pleasurable thing, both to herself and the baby; but if a scowl is given, or a hasty act is performed, such as a jerk, or a harsh or angry word is uttered, making it apparent to the infant that it is an unwelcome thing to give such notice, it will put it off as long as it can, with all the attendant mischiefs.

A soiled diaper should not be allowed to remain one instant day or night; and for fear there may be soiling and not noticed, there should be a frequent examination every day; but as soon as possible, and in every way possible, teach the child to wait until proper preparation is made for stooling.

EXERCISE

for the first month is not necessary, beyond the fatigue of dressing and bathing and nursing, with being carried across the floor a few minutes at a time, several times every day. The instinct of exercise is amazing. The author's youngest child, now a full-grown young lady, in perfect health, when placed in the arms the day after birth, would give a kind of push, as if to indicate a moving on.

After the first month, the child should be out of doors in the open air every dry day, especially every sunshiny day. If in the summer-time, when it is not cool enough for fires in the house, an hour in the forenoon, about eleven o'clock, and half an hour or more about four o'clock, not late enough for the damp of the evening, nor too early for the chills of the morning, while the middle of the day might be too hot.

In the late fall, and towards May, the middle of the day is best from eleven until two, say an hour or an hour and a half.

For the first month or two of this out-door airing, the child should be held pretty much in a horizontal position, so as not to put a strain upon the spine, for it might get an inclination which would last for life, to embitter it. The nurse should walk slowly, evenly; no jerking, jumping, running, jolting, or twisting round, for all such motions shock the child, and may cause permanent displacements. At the same time the nurse should never stand still, especially at the corner of a street or house, or in a draught of air, nor at an open door or window, or in the hall or passage.

If in cool or cold weather, especially when the wind is blowing, the face should be protected by a thin veil, but in such a way as not to interfere with the breathing of the child.

In the third month the infant indicates a desire to sit up; this should be gratified, but not over a few minutes at a time; three or four times a day at first, then a little longer every week; by degrees it can go out as early as ten o'clock in the morning, and remain out as long as two hours before sundown. Until a child is five years old, it should be required to be in the house, at the very least, an hour before sundown, winter and summer, even in the clearest weather; neglect of this has given fatal croups to multitudes, because there is always a heaviness and dampness, and more or less of a rawness in the sundown air, which, with the natural diminution of vitality and vigor, after a whole day's playing, very particularly exposes a child to the pernicious influences of cold.

Little carriages in cities for children are not advisable, as they are liable to jolts and jars, especially at the crossings; if not allowed to go over these, if confined to going round the block, they are to that extent admissible.

All tossing and swinging by the limbs should be regarded as a crime.

When carried in the arms, the child should be changed from arm to arm, every five or ten minutes, until two months old, so as to compel change of position frequently; it is of great importance, as it prevents obstruction of the circulation for any length of time. A child's leg or arm may get a permanent bend by being carried on one arm too long, or in any one position.

Not one hireling in a thousand is worthy of being trusted with a child out of its mother's sight for an hour out of the twenty-four, especially if out of the house. The more a mother can keep her child under her own eye the better and safer for both child and mother; and as so few nurses can be trusted, none ought to be wholly trusted; and that nurse ought to be dismissed on the instant who puts anything to a child's lips, solid or liquid, except by the direction of the parent at the time, for she will get into the way of giving things to keep the child quiet, in too many cases; if mothers do it sometimes, and thousands of them are tempted to do it every day, much more will an unprincipled hireling do it when out of sight.

It is a cruelty and a shame for any mother to keep a child in any one position longer than its own instinct leads it to do so. Hence, to make a child sit still for five minutes at a time is pernicious, or to lie down for five minutes at a time, unless it is asleep, or unless it chooses to do so, is a great wrong; hence, keeping them in cribs and cradles and tubs by the hour is an absurdity. The best plan ever devised for giving a child its first lessons in getting along in the world by its own exertions, is to put it in the middle of the floor, and let it take care of itself; let it learn to crawl, roll over, sit up, stand up, walk about of itself. This is the best possible method of preventing bow-legs, broken arms, and the multitude of other evils which befall little ones, in consequence of being watched too much at one time, and too little at another.

No one under fifteen years of age ought to be made the caretaker or watcher of an infant under two years, nor should the mother allow her child, under the first year, to lie on a bed, or floor or cradle, for an hour at a time, unless it is in a perfectly good humor. Little ones like change, and the mother ought to go to it the moment she perceives impatience, and play with it for a few minutes to divert it, to encourage it, to keep it company, to set it going again. We ourselves, grown up as we are, soon get tired of being alone. And to allow a child to worry and fret by the hour by itself lays the foundation for a sour, cross, ugly temper, to leave its baneful and wide-spreading influence in all after life.

All baby-jumpers ever invented are a bother and a pest, unnatural and absurd, and have ill and dangerous effects in various directions. There is no baby-jumper equal to a parent's arms, with a good-sized carpeted room, for a change of operations to its own forms of jumping.

In learning children to walk, it is better to leave them to themselves pretty much; first let them stand at a chair, next to go to a neighboring chair; parents often induce dislocation by holding the child's arms high above its head, in the efforts to steady it in walking.

SLEEP.

Proper sleeping habits for infants are of incalculable importance both to mother and child. With two or three repetitions, anything may become a habit to an infant. If it wakes up in the night, and is carried about the room for a few minutes a single time, it may wake up the next night at the same time. If it does wake up it is certain to want to be carried about again, and so on. Hence, there are children who will not go to sleep until they are rocked in the cradle, or are carried about the floor; or have their mothers sit beside them until they fall asleep, and the mother then steals away in the softest manner possible for fear of waking them. Others from mere habit wake up in the night to be nursed, do it regularly, infallibly, until they are weaned; all this is wrong, it is the result of mere vicious habits, formed because mothers have no firmness. It is best, then, to begin from the first day the child is born, from its very first sleep, thus: At its birth it is handed to the nurse, who lays it a short distance from the mother, on its right side, seeing that there are no obstructions in the mouth or nostrils to free breathing; it is next covered over, and allowed rest and quiet from one to four or five hours; it is then rubbed all over with some mild oil to soften a thin covering on the skin, which is washed off with warm water, say ninety degrees, more or less, soap and a soft sponge, special care being taken to get it from the eyelids, very gently, and all the creases and doublings or folds of skin, armpits, groins, and other places; wipe dry with a soft cloth, dress the child, and give it a teaspoonful of warm or cold water, put a little sugar on the nipple, place its little lips against it, and it will soon make its first meal; lay it down in a crib or cradle, cover it up warm, and let it take its first natural sleep; when it wakes up give it its second dinner, then lay it in the crib again. Let this go on for a week or two, never allowing it to go to sleep on its mother's arm or in its mother's bed. For the first month an infant sleeps two-thirds of its time; for the first week three-fourths of its time, but generally it sleeps less and less, and by the end of the second year, as it enters its third, it averages, if in health, about twelve hours' sleep in the twenty-four. Hence it is seen that infants sleep less and less from the first day; the plan is to let them sleep all they can, the more the better; never wake an infant up for any cause short of the house being on fire; if ever it has to be done, let it be in the gentlest manner possible, and not suddenly; the want of such care has brought convulsions and hopeless idiocy on many a babe. Even grown people, when waked suddenly from a sound sleep, seem at first scarcely to have their senses. A young wife waked her husband one night, saying the house was on fire. She further told him that there was a hogshead of water in the yard, under the spout; that he must get some of it very quickly; he found the backyard, found the hogshead of water, put his shoulder to it, turned it all afloat, came back to his wife and said there was no fire in the backyard that he could see. This shows how the brain is affected by sudden waking up; hence as to infants and children, it should be specially avoided.

Healthy infants, who have healthy mothers, want to be nursed as soon as they wake up, which is about every two hours; this may be done for the first seven days; then they do not sleep as long, the intervals are greater; so on the seventh day, when the child wakes up after its first nursing, it may be earlier than the day before, when, instead of giving it the breast as soon as it wakes up, make it wait; better to do it pleasantly by amusing it until three hours have passed since it was last fed; in this way the feeding will be regular; let it feed as much as it wants; thus will be brought about two important things by Nature's own operation: decreasing sleep, which is needed; increasing amount of food, which is needed, the decreasing and the increasing being regulated by the instincts.

Begin the very first night to nurse the child at ten o'clock, and as often as it wakes during the night, always laying it back in its crib; but at the end of a week, after giving the breast as long as it will take it at ten o'clock, make it wait until two o'clock next morning for its next feeding, and at the end of each week, half an hour longer, until the breast is given at five or six o'clock, thus allowing the mother to sleep full seven hours undisturbed out of every twenty-four; and then with half an hour's nap in the forenoon, not later than twelve, she will have all the sleep a nursing mother wants. What a heaven this would be to tens of thousands of nursing mothers this day; the very thought of the chance of sleeping one whole night undisturbed, would be like the promise of an elysium. There are tens of thousands of mothers who scarcely sleep one single night through undisturbed during the whole course of nursing; one of the saddest of all possible announcements, because it is an avoidable necessity, and if avoidable would add incalculably to the health of both mothers and children; would add to the lives and happiness of both, for all men can better do with less food than Nature requires, than less sleep. The sounder the sleep, the better for mother and child; when the two are in the same bed, the slightest motion of the one wakes up the other, and to be waked up out of sleep in the night-time is an injury and an insufferable annoyance. To allow a child to sleep on its mother's arm, to tug at her breast by the half hour, until it goes to sleep, is a folly that is scarcely to be spoken of with patience.

There is not the shadow of a doubt that every mother could train her infant in the way marked out, only if she makes up her mind to do it; if she fails to do this by saying "I can't," by being unwilling to let the child cry, just let her think of this one thing: suppose you were to die, what then? Certainly it would cry, and would have to cry, until the whole habit could be changed.

At two years of age the child should be made to go to bed at eight o'clock, winter and summer, and be allowed to sleep as long as it wants to sleep; but if this interferes with the breakfast-hour, so that the child cannot be washed and dressed by breakfast-time, then require an earlier and an earlier retiring, so that it shall get all its sleep out in time to be dressed for breakfast; but until six or eight years of age, and even longer in some cases, a nap of an hour should be taken in the middle of the forenoon, so as to be over by twelve o'clock. By no means allow a child over two years of age to sleep in the afternoon, if it is well, for this protracts the time for sleeping at night; it will soon not want to go to bed, will make it later and later every night, until, before the parent knows it, the child does not want to go to bed, in fact seems never ready to go to bed, and as a necessary result, never ready to get up; never ready for breakfast; breakfast has to be "saved," to the annoyance and discomfort of the servants, to say nothing of the injustice done to them in the deranging their work, putting it back, and increasing the amount, and all this for the bad habit of a child, a habit which is positively injurious to its health and well-being.

It is most earnestly requested that all young mothers especially look at this thing of children's sleep in all its bearings, and act wisely and conscientiously.

RECAPITULATION.

For the first five or six days immediately after confinement it is of incalculable importance to both mother and infant to have bodily rest and mental repose. Everything practicable should be done to give the mother peace of mind; remove everything which could either annoy or disturb; exclude all disagreeable intelligence; relieve her as much as possible from every domestic responsibility, propose nothing which requires deliberation; nothing which demands comparison, and important decision; the mind should be kept as perfectly at ease as possible, and in an encouraged, hopeful mood, all aiding greatly towards promoting sleep, and giving power to recuperate.

For similar reasons, all visitors should be absolutely excluded, except husband and nurse and physician, for at least four or five days; if any one should be allowed admission, it is the mother of the invalid, and not even she, unless she is of a calm temperament, and can be trusted for her prudence, consideration, and cheerful lovingness of disposition. After the first week, one or two at furthest may be admitted each day, and in a few days more; a gradual increase in numbers is admissible. But as to the

NEW-COMER,

more stringent rules should be observed. A new-born baby requires from the very first instant three things,

WARMTH, FOOD, SLEEP.

Keep it warm in a soft, fine blanket or flannel cloth for the first five or six hours, then, after feeding it, let it sleep; when it wakes up, feed it again, if not sooner than two hours; if it wakes up before the two hours, let it wait for dinner, like a grown person; it will soon get used to it, and be all the better for it; then lay it down to go to sleep again ; this secures two of the most important things in infantile life, regularity of eating, and abundant, sufficient sleep ; for only give the child a fair chance, and Nature will regulate that. But just here comes in a perfect nuisance : the baby has been put to sleep, some aunt or uncle or other privileged person calls, has but a moment to stay, but wants to see the baby ; admission is given, or the child is taken into another room ; in either case its

NAP IS BROKEN,

it may not be able to go to sleep again ; and failing of that, feels badly, frets, is put to the breast an hour before its time, and regularity in sleeping and eating is at once broken into. There is but one rational, humane plan : Never wake up a sleeping infant for anybody or anything ; if a neighbor happens to come in when its nap is out, when it has waked up of its own accord, then it may be shown to a visitor for two or three minutes, no longer, for the first week ; any woman who does not enforce this rule, considering its far-reaching consequences, does not really love her child. The husband who does not help his wife to enforce these reasonable observances, fails of a most important duty to himself, his wife, his child, and to society in general. If mother and child can be helped to the fullest quietude, to all the sleep they can get, to exemption from all excitement and solicitude and care, both will grow stronger and healthier and heartier every day, with a constantly accumulating force of vitality, circulation, and of resistance to all ordinary diseases. Nor is this all : the mother should not be put to the trouble of deciding whether this visitor, or that, or the other, should be admitted ; let it be sufficient for the servant to meet all callers at the door with the announcement that the doctor has given orders that no visitors should be admitted for the present on any account ; this is the easiest, best, and most direct method of securing the important ends desired.

THE APPETITES

are three in number : they are the passions, the propensities of our nature, and were intended to be gratified, to be satisfied. As they are equally essential to the life of man and the perpetuation of the race, it has been wisely arranged that their gratification is attended with satisfaction and pleasure. They are called passions, because all the energies of a man's nature are summoned to procure the means of their indulgence. The term propensity is used in reference to them in consequence of nature always seeking or calling for their gratification. The word appetite means a seeking for, as the bird is always in search of food. If either of these three propensities were to die out, the race would perish; but Revelation teaches that it was the end and aim of the creation of the material universe to perpetuate the human species for the purpose of peopling heaven with an innumerable company of the redeemed from all nations and kindred of the earth; and the more certainly to accomplish this great design, both eating and drinking and reproduction are made a duty and a pleasure; a duty to the Maker, a pleasure to the man. If these pleasures are too freely indulged in, disease comes on, premature decay and death. But here the Scripture comes in for our guide, and counsels us to be temperate in these indulgences, and warns us against being gluttonous and wine-bibbers, as being vices which bring their own punishment here, and " condemnation " hereafter. Here comes in the law of rational indulgence. We should not eat or drink more than we want, more than we need, more than is good for us; if we do, sickness and suffering are sure to follow.

Some require more drink than others; some require more food than others; one cannot be a law to another, each man must be a law to himself. His reason must be brought into requisition to enable him to decide as to the extent of his indulgence. Each man for himself is practically interested in the question, How much must I eat? how much must I drink? These inquiries are constantly made of the physician, but it is utterly impossible to make a rule which would meet all cases; for some work harder than others, and the more work, the more food; the nearest we can get to it is, we must eat and drink until we are satisfied, until the sense of hunger and thirst is appeased; if these are present to the extent of making themselves felt, giving rise to the desire to eat and drink, then we have not had enough and ought to have more. These statements have been made to give an idea of the analogies of things, in order to throw light upon that most important, personal, practical question which so nearly concerns the happiness and well-being of every married man, and which is so often proposed to the physician, and would be proposed millions of times oftener, did not certain feelings of delicacy prevent. Deficiencies and excesses in reproductive indulgences are productive of quite as much sin and sorrow and suffering as excesses and deficiencies in eating and drinking. Many starve to death because they have not enough to eat, and cannot get it; millions more die prematurely because they gluttonize. In a sense man is always ready for the performance of the reproductive function if in vigorous health; not one in a million is otherwise, and when such a one is found, it is because he is deficient. Some women, not a few, have no such desires; on the contrary, there is an abiding aversion, approaching to disgust; multitudes more have them only for a short time after each catamenial flow, when the system is prepared for impregnation, for the making of a new being, as if in obedience to the command to "multiply and replenish," from a sense of duty. At the same time it is the wife's duty to acquiesce whenever indulgence is desired; and as indulgence involves no drain on her system, and when no inclination is present she can be passive, refusal becomes a crime, because one of two things will always happen, will inevitably happen; nothing but a miracle can prevent their happening in any one case: the man will go elsewhere, or his health, moral and physical, will suffer, and he cannot prevent either, any more than he could take wings and fly beyond the ocean.

It would be altogether useless to introduce this subject, unless it was treated in a manner so plain and so specific, as to come before the reader's mind with sufficient clearness and definiteness to make it usefully practical; and yet it is of such a character that it is desirable, it is more agreeable, to express the ideas in an indirect manner or in roundabout phrase, for neither reader nor writer can be divested of the feeling, that there is a certain degree of privacy connected with it which calls for expressions which leave something to the imagination to do, in order to carry out the full idea. It would be otherwise, if what is written could meet the eyes only of those who are most directly concerned, those who are living in lawful wedlock.

This subject is treated more fully in the author's book on

36

sleep, but this volume would not fill a family want, unless some suggestions were made in reference to the matters in hand.

If a man is honorably faithful to his wife, and the reproductive functions are not performed to the extent of appeasing the appetite as to him, whether it is the result of her unwillingness, or his not being disposed to annoy; when, from any cause, real or imagined, it is so, he may maintain his integrity, he may honorably, from a high sense of principle and duty, and in consideration for his family, refuse outside gratifications, but Nature will not be appeased for all that, any more than a hungry man can be satisfied without food; and this result follows: Nature is, in a sense, always manufacturing the reproductive substance, as she is always manufacturing bile or urine, and when the bladder is full it must be emptied; if not, inflammation takes place, and death follows within a week; if there is no discharge voluntarily, by the will, Nature sends dreams, and there is a spontaneous emptying and involuntary evacuation, and the bed is soiled, as in children. When the reproductive fluid is not disposed of in the way Nature designed when marriage was instituted, it accumulates in the vessels made to receive it, over-distension follows, dreams are the result, and they evacuate; the name given to describe this is nocturnal emissions, and when this thing is once set up, once becomes a habit of the system, it becomes as perfectly uncontrollable as that of nocturnal urination in a child; it is a thing which takes place beyond any possible control, and can't be helped in any other way than by not going to sleep. There are medicines which will arrest this manufacture, but they endanger the destruction of the function, which would be just as much a crime as to cut off an arm or to destroy the sight. But these occurrences do not take place with impunity: they grow, increase in frequency, bringing on such debilities of body as sometimes destroy life, and so affecting the mind as sometimes to destroy it, making it idiotic; not always inducing such sad results, not often inducing them, but the tendencies are in that direction; the constitution is always injured and the moral character always impaired. Hence, it clearly follows, that any woman, who for a mere whim, in sheer ugliness, is willing to risk results like these, is unworthy of the sacred name of wife, and ought to be "cast out," because her life is a living lie and an habitual perjury, an accumulative crime, becoming more aggravated every day.

It is within a few years that ignorant, knavish, and unclean men and women were going through the country delivering indecent harangues, dignified by the name of " Lectures," with the announcement that they were only for ladies, the burden of them being that they were " made a convenience of," and that this was the cause, the great cause of their impaired health; that unless remedied, permanent disease and premature death would be an inevitable result. The more weak-minded were carried away with the shallow reasoning, with the result that in many cases discords were sown in families which had lived in harmony and love for five and ten and twenty years; no one seeming to have known the important fact that maiden women, on an average, die several years sooner than the married, all the asserted indignities and outrages, and hardships and perils of child-bearing to the contrary notwithstanding. But in this, as in all other cases, throughout the moral universe, wrong-doing, perverseness, always brings its own punishment. Comparatively few men hold fast their integrity; their reasoning is, they have a right; if this right is refused from a mere whim or caprice, they will seek it elsewhere; and when once the ice is broken in this direction, there is such a fascination in variety, a fascination first, then an unconquerable passion, that the path is never retraced this side the grave; the moral sense is perverted and the course is downwards forever. Thousands and tens of thousands of husbands are thus made vicious every year; thousands of divorces are sought for and tens of thousands of others would be, were it not for the discredit of it; for, however rightly a divorce may be obtained in some cases, there is, in the minds of all decent people, a stain left on both, carrying with it the feeling of contempt and disgust, and one which is ineradicable, however unjust that may be in some cases; the very fact of a divorce leaves an impression of degradation, for there is an instinctive feeling that both are to blame; that both had descended to a cat-and-dog life, and had lived in it for a long time before it came to the crisis of a separation. When the house is once left for an abandoned purpose, that house never becomes a home again; the fireside feeling never again enters that man's heart—the oneness, the unity, is gone;

THE LAST LINK IS BROKEN;

and he feels himself, ever after, an outsider.

These things have come to the author's knowledge in the course of many years' practice. The cases have been so numerous, the " confidences" have been so frequently made, that the broad facts cannot be disputed. Only a physician in a large city can come to the full knowledge of how these things work; and he judges not from the city merely: from all parts of the country also is he consulted, under the impression that his experience is more extensive and his counsel more valuable than under other circumstances. Hence it is the city physician only, who is an adequate judge of the propriety, the utility, and the wisdom of discussing such subjects in book form. But as many do wrong things unwittingly, and would promptly and gladly correct the wrongdoing the instant it is made palpable to them, the hope is that multitudes of married women, especially young wives, may escape the rock upon which the domestic bark has been so often dashed, by having had presented to their minds a clear idea of how these things work in practical, actual life, and of the value of one short lesson. Interpose no obstacle unless there is a clear necessity for it. If a sense of duty and love does not impel such a course, let that of cold policy avail, for it will certainly avert a world of

DOMESTIC WOES.

A more delicate subject is still to be discussed, it is that of frequency; and although no one can be a guide for another, any more than in quantity of food, yet it is capable of a satisfactory and accurate solution in the light of nature and instinct; in this, reason is no guide at all—as proof, a book has been written by one who has written much, teaching the doctrine of an annual consummation, which is so perfectly absurd, in fact, idiotic, that it is only named to show the truth of the statement just made, that human reason is not a safe guide in this respect. As the idea has never been presented in writing, as far as the author knows, and as with the advancing intelligence and inquisitiveness of the race, such things will sooner or later be inquired into while they are yet new, the reader is requested to bring his own rationality into requisition, and examine and decide every statement made on this abstruse and delicate point.

If a man does not get enough food for the wants of the system, he is made sensible of it by a certain feeling in the stomach, his attention is directed to the fact that he has a stomach; so in this other appetite, if not satisfied up to Nature's want and need, there is a constant reminder of this want, that there is a reproductive nature; when the propensity is fully fed, the mind goes off to something else. If a man is very hungry his attention is acutely and quickly attracted to everything eatable on the street; were he not hungry he would pass wagon-loads without even the knowledge of their existence. A countryman will walk the whole length of Broadway and never notice a book of all the thousands which are so temptingly displayed, as he passes Appleton's and Carter's and Randolph's, because his tastes, his feelings are not in that direction; but he would notice a

BIG PUMPKIN

or a good horse collar or a magnificent saddle, because these things are in his line, and he wants them, needs them, has not enough of them at home, his desires are not satisfied in that direction, hence he is fully alive to everything of the sort. The man who has not had the desires of his nature met, is committing adultery in his heart at the meeting of every fair form, and he cannot help its being said of him, he "looketh on a woman to lust after her;" of all such, of all unmarried men who are continent, it is most literally true, the imaginations of the thoughts of their hearts are evil, only evil, and that continually. A man could not be a man, were it otherwise, and it is utterly useless to blink the question. Hence he is constantly committing sin on the public streets; and in retiracy, unclean thoughts will run rampant, both in his day dreams as well as those of the night, and in time his mind becomes impure, his thoughts impure, and the association of his ideas will become impure to an extent that sights and even sounds will set up trains of thought which father imaginations very often little less than bestial. Hence it is that marriage is a great purifier of the thoughts and intents of the heart, as all conscientious persons well know who have passed from the single to the married state. Therefore it clearly follows that all these sins, all these demoralizations, are justly laid at the door of the unwilling wife. The whole subject merits the deliberate and serious and mature consideration of every intelligent, conscientious, and pure-minded woman. The law allows divorce on the ascertainment of such malformation as clearly makes reproduction impossible, because it is against Nature; moral malformation is in effect the same. Indifference is a moral deformity, let alone aversion to the act.

Besides all this, a woman of the class under consideration has married for a home, or for other unworthy reason, and not for love. She has perpetrated a deliberate fraud on her husband and on society, and has none of the rights of a wife; nor can she justly claim her husband's respect or sympathies. Then there is a consideration which sinks her into deeper depths. She allows a man to spend his waking existence at his shop, his office, his store, or his manufactory, in labor and in toil, to support his household respectably, in comfort and abundance, to supply the means for dress, and for all the other calls incident to social life; while in return there is not accorded that consideration, and the exercise of those claims which of right belong to him; or if accorded, it is grudgingly, with the interposition of such obstacles, and the exhibition of such indifference, such an unwillingness, and with such an ungracious manner, that the mind can come to no other conclusion than that there exists an intensity of selfishness, which degrades any human being who possesses it to the level of the meanest of the race. Of course there can be no love there.

There are other circumstances which show that the all-pervading appetite has not been appeased. Not only the debilitating occurrences already alluded to: the "looking after" others lustfully, and the evil, impure imaginations before spoken of; but in the early morning, on waking, there is a uniform rigidity of the reproductive parts, which shows the yearning of the instinct for its natural feeding, as a hungry man thinks of richly spread tables, just as the waking dream of the morning is breaking up the sleep of the night.

There is still another and a fifth indication that Nature has not had her satisfaction. When there is good bodily health, and the functions are vigorous and perfect, accompanied with honorable continence, there is always, in the earliest part of married life, an instantaneous completion of the consummation even before an accomplished introduction. A city physician is constantly consulted by letter or in person in reference to this, and always with considerable mental perturbation. There is, in the first place, an apprehensive impression of very serious defects of organization, with a very great annoyance at the consideration of reaching the acme alone; no time having been afforded, in the other direction, to come up to the point of enjoyment; causing, and justly too, very considerable dissatisfaction, felt, but not expressed; for there is an innate delicacy of sentiment in every true woman in these regards, which prevents expression of feeling. Hence, most of them cover it up, and patiently abide the cure of what is so undesirable, until time and practice bring about the rectification.

These considerations fully answer the important question as to the measure of frequency, and indicate a rule of conduct which can be clearly and satisfactorily applied to all, of whatever age, temperament, habit, or constitution. It is an unerring and perfectly safe principle of application in all possible cases, and to which, in healthy persons, there are no exceptions. To recapitulate: Marital consummations are to be accomplished to the extent—

First, of preventing the " looking on a woman to lust after her."

Second, of preventing lascivious dreams.

Third, of preventing the early morning rigidities.

Fourth, of preventing the tendency of the mind to run off into evil and impure imaginings on the instant the attention is directed by sight or sound to anything which can bring to it thoughts on the great, controlling, prevalent subject.

Fifth, of preventing instantaneous consummation, and,

Sixth, of preventing great debility or any discomfort following the act.

The frequency should be diminished until no discomfort whatever is experienced, even transient; just as in a dyspeptic condition of the stomach, a man should eat less and less each time, until no discomfort whatever is induced, and that is the proper measure for him; if that limited amount is continued for a while, the stomach becomes stronger, and more can be indulged in, and more and more, until the person can eat as much as others without any inconvenience. But if in increasing the amount of food he does it too fast, and discomfort begins to show itself, he must at once diminish the amount to a satisfactory quantity. This is precisely the line of conduct to be pursued as to the subject under discussion.

If hebdomadal, or even annual consummations are followed by debilities, or exhaustions, or other indications of a strain on nature, then they are to be demitted, howsoever great the misfortune in any particular case; pitiful though it be, and commanding the sincerest sympathies of all generous minds. As in a man losing his fortune undeservedly, it is a hard case, but it cannot be helped.

Many a man has married to-day, and to-morrow has shot himself through the head or hung himself on a nail behind the door. Thousands of marriage bells have been rung, and the next day the young bride has retreated to her mother's bosom and taken refuge there for the remainder of a blighted life. The author knew a man of great name, a statesman and a warrior of renown. At the height of his power and his fame, he married an accomplished woman, of high social position, educated, cultivated, refined, of commanding personal attractions, and of queenly bearing. The next morning he was missing. The executive mansion was closed, no sight nor sound of living thing was there, it was literally a

"BANQUET HALL DESERTED."

The lady had returned to her father's house, and the gentleman became by degrees more and more forgotten; at length, however, it was ascertained that he had made a home with savage tribes, not returning to civilized life for many years afterwards. An explanation was never vouchsafed, "no man can say, Doctor, that I ever said a word against her," and that was all that either of them would allow the great world outside to know; both have long since mouldered into dust.

At other times, and such things come only to the knowledge of physicians, the foundation is laid on the wedding night for life-long antipathies, estrangements, and disgusts, which make of the whole of married life thereafter a purgatory instead of a paradise, without any positive crime, or wrong, or fault on either side sometimes; but the result, in many cases, of the want of a little consideration, a little intelligence, a little common sense; was merely a little misapprehension; and if one such blighting and blasting and mildew shall be prevented by what is here written, it will be some compensation for having spent so much time in the consideration of a subject which bristles with aversions. Youth is impulsive, hasty, passionate, and has so much inconsideration, that it is rather complimentary to human nature that greater and graver evils are not more frequently fallen into, than there are; especially when it is taken into consideration how ignorant the young are in these matters, at least those who have been brought up virtuously.

The young husband has often murdered himself outright from a sheer misapprehension; the young wife runs home to her mother, or worries herself into an early grave, or into a place far more terrible, a mad-house, from hasty and groundless impressions. It is purposed here to give some practical suggestions for the avoidance of such calamities in a great many cases; the starting point for the lesson is the consideration that the animal pervades the man, the angelic the virgin, not literally true, but in a sense it is true; in effect it is true. At the marriage altar and in the bridal bedchamber, indulgence takes possession of the young man's whole nature; it is uppermost in every thought and feeling; there is no idea with which it is not associated. With the girl it is different, she wonders, she imagines, she covers her face, she shrinks away, would willingly sink through the floor, and a million of times she sincerely wishes there was a trap-door in it for escape from the ordeal, which otherwise has to be passed; and as this book is designed for parental use, the suggestion is here made, that both father and mother, in their appropriate spheres, should make such suggestions as their own experiences have brought to them; such as might be serviceable on an occasion as important as it is new and overpowering. The young man should bear in mind that he is approaching a tender flower, which a breath may scorch, which a rude touch may break from its stem; in an hour to be wilted and to die, metaphorically. For the first month of a first marriage, the husband should not feel himself to be any other than the betrothed; this single consideration would prevent the blight of many a married life, and the parent reader cannot take too much pains to impress the idea upon the mind of the child. It is meant that the young wife should be treated as if she were still a girl, a young lady, in respect to her wishes being implicitly deferred to in every conceivable thing. Before marriage it was only necessary for the very slightest intimation to be given on her part of what might be most agreeable to her; it was never requisite to repeat that intimation; it was never necessary to wait an instant; no demur was ever made; no objection interposed by any possibility, no undue urgency ever exhibited, except now and then for a stolen kiss, sweeter than the nectar of the skies; and then, what delicacy of deportment in all respects; what knightly courtesy, what ready attentions, what respectful lifting of the hat at every meeting and departure; what beseeching looks for the slightest favors desired! let these principles of conduct and action be carried out the first night, and the second, and for a month, asking nothing, insisting on nothing; patiently, generously, heroically waiting for intimation of will; gentle as in the handling of the tender infant, and deferential as the courtier at the reception of his Queen. In this way an initiation will be made, an entrance effected into the new life which will give it one of the most attractive colorings, and will throw a halo around it, beautiful to all beholders.

No disappointed surprises; no impatient gesture, or sign, or look, should ever escape from either; if never, better; but at least for one little month, that first month, that eventful month, let it be spent in the diligent practice of all these little amiabilities which so smooth enjoyable, social intercourse, which cost so little, which bear such a large fruitage for good.

A different course brings about the results a while ago intimated. Impatience alarms; roughness pains; impetuosity angers; brutality disgusts.

If the animal is seen to predominate; if it is shown to be the ruling passion, the young wife instinctively despises, and it may take long years even to efface the impression. Surely these are considerations which should outweigh a Chimborazo or a Cotopaxi.

But there are circumstances within himself, which often lead the young husband to groundless imaginings, and being cherished, grow to enormous dimensions, causing, often, the overshadowing of the intellect, or its total destruction; and all this from a misapprehension engendered by reading a certain class of books, which are unfortunately too sure to find their way into ands of young men, by reason of their, to them, attractive titles; promising revelations on subjects which the young mind has a most intense desire to investigate, and upon which it earnestly seeks information; but the information vouchsafed is not the kind which is instructive in what is true and useful; the whole intent is to mislead first, then to alarm, and then to fleece. All these publications open with expressions of a benevolent regard for the happiness and best interests of humanity, and of the young in particular. Next, with a show of learning, investigation, and research, braced with quotations from the most eminent authors, the way is thus prepared for the most outrageous falsehoods, falsehoods which the young have no available means of detecting. All these things are of a private nature, and there is an instinctive delicacy in comparing ideas, even with the nearest friends; these things the writers of these books are too old in sin and in the knowledge of the worst and weakest phases of human nature, not to take advantage of; hence they feel safe in their strongholds of falsehood and infamy. Their mode of procedure is to appeal to physical appearances in part; that such and such a thing looks so and so, or is so and so; the reader sees that this is the fact, and finding this to be a truth, his confidence is gained, but the next statement is a mere assertion, the most palpable falsehood, at least palpable to a professional mind; but the victim receives it as true, and here he is ensnared, led astray, and becomes an easy prey to imposture. As to the case in hand: These books give the information that instantaneousness of consummation is a sign of nervous debility, of absence of virile power, and that there is no manliness, no capability of perpetuation; that unless it is remedied, the infirmity becomes permanent, and that such a condition is dreadful to contemplate; this naturally excites the gravest apprehensions, and with assurances of certain and permanent rectification, the way is opened for charges measured by the ascertained ability of the victim to pay, ranging from fifty to a hundred or a thousand dollars. Remedies are given which are perfectly inert, but the information is vouchsafed, that it is better to run no risk, to impart to the system no shock, but to bring it gradually under the influence of the potent and costly drug, all of which requires time; meanwhile, by practice and habit, the instantaneousness diminishes, as a matter of course; the keen edge of desire wears off; the diminution is appealed to as a fact, but the fiction is not seen by the blinded victim; he is so carried away with the seeming success of the treatment, that he sometimes not only pays the charges, but, if flush of money, adds gratuities of jewelry or other costly presents.

The actual facts are, that this very instantaneousness is a demonstration of healthful vigor, that all is just as Nature would have it, and the change comes, as in the appetite for eating, the more frequently food is taken, the less urgent are the demands of the stomach, but more healthful and far safer. These, and other false teachings, abound in books about "Manhood," "Marriage," "Physiology," and the like, intended for boys of fourteen and over, offered at a trifling cost, and embellished with cuts and engravings to excite curiosity and lead to the consideration of subjects connected with the reproductive functions, with the express purpose of misleading them in the same manner as just detailed. These youths are led on from one thing to another in these publications, until in the same way they are persuaded that something is the matter with them; to a certain extent facts are appealed to; the facts are palpable to the youth's sight; he cannot help but believe them; and when he is told that such facts are proofs of an unnatural, a diseased condition, he receives this latter statement as gospel truth; the mind is misled, fears are excited, and money is gladly parted with on the promise that everything will be certainly and permanently remedied. But these appearances, these feelings, these occurrences, are natural, just as much so as in the case detailed above; but the youth has no means which he is willing to resort to to gain information; he is unwilling to consult his parents, or any physician of his acquaintance, because there is an impression that a degree of disgrace is attached to it, and this he wishes to hide from the eyes of those whom he knows. If it were only a loss of money, it might well be passed over; but a young reader of the books named is often thrown into a state of excitement, dread, and remorse, which becomes terrible. City physicians of any name or note are constantly receiving letters from youth in the country, which clearly show that they are on the very verge of insanity; and cases are on record showing that suicide has been committed as the shortest and easiest way of getting rid of the mental torments. In fact, many of these letter writers do not hesitate to say they would rather be dead than remain in their present condition; others say they would pay any amount of money possible in their circumstances for relief, and in many cases it requires a great deal of time and trouble to explain to them and show them that nothing is the matter with them, but their condition is natural and healthful. Sometimes neither letters nor references to standard books nor personal expostulations avail to dispossess them of their absurd opinions. Under these circumstances, parents will readily see that it is their duty to keep such books out of the hands of their boys, by explaining to them their true character; and further, it would be a great point gained to exclude all newspapers from the family which advertise these books for sale, under whatever title they may appear. These books have a greater influence on the mind of youth, from the professions of humanity which their writers indulge in, and their reference to Scripture.

Among the things harped on in these vile publications is, that a want of memory, a downcast look, an averted eye, not looking people in the face, are certain proofs of the habitual practice of such indulgences as induce nocturnals; as if to be brazen-faced, and to stare decent people out of countenance were proofs of purity and virtue. Being thus misled, a youth is prepared to pay any amount of money possible to him, on assurances of cure, which are glibly given; or, not having the means, he broods over these things from day to day, he is abashed, he considers himself a criminal, he feels disgraced in his own eyes, and imagines that everybody who looks at him knows all about it; hence, the impassioned appeals to city physicians for gratuitous aid from direful impendings; the letters many times blotted and blurred with the marks of tears, O how bitter! And all this without the slightest foundation in fact, because nocturnal emissions have no necessary connection with habits of self-indulgence, since they come on spontaneously, as naturally as hunger or thirst; they are really an indication of the healthful vigor of the parts; all have them up to marriage, unless there are natural defects; marriage is their only safe and healthful remedy; but after marriage they will inevitably return to the healthy, under two conditions: separation, even for a week or two, in cases of the vigorous, or an inadequate home supply, a supply which is not up to Nature's rightful demand. But it suits the writers of the books in question, that the whole subject should be made to take this turn ; hence, nocturnals are represented as the ruinous effects of self-abuse, and are the sure precursors of utter disqualification for honorable marriage.

It is easy to see what a disturbing effect these representations have on the susceptible minds of youth, and how willingly they would spend every dollar they could spare, to relieve themselves of what they consider not only a most deplorable, but a most disgraceful condition, second only to a venereal affection ; and this is precisely the state of mind intended to be induced ; a readiness to part with any amount of money they could raise to be cured of a thing which is no disease, and not only so, is an indisputable evidence of a healthy vigor of the parts, an overflow of vitality, having no natural connection with self-pollution, denominated " Onanism." This truth cannot be too distinctly placed before the mind of the reader and parents, with a view to their imparting the information to their boys when there is occasion for it.

As has been before stated, the fluid discharged in the nocturnals, is, in a sense, all the time in formation, as urine is all the time in formation ; not exactly so but practically so ; and it is just as necessary for the seminal vessels, reservoirs, to be emptied as the bladder ; the natural method is in the consummations of honorable marriage, and in its absence, if continence is observed, if promiscuous indulgence is not practised, Nature will find an outlet, for out it must come ; and she does it through the instrumentality of lascivious dreams in the light sleep of the early morning ; this fluid accumulates during the night, the vessels are congested, excess of blood is attracted to the parts, dreams are excited in that connection, and emission takes place, just as dreams are excited by an over-distended bladder, and urine is passed in the bed, for Nature will not be cheated.

These nocturnals occur with varied frequency ; the oftener, in proportion as the person is virtuous ; meaning thereby, abstinence from sexual intercourse ; and in proportion as the health is vigorous, and the manly powers are all right ; and yet, in the face of these known facts, the books referred to make it appear that these very nocturnals, which are the water-ways, escape pipes of a healthy nature, are unmistakable proofs of a disgracefully diseased condition of the reproductive functions ; they are simply the spontaneous efforts of Nature to relieve herself of an over-accumulation, and would occur if a youth had never seen a woman, nor ever conversed, or been permitted to associate with any human being; they would occur in all healthy youths as inevitably as a discharge from the bladder, the rectum, the ear, or the nostrils.

They appear as early as fourteen, and take place with increasing frequency, until they amount, on an average, to five or six or eight a month, for five or ten years, when they begin to abate, and by thirty, average two or three a month. It is the testimony of distinguished medical men, that they have occurred as often as six or eight times a month for successive years, the parties have married without any ill result traceable to that thing; children being born as numerous and as healthy as to others.

They are more or less debilitating when occurring in excess; when they are found to be so, then measures should be taken to bring them down to a safe average of four or five a month; this can be done in three ways:

By medicine.

By marriage.

By Hygienic measures.

There are medicines which seem to control them while they are taken, but they require to be given in increased quantities, even when they are efficient; endangering the destruction of the reproductive power; of course, no honorable physician could persuade himself for any price to risk, even remotely, such a serious result. Bromide of potash, in ten or fifteen grain doses, three times a day, has, in some cases, appeared to have a controlling effect, at least for the time being, but any one may know, that what represses for a day, may, by continuance or excess, control forever, which means to be no man for all after life.

But this is not the object of these book writers: they would not succeed in repressing if they could; and nine times in ten they fail, beyond a transient effect; so they lead along the patient until the close of the first term for which they have been paid; then they advise, that as it seems to be a stubborn case it would be best to take a second course of medicine, to complete what was begun; at the end of that time, if they find that the weak-minded youth has spent all his living, or from any cause is not willing to pay more, the statement is made that it is an extraordinary case, rarely one is ever met with so difficult of management, and that under the circumstances, there is no cure but marriage.

"But this is impossible for me at present."

"In that case it would be better to keep a woman."

Such are the morals of the persons who write the books already referred to, and who send their advertisements to family newspapers, under the headings of "Nervous Debility," "Benevolent Association," "Advice to Youth," and other taking titles.

But there is another form in which their deceptions are practised: ignorant and credulous and weak-minded persons are persuaded that certain glairy fluids which exude from parts after urination or defecation are sapping the very foundations of health; that it is nothing more or less than the involuntary loss of seminal fluid, a drawing away of the very life-blood, and unless arrested, incompetency is an inevitable and permanent result. This they promise to cure certainly and soon. But this glairy substance is what Nature prepares to lubricate the channels, as water is prepared to lubricate the eye. Sometimes this substance is greater than others, as the eye sometimes waters more than common; or the nose, in consequence of a cold or inflammation; it is simply, when in excess, a catarrh of the parts; the inflammation is sometimes caused by the urine being more feverish or irritating than usual. These oozing substances have been examined by professional men in the most careful manner, and are always found wholly destitute of those living things which are essential to the seminal fluid.

At another time they are told that proof of diseased conditions is present in the fact that one testicle is greatly more relaxed than the other; or that one has disappeared, or that they have failed to come down; the parties make an examination; find it is so, for they see it, and forthwith yield themselves willing captives to the falsities which are taught them. The facts of the case are, that these all are natural appearances, are natural conditions, depending on those natural contractions and relaxations which belong to the parts, under the varying conditions of heat and cold, of excitement and repose.

It is pitiful to think how men could become so degraded as to persuade themselves to follow, as a calling, such despicable practices; but they find it profitable. One individual, in the course of a very few years, rolled up a fortune of over a hundred thousand dollars; his charges in some cases amounting to five hundred dollars.

It is by these books that the minds of boys are corrupted, preparatory to engaging in depraved practices in some cases; and in others, where there is a living conscience, groundless fears, wearing apprehensions, and wasting remorses, make life a misery, and many times, a burden, too heavy to be borne, and rest is found only in suicide; and as no parent can tell that his boy may not fall into these wiles, it becomes the duty of fathers and mothers to make themselves acquainted with the whole subject, and devise measures appropriate to each particular case, temperament, and disposition; to warn, to instruct, and to save. But in approaching a boy in this connection, it will be found better not to make a great secret of it; not to go into some inner room, and lock the door and get at it in a most gingerly, roundabout manner, but to speak of it as a matter of fact, one of every day occurrence, and one that it is rather better to pay some attention to; and then occasions may be taken to suggest, in a very incidental way, that books treating of such subjects are not worth reading, were written by bad men, and that nothing they contain can be relied on.

The third method, the Hygienic plan of keeping nocturnals within what might be called natural, safe, and unhurtful bounds, averaging a hebdomadal occurrence, is simply to remember, first, that warmth promotes excitement of the parts; without warmth it is impossible to occur; hence sleep in a cool room; not on a feather-bed, but a mattress, or even on the floor, the very hardness of which draws attention away from desire; have but very little cover on the body; but have abundant bedclothes from above the middle of the thighs downwards, so as to keep the lower limbs extra warm, thus drawing the blood away from the parts in question.

As lascivious dreams come in the unsound sleep of the early morning, or in second naps, avoid going to sleep after having once waked up. If a person needs only seven hours' sound sleep, but spreads it over nine hours, none of the sleep will be very sound; hence dreams which attend unsound sleep will be very certain to take place; but suppose all the sleep is concentrated within the seven hours, then it is all sound, there is no time or opportunity for dreams; hence the trouble is avoided, in many cases, simply

37

by arranging to remain in bed only seven hours, not sleeping at any other time of the twenty-four.

The more full the bladder is, the greater the heat of the parts; and as it is heat which brings the dreams, much is gained by urinating the last thing on going to bed, and also if waked up during the night.

There have been various mechanical devices for waking up the person before much excitement can take place, such as rings or bands, with spikes in them, which press into the parts as soon as the enlargement of excitement takes place; these are objectionable, because they are dangerous. Suppose the person slept so soundly as not to be waked up, then the ring or band would obstruct the circulation, and the rupture of an important blood-vessel might take place. And then again, it must be borne in mind, that to a certain extent these nocturnals are necessary, and it is not desirable to suppress them altogether, even if it could be done. But there are times when a youth becomes so possessed with a falsity, that it is almost impossible for his mind to be set aright, and he broods over fancied ill conditions for a great part of his waking existence, until the mind becomes almost unbalanced, and he is a short remove from insanity. Such a case occurred within a year, the only son of a widowed mother, but death happily came to his rescue. It is the idea of incompetency. There is one short way of settling this question in any specified case. There is always competency where there is erection; it is only when the part never rises from a flaccid condition that incompetency is a demonstration; *never rises for an instant.* If, for the shortest second, the part can be made to be at right angles to the person without touching, simply by an effort of the will, all idea of incompetency is absolutely groundless.

Going back now, many pages, the subject branched from may be resumed. How each person may settle the point of frequency, natural, proper, safe, and healthful for him. It can be done as certainly as each one can determine how much sleep he requires, by simply going to bed at a regular hour, and getting up in the morning the moment he wakes up; or, which would be better, remaining in bed long enough to allow the whole system to wake up gradually, and the feeling of tiredness passes away from the limbs; only do not go to sleep again, nor sleep a moment in the daytime; in this way, any one can tell within a week how much sleep his system requires; and if he retires regularly, he will wake up within a very few minutes of the same time, except that in heavy, damp weather, or from unusual exercise or labor, he may sleep a little longer; so in the matter under consideration, what is needful can be ascertained, when both parties are healthy, and have no peculiarities of temperament or constitution; when this is the case, there is, in the act of reproduction, at least once in the month, during the child-bearing period, a synchronism in the consummation; and this should not be on the instant; if it is, the consummations must be increased in frequency, even if diurnally, and kept up, until at least a score or two of movements are necessary. If more than that, or if attended with perspiration and cessation for rest, before completion, then are the powers of Nature overtaxed; it is excess; the prostate gland is stimulated beyond its healthful abilities, debilities and congestions or sub-acute inflammations follow, to end in a disease connected with the water works, which is of frequent occurrence among men past fifty; a disease which comes along insidiously, but with the steady and irresistible advance of an avalanche, finally racking with pain, and embittering every moment of the waking existence. But men inflict these pains and penalties on themselves from the want of knowledge on the subject; a knowledge of the kind which has been communicated in the few past pages, and which never has been found in books before, and was never understood, except among professional men. And if, in the course of years, the circulation of this book shall be extensive enough to induce some thousands of men to study and understand the subject, and practise the precepts given, by abstinences to the extent of coming short of excess, and by indulgences to the extent of preventing the six occurrences or conditions named in a previous page, not only will health be improved, and the moral nature advanced and purified by the prevention of lustings, but the satisfactions of consummations will be as vivid at threescore, as at thirty, instead of incompetency and imbecility at forty, as was the case with one of the brightest minds of our country; one who made a notable mark on the times in which he lived, for he was as brilliant as he was powerful, but of unbridled animal passions: no reason, no sense of decency, no consideration of social position or family claims, could or did restrain him; he ran riot in his lusts, and before he was fifty he was a nihility, died an outcast, homeless and a driveller in his old age, after having been one of the most admired and honored men of his day and generation, the associate and the peer of the magnates of the land.

Yet men will recklessly brave these dangers and disgraces as they brave the dangers and disgraces which inevitably follow habitual drunkenness. Some would reform if they could; if the temptations or the opportunities were removed. Perhaps some may be saved by being shown how to avoid the hurtful indulgences alluded to. This is discussed more at length in the author's book on "Sleep," it being one of the subjects connected with the sleeping hours; but the main idea is, that if married persons slept in separate rooms, or at least in separate beds, as is the almost universal custom in Germany and Holland especially, several very great advantages would result, in regard to comfort and health.

It is known that if two persons, one healthy and one sickly, sleep in the same bed, the healthy one will become diseased, without the sickly one being benefited; this is notably so, when a little child sleeps with a feeble old person. Hence, as it seldom happens that both man and wife are in perfect health in all respects, at all times, at least one party would be saved from injury by sleeping alone.

Good, sound, refreshing sleep and abundant, is essential to the health and well-being of every one; how important to a nursing mother, to the toiling farmer, to the hard-worked mechanic, it is easy to imagine; how uncomfortable it is to be waked out of a sound sleep, and how very difficult it is, when thus roused, to get to sleep again, very many know by repeated experiences. It is easy to be waked up by one turning over in bed, by a cough, a groan, a nightmare yell or terror. Then, some of the worst forms of low fevers are induced by too many persons occupying the same room; terrible narrations of this kind are given in the book just named; and to that extent will injury be done by the bodily emanations of two in the same bed; besides breathing an atmosphere already contaminated by having been breathed by another.

Opportunity makes importunity. If a plate of cakes is always on the table where little children are playing about all day, as often as their eyes fall on it, there is a want and a request of the mother for one of them; but if out of sight, if there were no cakes there, they would only be thought of when natural hunger came. So, if married persons slept in different rooms, the indulgences would only be specially thought of, when there existed a natural, healthy appetite for the same; and as food is the more enjoyable from the longer interval of fasting, so here. In this way, troublesome temptations are escaped, and a rational temperance would be practised without inconvenience. The subject merits serious consideration, and every husband of intelligence and force of character who reads these lines will at once, for his own best interests, begin to make such observations and experiments as will enable him to decide what are his needs, to what extent does his temperament require the reproductive gratifications, and will habitually and rigidly adhere to the allowance, as all rational, well-balanced minds impose a limit to the gratification of the appetite for food and drink.

AMENORRHŒA

is an interruption or cessation of the monthly periods. Healthy cessation occurs temporarily on becoming pregnant, and at the turn of life permanently. Interruption is the result of colds, exposure to dampness, or nervous shock, or some great trouble; when it occurs in the progress of any disease, it is a dangerous indication, as in consumption; most commonly the interruption is the result of colds taken; hence mothers should begin early, to impress on the mind the utmost importance, during the monthlies to avoid the application of cold in any form. The daughter of a wealthy gentleman alighted from her carriage and stood on the grass for half an hour listening to the sweet music of a band at the Central Park; it was a beautiful summer afternoon, but an hour before there had been a shower, the grass was wet, the shoes were thin, the feet became damp, and cold; suppression took place, inflammation of the lungs set in, and she died in a few days, an only daughter. Any other means of dampening the feet, or of making them cold while the monthlies are present, will bring about the same results, and so will the cooling off too soon after taking exercise of any kind, sufficient to cause even a slight perspiration, in ways similar to those mentioned in other parts of this volume, which should be read in this connection, often ; and with special care and intelligent attention, many a valuable life would be saved, thereby.

Sometimes persons of a full habit have amenorrhœa as a permanent thing, and seem to have good health for years but investigation will show in such cases that the system has some other form of discharge, some running sore, some frequent loss of blood from the nose, from the stomach, bowels, lungs, from piles or other form of depletion. But in most cases of amenorrhœa lasting for months and years, it will be found to exist in those who have " Anæmia," which see. The first point to be determined is, and it ought to be done without an hour's delay, what is the cause ? is it the result of some other disease which is gradually destroying the system ? is it causing some other disease, or has it originated from a transient, accidental cause, as a bad cold, getting drenched in a shower of rain, or other exposure ? When the malady comes on gradually, it is the effect of some other disease in the system, in which case, the only mode of cure is to remove that other disease, and secure the good general health of the patient.

When cessation comes on suddenly, as in the midst of a " turn," there are marked symptoms, there is headache, flushed face, strong pulse, cold feet, with minor symptoms ; make the feet warm, take immediate measures to have a full and free action of the bowels, to do which, a teaspoonful of the tincture of aloes and myrrh three or four times a day, so as to produce the effect of at least two full, free, large actions of the bowels in the course of twenty-four hours, and then a less amount, so as to keep up one action every day ; the two most urgent points are to empty the bowels at once, by purgatives or injections ; put the feet in hot water with strong mustard in it, two tablespoons in a gallon, in a pan so as to keep the feet covered up to the ankles ; the object being to bring back warmth to the body, the absence of which has caused the attack, and to unload it in any other direction most quickly available, for the system was unloading itself of a surplus, and it was the interruption of it which has caused the trouble ; warmth may be promoted by covering up in bed, hot water-bottles to the arm-pits and warm poultices to the breasts, the dry kinds being best, as bags of salt, or hot ashes.

Multitudes of remedies have been advised from time to time, which are considered to have a forcing effect, but it is a dangerous loss of time to wait for the action of one of them; none of them are really efficient. After using the first efforts of warmth and purgation, take at bedtime three of Cook's pills, or one liver pill, and patiently wait for the reappearance. But in any case of the non-appearance of the monthlies, first determine whether it is the result of pregnancy, whether the person is married or not; this question must be investigated, for if there is active purgation or other means to make the monthlies reappear, when in reality there is a child, the life of mother and child are imminently endangered by a single purgative. The patient ought to know the facts of the case, and must take the responsibility of action.

DYSMENORRHŒA

is when the monthly turns are attended with difficulty, or pain and suffering; this is the case of some women all their lives; sometimes pregnancy is a permanent cure. Ordinary painful menstruation is either from some mechanical cause, or it is functional; in this latter case, the patient begins to feel badly, there are pains in the back, in the head, in the region of the womb, changing, darting, hurting pains; the belly is sometimes swollen, relieved by pressing the hand on it; all of these symptoms are relieved when the discharge takes place.

If the trouble is of mechanical origin, as swellings about the mouth of the womb, constriction, or its misplacement or its closure, wisdom directs to the skilful physician.

But from whatever cause, avoid being on the feet much for a day or two before the time; lie down as much as possible, have the bowels act daily, eat moderately, and go to bed as soon as the pain begins, keeping the whole body abundantly warm. Cloths dipped in hot water, or water and spirits, and after being wrung out, laid while hot on the belly, renewed often, give grateful relief. Sometimes large injections of hot water into the vagina give immediate relief, drinking hot tea the meanwhile; in severe cases, a dose of paregoric is advantageous.

MENORRHAGIA

is when there is too much or too frequent a flow, caused by a want of vigorous health, or brought on temporarily by overwork, great fatigue, a tendency to bleeding of various kinds, too great excitement of the genital organs, over-marital indulgence. All that is to be done is to avoid the causes and use the means to obtain more vigorous " general health," which see.

LEUCORRHŒA,

whites, Female weakness, or Fluor Albus is a discharge caused by falling of the womb, or by a want of good health; if the womb is misplaced or disarranged, a physician should be called in to rectify it; but this is seldom the cause in any one who has good general health, because that very health keeps the womb healthy and in its place, and prevents that relaxation of the parts which keep it in position; while their relaxation very naturally attends a want of general health. Hence it may be set down pretty certain, that when a profuse discharge from the parts is present, it arises from a want of good health, and means should be adopted to secure it, such as regular eating, warm feet. This " flow " is generally of a whitish color, sometimes yellowish or greenish; if there is any blood at all, it is not leucorrhœa, but the whites. It is a troublesome and very annoying affection, and becoming more and more common, as the habits of the people become more sedentary and self-indulgent. Multitudes of remedies have been advised for the whites, none of which are efficient or do any safe, permanent good; astringent remedies as white-oak bark, " ooze," as it is called in country places, being the water in which white-oak bark has been boiled; it acts as an astringent; alum water would do the same thing, or logwood water, or claret wine, but all remedies of this character, in proportion as they have the desired effect, do harm, because they do to that extent thwart Nature; she is trying to get rid of unhealthy humors; while these things tend to stop them up, to keep them in the body; but Nature will not be interfered with, with impunity, in this way; if there are cases in which these styptic remedies must be used, care ought always to be taken to have at least one action of the bowels during every twenty-four hours, if not two, the idea being that if you stop up a sluice which Nature is opening at one point, we must open another elsewhere. There are in reality only two things to be done in functional or constitutional menorrhagia, or female weakness : use all means possible to maintain the general health, and keep the parts as scrupulously and as perfectly clean as intelligent care can do; at least twice a day, in the morning and at night, the " vagina " (which see) should be most thoroughly syringed with cold or warm water. First get over a basin of water, cold, cool, or warm, and flap it up with the hand, rapidly, against all the surrounding parts ; then use the syringe with other water, clean and fresh, the last syringeful being cold water, if not very particularly disagreeable.

The most popular remedies in Homœopathy are Pulsatilla, Sepia, and Mercurius, requiring, as other pathies do, a simple nutritive diet, and a large exposure to the open air, avoiding fatigue, over-exertion, standing still, even for a moment, unnecessarily, using cocoa and arrow-root, instead of tea and coffee.

It ought to be known that the discharge in whites may become so acrid as to cause a diseased condition of the male member, such as inflammation and peeling off of the skin, but this will soon cure itself in a healthy person in a very few days; but, in order to prevent uneasiness of mind, it should be known that studious cleanliness and free use of the syringe, as above indicated, is an effectual guarantee against any annoyance.

The water-cure practice is to use hip baths and vaginal injections freely, four or five times a day; if cold water irritates, use warm ; in all cases begin with a temperature of ninety degrees, gradually falling to fifty. If there is any blood, water at forty should be thrown up, and cold cloths applied to the belly, and as a diet, brown bread, cracked wheat, fruits and vegetables, with as much out-door air as it is possible to secure. without that over fatigue which aggravates the malady.

There are, then, three forms of abnormal Catamenia :

Amenorrhœa, when they do not appear.

Dysmenorrhœa, when their appearance is attended with more or less pain or suffering.

Menorrhagia, when there is an excessive discharge from the parts.

Whether the Catamenia have never appeared, or whether having appeared for a time they have ceased, the great points to be kept in view are two :

First, improve the general health.

Second, attract the blood of the body to the parts.

The first is done by improving the general health ; secure a regular, daily action of the bowels; use all possible efforts to keep the feet always warm; dress warmly, avoid taking colds, be moderately busy all the time in work which does not over fatigue, exercising in some way, at least two hours in the fore-noon, and one hour in the afternoon in the open air, out of doors, in as joyous a mood as possible, using a fruit and coarse bread diet, which see. In this way good blood is made for the body, and when it comes to the sexual parts, its inevitable tendency is to stimulate them healthfully, and invite a steady flow in that direction. That is done by warmth, not by external or internal stimulants, but by securing to the parts a natural warmth, which sooner or later brings on natural action. Medicines are given for that purpose, called Emmenagogues, but it is extremely doubt-ful whether any of them ever had a healthful effect in bringing on the Catamenia; but securing that object through the improve-ment of the general health, is always safe, and will always be efficient in any case that could have been cured by other means.

The best way to bring warmth to the parts as a means of in-viting the catamenial flow is to take a sitz bath of ten minutes with both feet in hot water nearly up to the knees; at the same time, a bath of a hundred degrees, then about ten seconds sit in cold water, feet also. But if the feet are comfortable, sit half an hour at a time in water of ninety degrees, allowing it to cool down to eighty and even seventy, by the time the bath is ended; these baths should be taken twice a day, before breakfast and near bedtime. The best results may be expected from the above course, always keeping the bowels free, and when practicable, take an hour's horseback exercise daily.

A similar treatment is specially applicable to cases where the catamenial flow is attended with difficulty and suffering. But when they are excessive, it is often because the blood is poor; then the course already advised, which makes better blood, more healthy blood, is the best possible to remedy an excessive flow. To know when the discharge is excessive, is of importance. The healthful flow lasts from three to six days, on an average; the average is perhaps three days; if it lasts longer than six days it may be set down as excessive; if the flow leaves the person weak, dispirited, languid in mind and body, it is excessive, usually, al-most always, induced by one of three things: overwork, poor food, general ill-health. Quantity, duration, or frequency are not to be so much the guide, in deciding that any case is excessive; it is the effects; if there is debility, languor, exhaustion, in proportion, the flow is excessive in that case, for in a healthy condition the spirits rise, there is an increased alacrity of body and activity of mind and joyousness of spirits, which show that all is well.

The causes have already been reverted to in detail, but the almost universal cause is a want of vigorous health, induced generally by constipation, cold feet, irregular eating, want of out-door exercise, too close confinement in warm rooms and having little or nothing to employ mind or body actively and profitably. Leucorrhœa is, in many respects, in cause, conditions, manifestations, and effects, like menorrhagia; the latter may readily slide into the former, and the best and most certain and most enduring cure for both is to build up the general health; it is doubtful if anything has a tendency to cure, except in proportion as the general health is restored, together with vaginal washings most thoroughly done two or three times every day, for there is reason to suppose that there is a virus in the leucorrhœal discharge which keeps it up; all may be washed out except in some little nook or corner or fold of the skin, to infect the other parts which were cleansed, just as a little fire left anywhere may spread over the whole building again, making safety to consist in a complete putting out of the fire; the same principle is involved in vaginal washings. Let them be well done and the greater will be the promise of cure. Homœopathists give Pulsatilla when the discharge is cream-like, then Calcarea, four days after second dose of Puls. Sepia, to delicate, exhausted persons. Mercurius, when the discharge is thick, yellow matter, or greenish, or corrosive. Alumina, when profuse. Graphites, when watery and acrid; Acid Nit. when brown, slimy, offensive, corrosive.

ABORTION

means arising or coming up out of season; applied to humanity, it means a birth before the time.

It will best answer a practical purpose, and be more easily understood, to say that Abortion is accidental or artificial; it is accidental when it arises from causes in the mother or outside of her. It may be caused in the mother by malformation; by the death of the unborn; by excessive nervousness; great debility;

exhaustive employments; by the tilting of a chair from placing the foot too near its edge; by a misstep in coming down stairs; by the use of step-ladders in adjusting curtains or hanging paintings, or by efforts which require straining, lifting sideways, hoisting windows at arm's length, by working until fagged out, or until heated and wearied in the endeavor to finish up some work in hand; the loss of a child is of frequent occurrence in these various ways, as also on occasions of having "company," when a wife's pride is very apt to stimulate her to exertions beyond her strength; at other times servants leave unexpectedly; in short, whatever causes any great mental or bodily shock, or any great bodily or mental strain, especially if long continued, is capable of producing an abortion.

That which becomes the child healthfully born into the world at the end of nine months from the moment of its generation, by the effectual congress of the sexes, has different names, according to the time which has passed from the impregnating act, as Foetus, Embryo, Germ, etc. The term "unborn child" will be here used to express the whole duration of being, from the moment of impregnation or sexual congress to the moment of birth. From the first instant of successful impregnation, there must be life; there must be the germ both of body and of soul, having in it all the elements of a perfect body and a perfect soul, which only need to be let alone to grow into a full and perfect human being. To destroy it at any moment of its life, from the first, to the moment of birth, would be as certainly a murder as the killing of a full-grown man, because within that germ are all the elements of a man; which, had it been permitted to live, might have been a benefactor of the race. The moral code of physicians is stern and uncompromising on this subject; the destruction of the germ, at any age of its unborn life, is regarded as perfectly inexcusable on any other ground than that of its demonstrable necessity, as a means of preserving the life of the mother; the rule is this: if mother or child must die, clearly must, then let it be the child. But no honorable physician can ever bring himself to the point of sacrificing the unborn's life under any other pretence whatever; and so conscientious and high-minded are they on this subject, that a proposition to that effect for any other reason than to save the mother's life, is resented as an insult, however high the source from which so infamous a proposition comes. The teachings of the Roman Catholic Church (see a few pages after) on this subject have always been clear, explicit, and uncompromising; that the deliberate destruction of an unborn is a murderous deed, and it is to be hoped that the time is not far distant when all branches of the Christian Church shall be as outspoken, and will visit with their severest penalties all infractions of a law, whose violation is in such palpable opposition to the Divine precept, to " multiply and replenish the earth," that being one of the main objects of the marriage relation, which is as holy in its nature as it is Divine in its institution. Let every man and woman in these matters stand in their lot, and meet all life's responsibilities bravely, honorably, without shirking, without trickery, without manœuvring to outwit the Omniscient One, who wisely made man to perpetuate the race, in order eventually to people heaven with saved and glorified immortals.

If the germ is brought forth before the end of the seventh month by deliberate artificial means, it should be properly called an Abortion ; if from accidental causes, a Miscarriage ; if caused by any means before the ninth month, and after the beginning of the seventh month, it is a Premature Delivery. By whatever means abortion is intentionally induced, the same, and in many cases a thousand times worse effects are left on the constitution, than if it were an accidental occurrence.

In whatever way an abortion is induced, shocks are imparted, which are never rallied from ; but when intentional, life-long results follow which it is painful to contemplate, let alone endure ; a chronic menstrual flow often follows a single abortion, to be a source of life-long annoyance and debility, if not severe disease, and how often fatal, the city physician too well knows. If abortion takes place in the early months, a profuse and even fatal flooding is by no means an unlikely result ; is liable, very liable to take place in any case; but even if this does not take place, the uterus is left engorged with blood, inducing excessive menstruation, chronic congestion, enlargement or granulations, only to be recovered from, if at all, by a long, wearisome, baffling, and expensive course of treatment.

Nature's method is to deliver at the end of the ninth month ; the earlier this is done, the worse, the more dangerous under all circumstances ; a first month's abortion is more likely to be fatal than any later one, because the uterus is then small, and the removal of the placenta, or after-birth, is attended with great difficulty and hazard, and fatal flooding is likely to occur in any case until the removal is accomplished; or the placenta not coming away, has to rot within the womb, become absorbed, and thus poisons the whole constitution. Small wonder is it then, that abortions, especially early ones, are regarded by all experienced physicians as a most unfortunate event in every single case; even in the very few cases where no serious results are observed, it is only a seeming escape; sooner or later the penalty will be inflicted. But these are physical sins only, sins against the body; there is a moral guilt, a sin against the soul, against humanity, against the unborn, for which there is no self-atonement, for it is murder; a holy human life has been destroyed, and if that is done within a week after impregnation, it is a life destroyed, as truly as if "six months gone," or any later period. Although quickening does not occur until four and a half months, that does not indicate that there was no life; it only shows when the mother first noticed life; life was from the instant of the impregnating act.

Bearing children is a healthful process, if a proper course of living has been observed; actually increases the chances of living longer; where one woman's health suffers from child-bearing, many suffer immeasurably more from induced abortions.

It is not only a crime to procure an abortion; it is a crime, in lawful wedlock, to avoid impregnation, not only as shown in the after part of this chapter, but in the direction of leaving the natural passions ungratified; and when this is the case, it is inevitable that the mind shall be filled with unholy desires, lascivious imaginations, impure thoughts; and these moral adulteries of "looking on a woman to lust after her," making them daily adulteries, and the "lust" is the same in either sex. Then there is that terrible remorse for wrong-doing, which may never be washed from off the hands, to follow on in all after life, a cloud upon every happiness, a blight on every joy, a veil upon the sunshine of one's whole after existence.

IN THE DARKNESS

things are done which cause inscrutable diseases; and as every one who reads this article once will read it again, and perhaps many times, it is purposed to word it with great care, and make it plain enough to be understood fully by those whom it most concerns.

Whether in the palatial mansion of the city, or the hut of the forest, the little child is an angel of light and gladness; so ordained by Omnipotence, as the means of perpetuating the race, of peopling heaven with angels, gathered as redeemed ones from all of humankind that are born. There is an increasing number of husbands and wives who antagonize this design, on the ground that the expense, and trouble, and care of children make it necessary to limit the family.

All the means used impair the health of the wife; not a few endanger life. The wife suffers most, for she sins and is sinned against; not only is the body injured, but the moral sense is impaired.

The means oftenest employed are imperfect marital rights; cessation before the instant of completion, when the whole nature is aroused to the utmost tension, involving every fibre of the system. To arrest the progress instantaneously, throw back into the system and quench remorselessly what would have the next moment become a new life, and which in the lapse of time might have added glory to the race, is but a short remove from murder. The man must feel degraded in the act; the woman, in the aim to avoid the responsibilities for which she was created, must have remorse, at the moment the whole reproductive system is shocked in the disappointment of its appeasement.

In some of the Roman Catholic books of devotion there are many useful teachings in regard to such matters, and so delicately proposed, that only gross minds are excited wantonly. Two lessons are taught, which the whole Protestant world ought to know; lessons which, by being silently impressed on the mind by frequent reading and in devotional contemplation, come to have in time the preventive power of a direct revelation, attention to which is as beneficial to the physical nature as it is to the religious.

First: Whoever performs any act from the instant of conception, to destroy life, to blight and blast the flower, is guilty of

MURDER.

There is no prudish mincing of words; nothing is left indefinite, obscure; it is not a mere hint; it teaches that the destruction of a germ of immortality, whether it be a minute or a month old, whether before or after birth, is nothing less than

MURDER.

This is the true doctrine, because the motive and the effect is the same; it is simply thwarting the purposes of the Almighty Father of us all, as plainly declared in His revealed Word, in the very beginning of human existence,—" Multiply and replenish." To destroy what would have been a life, is doing as much to thwart Omnipotence as to kill at any moment after life began; hence the far-reaching prescription of the second lesson inculcated; a lesson universally needed, a lesson universally disregarded, violated, every night of the world (see our book on "Sleep"). It was foreshadowed, at least it was in the mind's eye of the poet, when he wrote the lines,—

" Linked sweetness long drawn out."

The idea is, that the marital right, the act of reproduction, should be continuous until completed; no cessation for protracting gratification, because it baffles Nature, it deranges the delicate machinery, and sometimes breaks it as effectually as a machine would be, which, revolving at the rate of a hundred revolutions in a second, is stopped still in an instant; it would break any mechanism to atoms. Nature cannot bear these violences with impunity, and hence are monstrosities of birth! The lesson is completed by announcing that the object should be, as much as possible, to comply with the requirement to "replenish," and as little as possible for the mere gratification of propensities.

This subject has been introduced thus into our pages with the utmost reluctance; but it has been so studiously avoided by the pulpit and the press, that a sentiment has actually grown up in the minds of many that if a child is destroyed any time before birth, there is no harm in it; that it is only murder when the full-born infant is strangled; while in reality, not only is that a murderous crime, but using means to prevent an immortal life, while indulging in the pleasures connected with it, is not less a murder, is not less a crime, a crime against the Infinite One, as its direct aim is to thwart His purposes.

It was not considered advisable to give the slightest intimation how an abortion might be designedly induced, because it would be putting murderous weapons in the hands of the morally weak, but it is of immense importance for every virtuous and conscientious wife to know how accidental abortions may occur, how they may be averted.

If an accidental abortion takes place, even once, there is an increased liability to it at every additional impregnation, and more likely to occur about the same time. If it happens in the tenth week, there is a liability that it will occur when the next tenth week of pregnancy arrives, and if a second occurs, then a third is still more likely to take place.

Of course the danger of a second abortion can be certainly avoided by abstaining from the marital right, but this is inconvenient, and it is a wrong to the other side of the house, a wrong to both, because ungratified desires lead inevitably and always to lasciviousness, to moral adulteries, and on the part of the men, in a proportion of cases so large that if mentioned it would be received with incredulity—for whatever may be said, men will feel that they have a right, and if that right is not obtained in one place they will have it in another, thus easily persuading themselves into the belief that what they want to do, it is right to do. Many a man has been honorably faithful to his wife up to this point, then has committed one fatal transgression, which opening his eyes to new fields of delight, they are never closed again, never ; the fence once broken down,

THE RUBICON

once crossed, there is no return forever to marital fidelity, for there is a fascination in promiscuousness a thousand times more resistless than the first winnings in a game or a lottery, and the first step becomes a fatal one. Literally, thousands of wives have themselves cast the die of marital infidelity by placing a barrier to marital rights, doing it thoughtlessly many times, never, perhaps, imagining the result, never intending such a result, but that result will follow for all that.

In nine cases out of ten, if the husband is not satisfied at home, he will obtain satisfaction elsewhere; in nine cases out of ten those satisfactions once obtained, they will continue to be thus procured. This matter is of incalculable importance, and there is scarcely in the whole range of married life a single subject which so imperatively claims a wife's attention as this, and the want of such attention has broken up the peace of many a hitherto happy family. The lesson to be conveyed is this: if you are hungry there may be an all-sufficient reason for not gratifying that hunger; you may be on a plank in mid ocean many a league from any human help; this is an all-sufficient reason for your not eating; at the same time you are just as hungry as if there was an abundant table set before you. If a man's natural desires are not appeased, there may be ever so good a reason for it, but the craving is as remorseless for all that, just as much so as that thirst can never be quenched without a liquid drink. On a subject of this sort, plainness of speech is essential to a proper understanding of the case, and yet plainness of speech is highly objectionable from several points of view, but for want of proper plainness the actual practical force of many a valuable lesson has been altogether lost.

This episode has been purposely made, as it was not thought advisable to have a separate heading, and may be carried out still further to very great advantage.

A very highly esteemed patient called the other day, and in the course of a consultation, made more free from an acquaintance of some years' standing, stated " I have been married over six years, and have never had the marital right. The first night there was an objection, and the second; in consideration of my respect and sincere love, it was deferred, and weeks passed, and months, and years. Educated, cultivated, refined, with a taste in dress, a manner in company, faultless in person and feature, the admiration of all, my fortune at command, I am supposed the happiest of men; waiting, waiting, in hope to this hour; I am proud of my fidelity. What shall I do? Divorce is a disgrace among respectable people; it would ruin one for whom I have lived and waited all these years."

This was a noble man. In a myriad of others, his like might not be found again.

Another gentleman aged thirty had been married five years,

averaging a right a year, because it gave physical pain from faulty formation; there was an intensity of love between them which was beautiful to see, and for the sacrifice of one, the other seemed willing to give the whole soul. But note the result; unappeased nature refused to be satisfied; there was too much force of character, too high a moral sense, to descend to corrupting third parties, yet the contemptible substitute of self was obtained, with the result of a ruined constitution and a grave within a year.

There can be no rule for the observance of marital rights, no more than there can be a rule making out how many ounces of solid food each man requires at a meal, for there are differences of age, temperament, constitution, and capabilities, and conditions which greatly modify circumstances. To understand the whole subject properly, some preliminary statements are necessary. During the impregnating period of life, it is perhaps more frequently so than otherwise, that there is no special sexual inclination in married women, except at that monthly recurring period, when the system is most capable of efficient impregnation, which is within a few hours after the complete cessation of the monthly flow; as to the domestic animals, it is termed being in "heat." Men in health are always prepared. Putting these two statements together, another one makes the whole condition of things more compact and concise, rendering it easier to take the whole situation in at a glance. Except at this time, the sex is passive in the act of right, there is no giving up of anything, no loss of bodily substance, hence no resulting debility or drain, hence no injury; there can be none under the circumstances, not even the injury of effort, of expended strength, because there is none where there is perfect impassiveness, indifference; then it follows that in this direction there is no reasonable limit to admissions, if rest and sleep are not infringed. But in the other direction there is an immense difference in capabilities, even when there is good health, as there is an immense difference in the strength of mind of any hundred men, all being in perfect health. The observant may tell for themselves; just as an observant man may tell for himself how much or how often he can eat. If weariness or debility or any other ill-feeling follows a man's eating, there is excess; so in speaking or singing; so in the other direction.

A secretary of state reported distressing exhaustion beyond a monthly right, but let every reader note the important lesson ; it was the result of years in the practice of cessations just the instant before completions, to prevent impregnation. Others have diurnal indulgences for years together ; but note the terrible lesson of this. A man called who had been over the world for relief, nor was he an old man. He had thus doubly indulged for five years, saving the time of catamenial presence. No injury seemed to result ; no abatement of satisfactions ; until, with the suddenness of an apoplectic shock, or the thunderbolt in a clear sky, all capability disappeared, there was a perfect powerlessness throughout the whole of the reproductive functions. A steady drain of the vitalities was set up to dribble and dribble and dribble, inflicting physical debilities and mental tortures which made social association distasteful, memory a remorse, and existence intolerable.

No sane man properly informed could possibly incur a risk like this ; but having no information of themselves, and no hints from books, kindred troubles have come to thousands, and thousands have been prematurely lost to themselves, their families, and to the world. And it is safe to say that tens of thousands would pay sums of money, large to them, to know the proper measure of marital indulgences as to themselves individually. But there is an innate repugnance to the only method of obtaining the information which could be had by personal conversation with individuals, and would not only be unsafe as a predicate for rules and regulations, as being on a restricted foundation, but to get from others you must impart yourselves, and there is a sacredness of secrecy as impenetrable as the Holy of Holies, in matters of this kind, which is open only to the All-seeing Eye. Hence, the effort in this volume to convey such information as may be barely necessary for the occasion, and even that in phrase which is a filmy foreshadowing of the fact. Taking a man in good health, at the age of twenty-five years, who has never in a single instance degraded himself by promiscuous gratifications, marrying a healthy woman, the great general rules should be observed to the extent of the preventions named in previous pages. But to be safe, tri-weekly until forty, semi-weekly until sixty, and hebdomadal thereafter ; with this measure, there may be at threescore and ten, satisfactions not inferior to twoscore, as if compensatory of the failure of many other sources of pleasure and enjoyment which are in full flow in the earlier parts of life's prime.

———— ∞ ————

GETTING UP.

WOMEN are usually required to remain in bed ten days after delivery. There can be only one safe rule for all: wait until you feel as if getting up would do you good; as if it would rest you; but do not remain up until you are tired; better limit it to five minutes; then if you feel all the better for it, repeat in a few hours, and thus feel your way along, always returning to bed before a sensation of weariness comes over you. Sometimes it is better to sit still in a chair; at others, to walk across the room a few times. But until the constitutions of our women become more robust, no one is advised to leave the bed, even for five minutes, or sit up in bed that long, sooner than the third day. The aim should be to exert the strength but very little in any way, and by the slowest degrees increase the time of sitting up, and of walking, always stopping short at the first intimation of fatigue or weariness, or even tiredness. In short, the patient must notice, and compare, and decide for herself, how much she can safely do.

PUERPERAL FEVER,

or child-bed fever, is of an inflammatory character, either of an active or typhoid type. The inflammation is in the peritoneum or covering of the bowels, and extends to the various organs within the abdomen, and sometimes to the womb itself. This comes on with a general shivering about the third day after delivery, or sometimes limited to the back; this is followed by a hot skin and a hard, full pulse, from a hundred and ten to a hundred and fifteen in a minute, with headache and restlessness. The abdomen is swollen, and the lochial discharges are checked. The breasts shrivel, the milk dries up. The patient lies on her back with the knees drawn up, this being the least painful position. The sooner it commences, the more dangerous it is. Sometimes it does not appear until the sixth or seventh day. As the patient gets better, the pain and swelling subside, the countenance is less anxious, it brightens up, and in a few days more all is well.

This dangerous ailment is brought on by violence during delivery, by a bad cold, by premature exertion, by agitation or mental shocks, by over-eating, or by the use of stimulants. In all cases where there is a decided feeling of shivering along the back, from the third to the eighth day after delivery, a physician should be sent for at whatever cost or trouble; for early attention is life; delay, death.

The causes of this affection have been stated in detail, that they may be studiously avoided. Only general treatment is advised until the physician arrives, such as an open condition of the bowels by enemas; warm compresses to the abdomen in case of pain and swelling, without heat or fever; if these are present, then cold compresses; and if relief is not prompt and decided, take a liver pill.

The principles of Homœopathic treatment require the administration of Aconitum if there is fever; of Belladonna for violent pain or cramp, or Hyoscyamus when swollen and sensitive; Bryonia, Rhus Tox., if there is a low fever, or typhoid. If there is great thirst or depression of spirits, Mercurius meets the case. Nux Vomica on the instant of the disappearance of the lochia, or diminution of the milk, and scalding urination.

If the abdomen is greatly distended and pain almost unendurable, sharp, cutting, lancinating, thighs drawn up, Colocynth will be valuable.

If breasts are flaccid, no milk, colorless discharges from the bowels, pains as if in labor, fever, red face, nervous, impatient, irritable, Chamomilla is given with confidence.

If sudden prostration, anguish of countenance, sunken features, livid face, feeble pulse, burning belly, use Arsenicum.

If the belly cannot endure the pressure of the clothing, and all the symptoms are worse after sleeping, take Lachesis, or Opium, or Secale, or Carbo Veg.

In addition, the utmost repose of body and mind should be secured in all forms of practice; darken the chamber, exclude all noises, and secure a well-ventilated chamber with a cool atmosphere. If thirsty, give bits of ice, or cold water by the spoonfuls. Flannels to abdomen, wrung out of boiling water, and also to genitals; tepid injections if constipated.

MILK LEG,

called Phlegmasia Dolens by physicians, an affection of the large veins of the leg in connection with a confinement; these veins are inflamed, enlarge the limb, and cause considerable discomfort.

Apply hot fomentations to the limb, or wring a blanket dipped in boiling water and wrap it round the entire limb, in such a way as not to wet the clothing or the bed; as soon as one becomes a little cool, apply another as hot as it can be borne. Do this for half an hour at a time and repeat it four or five times in twenty-four hours; the object of this is to convey away the extra heat from the limb by evaporation; hence, between these hot applications have the limb wrapped in a linen sheet, not wet enough to dribble, and a dry flannel around that, to keep it warm; at all these changes rub the skin with soft cloths and the hands, to promote the circulation, keeping the bowels lax every day by eating cooling, loosening food; if this does not avail, employ enemas, or castor-oil, Epsom salts, or a purgative pill. In bad cases a single liver pill will answer an admirable purpose.

Under any circumstances, it is specially important that the bowels should act freely and fully every day, after the birth of the child. If the patient is averse to taking medicine, an enema of tepid water may be used every morning in ordinary cases, or even a quart at a time if there is a decided tendency to constipation; meanwhile the bowels should be gently kneaded with the hands of the nurse, under the bedclothes for a quarter of an hour at a time several times a day, in order to wake up the intestines to a freer motion.

This free condition of the bowels tends to prevent and aids directly in curing many of the little ailments incident to the mother after delivery, because costiveness is the cause of most of them.

Sometimes piles are troublesome, but are readily removed by avoiding costiveness, and bathing the parts well in cold water several times a day, as elsewhere directed.

LOCHIAL DISCHARGE.

For about a month after confinement there is a discharge from the uterus, gradually ceasing as the system regains its strength ; a free daily action of the bowels is essential, so as to draw the drains of the system in that direction ; the parts are strengthened by a sitz bath of a quarter of an hour, two or three times a day ; begin with water at ninety degrees, reducing it five degrees every fifth day, not going lower than sixty, remaining in the bath a less time as it is colder ; employ vaginal injections of cold water three times a day. If the lochials are profuse, traceable to sitting up too soon after confinement, to hot rooms, mental emotions, or errors in eating, they should be rectified under whatever treatment ; in addition, Homœopaths give Crocus if there is dark-colored blood, Bryonia if the blood is red, with internal burning pains. Nux Vomica should be given if there is chill, pain in small of back, and fruitless efforts at stool. Those of full habit and protracted discharges or troublesome itching should take Calcarea. If pure blood comes with the lochial after every nursing, give Silicea. If the discharge is suppressed, give Pulsatilla. If from shocks, Aconitum is proper ; Opium, if there are convulsions. Dulcamara, if suppressed by cold ; Belladonna, if face is red ; and Colocynth, if there is colic and flatulence.

If offensive and thin discharges, exhibit Belladonna and Carbo V. in twelve hours after the third dose of Belladonna, and Creosote after the third dose of Carbo.

The Allopathic Treatment, until a physician can be had, is to keep the bowels free by enemas or small doses of castor-oil or salts, a light and nutritious diet, doing everything to soothe and quiet.

THE NIPPLES

occasionally give discomfort for weeks or months before confinement. In fact, soon after pregnancy, within a month, the breasts begin to full up, there are stinging pains, the nipples become more prominent, and sometimes sensitive, the colored circle broadens and becomes darker. If there is heat or pain or sensitiveness, they may be held in a bowl of cold water five or ten minutes at a time several times a day, and in the intervals wet compresses may be kept on them, frequently renewed so as to keep the surface of the skin moist, and this, by evaporation, carries off the extra heat of fever and inflammation ; at the same time be sure to keep the bowels free, and live largely on a fruit and coarse bread diet; with meat at dinner only, and that should be lean beef, mutton, or poultry, or fish.

There should be no compression about the breasts, not the very slightest; the clothing should hang from the shoulders; neglect of this has in thousands of instances laid the foundation for gathered breasts and cancers of the most dreadful character twenty years later. Words cannot express adequately the importance of causing every article of clothing about the body to hang from the shoulders on the very first intimation of pregnancy.

SORE NIPPLES

may be warded off in almost every case by a little wise care. Bathe them freely in cold water twice a day during the whole time of pregnancy, leaning over a bowl or basin for five or ten minutes, until there is a sense of relief from fever or other uncomfortableness; at the same time rub them patiently between the finger and the thumb after each bathing, and even between times; this helps to bring them out so that the infant can take hold of them; it should especially be done if they are inclined to lie flat on the breasts, as is sometimes the case. This operation also toughens and hardens the skin in a natural way; if astringents are used—oak-bark, alum, or tannin—the skin is contracted more, when the very object should be to soften and distend it; this is done by rolling the nipple between the thumb and finger, as above directed; nothing is so good as this to draw out the nipple from the breast; it is a much safer way than to use a breast-pump or other artificial drawing or suction by another, for these have been known to cause premature delivery.

If the nipple is actually sore or excoriated or fissured, put a grain of sulphate of zinc or half a teaspoonful of powdered alum in two tablespoons of water in a vial with a mouth large enough to receive a nipple, and apply it to the nipple by tilting up the bottle for five minutes at a time. If the nipple is tender and smooth, apply a borax mixture in the same way, three times a day; put fifteen grains of borax, six grains of tannin, and an ounce each of brandy and water; sometimes a level teaspoonful of powdered alum and two tablespoons of water will answer the purpose.

After the child is born, there is a sensitiveness about the nipples causing the mother to have a fear of nursing the baby; hence, she puts it off, allowing the breasts to become too full, inviting fever and inflammation, and thus increasing the tenderness of the nipple itself; and yet it cannot be let alone, and the child must be fed, each feeding aggravating the trouble; hence the great importance of taking means at an early stage of pregnancy to ward off the trouble; such means as have been already detailed are generally efficient. Nipple shields are of some benefit. After each nursing, wash the nipples freely with a level teaspoon of borax in two tablespoons each of glycerine and rain or rose water. If the fissures are deep, take a fine, small brush, dip it in nitrate of silver and water, 3 or 4 grains to the ounce, or strong enough to cause a little smarting; do this twice a day after nursing, and a cure usually results. If one thing does not answer, try another. If the bowels are kept acting every day, twice, the nipples will get well much sooner, especially if a fruit diet is adhered to. But the cure is sometimes so tedious, and the mother suffers so much, that additional remedies are here given: borax, one dram; water, three and a half ounces; spirit of wine (alcohol or other spirits), half an ounce; mix well, and use after each nursing, and shield the teat by an artificial one, or make a liniment of equal parts of oil of poppies and lime-water; mix, and apply as an ointment frequently.

Another. Three and a half parts of empyreumatic oil of juniper; oil of almonds, three parts; glycerine, three parts; mix it well and apply it every time the child has nursed, with a camel's-hair brush. It hurts a little at first, but the sore is healed in a few days. Take care that the nipple shall not stick to the clothing; protect it with a fresh green leaf or piece of oiled silk.

But it will generally be found that the application of nitrate of silver, with a camel's-hair brush, drawn through the cracks, although it smarts some, is the quickest and best cure; avoid touching the healthy skin, as it blackens it, but does no injury. But in all cases the cure is greatly expedited by having a shield made of wood, ivory, or silver, neatly covered with a prepared or artificial cow's teat; but the teat should extend but little over half an inch beyond the ivory piece, for then it gets between the child's teeth or gums and interferes with its nursing.

TEETHING.

In six or eight months the teeth begin to cut the gum, if the child is vigorous and healthy; if feeble, puny, or rickety, they do not appear for a year and a half. The two middle front teeth come first, and the other two in a month or six weeks; next, two side teeth, above and below. In about a year the first double teeth appear; the eighteenth month, the eye-teeth. In two years and a half the whole twenty have appeared. These remain until about the sixth or seventh year, when they begin to fall out and make room for the permanent ones.

Teething is a natural process, and ought not to be attended with discomfort or sickness; but owing to faulty habits of life, a great variety of symptoms and sufferings make their appearance during dentition. This would not be the case if children were properly fed, clothed, and watched over, for they have only to be kept clean, have plenty of out-door air, be regularly fed, have abundant sleep, and regular bowels, about two passages every day; this last should be had by enemas, or by syrup of senna or syrup of rhubarb; fever and irritation and general restlessness can be kept down by tepid baths. Sometimes the bowels are loose; this should be controlled by the diet, using boiled milk, and enemas with a few drops of laudanum.

The gums should never be lanced; or if at all, the cases are rare, and should be done only when a physician advises it, and the operation should be performed by him; if this is not possible, take a lancet or common penknife, very sharp, and carry it down to the tooth; to be sure that this is done, grate it on the tooth below; but if the bowels are kept sufficiently free, and the child is fed regularly and not too much or too often, lancing the gums will not be necessary, and in order to avoid any possible necessity, the mother should be watchful during the whole time of teething, against costiveness; let her see to it that the bowels are kept acting, at least twice in every twenty-four hours.

Another thing should be as imperatively avoided: never give an infant, for any ailment whatever, any anodyne, any preparation of hops or lupine, or morphia, opium, laudanum, paregoric, or anything else, the constituents of which are unknown. Whatever is sold under the name or pretence of being a soothing syrup for children, is a murderous preparation, and the parent who administers it, whatever may be the intention, endangers the life of the child. Whatever parents give these things for any ailment, on their own responsibility, should make a note of it, that if afterwards the child has died of

Convulsions,
Inflammation of the Brain,
Water on the Brain, or
" Fits,"

it is justly chargeable to the medicines given, which were named above.

Whatever diarrhœa is present during teething is a safety-valve, and should by no means be interfered with, in any way, unless the child seems to be falling away, getting weak, losing its appetite, or has nausea and blue finger-nails, and other indications of a feeble vitality. A third thing in connection with teething which should never be done except in the severest cases, and that by the direction of the physician, is the extraction of a tooth to make way for another under it. Nature has her own modes of doing things, and they should never be interfered with, unless there is an imperative need ; her plan is to push them upwards and outwards by the undergrowing tooth, which by its constant pressure occasions a gradual disruption of the greater part of the tooth. No intelligent dentist of skill, experience, and observation will advise the extraction of a first tooth, and very rarely of young persons, for the inevitable effect is the contraction of the jaw ; it is the well-developed jaw which indicates firmness of character, which gives expression to the face, and to do anything to operate against its development, is always unnatural and always unwise. By such interference one jaw becomes smaller than the other, and thus alters the whole contour and expression of the face, and always for the worse, never for the better, unless it may be for the better appearance of the teeth. These premature removals sometimes seriously impair the utterance or vocalization, make the voice and accent and tone unnatural. If a tooth is in an actual state of decay before the jaw is fully developed, it should be removed, but it is a misfortune, for all that.

NURSING INFANTS.

NATURE and reason point out the duty to the mother of nursing her own child, and nothing can ever compensate for the loss of it. There is an intercommunion of soul with soul, between the mother and her babe, which has a bliss in it for both, as it draws its sustenance from her bosom and looks up into her eye so lovingly, so confidingly, and at the same time sees in the expression of her countenance an affection and a tenderness which carry away in its own little heart a very heaven of sweetness. The mother alone can have that instinctive gentleness and tenderness of look, and handling, and telegraphic communication from eye to eye which are so necessary to complete calmness, quietness, repose, and happiness of mind, and which are essential to a healthful feeding and a good digestion. While nursing, an angry look, a frown, a harsh word, a sudden jerk of body or change of position, is tenfold more injurious to an infant than to a grown person; and yet all know what a shock it is to the feelings, how it discomposes the whole nature, how it utterly destroys appetite, to be enraged or shocked or scared in the midst of a meal, or soon after; but the tender nature of the infant must suffer more; infants are often thrown into convulsions by such things, and nothing short of a mother's love can be incessantly on guard against them; hence to commit the nursing to a stranger is, under the most favorable circumstances, even if it be an unavoidable necessity, a violation of the natural rights of the infant, and is a remorseless outrage upon its just claims. The mother who could willingly avoid nursing her own child, short of a necessity, is unworthy of a child, is unworthy the name of mother. In another place directions are given for the regular nursing of infants and feeding of children when the mother is in good health. But when she cannot nurse it with impunity, it will be indicated by some discomfort, by pains between the shoulders, and aversion to nursing amounting sometimes to a repugnance; there is a distressing and very general debility pervading the whole system, she is tired in the morning, she is tired at night, tired all over, and tired all the time; all the time more dead than alive; but long before this the infant should be turned over to be fed by other hands either wholly or in part.

If there is any milk, it should be suckled once a day, then fed artificially for the remainder of the twenty-four hours, and within a week or ten days it should be taken from the breast altogether.

If the mother is pregnant again, nursing endangers abortion; she cannot feed two besides herself. One stomach cannot do the work necessary for three persons. Therefore, when the catamenia return, immediate measures should be taken to wean the child, for the next thing is an impregnation. Besides, the drain of the catamenia is quite enough without that from giving milk at the same time; the mother would soon grow thin, and pale, and weak.

Under such circumstances, injustice is done the child, because its constitution will soon become impaired necessarily, from the fact that it cannot get enough nourishment, and what it does get is not pure and health-giving; it is weak, watery, sickly.

The best time for weaning is about May and October; mid-summer is dangerous, in proportion as the weather is warm, for a change of food is apt to induce indigestion and sourness; then follow loose bowels, summer complaint, and all its attendant ills and dangers.

Mid-winter is unpropitious, because the long nights make artificial feeding really dangerous, from having to get up in the cold, and for other reasons.

PREPARING TO WEAN.

It is best for mother and child to begin to wean in the day-time; first give the breast in the morning on waking up, then at noon, then at bedtime. In five days, omit the noon nursing; if the child will not take artificial food, make it wait until its hunger compels it. In five days more, omit the morning nursing; if this makes the child fretful, it need not interfere with the mother's sleep; in ten days more omit the bedtime nursing; if convenient, let the mother or child be in different and distant parts of the house, so that her sleep need not be interfered with, nor her presence encourage the child to stubbornness; besides, if the child cannot see the mother, it is not half as difficult for it to give up the nursing.

The advantage of this method is, the secretion of milk dries away by degrees; but by all means keep up at least one full, free action of the bowels every day, from the very first hour the weaning process commences, for it is always dangerous to stop one drain of the system unless another drain is kept free, a little freer than before; this gives time for the adaptation of things. Another precaution: do not eat as much; take meat but once a day, until the weaning is completed, and use fruits and berries more abundantly; and if these things do not avail to keep the bowels free, take salts, oil, or a dinner pill, or an injection.

FEEDING INFANTS.

If the breast has to be given up, a substitute must be provided, with the understanding that when a child is old enough to be weaned, it is old enough to be made to feed but four times between daylight and bedtime, the intervals never being less than four full hours; it is too frequent and irregular feeding that kills half the infants who die before two years of age. If when the child is born the mother is healthy and strong, the infant may be put to the breast for the first time in three or four hours. If the mother is feeble, she should defer the first nursing until next day. If in either case the milk does not come at first, the infant can make trials from time to time, and this tends to invite the flow of milk. Meanwhile, give the child a teaspoonful of sweetened warm water once or twice in the course of an hour or two; after that, feed with water a little sweetened, three parts, and milk one part, warmed; do not put a whole teaspoonful to the mouth at once, fifteen or twenty drops at a time, with intervals of a quarter or half a minute, interesting the little thing meanwhile, if possible, the object being to introduce the food very slowly at first, for the stomach the first day is not large enough to hold over an ounce or two, or three, at once; in a day or two, more may be fed at a time, but always very slowly indeed, so that the stomach may not be over-full before we know it, for then wind is generated from the souring of the milk, and colic follows with the crying and distress consequent. There is no such thing as colic, caused by sucking in wind; it is always brought on by a cold, by eating too much, too often, or too fast; this should be set down as an incontrovertible fact. There are various devices for imitating the mother's teat; each must decide according to the circumstances of the case.   As to

nothing can be said satisfactory or definite, but the difficulties in the way are so great and so numerous, that it would be best to lay down a rule seldom if ever to be deviated from : never get a woman to feed your baby as long as there is a cow to be had within fifty miles.   For the first ten days take the milk from a good healthy cow in the proportion named, and gradually increase the amount of milk so as to make it more substantial.

If the bowels become torpid, use a little brown sugar or molasses, but only a day or two at a time ; gruel answers a good purpose for a change, a tablespoonful of Graham flour, stirred well into three or four tablespoons of cold water; then stir it in a pint of boiling water; boil at least twenty minutes, stirring it well all the time to keep it from burning and to cook it regularly, add a pint of warm milk; if there is diarrhœa, boil the milk.   The diet should be changed from time to time to farina gruel or oatmeal gruel, or other preparations known by experience to be good for the purpose in that part of the country.   But do not change the diet, if the child seems to be doing well; only when it appears to be getting tired of it, as too great a variety is injurious ; and never forget at any time for a single day that regularity is essential to the comfort and health and well-being of the infant, feeding it at the same intervals day after day, and at no other time.   If the infant seems to be fretful for something to eat between times, amuse it by giving it a little warm water out of a spoon; sometimes cold water may be given it in the same way; that is best for it which it seems to relish best; the point is to divert it until the feeding time comes. Watch carefully against loose bowels in artificial feeding; it may be regulated generally by the use of arrow-root, corn-starch, or crackers powdered finely and put into boiled milk.   If the looseness seems to be weakening the babe, then give it some well-made soup or gruel or beef tea ; if the stomach retains nothing, use enemas containing some nutriment, as gruels, beef-tea, and the like.   It is best to teach the infant to take its food by sucking, because it is then introduced into the stomach gradually and regularly. At the end of the third month, a little chicken or veal broth or beef-tea thickened with oatmeal may be added to the milk diet; make the addition gradually, varying it with oatmeal, sago, or arrow-root, changing from time to time as the oatmeal may purge; if it does, it may be used to advantage when the bowels are confined. It is prepared by stirring two tablespoonfuls of oatmeal in a pint of cold water, let it stand ten minutes, pour off the liquid, which is to be boiled to a thin jelly. All food for the first six months should be thin, and sweetened only a little. After the front teeth are all cut, give more solid food, as rice puddings and the like, as children do best who have but very little animal food during childhood; it certainly is not a necessity for the first three years. When the first teeth are cut, soft-boiled eggs, calf's-foot jelly, and fresh milk with water are admirable, for one meal in the day. After the sixth month, four feedings during the twenty-four hours are abundant, the first one early in the morning, the last one about bedtime.

WEANING INFANTS.

It was stated that when the choice can be had, May and October are the best months for weaning. It should not be done suddenly; when all parties are in health, preparation should be made for it at the seventh month, by giving artificial food at one of the nursings; then in the course of two weeks, twice; then feed it from the breast only twice in twenty-four hours, night and morning, as already suggested. But these processes should be carried out regularly, steadily, firmly, without wavering, so that by the tenth month it shall cease to take food from its mother's bosom altogether. Never go back for an instant after once commencing to wean. Let the child cry ever so much, let it keep on crying until it is so tired that it falls to sleep, but don't give it the breast; it will scarcely ever repeat the crying over three times. It is not a favorable time to wean while cutting one or more front teeth, nor while the child is sick; the best time is when it is in good health; the best mode is regularity and firmness. After a few of the teeth are cut, the child may be allowed to suck fresh roasted beef or boiled potatoes; butter and gravies should not be allowed until the double teeth are cut, nor cakes or pastry of any kind.

If in this process of weaning the milk does not dry up readily,

39

the bowels should be kept acting once or twice a day, averaging three times in two days, by means of a fruit diet; if this does not answer, use castor-oil, Epsom salts, or enemas, but, by all or any means, have the bowels free.   If the breasts are painful and not hot, use warm compresses, changing them every four or five minutes until relieved, even if it requires hours, and to be renewed as soon as any hurting begins to return.   If there is heat or redness, use cold compresses in the same way, as often as needed.   In the intervals, the parts may be freely rubbed with soap liniment, or laudanum; if these things are well done, the milk will be removed in all cases, it being understood that the bowels are to be kept free.

INFANTILE DISEASES

are all cured, if the little sufferers are kept clean, have good air, are dressed loosely, fed regularly, and have the bowels kept free, twice a day at least, by enemas; medicines may be given for that purpose, castor-oil, a little Epsom salts, but they are not advised until the other measures have failed.   If the bowels are costive, the enemas should be at ninety-eight degrees, injected gently, slowly, and to cease the instant the little one begins to strain; the same injections are good for straining and griping; if the bowels are too loose, never give a drug; a little boiled milk with its food is better; or let it sit in a bath of ninety degrees, the skin of the back and bowels being rubbed with the hands all the time; this diverts the blood to the surface and gives delightful relief; if not, an enema of ten drops of laudanum in a tablespoonful of warm starch-water, and instantly press a warm napkin against the bowels for ten or fifteen minutes, strongly, so as to keep the injection in.   At the same time, keep the child in the open air as much as possible in the arms of the mother or nurse, because the slightest cold or jar is very injurious; and by all means, it is a necessity to keep it abundantly warm, for every instant, for a single chilliness or crawl will strike the blood in and increase the looseness.   This is one reason why the summer complaint is often so difficult to manage: the child is not kept warm enough about its body; cool, pure air to breathe for the lungs, and abundant warm clothing for the body.

If any mother wishes to be the murderer of her child, give it something to take into the stomach to stop the looseness, some soothing-syrup; even though it may have the commendations of every president and every clergyman ever born since the Declaration of Independence. Soothing-syrups are but another name for death by convulsions in a few days, or water on the brain, or other form of sudden arrest of all the powers of life.

DISEASES OF CHILDREN.

Many a child has died in consequence of the mother's vanity, beginning sometimes before it is two days old; waking it up out of its sleep to gratify some idle caller; often a mere complimentary call, and not for any real desire to see the baby. Abundant sleep is one of the first necessities of infant life; to be waked up out of a good sleep discomposes the gravest of grown persons, and makes many uncomfortable the remainder of the day; much more an infant. Not long afterwards there is another vanity exhibiting itself: to show off the baby in fine dress; and when it is taken into account how much pulling and hauling and twisting and turning it takes to dress a baby, it is easy to see how tiresome it must be to its tender frame to have to undergo it all, for full dress, to be repeated perhaps several times a day; with this full dress there are various bindings and pinnings and tyings and buttonings, all of them interfering with the circulation at a time so early that the slightest obstructions are liable to be followed by serious, permanent, and even fatal results, besides the liability to take colds, with all their attendant discomforts.

In the very beginning of child-life, it will be of immense importance to its future well-being for the mother to ascertain the predominant temperament of the child: whether it is excitable or dull; that is, nervous or phlegmatic; if the former, then it should be the habitual effort of the mother to curb that excitement, to avoid what tends to increase it, for that helps to bring on nervous diseases, affections of the brain, and various forms of fits and convulsions; hence, cultivate quietude, encourage sleep, abundant sleep, avoid as much as possible boisterous conduct of the other children, all sudden noises or shocks, everything, in fact, which tends to excite.

If the phlegmatic temperament abounds, if the infant is sleepy or stupid or inattentive, then it is well to pursue an opposite course, and encourage everything that is lively, animating; everything calculated to wake up into life and activity and joyousness; with such treatment the dullest children sometimes grow up to be the lights of the world. When a child,

SIR ISAAC NEWTON

was so frail and foolish that he was regarded as a dunce, was the butt of the school, and was imposed upon by the boys of a larger growth. One day an overgrown fellow insulted him and kicked him in the stomach; this aroused his whole nature; it waked him up to a determination to application which would place him ahead of his tormentor. He accomplished his purpose, and not only reached the head of his class in a country school, but stands in the very front ranks of all created men. This shows that mothers may do much towards bringing out the intellects of their dull children, by studying their temperaments from the week of their birth.

TEETHING

is a natural operation, and would go on healthfully and safely in all cases, if the mother and child lived naturally; but under present habits, it is accompanied with more or less irritation and inflammation. The great points to be aimed at are, to keep the bowels free, to keep the feet warm, so as to draw the blood from the head; this may be aided by noticing whenever the head is hot; then put on a linen cap and keep it wet, or lay wet compresses of cold water on the head, renewed every five minutes, or even less, until the head is cooled off; in addition, let the child sit in a warm bath of ninety degrees five or ten minutes at a time twice a day; this also draws blood to the surface and away from the head, and to that extent tends to prevent inflammation of the brain and convulsions. When there is considerable twitching of the muscles, or convulsive jerkings of the limbs, the irritation is very decided, and more active measures should be taken; for whether it arises from colic, or irritation, a more general warm bath should be taken than sitting in the water, preceded by an enema of warm water; they are always safe, always applicable, and have sometimes a marvellous power, by the relaxing influence of the warm water, internal and external, in removing spasms, and cooling and calming the whole system, body and mind. But in all cases of warm bath, it is important to have cold water compresses on the top of the head all the time; and it is also of special importance that food at such times be given regularly, slowly and warm; for a single mouthful of food, especially if hard, may induce spasms, convulsions, and fits.

It must be recollected, hence it is here distinctly repeated, that in all diseases of infancy and childhood certain things are always applicable, always safe, always beneficial, always efficient, always necessary, to wit:

Keep the bowels open;

Keep the extremities especially warm;

Have an abundant supply of fresh air.

Keep the skin clean, with abundant frictions of the hand besides. These directions are of special importance, and are often all that is needed in bad colds, serious coughs, and even croup and diphtheria. In these latter cases, especially where the breathing is at all labored, a linen cloth of three or four thicknesses, large enough to cover the whole chest, should be dipped in *warm* water; that is always safer and less liable to shock; lay it over the chest with a dry cotton or woollen cloth of two thicknesses, and a little larger every way, laid over the wet one so as to keep the steam in and the pores of the skin open and soft; as often as they become dry, especially in the night, wet and renew; if there is trouble in the throat make a similar application as high up the neck as possible. The object of these applications should be fully understood: it is to keep the skin warm, to draw the blood from the interior to the surface, thus relieving the more critical parts and affording an exit from the body of those humors, as they are called, which do so much to afflict it. If there is a tight, dry cough, hot fomentations should be kept over the whole chest and throat all the time, until there is perfect relief, ascertained by the increasing looseness of the phlegm. The fomentations are flannels dipped in very hot water, wrung out and laid on the chest, thin linen intervening, so as to avoid burning the tender skin of the child.

If the skin is burning, while the feet are cold, then endeavor to draw the blood to the surface and extremities by a hot foot-bath, by plentiful frictions with the hand or dry flannel over the skin, so as to redden it; and if judiciously applied, a broad girdle of dry flannel over a wet cotton one around the body, would help to cool off the skin.

If there are any swellings about the body, as in

MUMPS,

the same treatment is applicable as before named, and the swollen parts should have a plentiful application of hot fomentations in the daytime, and wet bandages covered with dry flannel at night.

The young mother should remember, that for all affections of the skin, of whatever name or in whatever part of the body, two things should always be avoided, for they often cause convulsions and death. These are:

1. Cold air or cold water to the skin.

2. Applications calculated to drive in the appearance on the skin.

On the other hand, it is always important, always applicable, and always curative to keep the skin clean and moist and soft and warm, with very free bowels; the main agencies being warm water to the skin, and warm enemas to the bowels, if at all confined.

Considering that it is difficult to get children, and especially infants, to take medicine, parents are advised to make themselves familiar with the principles and practice above referred to, for they are applicable, especially applicable, to *all* the ailments of children; to all affections of the skin, whether rashes or sores, boils, tetter, measles, anything and everything, they are not only applicable, but they are safer, better, and more efficient than medicines nine times out of ten.

It must be remembered that in all forms of sickness in infancy and early childhood, it is necessary to keep up the strength; it is necessary to give good, nourishing food, plain, simple, well prepared, warm and cooling, such as gruels, mush, bread, milk, ripe fruits, and when the teeth appear, lean meats sometimes. Nourishment, warmth, cleanliness, good air, these are the great saviours of young children.

MOTHER'S MILK.

When it is not sufficient for the wants of the child, it grows thin and weak; the circulation declines, the finger-nails turn blue, the ends of the fingers shrink or shrivel, whether the milk is poor in quality or scant in quantity. Much may be done under such circumstances to enrich the milk, or make it more abundant; in either case, it is necessary, and it is sufficient to improve the general health of the mother; this will not be done by the tonic effect of medicines and stimulants, but by the vigorous digestion of nourishing food. The too prevalent custom of causing mothers to drink abundantly of beer, ale, porter, wines, and the like, as a means of increasing the quantity of milk, is full of error; if the quantity of milk is increased, there is no increase in its substance, in bulk, not in nutriment, but it is the increase of nutriment that is especially desired; the mother is stimulated afterwards, and if during that stimulation the infant is nursed, its susceptible system is stimulated, but it is not a whit more fed, while its nervous system is excited, and the foundation is laid for the love of liquor, to be, in after life, in twenty, forty years more, or longer, developed into drivelling drunkenness, in sons and daughters. Twenty centuries ago these principles had become so obvious, that Plato, the greatest of Grecian philosophers, would not allow the newly married to drink wine, because it was believed that a child, begotten when the parent was under the influence of the stimulant, would have an injury done to the nervous system, which would have an evil bearing on its whole after life; much more then would this be the case if the mother took wine while she was nursing it, if she took wine while she was carrying it. The use which parents may make of stimulants at the time of impregnation, during gestation, and through nursing, is the hidden cause of that large class of men and women who are said, in a kind of sympathetic pity, to have

UNBALANCED MINDS.

Persons of no character, no force of will, no vim; without decision, neither sensible nor senseless, aiming at nothing, accomplishing nothing, or at least failing in everything, and when they pass from the world

THEY LEAVE NO SIGN,

and all apparently is as if they had never existed; and many times even worse than all this, they not only lived without doing anything for anybody, but they had to be helped through the world by others, had to be fed and clothed and housed, and at last buried by the charity of those who had the force which they had not, and for want of which their life was

WORSE THAN A FAILURE.

But the suggestions of Plato have been utilized within the last half century, and men of investigating power and of strength of mind have brought to light some of the most startling facts in this connection. In a report recently made to the Massachusetts Legislature, it was officially stated that very nearly one-half of all the pauper idiots of the State were the children of parents, one or both of whom were drunken; the father begat them in drunkenness, the mother carried them in the womb in drunkenness, and fed them after birth with milk made of drunken material. And bearing in the same direction is the ascertained statistical fact, that when drunken parents join temperance societies not only does their own health improve, not only is the physical condition of the children materially advanced, but they have better and brighter minds than those who were born while intemperate habits were indulged.

There is another important fact recently published in England, that where there was an insane tendency to burglary, to murder, and to arson, it was uniformly found that the parents were drunken.

The children of the drunken need not inherit exactly and always the same defects, moral and physical, of their parents, but combinations of the same, the result of a variety of elementary traits; just as in the face of a child sometimes we do not see the full features of either parent but a combination of the eye of one, the lip of the other. The child may not be a drunkard like the parent, but there will be some unfavorable oddity of character, or temperament, or disposition; or there will be some faulty mental characteristic or physical ailment, as hysterics, or neuralgia, or dyspepsia, or rheumatism. The house of correction, the jail, the penitentiary, and the insane asylum are mainly peopled by the children of drunken parents; not parents necessarily known to be drunkards, but who used liquor at the late dinner, the midnight supper, occasionally, and occasionally drank wine, and took bitters and tincture tonics during gestation and for the first year of nursing. The author has already recorded a confirmatory case in his

HALL'S JOURNAL OF HEALTH.

Most of the parties to whom reference in the narration was made he knew himself, attending the funeral and witnessing the burial of the victim.

THE WEDDING-DAY.

Two healthy persons, with trusting, loving hearts, having been united in marriage, immediate preparation should be made for housekeeping, following the beautiful instincts of the birds of the forest, whose greatest happiness seems to be in preparing a place in which they may nestle with their young. The very labor necessary may well be supposed to be one of love and delight.

For the young pair to enter a splendid mansion, completely and elegantly furnished by parental love the very day after marriage, does not afford the thousandth part of the pure, enduring, and healthful gratifications which attend those, seemingly less favored by fortune, whose home has to be selected with much previous calculation, and debating, and hesitancy; where every article of furniture has to be talked over; its style and quality to be considered; what amount of means can be afforded to procure this, that, and the other housekeeping necessity; can the money be spared to obtain that elegant pattern of carpet? would it not be better to take something less costly for a year or two; then move that upstairs, and have the more elegant one for the parlor? The very circumstance of having to stop for want of funds long before the furnishing is completed, when in a plain way, is not without its advantages, its springs of lovingness; for these things bring the young husband and wife to counselling together; the wife's native pride and fine taste, and the young man's prudence, balancing against each other; his devotion urging him to gratify the woman whose happiness is his highest aim, and his secret thought that a little more energy, a little more application, a little longer staying at his place of business, will enable him to make it up; then the fear of debt; of being hampered; of possible failure of this, that, or the other plan. On the other hand, the wife's fear that he cannot afford it; that it may require him to work too hard; and then comes the indefinite apprehension of sickness and suffering, and all to gratify her; and she resolves to do without it. He insists that she ought to have it; and then they begin to skirmish and make their little feints and falsities, and practise their filmy infinitesimal pretensions, to the end that the woman eventually has her way in the first battle of married life; she stoops to conquer; she governs in the future by yielding now, resolving that she can do without the coveted article for the present; telling him that in a short time it may be better and more safely afforded. The young man straightway looks upon the blossom before him with a greater devotion, a deeper, purer, warmer love, and resolves in his own mind that she is worthy of all the efforts he can make for her happiness, and that all the energies within him shall be exerted with a will to gratify every desire of her heart; and thus, before they know it, they have been wedded together in a closer, stronger bond than any clerical formula ever forged; for in this they have learned to " take counsel together," to defer to each other's views, and arguments, and wishes. Each has seen in the other a disposition to mutual sacrifices, and a habit of giving up one's own will for the gratification of the other is begun, and one of the broadest stones for the foundation of domestic happiness is laid; and then, the one who has given up is more than repaid by the conqueror, who feels within a purer life and a deeper emotion arising to go out in acts of lovingness which make both giver and receiver happier and better.

Working thus together, playing into each other's hands, striving to accomplish any commendable object, which is to make both happier; which is to add to the common store; making mutual sacrifices; bringing constantly into play each other's sympathies by labors, and efforts, and self-denials—these are things which bind young hearts together, and build up between them an affec-

tion, a love, a devotion, which passing years but purify and con-
solidate and sweeten until life's close.

This mode of beginning married life has other advantages. It
gives opportunity for the exercise of hospitalities towards friends.
This stimulates to greater industries; to tidiness in housekeeping; to neatness of attire; to the practice of little economies;
to the exhibition of courtesies; and to those little " praisings
up " to guests, which will involuntarily escape from the lips of
the new housekeepers, and which very things deepen attachments, fan anew the flame of love, and become another spring of
domestic beatitudes.

Another high advantage is, housekeeping keeps the young
wife's mind busy—a very important consideration. She is not
only busy thinking, but it is a thinking on practical matters, on
things necessary to be done promptly, yet with deliberation and
judgment. Thus the powers of the mind are evolved, responsibility is exercised, executive ability is brought into requisition,
self-reliance is cultivated, because the husband is not at hand
to be consulted; and when he comes home and finds she has
acted with judgment, with prudence, with wisdom, he shows his
appreciation of it by his cordial and affectionate commendations,
and the light breaks in upon her for the first time that she is not
a doll, a plaything, a baby or a child, but that she has capabilities. Then she feels stronger; there is a consciousness that she
can be a help in the family; that she is worth something; that
while she is a recipient, she can be an aid. The husband, seeing
this practical exhibition of her capacities, is gradually led to ask
her advice, to talk with her about his own business matters, for
the sake of possible advantages to be derived from her suggestions. Thus one leans on the other; they look up to each other;
mutual and additional confidences arise, and it is not long before
they find that, between the household affairs of the wife, in
which she sometimes wants her husband's counsel, and the more
important business matters of the husband, about which he is
quite willing to listen to her suggestions and hints, they have
plenty to talk about. There is no sitting in the room for half an
hour at a time, without the exchange of a single word; there is
no silent smoking of a cigar for a great part of the evening; no
poring over a novel by the hour; no burying the nose in a newspaper, until every column has been read, advertisements and all;

no sudden jumping up from a chair to take a solitary walk; to visit a friend; to meet a business appointment, the wife left alone all the while to brood over the mishaps, the annoyances, the disappointments of the day.   On the contrary, each has subjects of inquiry; each has points of information to communicate, and a mutual interest in each other's respective departments springs up, which still further tightens the marriage bond. Each hour and each day is filled with its own duties, and responsibilities, and satisfactions, and there is domestic happiness, more thoroughly cemented every day and every hour, giving the promise of a deeper and a purer enjoyment in the future.   A writer in the New York "Ledger" says under the head of

LIFE'S BRIGHTEST HOUR.

Not long since I met a gentleman who is assessed for more than half a million.   Silver was in his hair, care upon his brow, and he stooped beneath his burden of wealth.   We were speaking of that period of life when we had realized the most perfect enjoyment, or, rather, when we had found the happiness nearest to the unalloyed.   "I'll tell you," said the millionnaire, "when was the happiest hour of my life.   At the age of one-and-twenty I had saved up $800.   I was earning $500 a year, and my father did not take it from me, only requiring that I should pay for my board.   At the age of twenty-two I had secured a pretty cottage just outside of the city.   I was able to pay two-thirds of the value down, and also to furnish it respectably.   I was married on Sunday—a Sunday in June, at my father's house. My wife had come to me poor in purse, but rich in the wealth of her womanhood.   The Sabbath and the Sabbath night we passed beneath my father's roof, and on Monday morning I went to my work, leaving mother and sister to help in preparing my home. On Monday evening, when the labors of the day were done, I went not to the paternal shelters, as in the past, but to my own house—my own home.   The holy atmosphere of that hour seems to surround me now in memory.   I opened the door of my cottage and entered.   I laid my hat upon the little stand in the hall, and passed on to the kitchen—our kitchen and dining-room were all one then.   I pushed open the kitchen door and was—in heaven!   The table was set against the wall—the evening meal was ready—prepared by the hands of her who had come to be my helpmeet in deed as well as in name—and by the table, with a throbbing, expectant look upon her lovely, loving face, stood my wife. I tried to speak, and could not. I could only clasp the waiting angel to my bosom, thus showing the ecstatic burden of my heart. The years had passed—long, long years—and worldly wealth has flowed in upon me, and I am honored and envied; but—as true as heaven—I would give it all—every dollar—for the joy of the hour of that June evening in the long, long ago."

One of the great faults and dangers of the times, especially in cities, is the increasing custom of young married persons spending the first months or years of married life in boarding-houses and hotels, or in the family of one of the parents. Trouble may be saved by this, the trouble of housekeeping; money may be saved by it; but it is at the expense of domestic comfort, of domestic happiness; more, it is risking the bringing about of domestic discord and domestic ruin; discord, because the young wife has nothing to do but to eat and dress, and sleep, and lounge about, lolling on sofas, gazing out of front windows; frittering away the time in trifling conversation with callers as idle as herself; spending many hours in dreamy imaginings; in poring over worthless novels; making questionable acquaintances; at other times indulging in the vain ambitions which want of occupation and undesirable companionship engender; to say nothing of the bickerings, the suspicions, the envies, the jealousies, the misunderstandings, and the thousand other sources of disquietude and discontent which are found under any roof which covers more than one family.

Remembering that the prevailing condition of the mother's mind during gestation will be impressed upon the child to be born, the highest appeal possible is made to parental justice, humanity, and love, to cultivate those feelings and affections and sentiments and thoughts which most ennoble our nature, by avoiding idleness during gestation; by keeping the mind on the alert, as much as possible, in housekeeping and domestic duties; in callings which keep the wife out of doors at least two or three hours every day, so that she shall be engaged in pleasurable activities to the extent of having the mind fully occupied, and the body engaged in doing something profitable, useful, pleasurable, with absolutely not a moment's leisure for nurturing dissatisfactions, envyings, remorses, hurt feelings, supposed slights or animosities of any description.   But this is not half the duty; there is a positive obligation to engage in whatever may cherish and cultivate all the higher feelings of our nature—our magnanimity, our benevolence, our loves.   Contemplate nothing which is not agreeable, that does not wake up the better sentiments. Gaze by the hour upon paintings, upon sculpture, on the waterfall and the mountain-top, on landscapes of tree and fountain, of fields and flowers, of lake and river, of hill and valley, listening to the songs of birds, to the music of the sweetest instruments, and that, nearer the divine, the human voice itself.

In addition to these, give many thoughts to serious contemplations, inward reflections, to yearnings for human ameliorations, the relief of the poor, and the elevation of all.

The remarks made, and those to be made, are intended to be carried out in practice, not merely for the first, but for all subsequent gestations, during which periods it is the husband's highest duty, and without the performance of which, for every hour of every successive day he cannot be a man, to make his wife's happiness his constant study; and in no way can he do this better than by a prompt gratification of every reasonable desire. Anticipate her probable wants; do everything with a ready and cheerful alacrity; be quick in sympathies; plan pleasant surprises; make coming home, when the business of the day is done, an event lovingly looked for; come home full of news; bring messages from friends; never come empty-handed; a bunch of grapes to-day; a rare fruit to-morrow; next day a pink, or rose, or little flower; anything to show, without telling it, that the wife at home has been lovingly thought of.   But there is more to be done than all this.   The pregnant wife, in every word and tone and look and gesture, should see that her husband's heart is full of tenderness, that he has the chivalry of a lover, and that his whole deportment towards her is manliness itself.   By no possibility, whatever might be the provocation, should an impatient look, or cross word, or angry reply ever escape him; and let every one see that the wife is considered the queen of the table, the mistress of the mansion.   In these ways she will be kept occupied fully; will be kept hopeful, and will enjoy everything.   She will also become self-respectful, self-appreciating, self-asserting, fearing nothing, all the time full of implicit trustingness in her husband's confidence and sympathies, pouring out upon him, in turn, the full measure of a woman's love; thus will the mother mould the character of her first-born in a cast which is noble, generous, and beautiful.

WHEN EDUCATION BEGINS.

It should begin a year before the child is born, before marriage, and if twenty years earlier, so much the better; for then the chances would be greater that the youthful pair would meet at the marriage altar in physical health, vigorous and permanent, with all the bodily functions matured, regular, and perfect.

There should be no concealed malady, no burrowing disease, no ailments of even a month's or day's duration; should there be any sickness whatever, the marriage ceremony, or its consummation, should be deferred until the system has been restored to its natural healthy condition, because whatever may be its state, whether of body or brain, at the instant of efficient congress, that condition will be imposed on the child to be born therefrom.

Authentic cases are recorded where persons have been so enraged, that within half an hour or less, the eyes and face have been diffused with a yellow tinge, showing that the entire blood of the system has been transformed; and as out of this blood the materials for the new being are drawn, it is a physiological impossibility that an impress should not be made on the physical and mental and moral constitution, foreign to nature and to health, precisely as has been ascertained, that a child begotten in a drunken stupor will be idiotic, or will be prone to brain diseases or actual insanity, if begotten when the parent was "excited with liquor," having "taken a glass with a friend," a very little thing indeed, in the estimation of some, but capable, under the combinations stated, of laying the foundations for untold miseries, the misery of a mad-house for a lifetime, to a human being capable otherwise of the highest human achievements.

If a transient sensation of the parent may give to a child the impress of that parent's character, much more will feelings which have been indulged in for days and weeks and months together, be incorporated into the very being, physical, mental, and moral, of the child born after them.

If any intelligent pair, in any community, should become parents in the practical observance of the principles inculcated in these pages, their children would not die early, but would mature and fructify, and thus become living springs themselves, sending out healthful progenies far and near, until the whole land would be peopled with inhabitants healthy, happy, and good, because "Like produces like;" because the time is divinely decreed to come, when it shall no longer be said that "The fathers have eaten sour grapes, and the children's teeth are set on edge." That good time can never come until the fathers cease to eat sour grapes; until they cease to be vicious, until they cease to riot in animal appetites and passions for the enjoyment of them, but shall gratify them in temperance, as a means of fulfilling the eternal design of replenishing the earth with the highest type of manhood.

As an incentive to cultivate aspirations like these, there is the great truth that evil and disease are not eternal; they are destined to death; while goodness of heart and mental activity are immortal. The latter must "increase," while the former must "decrease." The tiny mustard-seed must grow and fructify, and give its cooling shade, indefinitely extending. The "little stone cut out of the mountain without hands," shall roll onward, increasing ever, until the world shall be brought beneath it. The cloud, no bigger than a man's hand, must cover the whole sky, and pour its living rain on all that grows. All evil is for a day; all good for unending ages. But while these considerations are written for our comfort and encouragement, it must not be forgotten that vice and disease are to be exterminated, are to be hunted from the world, by the aggressive action of good men and women, an action which begins at the root of the matter, an action which removes the cause; then the effect ceases by its own limitation, ceases in the very nature of things. It cannot be that evil will in the end triumph. In plainer phrase, if the children to be begotten are born healthy in body, mind, and morals, their descendants, in turn, will be like them, while the evil race now living perishes from the world. Such results will not come of themselves; they must be wrought out like every other good; they come by planning beforehand, and then carrying the plans into execution.

There must be a beginning somewhere; that beginning must be made in two human hearts, elevated, cultivated, conscientious. And infinite blessings must come for time and for aye upon that man and woman who, for the glory of God and the good of the race, shall set out to do all they can to make a beginning, to sow the first seed which will bear a fruitage so helpful to the world of mankind.

HEREDITARY INFLUENCES.

A single ear of red corn will sometimes be found in gathering the crop in the autumn, and if one grain of it be planted in the following spring, there will be other red ears. If the grains of all these be planted the next season, it will be a few years only before every grain of corn in the whole field will be red, like the original. By analogy, the same law prevails in living generations, among insects and birds, and animals and man, for "like begets like" throughout the universe of living things. By this general law it follows that if in any community a healthy, intelligent pair should marry, and should in their lives carry out the principles of healthful living laid down in these pages, they will have children; their children will be healthy, intelligent, and prolific, like themselves, each one becoming a centre of population, the progenitor of others, until, in a time not remote, the whole land would be peopled with a stalwart race, possessing physical vigor, active minds, and elevated sentiments; because in the nature of things, the healthy individuals among animals and men have ability to perpetuate themselves; while the diseased, the weakly, the vicious, die out; for the Scriptures say, "The wicked shall not live out half their days;" and just as explicit and positive is the announcement, "The righteous shall go down to his grave like a shock of corn, fully ripe in his season." Hence, the fundamental truth is founded on the eternal rock of Divine assertion, that goodness naturally spreads, perpetuates itself, has in itself the seeds of immortality; while vice and disease have within themselves the seeds of death. Thus far as to the physical man; and not less true is it of the spiritual nature; and on the same rock is the truth grounded, that covenant and

40

mercy would not only be kept towards the good man, but to his children also to thousands of "generations" after him, which means that good men not only transmit their qualities to their own immediate children, but to those born to them to remote ages in the future. And with such responsibilities, with such "exceeding great and precious promises" from the Infinite One, can any good man or woman, can any Christian pair, consistently beget children without any care, without any premeditation, without any arrangement of circumstances to give for good the first impress of physical, mental, and moral character? And yet, the very best men of all ages up to the present hour have habitually committed acts of parentage without the very first thought, without the very slightest deed, intended to have any bearing whatever on the character of the child, but everything has been left to the most perfect hap-hazard imaginable. No sermon has ever been preached, no book ever published, nor has any ever been written with the express object of enforcing a line of conduct which would give to those who come after us healthy bodies, good constitutions, and mental and moral qualities which would, in the highest sense, fit them for the duties of life. It is a historical fact that "descent," meaning thereby "hereditary influence," does more towards fashioning the physical constitution and the moral character of man than all things else besides, external or internal. And there is scarcely another truth in the whole range of human observation which has gained such a universal assent among thinking minds of past ages as that of the hereditary transmission of physical, mental, and moral qualities, and which at the same time has been so universally disregarded in practice, although it should be clear to every one that if a parent becomes addicted to any form of vice, is habitually vicious in any one thing, it cannot fail to leave a bad impress on the child's constitution, and that diseased physical constitutions affect the will and the conscience and the moral nature in such a way as to impair their vigor and their legitimate, pure, and right action. If any change is to be made in these directions, it must be done by those who have loftier thoughts, higher heroisms, and more transcendent aspirations than have yet influenced mankind. Yet the motives to these higher things may be cherished, may be cultivated in the humblest hearts where true love to God resides, until the morning dawns of a brighter and a better day. The following is an illustration of

HEREDITARY INFLUENCE.

Nearly a hundred years ago, a New York lawyer was travelling on horseback on Long Island, and coming to an inviting country inn, at the close of the day, he alighted for the purpose of spending the night. The family consisted of the father, mother, and daughter of eighteen, so retired in her manners; so comely in her person, and of a mind so cultivated and refined, that on leaving next morning the young man determined that he would repeat his visit before a great while, which he did. In due time they were married, went to housekeeping in New York, and set about the business of life in real earnest. The young lawyer rose in his profession, made a name, lived happily, temperately, and long, dying at a good old age, leaving a large fortune to two surviving sons, one of whom died within easy memory of the New York Knickerbocker, a besotted, drivelling drunkard, leaving two sons, both of whom

" TOOK TO DRINK "

early, and early died, childless. The other son of the lawyer married a beautiful and accomplished woman, himself a handsome man, of refinement and culture, but he fell into drinking habits, spent his own patrimony and a large share of his wife's fortune. His infirmity grew upon him to an extent which made it impossible for his wife to live with him longer, and taking her grown daughter with her, she left him, legally married again, and is now living happily with the second man of her choice, and another family of children growing up around her; all these things made such a profound impression on the mind of the forsaken father and husband, that he resolved he would never drink another drop of liquor again, and for twenty years has kept his resolution.

Was this turning to drink on the part of the children and grandchildren the result of enticements into bad habits or by inheritance ? The lawyer and his wife were strictly temperate in all their habits, and plain in their tastes and modes of living, but cultivated, hospitable, and refined. When the keeper of the Long Island country inn married, he was a well-to-do young man, fond of his wife, and fond of his home; but his occupation, particularly at that early day, led very naturally into habits of drinking; it was a common thing then to

"TREAT"

friends to a drink of grog when they happened to drop in during the day, and when night came, the neighbors would come in to learn the news from the city, as gathered from passing travellers; and this easily degenerated into sipping toddy and brandy and water during the evening chat, which by degrees extended into the night; the landlord, it is reported, generally going to bed full of liquor, rousing the "strong propensities" of nature, which would not be quieted without the fullest gratification. Under these influences a new being was made. But the leprosy of drunkenness did not break out in the first generation; the habits, the cultivation, and the refinement of the innkeeper's daughter were all antagonistic of what might foster the habit of drink, and so it skipped over a generation, the tinder being applied to the torch, to be kindled into flame under the greater susceptibilities of boyhood life and surroundings. It is precisely in this way that

INSANITY

overleaps a generation or two; thus also it is that a child bears no resemblance to its father or mother, but is often the exact resemblance to the grandparents or great grandparents. Doubtless in innumerable cases, the foundation of drunkenness in persons yet unborn has been laid by parents retiring after the sumptuous dinner, or the evening party, one or both saturated with wine, or worse. Let the terrible truth impress itself on the thoughtful reader's mind, that in a Massachusetts asylum for the care of idiotic children, three-fourths were born of parents one or both of whom were habitual drinkers of spirituous liquors. It is surely not necessary to state more clearly the inferences to be drawn from these observations, and yet men are so dull of comprehension sometimes as to require the plainest teachings; still the lesson is of importance but little less than infinite; it suggests the abeyance of perpetuative function when under alcoholic influence. The self-same lesson is powerfully taught in the facts recorded in standard medical works, showing that if a mother suckles her infant within half an hour of being in an ungovernable rage, it will be immediately thrown into convulsions. The great broad fact then remains, that mental and physical constitutions, appetites, and propensities, and passions, mould the physical condition of the infant nursed nnder their influences, fix the character of the being begotten at the time of their prevalence. And under this most important practical principle, having such a controlling power in forming the characters and fixing the destinies of the unborn, as well as the babe, are ranged that large class of what are regarded as

MYSTERIOUS CASES,

where children are so totally different from their parents in their mental and moral characteristics. Nothing can so well account for the character of

AARON BURR,

the first-born and only son of father and mother, models of humble piety, of Christian devotion, and of stern faith in Calvinistic doctrine, yet leaving that son, magnificent in his talents, but an infidel in religion, without moral principle, a *roué*, a traitor, and a murderer; the father or mother, or both, when he was begotten, laboring under the depressing influences of doubt and unbelief or temporary rebellion against the Divine government, which sometimes prevail for a transient period in the experiences of the wisest and best of men; for there were times in the lives of such as David and Knox and Chalmers and Cowper and Newton when the sirocco of unbelief would sweep across their hearts, scorching up all that was

GREEN AND GOODLY

to look upon in their moral and religious feeling and sentiment, tempting the mind to express itself in the words of the fool—

"THERE IS NO GOD."

Not only are physical defects and diseased conditions and moral depravities transmitted from parents to their immediate descendants, but as seen in the narration of the facts just made, even proclivities are imparted which affect subsequent generations even to the fourth degree ; a principle recognized as far back as Moses' time, for he was divinely instructed to write, fifteen centuries before the Advent, of " visiting the iniquity of the fathers upon the children unto the third and fourth generation of them that hate me," Exodus xx. 5. Meaning merely that the example which sinning parents set to their children does not cease to have its evil effects for several generations. Eighteen hundred years ago, Plutarch wrote of his own times, drunkards beget drunkards. And it is now admitted that the tendency to gluttony and gaming, and libertinism and vicious tempers, and animal passion, is often inherited. A writer in a British periodical states a fact coming under his own observation, where both parents died of drunkenness, and so did all the children. In another case both parents were drunkards, and the large family of children which they left, with one exception, died prematurely by drunkenness, suicide, or other violence.

In Norway all duty was taken off imported liquor for ten years ; at the end of that time insanity had increased fifty per cent., and the number of children born idiotic had increased one hundred and fifty per cent. This is a most fearful fact, and should indelibly impress upon every intelligent mind the extent to which a parent is responsible for the physical condition and moral character of the child, and that such condition depends, in the first place, on the physical and mental condition of the father at the moment of the impregnating act, and on the mental and moral and physical states of the mother during pregnancy.

M. Morel has recorded the history of a drunken father, extending to four generations of descendants.

First. The father was an habitual drunkard, and was killed in a public brawl.

Second. The son followed the drunken habits of his father, became subject to attacks of mania, which terminated in paralysis and premature death.

Third. The grandson was strictly temperate, was never drunk, but suffered with habitual depression of spirits, with imaginary fears of injury from others, and could scarcely restrain himself from killing other people.

Fourth. The great-grandson had but little intellect, had an attack of insanity at the age of sixteen, ending in an idiotic condition, and with him the family became extinct.

When we turn from these and contemplate the states of mind of the mothers of Samuel the prophet, of John the Baptist, and of our Lord, and the blessed results of having born to them children who became such exalted characters afterwards, we may have some faint idea of the honor and the responsibility put upon every mother in the arrangements of the Divine Ruler of the universe, making her but a little below the angels.

WASHING THE BABY.

AFTER delivery, lay the child on its right side, a short distance from the mother; cover it up well and warmly. Look at it now and then, to see if it breathes freely, and if the umbilical cord ceases to bleed at the end. As is elsewhere stated, rub a little oil all over the child, to soften the cohesions on the skin, with which it was born; then wash it with soap and water, not less than ninety degrees, using a soft sponge, to be rubbed hard enough to get off all the coating, especially all the places where the skin folds. After the umbilical cord detaches itself, there may be a little tenderness in the navel; lay over it a piece of soft linen, dipped in oil, and if necessary to stop any little bleeding, sprinkle finely powdered burnt alum on the place. After the washing and first dressing, give the child for its first swallow a teaspoonful of cold or tepid water. Notice particularly if the feet and hands are comfortably warm; if not, let each foot and each hand be held in some old, warm hand, even pressing a little; then rub the skin, and envelop with the hand again, to invite circulation and warmth.

All soiled diapers should be instantly dropped in cold water, and then, as soon as convenient, removed from the room.

Every time an infant is dressed or washed it should be held before the fire, if fire-time, or in the sun coming in at the window, and rubbed gently with the warm hands all over, especially over the back and abdomen: this promotes the circulation, imparts warmth, and is otherwise beneficial, especially to the skin, as it allows the air to come to it, and increases its softness and pliability.

An infant naturally dreads having a wet cloth flapped on any part of the body; it is intensely disagreeable. On the other hand, if it has not been cheated by being put into water too hot or too cold, it will surely delight in paddling in it;—for a minute or two or more, once every day, increasing the time as the child grows older, but never allow the water to be colder than seventy-five degrees, at least until it is two years old; and then not under sixty at any time. One such bath a day is enough, if a child is strong and vigorous; if weakly, two or three times a week. Baths should be taken in the forenoon. For the first year the water should range from seventy to eighty degrees or over, according to the vigor of the child; but always avoid allowing the water to get cold enough to chill, or give a bluish appearance to the finger-nails. As a general rule, an infant should be washed night and morning for three months; then, until the sixth month, once a day; and after that two or three times a week until four years old, always using tepid water; but when entering the fourth year, cool water of the temperature of the air may be used in summer. In winter-time the water should not be colder than sixty degrees, and the room where the bathing is performed should be as warm as sixty-five or seventy, so that there should not be a feeling of coldness when the skin emerges from the water.

After the fourth year the mother should give her special attention to the personal cleanliness of her children. She should consider them under her own supervision, giving them repeated instruction as to the importance of cleanliness, as associated with purity of mind and morals. Means should be used to inspire contempt for untidiness and filth and dirt in clothing or skin. And until a child has imbibed her own notions, and would feel miserable and degraded at the consciousness of having the slightest soiling of foot or finger or inner garment, no pains should be spared in judicious, kindly, and imperative teachings in this direction. Occasion should frequently be taken at bed-time, and in the mornings and while asleep, for personal inspection, so that the child may feel that any dereliction will certainly be discovered and punished. And washings and bathings should be required to be done every day, if they are needed, to keep the feet, the toes, the armpits, and every part of the skin in neck and groin and elsewhere, as perfectly and as habitually clean as the face itself. As consciousness of dirt debases, so consciousness of perfect cleanliness elevates, refines, gives power and courage and self-assertion. It is scarcely possible to give too much attention to impressive lessons of the most special cleanliness of person and dress and habit upon all young minds, as it is rightly associated with godliness and every high trait of character; it is a safeguard against many a vice; it is an irresistible power against many a temptation.

LIFE'S PERIODS.

Whether it be a mere whim or not, there is a general impression that there are certain periods or crises in human life at which great and important changes take place in the human economy for good or ill; these stations are about seven years apart; seven for teething, fourteen for the beginning of the change to manhood and womanhood. Twenty-one exempts from parental rule. Seven years later usually finds a man a husband and father, and the head of a family. At thirty-five, in all the prime of manhood, the world opens in its fulness to the highest aims, to the loftiest ambitions, to the grandest achievements. At forty-two, sobriety comes; it is at that age the man is a fool or a physician as to himself; at that age, it is supposed that if he has not made a fortune, or at least has not laid a solid and broad foundation for it, he will never secure one, and will be thriftless all his days. It is also said that if a man ever fails, it should be before he is forty, for then he may get on his feet again and will be careful enough not to hazard his means a second time. But if forty finds him poor, poor he will remain until the end of the chapter.

As to women, the great change of life begins to be prepared for; if the bridge is safely crossed, they may safely calculate on two or three periods more. At sixty-three, multitudes die; the downhill of life has been taken; a false step, a slight mistake, a trifling inconsideration, a little injudiciousness, there is a stumble on the steep incline, and a headlong plunge into the grave. If this is survived, one more period brings us to the threescore and ten, which few ever pass.

Having given the lessons applicable to the preparation for impregnation, for the whole period of gestation, the birth, the bathing, the feeding, the nursing, the weaning, the dress, the teething and the habitual cleanliness of person and apparel so necessary to the body, so purifying to the heart, so elevating to the mind; the second station, the second mile-post is reached, the tuition period, the beginning of learning and of

SCHOOLING CHILDREN.

Only general principles can be laid down, until the child, boy or girl, has entered the seventh year, when the permanent teeth begin to appear, as if nature were now intending a new effort, laying the first solid foundation for the great work of life, the discipline of the mind. No study should be required beyond learning the alphabet, and some of the first general principles of our holy religion. On entering the seventh year, two hours should be set apart in the forenoon, and one in the afternoon in learning to read, write and cipher. Until entering the tenth year no study connected with books should be allowed, no recitations, no tasks of any kind out of those hours; only three hours in the twenty-four for such things; at least twelve to sleeping and eating, and the remainder in muscular activities, either in work or play; every second of them possible should be out of doors in the open air, that is, every second before sundown, for at sundown every child, boy or girl, should be required to come into the house and stay there up to fourteen years of age, unless under a parent's eye or within a parent's call. Stay in the house from sundown until bed-time, winter or summer, in the city or in the country, at home or abroad. "It is outside of their father's door after sundown, from eight to sixteen, that nine-tenths of all the criminals are made who come before me," was the announcement from the bench, of one of the greatest and best of England's Judges. Before the seventh year, girls and boys are naturally within doors after sundown; but then they begin to want greater liberties, their natural restlessness becomes harder to control, and they yearn for the rompings of the street. And here it is that the tight rein of parental authority should begin to be drawn—stern, imperative, absolute. "Never outside of my door after sundown for one brief five minutes, unless under my eye." How would such a precept, irreversible as any Medo-Persian law, depopulate the penitentiaries in twenty years, and rid the gallows of half its victima. But there must be a substitute for the enlivenment of the street.

HOME MADE HAPPY.

This is the panacea; it is here that splendid women and magnificent men are made; in a happy home, a home of unity and peace between father and mother, where there is always and under all circumstances a reciprocity of courtly and affectionate attentions, a constant exhibition of deference, of self-abnegations; a mutual, watchful care and solicitude and sympathy; of quiet deportment, of gentle words and tender tones, the youngest child, the tiniest infant of a month, servants, the guest, the transient caller, the very atmosphere of the mansion, all will catch it, will instinctively adopt it, and there will reign inevitably and always whatever there is on earth of loveliness, of goodness, of purity and exaltedness of aim and end in life which makes of men the kinsfolk of the angels.

When children get toward the fourteenth year, three hours in the forenoon and two in the afternoon should be spent in severe study; the remainder of the day-light in outdoor activities in part; in the acquisition of the first general principles of botany, in the cultivation of the garden, the orchard, the field, and the forest. Nothing can be as delightful for the present, and so full of interest and pleasure in the future, as the study of the plants and flowers, with the objects before you, which you can see, feel and handle, and better comprehend with the aid of a competent instructor in one hour, than in a week or even in a month by the help of a book and the play of the imagination, with the waste of nervous and brain power involved. At the very least, one-half the study, one-half the vital force of childhood is worse than squandered and lost, by the mere effort to catch at and imagine what a book means and teaches; all of which might be saved, besides a corresponding loss of precious time, with a competent instructor and the object in view.

The same may be said of the principles of geology; out of the hours of study the teachers could go out into "the highways and hedges, to the spring bed and the branch," the trout-brook and the creek or river side; or scale the mountain, or delve into the valley, and with hammer and trowel could teach the histories of the rocks—how long they had lain there, whence they came, what their constituents, through what they had passed, and what their probable destiny in the lapse of ages to come, so that there would be not a rod of earth, of stony bed, or grass-green level, or tangled bush, wherein might not be found by an inquiring boy or girl, ever-gushing fountains of amusement, instruction, and acquisition.

It might take a little longer to educate boys and girls thus, but, if so much was not learned, what was studied would be more satisfactorily known, would be longer remembered, would be more thoroughly utilized and enjoyed in all the life thereafter. At the same time, when the weather was unpropitious, or the hour of the day was unsuitable for these out-door employments, with lessons in sowing seed and setting-out plants, in trimming and in pruning, in hoeing, in ploughing and harvesting; then, in-door lessons in music could be taken; music on the harp, the piano, the bass-viol, or the beautiful flute; or in sketching, and painting, and designing—all equally proper for girls and boys, equally elevating, equally refined, and equally full of saving amusement —amusement in the family which will invite from the street, from the low taverns, and from the corrupting theatre. By thus utilizing the time of children at home, losing no hour of any day, but having every one filled up fully between solid study and the study of amusement, making it at the same time a glad recreation and a pastime of intense, absorbing interest, more would be learned by the time boys and girls became of age—learned more thoroughly, and in a manner to be made more practically useful, with the saving of health, and with half the expenditure of mental and nervous power than is now incurred by the very best systems of education. This was the programme carried out by the Queen of England, to the end of raising a large family of children in vigorous health, without a death, and nearly all of them, at this writing, themselves healthy fathers and mothers, heirs to the proudest thrones in Christendom.

In reference to the whole subject of boy and girl education up to this date, it must be acknowledged that less progress has been made than in almost any other branch of human investigation.

School-teaching is yet a barbarism, a cruelty, a curse. Three-fourths of all the children who enter school-rooms this day literally despise school; it is their utter abomination, and in their deep execrations of it, they take their first lessons, in too many cases, in fraud and deceit and pretence and actual lying. They easily learn to feign sickness not felt, to invent excuses without foundation, and to play truant without remorse, only if they can avoid the hated, hateful task; a task which might have been made a pleasure and a life-long profit. In few words,

OBJECT-TEACHING

only ought to be recognized in any civilized land, in any humane community, at least until the foundation of the first elementary studies have been laid.

Meanwhile, we must go back to the eventful age of fourteen, the boundary-line between youth and womanhood and manhood, with all their high responsibilities, when the mind peers with such intense interest into the mysteries of reproduction; when the whole nature is on the eve of change, and a new world opens to the inquiring eye, waking up new sentiments, new passions, new aspirations; all wonderful, all absorbing, called the age of

PUBERTY,

From the Roman word " pubertas," derived from " puber " or " pubes," adult, entering man's estate. This comes earlier to girls than to boys, but there is a danger to both, arising from neglect or evil associations; a danger to girls now and then, but to boys always; a danger which parents remember they were exposed to, but which, somehow or other they fail to caution their children against; excusing themselves by shutting their eyes, glossing it over, and cherishing the hope that in some indefinite kind of way or other their children may not fall into it, or may make their way out of it without their troubling themselves about it. But this never happens. The appetite connected with the subject is inappeasable—nature calls as imperatively as for food and drink, and together with the curiosity engendered in connection with it, it winds its serpent coil around every boy, from which deliverance is never had without loss of youthful ingenuousness, and sometimes youthful conscience, youthful moral sense; now and then there is a loss of health, of life, and worse, of reason. Sometimes the young get into the circuit of the maelstrom, and presently wake up as from a horrid dream, and utter appeals so piteous as to move a heart of stone—appeals which, in some way or other, come to the city physician from one year's end to another, one of them, with a fee, while writing this very line, in an almost copper-plate handwriting, in faultless grammar, and in a perfection of composition which speaks for the writer as cultivated, educated, refined:

"JUNE, '72.

"DEAR SIR:—I trust you will not consider me impertinent in thus addressing you, for I know of no one with whom to advise, and whose advice I could trust as I do yours.

"I am suffering with a disease brought on by early indiscretion, a disease that is gradually sapping up my vitality. I should have advised with private physicians of this city; but they advertise so like quacks that I take them for such, and dare not trust myself in their hands. I should have consulted with our family physician, or other physicians of the city; but am known to them all, and I cannot bring myself to do so on account of shame. Hampered in this way, bound hand and foot, my only hope is in you, and in you I put my trust and pray you not to lay this carelessly aside, but give me your best counsel; for it is either a cure, or by my own hands I die.

"Six years ago, as near as I can guess, I learned through a companion what afterward became a habit, practised at first as often as once a day, for a week or two at a time, and then twice or thrice a week; and then as I became aware of its injuriousness, I with great exertion would lay it aside for a month or two; and once six months passed away without debasement, when the old habit returned, until I found that at night I would wake from lascivious dreams, with the results. That I should have fallen so low horrified me, and I swore never to err again. The debilitations ceased for two or three months, when I fell again, with consequences worse than before and with augmented force. It is now ten or more months since I degraded myself of my own free will. I can control my mind and thoughts during the day, and I would not have a thought or desire which I would be ashamed for my mother to know. But if I over-exert myself, or take a hearty supper, I have an exhaustion by the morning for two or three times in the week, undermining my health and impairing my memory. I am temperate in all things, and have never stepped out of the bounds of propriety and virtue."

See other remarks under head of " Nocturnals." In reference to one of the remarks above, the habit of secret vice is fallen into spontaneously without any teaching whatever, and nocturnals will come whether it is practised or not, and, as explained elsewhere, will continue to occur although the vice has been discontinued years before ; but let it be distinctly remembered, and it is repeated here in order to make a deeper impression, that they do not occur as an effect of the vice, they have no necessary connection with it ; and instead of taking remedies to cure nocturnals as a diseased result of secret vice, they ought not to be suppressed at all, cannot be healthfully and safely suppressed any more than the suppression of urine, which is always certain death within a week. The only method of getting rid of them is in honorable marriage and the indulgence of its rights, in accordance with the general principles enunciated in a previous page, when a healthful condition of the reproductive system will continue, until the clock of life runs down and the fires of youth are put out forever in sight of the century. Sometimes such excesses in secret indulgence are committed as to end in idiocy. Medical works record such instances, and as there can be no telling in the case of any child that there shall not be such excess, each parent owes it to the children to have a wise and intelligent eye to these things, and when there is reason to suppose the existence of such a habit, to plainly state its sin and danger, and, by appeals to the moral sense and to conscience, endeavor to implant resolves firm enough to break up the habit. Much might be done by teaching children that the hands should never be allowed to be carried to the parts a single instant, except what is requisite for bathing purposes ; teach them that it is degrading to do so ; that the good and refined would look upon it with the utmost contempt in case of its ever being ascertained, impressing their young minds with an utter loathing of such handlings. If there is such a degree of reprobacy in any case that no impression can be made on the mind, and there is seen every indication of a determination to persist in indulgence, the surgeon should be called to the girl, and the whole thing can be rectified in a moment, and ought to be ; as to boys, a discreet physician should be consulted.

Reference was made in the letter to having learned these practices from others. Two cautions are here given to parents : that in countless cases these things are taught children and youth by the servants in the kitchen, boy and men waiters, coachmen, apprentices, young clerks, and unmarried journeymen. Boys and girls should be early learned and drilled into the idea never to be alone in a room with only one person. Seek to impress on their minds, in proper ways, an idea of indefinable horrors resulting from such things. In addition, let it be a fixed thing, as irresistible as the fiat of a despot, never to allow one child to sleep in the same bed with another after entering the third year; never, after entering the fourth year, allow a boy and girl to undress in the same room, let alone enter the same bed, simply because of the acknowledged fact known to all physicians, that the sexual instinct has manifested itself before five years of age; hence it is better to begin early, and thus be on the safe side, so as to prevent an early shock of the moral sense of the young.

ENTERING WOMANHOOD.

When the young girl's nature first begins the great change, or even previous to the time, her mother should make it her business to give the proper information, not with a great ado, but with such an indifference, in such a matter-of-fact way, that it shall be regarded as a business, as an elevating occurrence, rather than one of shamefulness—that it is womanly—that it is exalting—a thing rather to be proud of. In this way the young girl will not hesitate to make the mother her confidant, and the door is open for a co-operation and a course of instructions which will lead to safe and happy results. If, on the other hand, the girl has no instruction, she will learn by degrees from schoolmates that something may be expected, and of a character that no one ought to know anything about. And many times, in their efforts at concealment, dangerous washings and bathings have been resorted to, causing repressions which impair the health, and lead the way to a life-long invalidism.

Girls should be taught the importance at such times to guard against all causes of suppression, to give instant information of any stoppage, or death may occur in a very short time; that cold feet, that wet feet, that getting out of bed on a cold floor, or with the feet on an oil-cloth in a bath-room, or sitting upon stones, on marble seats or damp benches, or standing on the wet grass even for five minutes; that having a garment wetted by the rain, that sitting in a door or at an open window, at home or in a carriage or other vehicle while the wind is blowing, especially after exercise has been taken—that all these things are positively dangerous to life.   Such should be the instructions given to girls by every mother, with such repetitions and explanations as are necessary to make a clear, distinct, and definite impression on the mind—one that cannot be forgotten.   Without these confidences between mother and child, there will be more or less of concealment, especially about the development of the breasts ; the little girl will seek to hide it, just as the youth shuts the door, locks and bolts it, and puts a chair in front of it and a basin on the chair, and closes every window, draws down every blind, when he is going to shave himself for the first time.   In these efforts she fails to let out her dress, if anything tightens it.   This compression of course arrests the proper and healthful flow of the blood through the minute blood-vessels and causes hard lumps, which in after-life, sometimes are sure to result in cancer of the breast, one of the most horrible of all human maladies ; hence the conscientious mother, as she values her child's best interests, will begin early to impress these lessons on the mind, that under no conceivable circumstance should any pressure be made on the bosoms for even five minutes, but that the clothing should be as loose and free as possible, not less necessary during gestation and until the change of life.

Great injury is done to the moral and physical nature of girls by tight and heavy clothing over the hips ; by dancing, jumping down from heights, by excessive exertions, false steps, as in coming down-stairs.   Falling of the womb and other misplacements have often taken place from these things.   Girls should be early taught that in getting out of carriages, in stepping from chairs, in being helped over fences, it is always better to be deliberate, to alight on the toes as much as possible and as little as may be on the heel ; that all running up-stairs has a dangerous tendency, and all protracted efforts of every description should be avoided. Girls, in their ambition to jump a rope a certain number of times, have succeeded, and the next moment have fallen dead, in one case after two hundred jumps.

As early as fourteen the girls of a family ought to be taught to take their turns in the management of certain household duties, of clearing up rooms, of making their own beds, of sweeping and

41

dusting, of baking, of making cakes and pies and puddings, and other desserts and delicacies, of washing up the tea-things, of setting the table with taste and elegance, of darning and mending, and by degrees to sew on buttons, to cut and fit dresses and make them, to trim bonnets, and make shirts and work button-holes. Bring them up in these things, encourage them, lead them along pleasantly, patiently, firmly. Bear in mind two things: First, children have a pride in feeling that they are useful. Second, that they will take more pains to keep up their name for anything, to maintain their character for a specified thing, whether it be good or bad, than they will to get that character. There is a pride in excelling in the bad as well as the good. If you give a child the reputation of being the greatest dunce, he will feign being a dunce rather than lose his credit. Many an evil trait has been grafted in children by the injudiciousness of parents in giving them a reputation for superiority. In plain terms, if you give your child the credit of his being the noisiest in the family, he will soon be found working hard to keep up his standing, to add to his credit. But give your daughter a name for being the tidiest in her dress, the most orderly in her room, the readiest in her services or other good quality, and she will work hard thereafter to retain her standing.

TRAINING GIRLS.

Training girls for household duties ought to be considered as necessary as instruction in reading, writing and arithmetic, and quite as universal. We are in our houses more than half our existence, and it is the household surroundings which affect most largely the happiness or misery of domestic life. If the wife knows how to "keep house," if she understands how to "set a table," if she has learned how things ought to be cooked, how beds should be made, how carpets should be swept, how furniture should be dusted, how the clothes should be repaired, and turned, and altered, and renovated; if she knows how purchases can be made to the best advantage, and understands the laying in of provisions, how to make them go farthest and last longest; if she appreciates the importance of system, order, tidiness, and the quiet management of children and servants, then she knows how to make a little heaven of home—how to win her children from the street; how to keep her husband from the club-house, the gaming-table, and the wine-cup. Such a family will be trained to social respectability, to business success, and to efficiency and usefulness in whatever position may be allotted to them.

It may be safe to say, that not one girl in ten in our large towns and cities enters into married life who has learned to bake a loaf of bread, to purchase a roast, to dust a painting, to sweep a carpet, or to cut and fit, and make her own dress. How much the perfect knowledge of these things bears upon the thrift, the comfort and health of families, may be conjectured, but not calculated by figures. It would be an immeasurable advantage to make a beginning by attaching a kitchen to every girls' school in the nation, and have lessons given daily in the preparation of all the ordinary articles of food and drink for the table, and how to purchase them in the market to the best advantage, with the result of a large saving of money, an increase of comfort, and higher health in every family in the land.

Mothers should be encouraged to take pains to initiate their children when very young into the mysteries of the household, not only as a matter of duty, but of policy and humanity; of duty to the child, of policy to themselves, and of humanity to her own family. It is said of the wife of the munificent founder of Vassar College, at Poughkeepsie, New York, on the Hudson, which admirable establishment has in course of preparation for domestic duties, as well for the dining-room as the salon, several hundred young girls, going out one class after another to happify society as well as to elevate it, that she was left motherless at the age of ten years, and had to take charge of the large family of her father's children; to these she consecrated her youthful energies, and with all the disadvantages of want of schooling and a very limited knowledge of household affairs. She sacrificed her education, she sacrificed society, and through long years of care and toil, and anxiety and hard, hard work, she completed her task and did it well; and no doubt these experiences, in talking over them in after-life with her husband, led him, with her co-operation and her counsel, to establish at the expense of several hundred thousand dollars, an institution which shall continue to send out its benign influences all over the land for ages to come; its object being to qualify girls to become wives, mothers, housekeepers in the best sense of the word.

In reference to the subject of generally initiating girls into the knowledge and practice of household duties, a woman who has had experience of it all, and speaks from that experience with a practical clearness which well befits such an one as she is, and her name is given to add weight to her authority, Mrs. Henry Ward Beecher, says: "Little by little, as the child grows toward womanhood, let the mother throw off some portion of her cares, teaching her daughters to oversee or perform them correctly, and by so doing not only lighten her own labors, but make such duties easy for her children in after-years, or if they should be called prematurely to the entire charge. When daughters are old enough to become their mother's companions, they should also become joint partners in home and household responsibilities. When out of school divide the work so that every other week the mother shall be entirely free from all care—a guest in the family —or if that is at first too great a tax on the young partner, 'take turns' in dividing the work, the daughter one week having the charge of the cooking, marketing, and arranging for each meal entirely herself; the next week, of the dairy, if on a farm, or the laundry or chamber-work. When each week is ended, the mother can point out the failures or recommend a better or easier way of doing some particular thing; but unless advice or directions are asked, it is far better that the young housekeeper should be left to her own skill and judgment. · For a few times this may not prove the best economy, but in the end 'it pays,' and with good interest. Of course, before this plan can be carried into execution to any extent, the young lady has served an apprenticeship so far as to know herself that part of the work which comes under her jurisdiction each week; and when practice shall have made perfect, and the term of apprenticeship expires, it is excellent discipline for a daughter to assume the reins entirely, for a shorter or longer time, as health or pleasure may determine, subject to such suggestions as may be deemed advisable. This arrangement gives rest and liberty, if all her children are grown up, for the mother to read, travel, or enjoy social life, as she could not do when they were young and needing the care which should never be delegated to another, unless compelled by ill-health."

FRAIL CHILDREN

Need not die early; judicious care may educate into active bodies and vigorous minds, to become useful and renowned in later years. Dr. Farr wisely says: If weakly children are tided over infancy, the result, it may be said, will be an increase of sickly adults and degeneration of race. All breeders of animals throw aside bad specimens. The Spartans did not allow the father to dispose of his child as he thought fit, for he was obliged to take it to the triers, who, if they found it puny and ill-shaped, ordered it to be carried to a sort of chasm under Taygetus; of this course Socrates and Plato approved. At Athens and Rome the infant at birth was laid upon the ground, and was abandoned to its fate if the father did not lift his child from mother earth, who was assumed to have claims upon its fragile body. The Romans were reproached by the Christian fathers for their inhumanity. "Which of you," says Tertullian, upbraiding the Gentiles in rude eloquence, "has not slain a child at birth?" Thus the right of a child to life was questioned at its very threshold, and he only won it after examination. Children were dipped, like Achilles, in cold water to harden or to kill them, as the case might be. Through Christianity, through one of the leading races of mankind—the Jews—and through the manly sense of the Anglo-Saxons, we have been led to look upon children in another light, and be they weak or strong their lives are sacred in the eyes of English law. Experience has justified this policy. Great qualities of soul are often hidden in the frailest child. One Christmas day a premature posthumous son was born in England, of such an extremely diminutive size, and apparently of so perishable a frame, that two women who were sent to Lady Pakenham, at North Witham, to bring some medicine to strengthen him, did not expect to find him alive on their return. He would inevitably have been consigned to the caverns of Taygetus if the two women had carried him to Spartan triers. As it was, the frail boy grew up into Newton, lived more than fourscore years, and revealed to mankind the laws of the universe. If he had perished, England would not have been what it is in the world. In Paris one evening a puny child in a neat little basket was picked up: he had been left at the church door; the commissary of the police was about to carry him to the foundling hospital, when a glazier's wife exclaimed: "You will kill the child in your hospital, give him to me; I have no children, I will take care of him." She cherished the boy, poor as she was, until some one, perhaps his father, settled a small annuity on his life, with which he was educated at the Mazarin College, where he displayed the early genius of a Pascal; it was D'Alembert, to whom we are indebted for a new calculus, for the grand introduction to the Cyclopædia, and for innumerable physical discoveries. He was offered 100,000 francs a year by Catharine of Russia, but refused to leave his mother by adoption—the glazier's wife—and his country. While pagan Greece and Rome, and barbarous nations of a later date, have regarded infant life with such indifference, Christianity comes in with a more humane evangel and says, in the person of its Founder, "Of such is the kingdom of heaven," and the precept and the encouragement go together. "Be given to hospitality," and in doing so we may "entertain angels unawares."

CITY AND COUNTRY CHILDREN

Are exposed to their peculiar temptations. But as there is more elevation in the city, greater intelligence and more breadth of view on all subjects, the probabilities are that those bred in the city are more likely to live to purpose, to have higher ideas, more exalted ambitions, and, as a result, to attain greater achievements. The millions of money given to objects calculated to improve the condition of the poor and to advance society, by such men as the Astors, and Coopers, and Drews, and Greens, and Lenoxes, and McCormicks, and Roberts, the Stuart Brothers, and A. T. Stewart, the merchant prince, show clearly that it is the city which educates the mind to magnificent deeds.

In the country town, the village, the farm-house, there is a certain narrowness of life, a contractedness of observation and experience, with a general want of knowledge of the nature of things, of oneself, and of the human heart, all of which combined give less character, less firmness of mind, less fixedness of purpose, choosing the enjoyment of to-day rather than wait for the greater one in the future. Thus it is that they more readily yield to temptation, more readily fall into crime. The greatest crimes of the century have been committed in the country by country people; our penitentiaries and our asylums are peopled from the farm. There is a certain roughness of deportment, a certain low and contracted form of shrewdness common in village life, which make it easy to slide into wrong-doing. A nameless writer well says that "girls brought up in the city are less apt to be led astray than those reared in the country, and gives as the chief reason for it that they are educated into a higher delicacy with regard to all those forms of personal freedom, which serve as an entering wedge for the more dangerous liberties which may be attempted by the other sex. The country girl, on the contrary, is, by the ruder license of close neighborhood association, and the confidence inspired by intimate acquaintance in the school and social circle, from actual infancy positively educated into utter thoughtlessness with regard to manifold rough and boisterous personal freedoms, which, with equal thoughtlessness allowed in association with the more shrewd and unscrupulous character of the city, furnish all the initiative advantage desired by it for effecting her destruction. From the simple absence of culture and refinement, much is tolerated both in speech and action, among the reputable classes in the country, that is never thought of being practised among the corresponding classes in the city."

A writer in reference to the domestic habits of English families, says: "Having lived in different castles and manor-houses of Great Britain, and been accustomed to the industrious habits of Duchesses and Countesses, I was utterly astonished at the idleness of American fine ladies. No Englishwoman of rank (with the exception of a few) from the Queen downward, will remain for one half-hour unemployed, or sit in a rocking-chair, unless seriously ill. They almost all copy the letters of business of their husbands, fathers, or brothers; attend minutely to the poor around them, and even take part in their amusements, and sympathize with their sorrows; visit and superintend the schools; work in their own gardens; see to their household concerns; and with all these occupations, by early hours they keep up their acquaintance with the literature and politics of the day, and cultivate the accomplishments of music and drawing, and often acquire besides some knowledge of scientific pursuits."

Letter-writers of the olden time were charmed with the wife of Washington, whose busy fingers kept going in knitting and sewing while conversing with her most distinguished visitors at Mount

Vernon, or at the Executive Mansion in the Federal City. Parents
in later days should inculcate on their daughters especially that

IDLENESS IS WICKEDNESS:

That the odds and ends of time should be saved; that there is no
time to be wasted in trifling conversation, in spiritless lolling and
lounging about the house, in waiting for things or persons; rather
have something in hand all the time; either be crocheting, or
romping, or studying, or engaged in an occupation which leaves
less for the other members of the family to do, for servants, for
mother. That too many mothers are overworked, the more so,
that daughters who might help them fail to do so, is·known to
all observant minds. It is not putting the case too strongly to say
that many a toiling mother is hurried into her grave by lazy,
selfish daughters who sit idly by and see her toil without ever
offering to lend a helping hand, for fear their hands or dress
might suffer.

NO MORE GIRLS.

All are young ladies now, because injudicious mothers push their
children on too rapidly. Girls wear kid gloves and sport parasols
at six years of age; at so early a time, do they receive instructions
about being lady-like and womanly? The sequel is that our children
lose their pretty, childish, unaffected ways; early learn to be prudish and deceitful, and assume manners constrained and unnatural; too early do they cease to roll over the floor and run and sing
about the house, as the spirit of childhood would promp them to
do; the restrictions of propriety are forever held over them; instead of the sun-bonnet of the olden time, which they could throw
over their heads in a second, they seldom go outside the door
without the modern "hat," with its ribbons and its French flowers and other expensive ornaments; and the waist must be drawn
in and girded tight; the shoes must fit closely, and the gloves must
be drawn over the hand; and we look in vain for the unsophisti-
cated manners of innocent childhood. Our children will get old
soon enough, too soon, alas! and before we are fifty we will sigh
for the olden time when their ringing laugh and pattering feet
and noisy voices made the whole house

A BEDLAM,

as we thought then, and hoped for the time when we would be

delivered from it, and lo! now, we would give half we have to have those sunshiny days return.

GIRLS AT HOME

From fifteen to the marriageable age of twenty or over, and better over, being a great deal about the house, are very apt to lay the foundation of lives of wretchedness by inadvertently falling into personal habits which undermine the health irretrievably. Medical books assure us that the large majority of cases of

DYSPEPSIA AND CONSUMPTION

have their foundation laid in the "teens" of life, ailments which are easily avoidable in nine cases out of ten.

NIBBLING.

Girls going round the house easily fall into the habit of nibbling at every eatable their eyes happen to light upon. Everything eaten has to be digested, even if it be but a single pea or strawberry or apple; this requires the work of the stomach. Very few articles of food are digested, worked up into nutriment in a shorter time than from two to five hours; if something is eaten every hour or two, the stomach is kept on working, has no time for rest during the whole day; it may keep up for a while, but not long; it will give out; it loses its tone, its power of digestion; the food taken into it remains to a certain extent unaltered, the nourishment is not drawn from it, the proper quality and quantity of blood is not made; the blood is our life and strength; there is less vigor, less animation, less activity; the blood becomes thin and poor and watery and cold; chilliness is easily induced, bad colds easily taken, and these following after one another, it soon comes about that one bad cold comes before another has disappeared. They run into one another until there is at first a constant clearing of the throat, then a hack and a hem, and in due time a slight cough, often in the morning when rising from the bed or soon after—a fruitless cough, just enough to remove a little tickle from the throat, no phlegm, no expectoration. Feel the pulse; it is seventy-five or eighty or more in a minute. This is consumption. But suppose it took another direction, and the disease fixed itself on the stomach instead of the lungs, it soon develops itself into confirmed dyspepsia. The appetite at meal-times is irregular; sometimes there is none, at others it is voracious. There is more or less discomfort sooner or later after each meal. Sometimes the hunger is so great that it seems impossible to wait for the regular dinner hour. Occasionally it is found out that a swallow or two of food quiets this craving hunger. That spoils the desire; there is no relish for food for several hours after. Thus there is no regularity in eating, the whole system is deranged in its functions, the poor chilled blood cannot keep the feet warm; it is so watery that it fails to redden the cheek, and there is a pallor upon it, indicating too plainly that the health is waning. Long before now, perhaps, it has been noticed that the bowels fail to act every day, and there is more or less of headache; irregularities, delays, scantiness or excess, is observed in connection with the peculiar functions, and the young lady of eighteen is a confirmed invalid. What pertains to proper eating and drinking is fully treated in the author's book on "Health by Good Living," while the whole subject is fully discussed in the volume entitled "Health and Disease," pertaining to the proper regulation of the bowels, and the rectification of their various irregularities, and the wise management of the eating. It is sufficient here to direct the attention of mothers especially, to a few of the most important points in the healthful education of daughters.

EATING.

From four years of age until the end of life, without some peculiar modifying circumstances, three meals a day should be inculcated as a habit. Breakfast in the morning, dinner at noon, supper about sundown, with nothing whatever between meals, not an apple, not an orange, not a cake or a pie, nothing whatever. As to drinking pure cool water when thirsty, there is no restriction. At breakfast and dinner there need not be any restriction of the young in the eating of plain, nourishing food. They will seldom eat too much; not over a tea-cupful of warm drink, nor over half a glass of cold drink, never both at the same meal. Warm drink, in the quantity above named, is always the best for the young, sedentary, and invalids. Cold water in large quantities at meal-time, or within half an hour after, is positively injurious.

The supper should be always light from childhood to the grave, limiting it positively to a cup of warm drink, not sweet milk, and some cold bread and butter; an imperative rule of this sort for the young, for all that live, would be an inconceivable good for every human being, a life-long benefit, and it is greatly to be deplored that families will persist in having a little

" RELISH "

on the table, a little smoked beef or cake, or pie, or sweetmeats of some kind, the effect being that a person sitting down and not feeling hungry will take a bit of one or the other, then another bit, and before he knows it, a considerable meal has been taken, forced upon the system when it did not call for it, the result many times being, half a night of coughing, or nausea, or fulness or other discomfort, with a waking up in the midnight of weariness and weakness and unrestedness which leaves one more dead than alive, and scarcely any appetite for breakfast. If light suppers were taken, it would generally be found that the system would soon call for breakfast, would relish it, would enjoy it, and the exercise of the whole of the day following would go to its conversion into healthful, life giving blood.

The regular meals should be at least five hours apart, for they are not usually digested and passed out of the stomach in a shorter time; it is thus enabled to clear itself, and get a little rest; it is the want of that rest, occasioned by the habit of eating a little something between meals, which makes us a

NATION OF DYSPEPTICS,

with the aid of eating with headlong haste, gulping our food in lumps and chunks, large enough to choke an elephant to death.

The next most important thing for mothers to teach their children is the proper

REGULATION OF THE BOWELS

to one regular action every twenty-four hours, the best time being soon after breakfast. Without this there can be no good health, for one single week, to any human being. This want of regularity is more or less connected with every malady of man. Three times out of four, if you hear persons complaining, it will be found, on close inquiry, that for a day or two their bowels have not acted with regularity. This is an excellent plan for impressing it on the minds of children, that almost all sickness has, as an attendant, a failure of the bowels to act properly; show them, also, that as they are getting well, they begin to act more naturally. We are born with regularly acting bowels; this regularity is generally first broken into by putting off the inclination, if something is in hand to make it inconvenient, such as the calling of a visitor, the wish to complete a task, the hurry of preparing to go to school, or the waiting for other persons. The reason for deferring a call of nature may be ever so good, but the effect is always the same —she is baffled, is quiet for a while, then makes complaint again, but never with impunity, for the foundation is laid for a later and feebler call next day, until after a while a whole day passes, and there is no evacuation of the bowels; then comes other symptoms of headache, of cold feet and hands, irregular appetite, bad taste in the mouth, of vomitings, chilliness, and various other discomforts, ending oftentimes in life-long piles, and dangerous, expensive, and even fatal fistulas.

Daughters should be taught early, that delaying urination too long brings on inflammation of the bladder, water cannot be made, and death follows in four or five days. Four or five hours are too long in the day-time; but at night, because being kept warm in bed, the water in the system escapes more freely in the form of insensible perspiration. Urination ought to be attended to always, the last thing on going to bed, and before leaving home, especially for public gatherings, where there is liability to be kept longer than expected. If it should be so that water cannot be made, when there is a desire to do so, send for a physician at once; but don't excite or alarm the patient; rather attempt to divert the mind, and if left alone, the sound of water being made in an adjoining room has brought on urination, as the sound of it often induces animals to perform the function.

Great pains should be taken to teach girls the high importance of keeping their feet warm, never to go to bed with

COLD FEET;

That sitting or standing still five minutes with damp feet, endangers life ; or that being still for that time with damp clothing or skirt is not less dangerous ; and that nothing can be a sufficient excuse for not changing the clothing or stockings and shoes when noticed to be at all damp, especially during the catamenial flow ; that such neglect becomes a crime, because it unnecessarily endangers life, to say nothing of the trouble and expense of having one sick in the house for weeks possibly.

CHANGING CLOTHING

From a heavier to a lighter dress should never be done without consulting the mother. The change should be gradual, and north of Virginia should not be attempted sooner than the last of May. It is dangerous even to pull off a dress after a visit or drive or shopping, the moment one gets into the house, even in summer-time, and then put on a cold one. A cold silk dress at noon of a summer day in place of a warm one has often given a dangerous cold.

Mothers should begin early to impress on their daughters' minds the manifold forms of disease which have been brought on by

COOLING OFF TOO SOON,

After any form of exercise or work, by sitting at an open door or window, or hall, or anywhere if there is a draught of air ; that health is endangered at any time, more especially during the periods, hence a girl should never sit on a cold stone.

Never stand on the damp grass, or wet earth, or moist pavement for a single five minutes.

Never allow a damp stocking to remain on the foot for a minute, unless it is possible to walk fast until home is reached.

Never go to bed with cold feet, even if it is midsummer. Go to the kitchen, draw off the stockings and hold the naked feet to the fire and rub them all the time with the hands—soles, between the toes, everywhere, until agreeably warm in every part ; then draw on a clean pair of stockings; by no means walk to the bed-chamber over the floor, even if it has a carpet on it.

Never change an under-vest, the flannel or knit shirt which is worn next the skin, to a lighter one, from the time it is put on about the first of December until the first of June north of the thirty-sixth parallel; for the mornings are sometimes chilly when May has gone, and it is much safer to be a little too warm for a few days, than to run the risk of a cold which may bring weeks' discomfort. When a change is made, it should be to a material but a little thinner, should be made when dressing for breakfast and a few days after a sickness. Attention to these suggestions purposely made specific, plain, and definite, would prevent many a lingering cold, or alarming sore throat, or fatal pneumonia or lung fever, hurrying to the grave within a week.

Never lie down for a day nap without having some slight covering, even if it be in the middle of the hottest day of summer; for the body is peculiarly susceptible of cold during sleep, at the same time is liable to perspire, when the slightest draught gives a cold unless there is some covering.

In wetting the head or washing the hair, never allow it to dry of itself, but press upon it a soft cotton cloth or towel, and rub it over the scalp well; do this a number of times, a dry cloth each time, then comb the hair gently, with a very coarse comb, so that it shall fall over the face and shoulders, spreading out as much as possible so as to allow the air to get around each hair if practicable; or if you lie down spread it abroad over the pillow. In either case, every once in a while flap it up with the hand, carrying it away from the neck and forehead, the more perfectly admitting the air all around it. The want of these precautions has given colds and fevers in the head which have lasted for weeks and months, and sometimes caused the hair to fall off, requiring months for a re-growth.

Impress upon the daughter's mind this one great important practical truth: notice what is most apt to give you a cold, and then for a lifetime afterwards take special pains to guard against it. By these simple methods persons may live for months and years, without ever taking a serious cold even, with a reasonably careful attention to them. Many persons are all the time taking cold, and are all the time complaining, are never well, never happy.

Within twenty years, the constitutions of our women would be renovated and our girls would be found models of healthfulness if what has been proposed in this chapter was carried out judiciously in reference to our children.

Dressing loosely and warm, eating systematically and slow, sleeping abundantly at night, exercising regularly and often, studying how to avoid colds and secure the regular performance of the bodily functions, without a grain or a drop of physic being necessary for the accomplishment of any one of them. And if in addition the suggestions were carried out as to the mode of pursuing studies at school, of taking turns in household management, and of regulating the general conduct of life, it is impossible that there should not be a marked improvement in the quality of the wives of the country, and their capabilities for improving, elevating, and happifying home life.

THE BEST BREAD

Has never yet been made, for the want of the best materials out of which to make it. Considering that bread is the staff of life, that it is eaten at every meal, by every member of the family, that no meal is complete without it, it is of the very highest importance in connection with health to know what good bread is, and how to make it, premising that multitudes owe their dyspepsia and neuralgias to bad bread, and that the principal constituents of the bones and their strength, and of the teeth and their beauty and durability, are derived from the bread we eat, and mainly of wheat bread.

In ancient times the whole of the grain, whether of rye or oats or barley or corn or wheat, was made into bread, after a rude breaking it into small pieces, including the outer coat or jacket or husk or skin, by whatever name it may be called; but this is indigestible and innutritious, being made of sand and wood. We call this skin of the wheat " Bran," which has been fed to four animals in succession without losing any of its weight, showing that there is not one particle of nutriment in it; hence as a constituent of food in health it must be useless, and as it makes the bread more or less dark, modern ingenuity has been employed in separating the bran from the flour most perfectly, but in doing this, in the best way ever yet devised, one-fifth of the nutriment, and that its best portion, is lost with the bran, and thus lost as human food, because it is fed to cattle. That is, in plain terms, if wheat were properly ground, four barrels of flour would

GO AS FAR,

that is, would feed as many men for a specified time, as five barrels now do. Hence the man who discovers a method of converting wheat into flour without the loss of any of its nutritious portion in separating the bran, will be a greater benefactor to his race than Alexander, or Cæsar, or Napoleon. The problem will perhaps be brought to a practical and practicable solution within a year, as a patent has been secured for the same, that is, for taking the bran from the wheat-grain before it is ground. An inventor has procured it to be done, but whether it can be accomplished, perfectly and inexpensively on a large scale, is yet to be determined.

A GRAIN OF WHEAT

has three constituents, its covering or "bran," its gluten, and its starch. The covering, as seen, has no nutriment whatever; the starch has none, it gives only warmth; hence it is the glutinous portion of the grain which is really valuable as nourishing food; it is the gluten which makes flour "rise," it is the gluten that makes flesh, that gives strength to the bones, durability and beauty to the teeth; it is the gluten which feeds the brain.

Fig. 1.

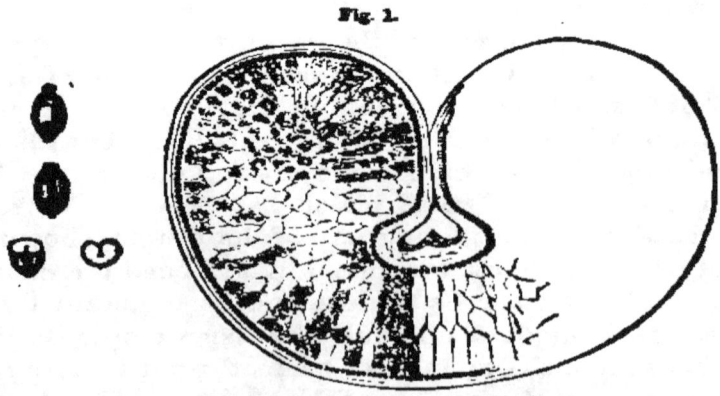

COMPOSITION OF THE WHEAT-GRAIN.

The small figure at the top, left hand side, shows a wheat-grain of the natural size in a position at right angles with the horizon, the rounded part facing the eye. The figure below it represents the wheat grain with the grooved part facing the eye. The smaller figure below and to the left represents the one above it cut in two; the other figure to its right shows how a wheat-grain looks endways, when thus cut in two. The large figure is a magnified wheat-grain cut in two, facing the eye, endways. The very outer rim, represented by the dotted line on the right-hand side, shows the jacket of the wheat-grain, its bran coat made up of silex and lignite, that is, it is nothing but sand and wood, and has no more nutriment than the splinter of a fence-rail which has been exposed to the sun for a dozen years.

This bran-coat is three and a half per cent. of the whole grain, according to the analysis of Professor E. N. Horsford, of Cambridge, Mass.

Within the bran-coat and next to it, as seen on the left-hand side of Fig. 1, there is a line of dark dots like a necklace, representing the cells which contain the gluten; inside this necklace is the starch of the grain, constituting, in bulk, the largest part of the wheat; this starch is found in all grains; it is found in potatoes, it is in the arrow-root, the starch of which root we feed to children and infants; all starch is granular, crisp; gluten is sticky, tough, tenacious; starch keeps us warm; gluten makes us grow, and after we have grown, gives us bones and covers them with flesh; the chief constituent of gluten is nitrogen, which alone can make flesh; the chief constituent of starch is carbon, to keep up the fires of life, for where no warmth comes, there is death.

Fig. 1.

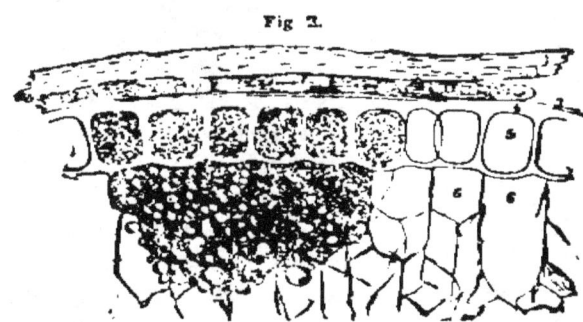

No. 1, 1. The outer coats of the bran.
"   2. The inner coat.
"   3 is a filmy material separating the bran from the gluten; it covers the gluten.
"   4 is an interval of cellular matter, which is essentially gluten.
"   5,   little bags full of gluten, all inside of them. The sixes, starch, with a very small amount of gluten.
42

After the whole wheat-grain is ground, the miller takes out the bran and gives us flour, made of gluten and starch; put that flour in cold water, make a dough of it, and work it between your fingers as long as it will whiten the water, what is left is pure gluten; boil the water until it is all gone, and the remnant is starch; or let it stand in a glass, and the starch falls to the bottom.

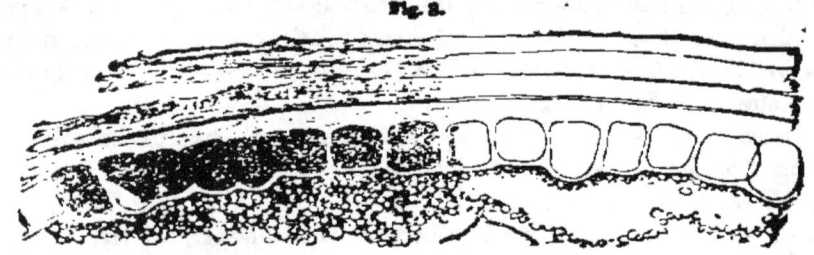

Fig. 3.

Fig. 3 shows a scale of miller's bran cut in two, the edge facing you, by which it is seen how the gluten will more or less adhere to the bran, and even some of the starch. In fact, a grain

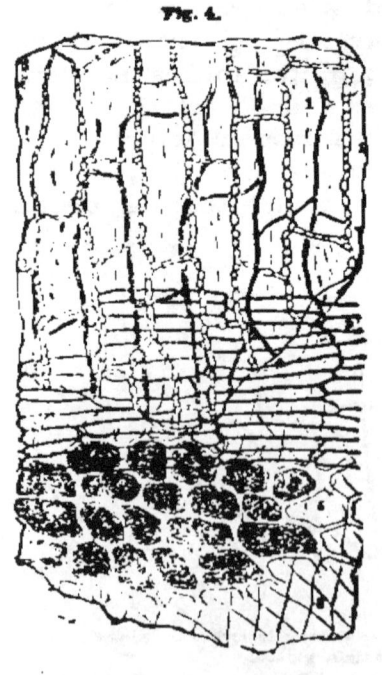

Fig. 4.

of wheat is very much like a potato, which contains almost its whole nutriment immediately under the outer skin, which is really thinner than paper; you can see how thin it is when you boil a new potato, thus it is that in peeling potatoes, as usually done, nearly the entire nutritious, strengthening part is thrown away, the starchy portion being retained, the warming portion used, while the strength-giving and flesh-making material is fed to the pigs, or thrown into the street. If potatoes must be peeled, feed the peeling to the cows or to some other domestic animal. Any reader who has the curiosity to pursue these details more minutely would do well to consult a prominent publication of Mr. Thomas J. Hand, of New York City, who has been enthusiastic in his investigations of the whole subject.

In figure 4 the entire gluten product of a wheat-grain is exhibited. The covering of the gluten, before spoken of as being very thin, is made of two layers, 1, 1 and 2, which can be separated with a moist cloth.

4–5 show the gluten bags, or necklace, containing the largest proportion of gluten.

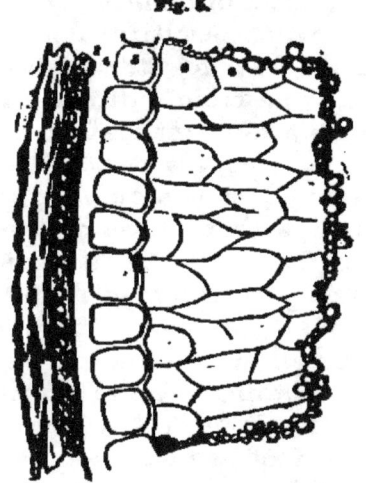

Fig. 5.

3 shows the beginning of the starch of the wheat-grain.

This figure 5 is to show how much of the real nutritive part of the wheat is lost in the bran, for the gluten will stick to the bran even down to a part of No. 5.

The most important part of the gluten of wheat is its phosphoric acid; it is the phosphorus which feeds the brain and helps to constitute the bones. If you burn wheat into ashes, and take a hundred pounds of these ashes, separating each quality as the chemist does, it will read thus: — In a hundred pounds of the ashes of wheat there

No. 1. The outer layer of bran.
" 2. The inner layer.
" 3. A membranous coat.
" 4. A layer of gluten cells.
" 5. The gluten bags.
Nos. 6, 6. Starch cells.

will be the third of one pound of sulphuric acid. Thus :—

Chloride of sodium..........................	a trace.
Sulphuric acid	.33
Oxide of iron..............................	.79
Silica or sand..............................	3.35
Soda	3.44
Lime......................................	3.90
Magnesia.................................	12.20
Potassa...................................	29.97
Phosphoric acid...........................	46.02
	100.00

The bran of wheat is about three and a half per cent. of the entire grain. This bran contains 3.82 per cent. of phosphoric acid. Fine wheat flour contains only the twentieth part of 1 per cent.; that is, the bran of wheat contains fourteen times as much phosphoric acid as superfine flour. The author knows personally that the largest flour-maker within fifty miles of New York City has taken the premium for the most beautiful flour at various fairs, of high-sounding names, which had no phosphoric acid in it or anything else, but simply starch ; he keeps it in his establishment to show what beautiful flour he can turn out. He asks eighteen dollars a barrel for it, says it costs that ; the object being to prevent any one from purchasing it, for a whole barrel of it would not make a ten-cent loaf of bread. As it has no gluten in it, it would not rise, nor would it contain any nourishment in it, being pure starch ; the common people valuing flour by its whiteness. Hence it is that Graham bread, the black, unsightly, and sour bread of Germany, made of the whole grain of the wheat, and the ugly, heavy, sour loaves found in the sacks of Russian soldiers in the Crimea, are each more nutritious than the most beautiful white bread ever found on an American table, because the bread named contains all the phosphates of the wheat. During the siege of Paris, in 1871, it was of vital importance to save every ounce of food, when even horses, dogs, and the very rats of the sewers had to be carefully preserved and cooked for food. Under such circumstances, all the appliances of science and art and skill were brought into requisition to prevent the loss of a single pound of food, and to devise ways and means to make it go as far as possible.

It was found that there were in Paris eleven million pounds of grain, which, in the ordinary way of conversion into bread, would undergo a clear loss of three million two hundred and thirty thousand pounds of human nutriment. Nineteen hundred years ago the Romans considered the grinding of wheat to be wasteful, so they roasted the grain entire, ground it, and made it into a paste. The Arabs of this day hull the wheat first by boiling or steaming. In England brown bread made of the whole product of the grain is considered a luxury ; they bake it twice a week.

Four pounds of grain yield three pounds of flour, entailing a loss of twenty to thirty per cent.

If the wheat-kernel is moistened the hull can be rubbed off at a loss of only five per cent. ; then soak the kernel eight hours in tepid water, or until it can be crushed between the fingers easily. In this condition it takes up fifty per cent. of water. Run this through rollers to make a paste, cause this to ferment and make into bread in the usual way; then all the nutriment of the bread is saved.

CRACKED WHEAT,

or wheaten grits, is essentially the same material, only with the hull on; it is wheat broken up, each grain into several pieces; but, whether broken or not, let it be soaked several hours, then boiled until as soft as boiled rice, and eat with salt, or butter, or sugar, or syrup, or sweet milk. The whole grain requires a whole day's boiling.

All grains can be prepared in the same way, whether oats, barley, rye, or others; the point being to boil them to a proper softness; boil slow, take several hours; all may be termed

MUSH,

as rye mush, wheat mush, etc.

ELEMENTS OF GRAIN.

	Wheat.	Rye.	Oats.
Carbon	46	46	50
Oxygen	43	44	37
Hydrogen	6	6	6
Nitrogen	2+	2—	2
Ashes	2+	2	4

It will be thus seen that the grains are pretty much of the same elements. The nitrogen is the flesh-forming principle; the carbon gives warmth, but no actual nourishment, hence half of the grain warms us. Corn (Indian) has more carbon than wheat, hence is more appropriate for cold weather.

A very healthful bread for all persons with weak stomachs is to beat up flour in cold water to a proper consistence, put it into little pans, an inch deep of the batter, put in a hot stove and bake; it cannot sour, cannot get heavy, can be eaten cold or hot, and will keep for weeks in a dry cool place. The following remarks on good bread, from a writer who understands the subject fully, merit special attention. It is sadly true that multitudes of people in the United States, at least half the population, do not know what good bread and butter are.

GOOD YEAST.

Boil in a porcelain or copper-tinned kettle two large handfuls of hops, tied in a cloth, six large potatoes sliced thin in six quarts of water. When the potatoes are very soft skin them, and either rub through a colander or mash fine on a plate. Take out the hops; squeeze dry, and hang away for another time, as they can be used twice. Keep the water boiling, mix one and one-half pints of wheat flour to a smooth batter with cold water, and one tablespoonful of vinegar, two of brown sugar, and one teaspoonful of salt; mix in the mashed potatoes, stir all into the boiling water, and boil ten minutes. Turn into a six-quart tin pan. When milk-warm to the touch add one teacup of yeast. Let it rise over night, then put into a stone jug.

This yeast will keep in a cellar, perfectly good, for six weeks. A large teacupful will make two large loaves of bread. Be sure to reserve a teacupful to raise the yeast with the next time. Always scald the jug thoroughly and keep water in it overnight, with a tablespoonful of saleratus stirred into it. This will sweeten the jug. It takes a larger quantity of this yeast to raise bread, biscuit, or muffins than of distillery yeast, but the effect is quite as good.

To make bread of first-rate quality, the sponge should be made overnight. Bread that has been raised three times is much the best. It is of a firm, even texture, has no fissures or cracks, and the slice presents an even surface. Here is a recipe that rarely fails: Take one quart of new milk, and add boiling water sufficient to make it warm to the touch. (Water can be substituted for the milk, but bread made without milk dries more rapidly.) Add one teaspoonful of salt, stir in three quarts of flour and one teacup of home-made yeast, or three tablespoonfuls of distillery yeast. Mix well together, then sprinkle flour all around the edges of the batter or sponge, leaving a small space in the middle uncovered. Set in a warm place to rise, covering with a pan. In summer the sponge will be ready to mould over before breakfast. Mix it up thick so that it can be kneaded well, and knead it half an hour or more. Chopping it with a chopping-knife adds to its lightness and porosity. When well-kneaded sprinkle flour on the bottom of the pan thickly, put in the dough, and set it away for half an hour or more, but watch it closely. (Bread-making should be most carefully tended, as any neglect ruins the whole. If allowed to rise too much its sweetness is gone, and though saleratus will take away the acidity, its aroma and flavor are destroyed.) When light, turn out on the moulding-board and knead thoroughly ; divide into two loaves, reserving a portion for biscuit, so that the new-made loaves may not be cut that day. Mould well, put into the pans, let it rise in a warm place fifteen minutes, then bake in a hot oven. If the oven be hot, the bread will lose less weight in baking than when the oven is slack. The batter can be baked in the morning in the muffin-rings, and makes delicious breakfast, better than hot biscuit.

Bread made with potatoes is very good. Boil three large potatoes, well pared, or six good-sized ones ; rub them through a colander into your bread-pan. Rinse them through the colander with a pint of boiling water ; add one quart of milk. Stir in half a pint of flour, and when the liquor is cool enough add a teacup of home-made yeast ; set it in a warm place. If this is done after dinner—using the potatoes left from the table—the sponge will be ready for more flour by eight or nine o'clock in the evening. Now mix to a stiff batter, sprinkle flour over it, set to rise. In the morning knead into a stiff dough, let it rise well, then knead again, put into pans, let it rise fifteen or twenty minutes, and bake in a hot oven.

All bread, biscuit, and doughnuts raised with yeast should rise after being kneaded before they are baked. If put in the oven or fried directly they are never light. The dough has had no opportunity to recover its elasticity, and cannot be as good. Common-sized loaves of bread will bake in three-quarters of an hour, provided the oven is of proper heat.

Palatable as good wheat-bread is, there is no doubt that eating it only is not conducive to health. Rye, Indian meal, and coarse flour make bread that is better adapted to the development of the muscles. Boston brown bread is much used, and is far better for young children than bread made of superfine flour. It is easily made : Take two quarts of Indian meal, sifted, one quart of rye meal or Graham flour, one large spoonful of salt, one teacup of molasses, one teacup of home-made yeast, or half the quantity of brewers' yeast. Mix with hot water as stiff as one can stir it, let it rise one hour, bake in deep earthen or iron pots, which are made purposely. To avoid the thick crust produced by baking so long, boil it four hours and bake one, removing the cover before setting it into the oven.

Good bread can never be made, however perfect all the materials are, without three things: First, abundant kneading, or working; the best bread-makers work the dough the longest, or with the most vigorous use of the arm and knuckles. Second, the oven should be steadily hot, kept at about the same heat; this is the chief reason why the French bread is the best in the world; they regulate the heat with a thermometer.

ERYSIPELAS,

Or St. Anthony's Fire, is Rose Fever, and depends on a bad state of the blood. It comes on with a chill, followed with fever, with a red eruption on the face, spreading like a slow fire, with soreness to the touch. There is some heat and some swelling. These may be limited or may extend all over the body, with pimples which may break and eat away as in an eating sore or sloughing. If in the scalp, it induces inflammation of the brain and stupor and death. It seems to arise in many cases from breathing the effluvia of human bodies, as in jails, barracks, tenement-houses, and the like, in connection with inflammation. But always it is caused by bad blood. Treat it precisely as bilious fever. Lard, tallow, cold cream may be rubbed freely on the skin, not only on the erupted part, but several inches beyond; slippery-elm bark, or gum-arabic mucilage, or flax-seed tea, may also be used thus; these soothe; to drive in, to suppress, is certain death; if it is on the face, it is desirable to prevent it from reaching the scalp; then interpose a blister plaster half an inch broad, or paint that much of the skin between the eruption and the scalp with nitrate of silver or collodion and live mainly on milk and rice. The water-cure treatment is to unload the rectum with an injection; stop eating; wet pack; then wash all over with tepid water;

then cool; keep tepid compresses over the erupted parts; in a day or two live on fruits, berries, and coarse bread.

Homœopathy gives aconite when there is much fever; if the eruption spreads like the rays of a star, give belladonna; rhus tox., if it tends to go towards the scalp; arsenicum, if strength declines; pulsatilla, if the spots are of a bluish red; nux vom., if in knee or joint; bryonia, if the joints are affected; sulphur, if the case is obstinate; sulphur and arsenicum, when there are ulcerations.

------------∞------------

FEVERS.

FEVER is increased heat of the body, with dry skin, quick pulse, diminution of all discharges from the body, weakness, failure of appetite, and in many cases a disturbed brain. It is essentially a poison of the blood; there are matters in it which ought not to be there, and the general remedy is to get rid of that poison by diminishing the quantity of the blood as soon as possible, for the less poison there is in the system, the less injury; and if the whole blood contains a pint of poison, the loss of half the blood would leave but half a pint of poison. This is done by

Laxative medicines, as salts and castor oil.

Purgatives, as by calomel, aloes, rhubarb, etc.

Diaphoretics, or sweating remedies.

Cold drinks.

Warm baths.

Emetics.

The principal forms of fever are:—

Bilious.	Relapsing.
Cerebro-spinal.	Scarlet.
Fever and ague, or	Spotted.
Intermittent.	Typhoid.
Malarial.	Typhus.
Pernicious.	Yellow.
Remittent.	Dengue.

BILIOUS FEVER,

or remittent, is accompanied by headache, sick stomach, quick pulse, hot dry skin, coated tongue, and a great variety of other minor symptoms; these symptoms increase in violence, then abate in the course of twenty hours; after an interval they become more severe, hence called remittent or mitigating. If the system is in an exhausted condition, the constitution radically impaired, the tendency is to fall into the typhoid type. The best treatment in the Allopathic system is to give at first a dose of Epsom salts, an ounce at least, in a pint of warm water, or two ounces of castor oil, and repeat every three hours until the bowels are freely acted on; then give a liver pill.

If at any time there is much distress at the stomach, as nausea or vomiting, if it is bitter, drink warm water, a teacupful every five minutes until the vomiting is increased, and continue this as long as what is vomited is bitter; if no bitterness in the vomiting, place a mustard plaster over the stomach and let it remain until relieved. In eight hours after the liver pill has been given take a grain of quinine every hour in two or three tablespoons of water, with a teaspoonful of vinegar; stir it well and give it time to dissolve thoroughly; a good plan would be to put sixteen grains of quinine in half a pint of water, with a tablespoonful of vinegar, which is used to dissolve the quinine more thoroughly. Take this quinine every hour for two days, except when sleeping; do not wake the patient to give it, but when he has slept give two or three tablespoons, if he has slept two or three hours, at the first dose after sleeping. If at the end of two days the appetite is not returning and the tongue is not clearing off and the fever is not lessening to a hundred beats of the pulse or less in a minute, take a liver pill and proceed as before.

When the patient begins to get well, indicated by returning appetite, the diet should be light, at five hours' interval, bread and butter and tea, or soup with the grease skimmed off, and bread crusts broken into it, or gruel and bread; as dessert, some fruits or berries, stewed if raw cannot be had, with lean meat or poultry once a day. During the fever ice can be eaten as freely as desired at any time. If ice cannot be had, drink the coldest water, a swallow at a time, an interval of half a minute at each swallow. If half a glass is drunk continuously the thirst is not so much assuaged as by four or five swallows, and the stomach becomes full and uneasy; sometimes it is better to satiate the thirst with some hot tea, when ice cannot be had.

If there is headache with high fever, put cold compresses on the forehead, renewed every three minutes until relieved; if hands burn, dabble them in cold water; if the feet are hot, let wet cloths be drawn over them, or dip them in water cold or warm, and let them be exposed to the air; the evaporation cools them rapidly and is very grateful. Sometimes it is very comforting to let the patient slowly suck a lemon, or to have a glass of lemonade, or vinegar and water sweetened.

HYDROPATHIC TREATMENT.

If the skin is hot take the cold wet sheet pack, and repeat until the temperature is natural, and repeat as often as the fever begins to rise. Keep hot-water bottles to cold feet, or keep them in hot water if necessary; if there is prostration, sponge the body with tepid water; but a cold pack. If pain anywhere apply cold compresses or hot fomentations, as may be most agreeable, until relieved. Cold compresses on scalp, if the head aches, or pour cold water, if severe or hard to remove. The great general principle in the hydropathic treatment in all fevers is to bathe when the fever is at the highest, or a few minutes before. If the fever is abating, note the time and wait until it returns, eating nothing meanwhile. Some prefer getting into a hogshead of cold water, keeping the head under as long as the breath can be held, and repeating the process every few minutes. Let the patient keep dabbling in the water all the time, until he feels comfortable; then get out, be wiped dry quickly, dress, and walk about or go to some light work, to keep up the circulation; or pour water on the patient's head as it is extended over the edge of the bed, a large tub being under; pour from a pitcher or bucket, a foot above the head, and keep it up until the patient feels comfortable, pouring from one part to another; not all the time on the same spot; but if the fever tends to return, renew the pouring until it is effectually dissipated.

This pouring removes congestion, it equalizes the circulation, the glands of the body are relieved of their load, so as to be capable of working, when they begin at once to carry off the wastes of the system as effectively as if worked off by medicines. Common bilious or gastric fever, as it is called, is treated by the homœopathic system with belladonna, alternated with aconite; nux vomica, when there is a bitter taste in the mouth; chamomilla, if the tongue is red at the edges ; pulsatilla, if the tongue is whitish ; ipecacuanha, if there is nausea ; digitalis, if there is debility ; arsenicum, if the preceding fail or the case is a severe one at the first.   Diet should be of soft food, no hard meats or vegetables ; gruels, farina, starch, beef-tea, and the like.   Carefully avoid exposure to heat or cold or fatigue or sudden changes. Let all forms of exercise be quiet, deliberate, never carried to fatigue in any event ; be regular in eating and sleeping ; use no stimulants in any form whatever.   .

CEREBRO-SPINAL FEVER,

sometimes called cerebro-spinal meningitis or spotted fever, or petechial fever, because little pimples are sometimes seen on the skin similar to the spots in typhus fever.   This disease appeared in France in 1310, next in 1482, very fatal in Rome and Madrid in 1580.   Sydenham described it in 1661.   In Paris in 1814.   In 1832 it was first spoken of in France as an epidemic cerebro-spinal meningitis.   It first appeared in the United States in Massachusetts in 1806, gradually extending to New York and Philadelphia.   Between 1840 and 1850 it spread over large tracts of country in the Southern and Western States.   It became prevalent again in New York and Pennsylvania in 1863.

SYMPTOMS.

It comes on suddenly, with chilliness and terrible pain in the head, extending to the back of the head, with nausea and vomiting, delirium, spasms of the muscles of the back and neck, and death when not relieved.   The young have general convulsions. The whole surface of the body is painful to the touch ; the tongue may continue natural, but grows yellow.   Sometimes there is a breaking out on the lips, skin from 104 to 110 ; some die within three or four hours, many in twelve or fifteen ; the danger lessens after that ; exudations are found at the base of the brain after death, showing that it is a disease of "congestion," which see.   It is not contagious, and seems to result from a bad atmosphere, made bad by human emanations and miasmatic influences ; the tendency is to a typhoid type of disease.   Empty the bowels at once with an enema, then give a liver pill ; if debility is a prominent symptom give two grains of quinine every two hours until the pill has acted two or three times; if it does not act itself in twelve hours, give a tablespoonful of salts or castor-oil every hour until it does act, then two grains of quinine every hour for eight hours. Leeching behind the ears, or a mustard plaster, four inches by six, over the back of the neck, lengthways downwards; rub the body well, rapidly and persistently, with red pepper and brandy, keep hot bottles to the feet if cold, do all that is possible to keep the whole skin soft and warm. If the quinine does not seem to rouse the circulation and strength, give from thirty drops to a teaspoonful of tincture of cantharides every hour, or tincture of camphor; remember that unless the system is aroused the patient will die.

PERNICIOUS FEVER.

Congestive fever, malignant fever, malarial fever, are really but more virulent forms of fever arising from miasm; yellow fever being a still higher grade. The fundamental principles of treatment are essentially the same—to remove the congestion of parts, to equalize the circulation, to relieve the system of its load of poison: the chief attention should be directed to these things first of all. In all the forms of fever above named, as in bilious fever, first unload the bowels by an enema or laxative, give two of the liver pills, and, two hours after, give from one to four grains of quinine every two hours; when the body is cold and chilly, give hot baths; when burning with fever, cool off with wet compresses; if great pain anywhere and no fever, apply mustard plasters; if pain and fever, apply compresses to the fullest extent possible, so as to reduce the symptoms, and bring about a natural condition. Malarial fever, and that with typhoid symptoms, are successfully treated as bilious fever—only a grain more of quinine at each dose.

YELLOW FEVER

is essentially bilious fever aggravated, and should be treated on the same general principles: unload the rectum by enemas; clear out the bowels with salts or oil, and then give two liver pills, followed every hour by three grains of quinine for two or three days, if the patient is improving; if not, give two more liver pills, and continue the quinine; the object being to unload the system of the excessive bile, and to support it with the quinine and a " light diet."

RELAPSING

Fever is recently known by that name: it is bilious fever modified, and to be treated on the same general principles. It is a continued fever, attended with chills, shivers, headache, nausea, vomiting, and yellow eyes and skin, stomach tender, bowels costive, urine high-colored; full, fast, jumping pulse; pains, restlessness, and sometimes delirium. First described in Scotland in 1817; but it appeared in Dublin in 1739, in the Crimea in 1855, and in 1870 in New York and Philadelphia. Ten out of a hundred died of it in Russia, three per cent. in England. To be treated as bilious fever.

DENGUE,

or Break-bone fever, so affects the system as to make a person feel as if every bone or joint in his body was sore, or broken. Dr. Rush first noticed it in 1780. It is bilious fever, with a cold settling in the joints, a combination of fever and rheumatism, and is readily cured as bilious fever.

HEADACHE

Is from a great variety of causes, hence the means of cure are various; in children it should be promptly attended to, as it may soon result in water on the brain or other form of dangerous inflammation. If it is a throbbing headache there is high fever; if sharp pains, it is inflammation, showing the congestion of the small arteries; if a dull heavy sensation, the veins are congested; in either case notice the feet first, and if they are cold put them in warm water, making it hotter and hotter from time to time, until it is nearly as hot as can be well borne. The vessel should be deep enough to allow the water to come well up towards the knees; have a blanket around the body, as with the hot foot-bath, perspiration may be induced. If the bowels are costive, give an enema or two tablespoons of castor-oil.

If the head is hot, apply ice-cold compresses freely.

Take pounded ice one part, fine salt half a part, put it in a little silk bag, lay it on the aching part for a minute; it makes the skin excessively cold, whitens it. Put two tablespoonfuls each of spirits of hartshorn and spirits of camphor on two tablespoons of salt, put them in a bottle, and keep closed; pour a little into the bottom of a teacup on a rag, and apply the rag to the head; wet it again as soon as dry.

If from an acid stomach, or where there is much wind, put two teaspoonfuls of powdered charcoal in half a glass of water, stir quickly, and drink it down. In most cases a warm-water emetic is the best remedy, as it empties the stomach, which is nearly always the cause. Drink a teacupful of tepid water, until the stomach is so full that a feather or finger will induce vomiting; then take an injection, followed by a liver pill; eat nothing until very hungry, and then for a day or two live mostly on coarse bread and fruits, or follow the fruit diet.

Homœopaths give belladonna for periodical headache, followed with platina when the pain is in the temples; mercurius when belladonna fails; sepia, in the worst forms; glonoine when from exposure to the sun; silicea when the eyes seem to be ready to protrude; rhus tox., when pains are shooting, tearing; veratrum, when there is chilliness; colocynth, in nervous headache; thuja, if chronic; cimicifuga, if there is a bursting feeling in the head.

The water-cure remedy, and which will relieve almost all cases, is to put the feet in warm or hot water, cold compresses to the head, an enema with hot fomentations to the abdomen, which are flannels dipped in hot water; squeeze out a little, and lay on the part; renewed every five or ten minutes.

If there has been suppression give warm hip-baths effectively, and keep the feet warm; if nausea, drink warm water freely, or pour cold water on the head and neck. If from sudden disuse of any stimulants, keep quiet; use hot foot-baths several times a day, with cold compresses to the head at the same moment, with a diet of fruits, berries, and coarse bread.

SICK HEADACHE

is always a distressing malady, occurring at intervals. The first and best cure is to put the feet and legs in hot water; after having taken an enema, drink warm water until copious vomiting has been induced; go to bed, and take a liver pill, as it is always connected with biliousness or a torpid liver. You are sick at stomach, and the head aches; almost always there are cold feet and constipation. The hydropathic and homœopathic remedies are those mainly for common headache. The wisdom of those who are subject to this malady is to notice what, in them, is the very first symptom of its approach, and attack it at once, thus preventing it, to a considerable extent. The quickest plan is to eat nothing, and at the end of five hours take a liver pill, go to bed, and wake up well enough to feel hungry, then follow a fruit diet for several days. Sometimes an attack is cut short by two or three teaspoonfuls of spirits of turpentine. Some forms are cured by putting both hands of another person on the head, carrying them down to the shoulders, and then slanting them off from the body, bringing the hands back to the top of the head, farther away from the body than when they went downwards; toothache has been cured in this way. It costs nothing but faith to try it.

A HEADACHE SNUFF.

Take snuff, common black rappee, half an ounce; powdered asarabacca, two drachms; a dozen drops of water; mix well, put in a bottle with a Tonquin bean, and let it rest for a few days; take out a spoonful or two at a time, crush it to a powder with a knife on a piece of paper, and put it in a box to use as a pinch several times a day; it frequently relieves headache and other discomforts about the eyes and nose, causing them to water freely; or take a teaspoonful of the ammoniated tincture of valerian every few hours until relieved; or

Take one-twelfth of a grain of the alcoholic extract of nux vomica, twice a day, increased to a fourth of a grain in the course of a week; continue that for one week, then diminish in the same way.

The tartrate of iron and potash, twenty grains twice a day, in mint water, with chloroform liniment rubbed on the sides of the temples twice a day, has cured cases of half a dozen or more years' standing.

DYSENTERY

Is an inflammation of the lining of the lower bowels, the rectum mainly, the minute arteries are so congested that they throw out blood which is discharged with tormina, and tenesmus, as the physicians term it, meaning a very distressing straining. There is a feeling as if you wanted to go to stool, but when you get there there is nothing to come away but a little blood with a painful bearing down. Sometimes there is nausea and vomiting. It is brought on by indigestible food, by sudden changes from heat to cold, by rapid checking of perspiration, and by miasmatic and other bad airs. Sometimes whole neighborhoods suffer with it.

There are a great variety of cures for this distressing complaint, and often all are unavailing. Some of the more reliable follow: Go to bed, take one of the liver pills, and repeat every two hours until the actions and straining cease; at the same time, if the distress at the rectum is great, give an injection of thirty grains of laudanum in half a glass of cool water, and retain it. Take sixty drops or a teaspoonful of the following: laudanum, essence of ginger, tincture of camphor, capsicum, and rhubarb; or take twenty drops every half hour until relieved.

Clarify over the fire, like honey, some butter which has just been gathered from the churn, without salt or washing. Skim off the milky particles after melting, take two tablespoons every six hours until relieved; or,

Drink strong tea made of the root of the blackberry bush, a teacupful every three hours. Add a tablespoonful of loaf sugar and half a teaspoonful of ground spice to a fresh egg which has been well beaten up in a bowl, then add a teacupful of sweet milk, stir it well, and take a teaspoonful every ten minutes; or,

One tablespoonful of common salt, two of vinegar in half a pint of water, take a wine-glass of it every half hour; if there is much nausea, put a mustard plaster over the stomach so as to enable the patient to retain it.

48

Dysentery has been cured by swallowing ice in as large pieces as practicable, to the fullest extent; to preserve the ice during hot nights, when it is scarce or has to be brought from a distance, put it in a large pitcher or china or stone vessel, in as large pieces as convenient, cover the mouth with a clean cloth and put the vessel between two large feather pillows. When some ice is wanted, obtain it with as short exposure to the air as possible.

Families in the country, who-have no ice-houses of their own, would do well to have on hand a flannel bag holding a peck or more, have another one larger, so that three inches thickness of bird or chicken feathers can be stuffed in between the two. The tops may be closed like the draw of a reticule; fill this with ice, and in a cool cellar it will keep a week.

Creosote is a valuable remedy: ten drops with thirty drops or half a teaspoonful of vinegar, two grains of quinine, well mixed in two tablespoons of water; one teaspoonful every three hours until relieved. It is almost a specific.

Raw beef, minced up fine, a tablespoon every three hours, eating nothing else but ice; it is also good in the diarrhœa of children; has been thus used in Russia since 1845, and recently with success in this country; or,

Take pussy wood, called Indian clover, boil the leaves, which abound in August and September, in new milk, and drink half a pint every three hours, eating and drinking nothing else; or,

Take Indian corn, burn it like coffee, grind it, then prepare as coffee and drink one teacupful every three hours until relieved; or,

One ounce of glycerine in five ounces of flax-seed tea, or gum-arabic water, as an enema, twice a day; besides, take it internally thus: one and a half ounces of glycerine in four ounces of water; give a tablespoon every three hours; or,

Chimaphila maculata, or spotted winter-green, formerly called pyrola maculata, or pipsissewa or wild arsenic; the leaves have a white, longitudinal stripe; make a strong decoction of the leaves and take one or two tablespoons every two or three hours, according to the violence of the disease.

Some prefer one drachm of sulphate of soda, forty drops of laudanum, in eight tablespoonfuls of water—cinnamon water is better; give a tablespoonful every three hours.

Homœopathy gives aconite if there is inflammatory fever;

then chamomilla if the heat and thirst are great, with restlessness; pulsatilla, if there is a disturbed stomach; ipecac, if stools are slimy; if there is violent colic, colocynth; carbo veg. in desperate cases, and phosphorus during convalescence.

At water-cures reliance is had on injections first, then a wet sheet pack when there is high fever; drink moderately of cold water; keep the whole abdomen constantly covered with a cold compress, renewed every ten minutes, until the heat and swelling subside. Ice-water injections may be repeated if grateful to the patient. If the fever is very high, take a hip-bath of fifty degrees.

Children take an injection and are then washed with tepid water three times a day, with constant cold compresses on the abdomen until the heat becomes natural; drinking cold or iced water or ice, two tablespoons at a time. Keep the bowels free with injections every twelve hours.

MALIGNANT PUSTULE

Is a little pimple which sometimes appears instantaneously about the head, face, or lip, or eyelids, or nose; it comes with an instantaneous, sharp, stinging sensation, as if from the bite of some insect, which it most probably is; for four or five hours there is but little change; meanwhile a little vesicle appears around the bottom of the pimple, breaks inside, sends the poison into the system, the skin swells, inflames, becomes discolored, and death ensues in a day or two, sometimes in a few hours, with all the symptoms of erysipelas in the head.

This malady is rare; only a few cases have occurred in this country; the life might be saved if the pimple was cut out with a knife, with a scoop of half an inch in diameter; or if a red-hot iron or knitting-needle were plunged into the pimple and pushed down half an inch.

As soon as the smart or sting is felt, it should be dabbled with a soft rag dipped in hartshorn, kept up for an hour.

QUINSY

Is inflammatory sore throat, causing the tonsils to swell and soon become painful, with difficulty of swallowing; pains dart about the ears, and there is headache and thirst, caused by cold, by cooling off too soon after being heated, or having a cold wind blow on the head for some time; it often destroys life. Give an enema at once, and then a brisk cathartic of two full tablespoons of salts repeated every two hours, until the bowels act freely; or three or four tablespoons of castor-oil.

Keep the body warm, drink all the hot teas needed, but eat nothing for a day or two; keep the feet warm, or bathe them in hot water freely; gargles may be used, such as alum water, infusion of white-oak bark, but free purgation ought to be promptly employed.

Hydropathists rely on wet linen compresses applied closely around the throat, without dribbling, renewed every five minutes or less, according to the severity of the attack; take also frequent small draughts of ice-water, a sitz-bath or a dripping sheet, in either case followed by being wrapped up in a warm dry blanket to cause perspiration, and then the patient is safe; if the heat about the throat is very great, use pounded ice, so as to make a pad, and apply it to the throat. Homœopathy regards as one disease ulcerated sore throat, quinsy, malignant, putrid, gangrenous sore throat, and malignant scarlatina; give aconite and follow with belladonna. Pulsatilla will answer in mild cases; nux vomica, if there are large amounts of phlegm; mercurius, if ulcers are seen; acid nit., if these ulcers are painful; arsenicum, if there is great prostration; rhus, in extreme cases. The diet should be of sago, gruel, boiled rice; if weak, give beef-tea.

Other remedies are used beneficially, from ten to thirty drops of tincture of belladonna every three or four hours, until relieved.

Others grease the throat well and keep it covered with a thick coat of common tar plastered over a cloth, to within a quarter of an inch of the edge; the oil is beneficial, besides preventing the tar from sticking.

HOARSENESS

Is caused by phlegm attached to the voice organs; if that phlegm is tenacious, it sticks close, and the person can scarcely speak above the breath without a great effort; making public speeches, under such circumstances, has often put such a strain on the fragile vocal cords, or rather plates, as to induce inflammation, and strainings which have ruined the voice for life, if not followed by fatal results; the same also with singers; no one should ever speak or sing when every word is an effort. If the phlegm is loose as in the breaking up of a cold, there is the hoarseness proper; it is sometimes relieved by cutting off a lemon at the end, then work a little loaf sugar into it with· a spoon-handle, making a kind of strong lemon syrup; in default of the lemon, honey and vinegar, half and half, is a good substitute. Or a teaspoonful of freshly-scraped horse-radish root, four ounces of warm water, let it stand four hours, add equal quantities of syrup and vinegar, stir, and take one teaspoonful at a time. Sometimes hoarseness is speedily relieved by breathing the fumes of warm vinegar and water; or hot water from a teapot spout; be careful not to draw the hot water into the throat. Homœopaths give for temporary hoarseness, pulsatilla if voice is almost lost; mercurius afterwards, or if there is sweating at night; nux vom. if ever there is a dry, tiresome cough; rhus tox., if difficult breathing and burning in throat; chamomilla, if phlegm is profuse; chronic hoarseness, hepar sulphuris. Sometimes hoarseness is relieved thus:—Take the whites of two eggs, beat them thoroughly with one table-spoonful of powdered loaf sugar, grate in some nutmeg, add a pint of tepid water, stir it well and drink one or two tablespoons every hour until relieved. In addition keep warm, with free bowels. The lemon and white sugar above-named was a favorite prescription with General Jackson in his last illness, when he was troubled greatly with hoarseness and cough.

EYES

ARE prematurely ruined by using them too much after sundown, by artificial light, especially in scrofulous persons. Children under twelve years of age should never be allowed to read or sew after sundown; nor persons of any age over an hour or two at a time, nor until after sunrise in the morning.

1. Never sit with the light directly opposite the eyes; let it come slantingly over the left shoulder.

2. Strain the eyes as little as possible; the instant you find that you have to wink your eyes in order to see clearly, that instant get up and do something which either requires you to look at things a great distance off, or at comparatively large objects near at hand.

3. When the eyes are weary, a great relief is experienced by closing them five or ten minutes, or even by looking at objects for that time a hundred yards or mile away, or at the clouds.

4. Never use the eyes in reading or sewing before day in the morning; the glare of the artificial light from the darkness of the long hours of sleep is most pernicious.

5. Never look at a glaring object for a second; many persons have injured their eyes for life by attempting to look at the shining sun.

6. Never sleep so that when you first open your eyes in the morning a window will face them with the full light of day.

7. The instant you find there is a strain on the eye sufficient to attract your attention, at any age or any time of day, lay down your book or your work.

WHEN TO USE SPECTACLES.

It does immeasurably more harm to try and put off the evil day of using spectacles, than to employ them promptly as soon as nature calls for them.

When you find yourself instinctively adjusting your paper or book so as to receive a better light, you need spectacles.

When you find that habitually you put yourself near an open window or door to read more comfortably, you need glasses.

If the eyes are easily fatigued, requiring you to shut them for rest, or there is a sense of effort to make out the letters in print, or to take the stitches in sewing, spectacles are needed.

CHOICE OF GLASSES.

Some think one pair of glasses is as good as another. It is a great mistake; some glass is more easily scratched than another kind, being softer. Never purchase glasses on the street; they are mostly discarded ones from a variety of imperfections.

Glasses are the last thing to be bought for cheapness.

Brazilian glasses or pebbles are best, because they are of nature's make, and are the hardest in the world, most difficult to be scratched, hence you will not want a higher power so soon.

Always note the number of your glass and the date of first using it; if lost, then you can easily tell the seller what number you want.

Get a lower number, one with a nearer focus, one more bulging, on the same conditions of getting the first, weariness or winking the eyes so as to see more clearly.

Glasses should be washed in cold water once a day, wiped with a linen fabric and then with buckskin, never with paper; it is hard and scratches them.

If the eyes are matted in the morning, endeavor to open them in warm water; if not to be had, apply the saliva to the lids, it dissolves the hard matter instantly, when it should be rubbed off with the balls of the fingers; the nail should never touch it, nor be required to free any accumulation on the eyelids or in their corners, as it tears the most tender surface of the lashes and lids.

If the eye is blackened by a blow and the parts are discolored, apply warm fomentations, renewing the cloths every three minutes; if there is inflammation, use cold compresses; in either case until entire relief.

Sty on the eye; never touch it; do nothing for it, but begin at once to adopt a fruit diet; it may expedite a cure by taking an enema, or swallowing a good dose of salts or oil.

A multitude of washes and ointments are used to cure sore eyes. Unless you are under the special care of a professed oculist, never allow anything to go near your eye, let alone into it, stronger than your own saliva, or tepid, soft or rain water; but keep the bowels active, three times in two days; follow the fruit diet; be out of doors a great deal, keep a clean skin, feet warm, and avoid all reading and sewing until the eyes get well; this is intended to apply to common

SORE EYES,

which are always a sign of bad blood. The only rational mode of cure is to purify the blood, to get up a high state of general health; any different course is always unwise, and is a waste of time. If the eyes have to be used at night, and there is a sense of feverishness or weakness, or if they water, bathe them freely in cold water; either put the whole face in the water, or flap up the water against the closed eye with the hand, not striking the ball with the hand or fingers, but making a cup of the palm of the hand, striking the ends of the fingers against the corner of the eye-bone.

The eyesight is impaired for life, and sometimes fatal amaurosis is induced by the instinctive effort of the eye to maintain a steady focus when the person is reading, while walking, or on horseback, or in vehicles. The simple fact should restrain every intelligent person from such a ruinous practice, or from doing such a thing for ten minutes in any day.

STAMMERING.

ANY person of small force of character can cure himself of stammering in a very short time, as it is a purely nervous disease, a kind of St. Vitus' dance of the tongue; more nervous power is sent there than it can use up.

The veriest stammerer can commit to memory a speech or piece of poetry, and, getting up before an audience, can repeat it accurately without hesitation, because, while part of the nervous energy is used in enunciation, another part is expended in the attempt to remember.

A stammerer can speak without halting in five minutes if at every syllable he will strike his finger or foot against an object, because the nervous current is sent out in two directions, not in one strong flow; or he can read or talk without difficulty if he will aim to enunciate every syllable, nay every letter, vowel and consonant, after the manner of the beautiful Spanish tongue. It is simply the practice of deliberation; begin by tapping the finger against the person at each syllable and at the instant of its enunciation. If a knitting-needle is thrust through a stammerer's tongue he is cured in an instant, but remains cured only until the tongue gets well.

COLD FEET.

IF the feet are habitually cold, or are easily made cold enough to attract the attention unpleasantly, the general health is not good, and never can be good until the defect is remedied; it shows that the circulation is not vigorous enough to carry the blood to the farthest extremity of the system. The gnarled oak of a century begins to die at the farthest twig, and so does man.

The feet must be kept heated by the fire within; holding them to the fire or over a register, or having them on a hot brick or footstone habitually, is only a temporary expedient.

In the first place, aim to keep up the "general health," which article turn to. The feet must be kept scrupulously clean, should be washed every morning in cold water, that is, dipped in cold water for an instant, both at once, then wipe well, the soles especially wipe hard and fast; at night dip them both in warm water for five minutes, ankle deep, then in cold, to come above the toes for a quarter of a minute, rub as before, put the feet in warmed slippers and get into bed, having the soles rubbed most vigorously; the cold water promotes reaction, while the frequent wetting and rubbing the soles keeps the pores from being closed up, and there they are much the largest of the whole body.

Some feet are kept more comfortably warm with woollen socks, others with cotton, others again with two thin pair; each must notice for himself.

Some wear ground mustard or red pepper next the soles, but the only real remedy is to obtain better general health. Whenever the feet are noticed to be uncomfortably cold in the house, go direct to the fire; the quickest and best way to warm cold feet is to draw off the stockings and hold them to a hot stove or blazing fire, rubbing the soles and between the toes until most perfectly dry. This should be done by all men who are out of doors and from home most of the day, first washing them, then wear another pair of socks for the remainder of the evening.

It is a filthy practice and most hurtful to sit around the fire for a whole evening in the same boots and shoes worn for several hours before; this makes

STINKING FEET,

because the perspiration condenses, is mixed with the dirt that will get in while walking, and then there is decomposition, a rotting and a noisome smell. Bad colds are often got and a habit of cold feet set up, by persons walking to their stores, then sitting down with their feet on a plank floor or thin bit of carpet; the feet should be always well wiped and rest on a soft woollen rug of some kind; it greatly aids in keeping warmth to the feet.

Another mischievous plan is to pull off a shoe and thrust it into a cold slipper. In fire-time of year the slippers should be always well warmed; at other times, they should be placed in the sun, or should not be put on for a moment or two after the shoe is pulled off, to allow some of the dampness of perspiration to escape by evaporation. These seem small things and may be called old womanish, but it is better to spend a few minutes every day in attention to these things than to have cold feet for the remainder of life, or be troubled with rheumatism and limping and hobbling about the house in one's old age. Besides, persons who have cold feet habitually are greatly more liable to take colds, and are greatly more susceptible to any form of disease which may be prevalent at the time. When any person's feet are habitually cold he may be said, with literal truth, to have begun to die.

Habitually cold feet indicate always a serious want of good general health, and the most certain and efficient means to get rid of so uncomfortable a symptom is to build up the general health, as pointed out in that article.

DIARRHŒA

Is so common a disease that it is desirable to give several remedies, as the attendant circumstances are different in different persons.   The first best remedy is quietude; every step taken aggravates the malady; if persons must be on their feet, a piece of
woollen flannel, over a foot broad and long enough to be double
in front, so as to keep the abdomen warm, should be bound
tightly around the body; this is a great support, and keeps the
intestines more quiet, their incessant and active motion being the
essence of the disease; this, with rest in bed and a diet of boiled
rice and boiled milk every five hours, and nothing else, will cure
ordinary looseness of bowels.

In more decided or urgent cases, go to bed, eat nothing, and
take a liver pill; if the bowels do not cease to act in three hours
take another.

In milder cases a teaspoonful each of salt and vinegar in a
tablespoon of water, repeated every hour until relieved, is all-sufficient.

Blackberry cordial, or tea made of the blackberry root, made
strong and drunk freely at two hours' interval, is a good household
remedy; or one ounce each of rhubarb root powdered and cinnamon leaves, sixty grains of capsicum, that is, pulverized red
pepper, pour on a pint of boiling water, let it soak four hours,
strain through a cloth, add half an ounce of bicarbonate of potash and as much essence of cinnamon, stir in four heaping tablespoonfuls of pulverized loaf sugar, then add as much brandy as will
equal the whole; one or two tablespoonfuls every three hours
until relieved.

Homœopaths give dulcamara in summer from cold; if not
effectual, bryonia, followed with antimo. crud. in six hours;
china, if the looseness arises from indigestion or too much fruit,
or drinking fluids soon after eating berries, especially if attacked
in the night.   Give rheum, if there is a sour smell from the defecations; mercurius, if from a chill.   Diet, avoid all acids and sour
or hard food—beef-tea, rice, sago, arrowroot, tapioca, flax-seed
tea, etc.

Hydropathy advises abstinence from all food except farinas and boiled rice, with sitz-baths, cold compresses, or hot fomentations to the abdomen, cold injections, and all means calculated to keep up the general health.

Some give, twice a day, one teaspoonful of the following mixture: Rhubarb, saleratus, and pulverized peppermint, five grains each in a tablespoon of brandy; or, an ounce and a half of tincture of camphor, half an ounce of the tincture of capsicum, one ounce of compound spirits of lavender—half a teaspoonful thrice a day in water or flax-seed tea; or, one pound of elixir vitriol to seven pounds of water; of this take half an ounce to twelve ounces of water; then of this, one tablespoonful in some mucilage or a wineglass of water every time the bowels act, and once every three hours after, for a day or longer, or every time the looseness returns; or, ten drops of creasote, twenty drops of acetic acid, in two tablespoonfuls of rain or boiled water, one teaspoonful every two hours; give it to children in some mucilage.

All the remedies for diarrhœa of the common kind are good for chronic diarrhœa and for dysentery. It should be always borne in mind that whatever tends to stop any form of loose bowels at once endangers a variety of fatal forms of disease; especially in children the liability to water on the brain is very great. Hence no medicine containing opium, in any form, ought to be given for loose bowels or dysentery until other means have failed. Chronic diarrhœa—quietude, the flannel bandage, diet mainly of boiled rice in boiled milk, farina, sago, tapioca, and lean meats, nothing else as food. Take before each meal, in a little rice or soft bread, twenty grains of subnitrate of bismuth, which darkens and thickens the passages. The drinks should be mucilaginous altogether, such as flax-seed tea, slippery-elm bark tea, gum-arabic water, with an occasional injection of a pint each of sweet oil and thick flax-seed or other mucilage, half a pint of common molasses, a tablespoonful of salt and a teaspoonful of laudanum. Mix well; use as much at one time as the bowels will retain, three or four tablespoonfuls generally.

Both homœopaths and hydropaths advise the use of the remedies for common diarrhœa should be persisted in, in the chronic form.

COUGHS AND COLDS.

A COMMON cold is a slight inflammation of the lungs, more blood there than is natural; this excess of blood increases the amount of lubricating fluid which nature prepares for all the internal portions of the body to keep the machinery in easy working order; this fluid or mucus is also thicker and becomes yellow; we call it

PHLEGM.

As fast as it forms in the lungs, a tickling sensation is experienced at the little hollow in front at the bottom of the neck, or top of the breast-bone; this tickling excites cough, which is a forcible expulsion of air from the very bottom of the lungs, or branches of the windpipe, carrying everything before it into the throat, and with a hawk it is brought into the mouth, from which it is expectorated. This is nature's method of diminishing the excess of blood in the lungs, and getting it outside of the body; if not brought away by the cough it would remain in the lungs, and we should soon suffocate, or it would be re-absorbed as in consumption, bringing on hectic fever, night-sweats, and death. Hence to "quiet" the cough, to "cure" the cough, by which is meant to get rid of it, to prevent it, is suicidal.

All patent medicines for coughs, colds, and consumptions, contain opium, laudanum, paregoric, or morphia, all of which are different preparations of opium; they all lessen cough by obtunding the sensibilities of the parts, they put to sleep the whole body and every part of it in proportion, so that all feeling is taken away, and in this case the lungs are so stupefied, their nerves are so drunk, that they are not sensible of the presence of the phlegm, no tickling is experienced, no cough is excited, and the phlegm remains, with the results above stated, always and inevitably; hence the

INFAMY

attached to the names of the men who have made large fortunes by the sale of cough medicines, expectorants, soothing syrups, and

every other balsam, balm, or other name for medicines to affect
the lungs. Educated physicians everywhere regard these persons
as unprincipled swindlers, and in effect murderers, as much so as
the makers and vendors of made liquors. The direct tendency of
all cough medicines and soothing syrups sold in drug-stores is to
kill the persons who take them. All that ought to be done is to
loosen the phlegm, increase the cough, and thus hasten the rid-
dance from the system. The most direct method of doing this
is to keep warm, have woollen flannel next the skin, have the
bowels act freely at least once a day, and live on a strict "fruit
diet" until relieved.

A COMMON COLD

can always be cured in twenty-four hours, if within twelve hours
after it is known to have been taken, and most persons of any
observation can tell in an hour when they have taken cold; but if it
is allowed to settle on some weak part for two or three days, it
will run its course of a fortnight or longer, as measles or any
similar disease; liable, however, to be indefinitely protracted, by
renewing the cold, which is done by the slightest possible causes,
and the person begins to feel as if he would never get rid of his
cold.

All colds are preceded with more or less chilliness, for that is
the universal cause, although it may be so slight as not to have
been noticed; then comes the reaction of fever, next loss of appetite, with a dry cough in two or three days; after a while it
loosens, and the cold wears away.

When a cold settles in the system something is taken for it;
it does no good; then, something else; in the course of a week or
ten days half a dozen things have been taken; then a seventh is
"tried," the cough loosens, and the man gets well; and as long
as he lives, he is a great admirer of the seventh remedy, and in
the course of a lifetime recommends it to fifty or a hundred
people; but it never did any one of them a particle of good, nor
did it do him any good; he only happened to take it when the
cold was "breaking." Nature had performed the cure, but in
this and other ailments it is the last thing done which bears the
palm; this is the way in which so many cures for colds have
arisen. A cold settling on any part means a congestion in that

part, too much blood; the only method of relief is to diminish the quantity of blood by not eating anything, then taking a large dose of castor-oil or salts, or a liver pill or other purgative; this relieves the system of one or two pounds of matter; keep warm in bed; eat nothing, not an atom, until the phlegm begins to loosen, then adhere strictly to a " fruit diet," keeping in the house all the time, in a room as warm as sixty-five or seventy degrees, until you are hungry, and there is no cough, except a loose one, two or three times a day. This process will cut any cold short off in twenty-four hours, if adopted as soon as the cold has been taken. It is the proper treatment in later stages, but its good effects will not appear so speedily.

A slight cold can always be cured, if taken in hand promptly, by going to bed at once in a warm room, well ventilated, taking an injection, drinking largely of hot teas, ginger, red pepper; plain water is just as effective but not so readily taken, wrap up warm, get into a profuse perspiration for an hour, cool off in another hour, keep in the house, and be confined to a fruit diet. Hydropathy relies on enemas, warm and hot baths, packs, and fruit and coarse bread diet.

Homœopathy prefers dulcamara, in loose cough; belladonna, if dry; hyoscyamus, if that fails; ignatia amara, in tickling coughs; conium maculatum, for severe night cough; nux vomica, in catarrhal or nervous cough; pulsatilla in hard, retching cough; chamomilla in a dry night cough; carbo veg. when attended with a harsh burning in the throat and chest; sulphur is best in obstinate dry coughs, used persistently; the diet should be nourishing, plain, and easy of digestion; avoid cold and damp air, especially east winds.

COSTIVENESS.

A PERSON may be costive and yet have an action of the bowels every day, and may not be costive with an action every other day. Costiveness really is small, scant, hard passages, or hard lumps or balls, passed with difficulty; if the passages are of the consistence of mason's mortar or thinner, it is not costiveness, if there be but one action every two or three days. But usually a person is costive when the bowels fail to act once in twenty-four hours; this seems to be the natural arrangement. If one goes several days without an action, it becomes

CONSTIPATION.

Costiveness attends almost every sickness, usually precedes it, sometimes follows. Whatever may be the ailment, an alleviation is almost sure to follow a large, free action of the bowels; hence the practice of a large class of persons in the lower walks of life to take salts or oil for everything that happens to them. Hence the popularity of all pills which are purgative.

Generally costiveness is attended with cold feet, headache, and variable appetite, and when these are present, two other symptoms almost always appear—a bad taste in the mouth of mornings, and great chilliness, when "the least thing in the world gives a cold."

Costiveness is often caused by resisting the calls of nature for trifling reasons, often repeated; next to that as to frequency of cause is a sedentary habit of life, sitting too much, staying in the house most of the time, omitting daily walks, and irregularity in the hours for evacuating the bowels.

Many persons bring on costive habits by taking medicines for every irregularity, or using injections. It is the tendency of all medicines which act on the bowels to leave them more costive than before, especially if more than one action is induced; if persons find they must take something to move the bowels, it should be just enough to move them once moderately, and it is better still to take it at two doses than all at once, for then the action will be more gentle, and its influence more protracted; if a tablespoon of castor oil is required to move the bowels, take half a tablespoon at night on going to bed, and the other half on rising, and so with all other remedies taken to relieve costiveness.

Slow bowels is such a common infirmity, and stands between so many persons and enjoyable health, that the subject merits intelligent consideration, especially as good health is rarely if ever enjoyed without a full free action of the bowels every morning. The author's book on Health and Disease is entirely devoted to the exposition of this subject. To prevent costiveness several things should be invariably attended to:—

First. Yield instantly to nature's call.

Second. If it does not come within half an hour of the usual time, go to the privy, have a paper or book, and wait and even solicit, invite, by a little straining, not much. If the mind is occupied with reading, the inclination is more likely to be felt than if there is a nervous anxiety on the subject; it is not advised to wait longer than half an hour, for the position invites the formation of piles.

Third. The best time for the bowels to act is after breakfast, in the morning; if it passes, then eat nothing until they do act, at least nothing until breakfast next morning, for it is self-evident that if food is crowded into the system when there is no outlet, there must be accumulations and hurtful oppressions or overloadings somewhere, and the system must suffer; while nothing should be eaten, the utmost fill may be taken of cold water or hot teas.

Fourth. Walk or work in the open air, in moderation; this is one of the best means possible for inviting the natural action of the system.

Fifth. If these means do not avail, make a breakfast of cracked wheat, or other form of bread or mush, as coarse as you can get, with a little salt or butter on it and fresh fruits, berries, cherries, or currants; or if not in season, use them stewed; in either case with but very little sugar, no milk or other fluid, and nothing else.

Dinner same, with lean meat and boiled turnips, or in their place potatoes. Supper same as breakfast, nothing between; the object of these articles of food is to keep the bowels free; if fluids are taken with fruits, acidity is likely to result; but an hour after eating them, as much water may be drank as is wanted. If cracked wheat cannot be had, common wheat may be ground very coarse and boiled thoroughly until very soft, as soft as boiled rice. Sometimes the flour made of the whole grain may be used in the form of bread. The effects of this diet will be greatly intensified if the person walks or works two hours in the forenoon in the open air, and an hour in the afternoon; or, if in mid-winter, two or three hours about two o'clock.

Injections are often resorted to with benefit at the usual hour of going to stool, but the great objection to them is that the need for them increases with time until the system gets into such a condition that the bowels never act without their aid, which is a very great inconvenience. The better plan is to keep the system regular by natural means, by the use of such food as each one observes for himself to have the effect of loosening the bowels.

One or more tablespoons of white mustard seed swallowed whole in half a glass of water on rising and retiring is efficient in some cases. Others take figs or tomatoes, or other food which contains little seeds, their mechanical effect being to irritate the surface of the bowels, as a speck irritates the eye, causing a flow of water, which washes out all before it.

The coarser the food, the less nutriment and the more waste, the more likely to move the bowels, as the accumulation of this waste in the rectum causes that amount of distention which is necessary to induce an inclination to expulsion; among these are the boiled grains, cracked wheat, hominy, boiled turnips; these last have five per cent. of nutriment, all the other is waste; stewed prunes, a glass of cold or salt water on rising, eating freely of parched corn. But the great point after all is to aim at regulating the bowels by the food, next use enemas and laxatives, castor oil, and the like, alternately and as seldom as possible; in all cases adding outdoor exercise. Hydropathy relies on enemas and a diet of fruits, berries, melons, and coarse breads, with abundant walking or working in the open air.

Homœopathy, on the principle that like cures like, gives opium in recent cases; nux vomica, when recent, as from a heavy meal; pulsatilla, when from indigestion; platina, if brought on by travelling; mercurius, when there is a bitter taste in the mouth, or the passages are hard and bally; plumbum metallicum, if obstinate; lachesis, if the rectum is torpid; lycopodium, when there is colic, wind, or sense of weight in lower part of the belly; rhus tox., if alternating with looseness.

Baryta C., in the constipation of old persons; belladonna, if there is headache; china, in pregnancy four globules in a tablespoon of water, night and morning.

One-fifth grain of belladonna, three grains of pulverized rhubarb, one grain of ipecac, take one three times a day.

One teaspoonful each of salt and black pepper in a tablespoonful of vinegar, night and morning.

Apples and pears pealed, cut into quarters, with a little sugar and water, eaten with boiled rice thrice a day at meal times the beginning of the meal, with nothing else for supper, is admirable for children and old or feeble persons.

Half a drachm of the alcoholic extract of henbane, one scruple of the compound extract of colocynth, three grains of nux vomica, made into twelve pills, one every night.

Four grains each of watery extract of aloes and extract of rhubarb, made into a pill, once a day, with an occasional enema.

One-sixteenth of a grain of acetate of strychnine, three times a day. is efficient in very obstinate cases.

------- ⚬⚬ -------

WHOOPING-COUGH,

CALLED Pertussis by physicians, is a "catching disease," and is had but once in a lifetime—the earlier in life the better.   Its distinctive symptom is, the coughing is so quick, spiteful, and urgent, the child keeps at it until the breath is so entirely exhausted, that in the effort to draw in the needed air with sufficient rapidity, the top of the windpipe seems to close and a whooping sound or a long-drawn breath with a whoop is drawn in.   It generally gets well of itself; keep the child warm, have the bowels act every day, and live on fruits, coarse bread, boiled rice, sago, tapioca, lean meat once a day.   If the cough is tight give syrup of squills or ipecac, not enough to vomit; or tincture of assafœtida.   Perhaps the best medicine is about four drops of the fluid extract of hyoscyamus to a child ten years old.   The air of gas-works seems to have had a beneficial effect in some cases. A blister to the back of the neck has given great relief; also free frictions to the spine twice a day with onion juice.

Homœopathy gives dulcamara when the cough is loose; pulsatilla when there is sneezing and hoarseness; mercurius when there is a dry cough; belladonna when the cough is dry about the middle of the disease.   Hepar sul. at that time if the cough is loose; arnica, if there is a bloody discharge from the mouth or nose.

From fifteen to thirty drops of diluted nitric acid, in some syrup, thrice a day, is said to have cured hundreds of cases. Dr. Gibb, of London, gives one hundred grains of bicarbonate of soda, as much cochineal powder, twenty grains of belladonna powder in ten grains of sugar, divide into ten doses; take one dose thrice a day during the whole progress of the disease; or,

Elixir vitriol twelve drachms, tincture of cardamom compound three drachms, one half ounce of syrup, one ounce of water; one teaspoonful every two hours of daylight until cured; or,

Beat a fresh egg in half a pint of vinegar, then add half a pound of rock candy. Take two tablespoonfuls every four hours during the day.

One gill each of sliced garlic and onions, or double the amount of either, stew with a gill of sweet oil for an hour, then add a gill of honey and half an ounce of camphor. One or two teaspoonfuls every three or four hours.

Into half a pint each of strained honey and water add a quarter of a pound of elecampane root, in a glazed vessel or stone ware, place in a hot oven, and when it gets as thick as honey, give one teaspoonful to a child before each meal.

INFLUENZA

Is a kind of cold in the head, seeming to combine with some ingredient in the atmosphere which causes it to spread among whole communities, even killing great numbers; hence is sometimes called

EPIDEMIC CATARRH.

Red patches appear on the skin; pustules arise in successive crops on the face and skin; sometimes the throat is seriously involved. It is really a combination of cold and liver derangement. Keep in the house, take a liver pill as directed under that heading, with a "fruit diet;" if particularly weak from cold or debility, take one or two grains of quinine every three hours during the day. Homœopathy gives aconitum when there is inflammation; arsenicum, if pain in the head and much watering at the nose; mercurius, when there are chills and heats and profuse perspiration; belladonna, if the tonsils are inflamed and swollen; phosphorus, if there is hoarseness or pain in speaking or swallowing; bryonia, when there is hot skin and "bursting" headache and cough, day and night; carbo v. if there is oppression in the chest. If there is nausea give ipecac.

Hydropathy treats this ailment as a common cold with great success.

BILIOUS COLIC

.

Is a frequent, painful, and dangerous malady; there is about the navel, and sometimes over the whole abdomen, a twisting, tearing, griping pain, coming and going by turns. Inflammation soon comes on—known by pain on pressure; the abdomen is sometimes much swollen, at others drawn in and lank. Bitter, bilious matter is vomited; the face is pale and clammy, extending to the whole body; these symptoms arise from various causes, all ending in congestion of the liver; sudden checking of perspiration, accumulation of bile, exposure to great heat; standing in the water for a great while, part of the body in and part out; sometimes working and sometimes still. An enema should be administered at once; a large mustard plaster should be spread over the abdomen. If there is sickness at stomach, apply hot fomentations. If no sickness, give two tablespoonfuls of Epsom salts, or as much castor oil, having added to it a tablespoonful of spirits of turpentine, and repeat in two hours if there is no operation. If the pain is very severe take a hot bath, eighty degrees at first, gradually adding hotter water; if the bath is not necessary, or not available, keep the body warm, and do all that is possible to get up a copious perspiration, by hot bottles to the feet, the arm-pits, and sides. As soon as the bowels act, give two liver pills; as soon as they begin to take effect, which will be in two or three hours, or as soon as perspiration is induced, the disease is conquered, and the patient is safe.

Homœopaths give nux vom.; if not efficient, carbo veg.; chamomile, if there is a feeling as if there were a stone at the stomach; if no relief in two hours, give colocynth or belladonna; lycopodium, when there is a sense of twisting; calcarea, in persons of drunken habits.

Hydropathy administers warm-water injections promptly and most freely, until the bowels are entirely unloaded; give frequent sitz, hip or half baths, warm or hot, as may be required; when these do not give relief, take the same baths of cold water as when the skin is hot and feverish, the pain being at one point, coming and going. Drink largely of tepid water; during all the bathings keep up a vigorous friction to the whole back with the hands; follow hot fomentations with cold compresses.

DELIRIUM TREMENS,

OR mania à potu, from drinking too much liquor, or taking too freely of any stimulants, is known chiefly by inability to sleep, and the apprehension of the most horrible things imaginable, with tremblings of the limbs in most cases; sometimes the hallucinations are of the amusing or ridiculous kind. Give hop-tea with a grain of opium every three hours. Give beef-tea or broth or gruel, very freely seasoned with the strongest red pepper; or put a blister on the back of the neck; or take valerian instead of opium; or a tablespoonful of digitalis tincture every two hours, or a teaspoonful every half hour. Make sixty grains of red pepper into pills, and swallow them at a dose; the result is immediate, there is a sense of warmth throughout the system, the patient falling into a sound sleep within an hour. Sleep is the cure. The capsicum might be taken in water or syrup or mucilage, putting the cup far back on the tongue. A wet sheet-pack is an admirable remedy in some cases, and should be first tried on all; it is the safest, cheapest, and best. Third and fourth attacks are often fatal. Some give thirty-grain doses of capsicum every hour. Homœopathy gives nux vom. in the first stages; opium if later; in the young and vigorous, aconite or belladonna or coffee.

POISONS.

In this table the poisons, symptoms, and antidotes are given in alphabetical order, so as to be found instantly, for the quicker they are given the greater chance for life ; five minutes' delay sometimes settles the question of life or death. But in many cases the poison is not known, hence the reader must act on general principles. Poisons are of two kinds : corrosive or insensible. The corrosive eat up, burn, destroy the lining of tongue, throat, and stomach, and are the most fatal ; they all cause a terrible scalding pain, vomiting, and purging ; most of them shrivel up the lips and tongue, and make them white or yellow, and constrict the throat ; countenance dreadfully anxious. The point is to know what thing will soonest cause vomiting, so as to bring it up out of the stomach the quickest, and which will at the same time dilute it. Warm sweet milk, a very little warm—for if hot it scalds more—is the very best of all the things which are most likely to be had ; if not, warm water is best, even cold will do, if there is no time to wait ; the milk soothes the irritated parts. As the two points to be aimed at are dilution and to empty the stomach, if milk is not to be had use the water ; both are to be used in the same way—drink a teacupful at once, in two minutes another, and so on until the stomach is so full that a feather or finger will cause vomiting. Then swallow the whites of half a dozen eggs or a half pint of sweet or other oil, this will antagonize any remnants of poison left.

The same remedies are still more applicable for the insensible poisons, that is, such as can be swallowed, and the person not be sensible of it, and which tend to produce insensibility after they get into the stomach, as laudanum, morphia, etc. But after causing free vomiting, instead of taking the white of eggs, drink strong coffee, and unless the patient is lively and wide awake don't hesitate a moment to pour a steady stream of cold water from a height of five or more feet from a pail, on the head and shoulders and back until all stupor or dulness is gone, and repeat if insensibility begins to return, for the system must be thoroughly waked up. A quicker way to empty the stomach of this class of poisons is to stir a tablespoonful each of common salt and ground mustard in a glass of water, stir and drink quickly; as soon almost as it touches the stomach vomiting commences; encourage. it with copious draughts of warm water or milk, and then drink strong coffee, and use the pour-bath if necessary.

READ THIS ONCE A YEAR

so as to have a general understanding of the whole subject; then if a parent has occasion to use this knowledge in the case of any member of the family, it will greatly aid him in acting with the necessary presence of mind and coolness and deliberation in any emergency.

But when all appliances are at hand, and the poison taken is known, the following table will be of great value :—

Aconite. See Monk's-hood.

Alcohol. Symptom, can't stand or walk, stupid, no sense. Give large draughts, even whole quarts of warm water until all is vomited enough. If too drunk to swallow, use stomach-pump, or set the patient up and let a stream of cold water fall on the head and back of the neck continuously from a yard high, no matter about wetting anything; if this does not seem to have some effect speedily, shake him, whip him with switches smartly, even to blood.

Ammonia or hartshorn. Great burning in mouth, throat, and stomach, and prostration; give vinegar and water, or lemon-juice diluted, or butter-milk, followed by warm-water emetic as above.

Antimony. See Tartar Emetic.

Aquafortis or nitric acid. It turns lips and everything yellow, burning throat, vomiting up shreds. Take any form of magnesia, chalk or whiting, or strong soapsuds, or soap and water, or wood ashes and water, or milk, or white of eggs, or sweet oil, then wash out with warm-water emetics.

Arsenic. Nausea, vomiting, pain in stomach, excessive thirst, tight dry throat; any kind of emetic, salt and mustard with water, or a teaspoonful of ipecac in a pint of warm water; then keep on drinking warm water until copious vomiting, then swallow the whites of several eggs, or magnesia, and use stomach-pump.

Baryta, Muriate of; now called Chloride of Barium. See Muriate of Baryta.

Belladonna. See Deadly Nightshade.

Bismuth. Metallic taste, hot and dry throat, burning in stomach and bowels, vomiting blood. Drink all the sweet milk you can swallow, or eat white of five or six or more eggs; stomach-pump.

Blisterers. See Cantharides.

Blue Vitriol (Sulphate of Copper), and Verdigris (Acetate of Copper). Metallic taste, vomiting, purging, cramps in thighs and legs, foams at mouth. Warm-water emetics to fullest extent, then drink strong coffee, take whites of eggs, flour and water, or stomach-pump.

Cantharides, or Spanish flies; intended to have been used for a plaster. Burning in throat, pain in stomach and bowels, vomits bloody mucus and may pass bloody water. Take warm milk and warm-water emetics to fullest extent, or stomach-pump.

Carbolic Acid. Use stomach-pump if possible; if not, warm-water emetics, followed by half a cup of sweet oil, or two table-spoons of castor oil.

Carbonic Acid Gas in wells, sinks, or privies, or from burning charcoal in close rooms. Drowsiness, slow breathing, discolored face, immovable. Get out in the open air on the instant, rub the hands rapidly over the chest, pour cold water from a height on the head, blow air into nose or throat with a bellows, with harts-horn rubbed under the nose.

Caustic, Lunar. See lunar caustic.—Cedar, Oil of. See oil of cedar.

Cobalt, used as fly poison, also kills children who eat it. Heat and pain in throat and stomach, retching, heaving, vomiting, anxious look, quick breathing, loose bowels. Swallow all the warm water or sweet oil or milk, or white of eggs, possible.

Colchicum. See Meadow Saffron.

Conium maculatum. See Hemlock.—Copper. See blue vitriol.

Corrosive Sublimate (Bichloride of Mercury), mixed with the whites of eggs to kill bed-bugs, has often been left about in unmarked bottles, and taken by mistake. Metallic, coppery taste; burning heat and binding feeling in the throat; pain in stomach and bowels, vomiting, purging, countenance swollen and anxious, with a white and shrivelled tongue. Swallow instantly the whites of half a dozen eggs. Next best is wheat flour in water; milk or warm-water emetics, and washing out.

Deadly Nightshade, or Belladonna (Atropa Belladonna). Swelled veins, dry throat, constricted; swimming in the head, nausea, blindness, hysteric laughter, the pupils of the eyes are enlarged, finally insensible. Take at once an emetic of fifteen grains of sulphate of zinc or five grains of sulphate of copper dissolved in a teacup of warm water; drink vinegar and water or lemon-juice freely; take an enema and a large dose of castor oil; then, if not fully sensible, pour a stream of cold water to fall on the head and nape of the neck, until fully roused.

Digitalis. See Foxglove.—Dogwood, Poison. See poison dogwood.

Fly Poison. See Cobalt.

Fool's Parsley (Æthusa cynapium), resembling the common kind. Heat in throat, thirst, headache, purging, swimming in the head and delirium. Salt and mustard water emetic, then of milk; next drink flaxseed tea and take three or four tablespoons of castor oil.

Foxglove, or Digitalis. Swimming of head, can't see distinctly, hiccough, senseless. Give brandy freely and largely, with mustard plaster over the pit of stomach. Pour cold water over the body.

Green Paint. See Paris Green, and Verdigris.

Hartshorn. See Ammonia.

Hellebore or Pokeberry Plant (Veratrum viride). Vomiting, bloody stools, tremors, shaking of limbs, fainting, anxious countenance, cold sweats. Take salt-mustard-water emetic, then warm-water emetics most freely; then purge with four tablespoons or more of castor oil, and in an hour drink strong coffee.

Hemlock, or Poison Hemlock (Conium maculatum). Dim sight, swelling and pain in abdomen, vomiting and purging. Take a salt-mustard-water emetic, then large warm-water emetics, then a glass of milk every half hour; pour cold water continuously from a height of six feet on head and back.

Henbane, or Hyoscyamus. Seems drunk, stupid, delirious, pupils of the eyes greatly enlarged. Vomit freely with tartar emetic, ipecac, sulphate of zinc or sulphate of copper, five grains of the latter in a teacup of warm water. Drink brandy freely, and rouse to life by pouring cold water in a constant large stream over head and shoulders.

Hydrochloric Acid. See Muriatic Acid.

Hydrocyanic Acid. See Prussic Acid.

Hyoscyamus. See Henbane.—Ivy. See Poison Ivy.

Jamestown Weed. See Thorn-apple.

Kalmia. See Mountain Laurel.—Laudanum. See Opium.

Lead. See Sugar of Lead, and White Lead.

Lime. Throat burns, stomach pains, vomiting, sometimes diarrhœa, at others constipation. Drink vinegar and water, lemon juice, anything sour which is nearest at hand, then a warm bath ; afterwards slippery-elm bark tea.

Lunar Caustic. See Nitrate of Silver.

Meadow Saffron or Colchicum. Sick stomach, griping pains, cold skin, pulse irregular. Vomit instantly with salt, mustard and water, then use warm-water emetics largely, then give brandy freely in flaxseed tea, or slippery-elm-bark water.

Mercury. See Corrosive Sublimate.

Monk's-hood, or Aconite. Nausea, vomiting, swimming in the head, convulsions. Take any kind of emetic as soon as possible ; then warm-water emetic, afterwards give brandy and water.

Morphia, or Morphine. See Opium.

Mountain Laurel (Kalmia latifolia), the ingredient in poisonous honey ; its buds are eaten by birds, the flesh of which is poison. The first symptoms are giddiness, constant and sudden flashes of heat and cold ; sick stomach, vomiting and purging constantly ; delirious ; the pulse is fast, a hundred in a minute, beats very feebly ; there is the perspiration of debility, and finally convulsions. First take an emetic of a tablespoon each of salt and mustard in flaxseed tea, or gum-arabic water ; then free vomiting with warm milk, if not at hand, warm water ; after the vomiting ceases take four or five tablespoons of castor oil, to clear out the bowels more thoroughly. If there is a tendency to unconsciousness, pour cold water on the shoulders and back, and give strong brandy and water, and keep up the pourings until the stupor has disappeared. This cause of poisoning is not unfrequent. Birds killed in the winter, from eating the seed, have their flesh impregnated with the poison, causing most distressing symptoms and long-continued illness. Sportsmen, gentlemen, and farmers' families, and persons in cities fond of game, are at any time liable to poisoning from this cause, hence instructions are given at length.

Muriate of Baryta (Chloride of Barium). Burning pain and heaviness in the stomach, blindness, swimming in the head, ears ring, temples pain, and convulsions. Tablespoon of Glauber's or Epsom salts, then drink largely of warm water to induce free vomiting, then take flaxseed tea, next a quarter grain of morphia or thirty drops of laudanum to quiet the system.

Muriate (Chloride) of Tin. Coppery taste in mouth, stricture in throat, difficult breathing, stomach-cramps, purging, quick pulse, and convulsions. Give milk or water to the fullest extent, so as to cause vomiting. Dip flannels in boiling water, wring out and lay over the stomach, renew every ten minutes; an enema of teaspoon of laudanum in a half pint of water, retain it as long as possible.

Muriatic (or Hydrochloric) Acid. Burning in throat, strangles to swallow, throat swells, breathes hard. Stir magnesia, or chalk, or whiting, or lime in water and drink it down, or soap-suds, or tear the plastering from the wall, beat it up and stir it in water, settle a minute and drink it down, or stir a teaspoonful of saleratus in a cup of warm water and drink it, then take a sweet milk emetic.

Mushrooms are healthy, but toad-stools are often mistaken for them, and are of a deadly poisonous character. Toad-stools have a bad smell, noisome, their taste is bitter or sour, or acid, draw up the throat when swallowed. Toad-stools, when bruised, have a bluish tint and give out a milky juice very acid, drawing up the mouth. Toad-stools grow in moist places; mushrooms growing in moist places are poisonous. The symptoms are nausea, vomiting, faintness, anxiety, pulse jerks, abdomen swells, cold feet and hands, livid skin, and death in forty-eight hours. Severe vomiting and purging sometimes save the patient. The symptoms do not come on until several hours after eating. As soon as nausea comes on, give an emetic of salt, mustard, and warm water; or if not at hand, warm milk or water, every five minutes until the freest vomiting occurs; then give three or four tablespoons of castor oil, and repeat every two hours until the bowels are freely acted on; then drink freely of flaxseed tea and a tablespoon of brandy, every hour until the symptoms have abated and the system is calmed down.—Nightshade, Deadly. See Deadly Nightshade.

Nitrate of Potassa or of Potash. See Nitre.

Nitrate of Silver in solution, or Lunar Caustic. Burning pain in stomach, vomiting and purging, irregular and weak pulse, and fainting. Drink instantly a tablespoonful of salt in a glass of water, stir quickly and don't wait until it dissolves. Then a milk emetic, next 30 drops of laudanum or morphia, or a grain of opium.

Nitre, or Saltpetre (Nitrate of Potassa). Intense bodily suffering, purging, vomiting, pain in bowels, bloody discharges, intense debility, and faintness. Molasses and warm water until full vomiting is induced; or milk vomit; or drink flaxseed tea or gum-arabic water, or syrup and water, half and half, then a milk or warm-water emetic; and when it is over, a tablespoonful of brandy in two or three tablespoons of water.

Nitric Acid. See Aquafortis.—Nux Vomica. See Strychnine.

Oil of Cedar. Convulsions, mouth froths, burning in throat, heat in stomach, pulse quickly ceases to beat, yet in case of death the body remains warm for a long time. Take promptly a salt-mustard-water emetic, then drink a cup of warm milk or warm water every five minutes, until stomach is free enough to excite vomiting by feather or finger in throat.

Oil of Rue. Headache, incoherency, even delirium, mouth dry, intense thirst, burning in throat, stomach, and bowels. Mustard emetic, then warm-milk emetic, then vinegar or lemon-juice.

Oil of Savin. Headache, delirium, pain, vomiting, purging, convulsions. Milk and water, mustard, or other emetic; glass of lemonade, or of flaxseed tea, or slippery-elm bark.

Oil of Tansy. Stomach burns, mouth froths, convulsions, pulse soon dies away. Milk, or water, or salt and mustard emetic, promptly, then drink largely of flaxseed or slippery-elm-bark tea.

Oil of Tar. Insensible instantly, breath rattles as in apoplexy, chest heaves, pupils contracted, eyes water, pulse small and low. Milk and water emetics instantly, then vinegar or lemon-juice.

Oil of Vitriol (Sulphuric Acid). Pain, burning, strangulation, vomits a dark-colored fluid and little stringy particles from destruction of mucous membrane of throat. Stir whiting, magnesia, chalk, lime, or plaster in water, and drink it down; then warm-milk emetic.

Opium, whether in form of Morphia, Laudanum, or Paregoric. Drowsy, insensible, stupor, slow and loud breathing. Give instantly a level tablespoon each of salt and mustard in half a glass of warm water; next a teaspoon of brandy in half a tablespoon of water, every five minutes, with pouring water from a pail, five or more feet high on head, shoulders, and back, until the person is roused to life; drink largely of very strong coffee, or tea; do everything possible to wake up the patient; keep him walking about by all means, until the drowsiness has passed off; never safe until then. The quickest way is to use a stomach-pump, if one is at hand.

Oxalic Acid looks like Epsom salts, and is used in kitchens to clean copper boilers, etc. Gives instant heat in mouth and throat, with vomiting persistently a greenish or brownish acid matter, great pain, small pulse, spasms, and numbness. Take in water magnesia, or chalk, or whiting, thick as syrup; or tear plaster from the walls, and stir it in water; or swallow common lime-water and sweet oil, half and half; then emetics of milk, then flaxseed or slippery elm tea.—Paregoric. See Opium.

Paris Green. The most perfect antidote is the hydrated ses-quioxide of iron, found in all good drug stores; but it can be made thus: Dissolve copperas in hot water, keep warm, and add nitric acid until the solution becomes yellow; then pour in ammonia water—common hartshorn—or a solution of carbonate of ammo-nia until a brown precipitate falls. Keep this precipitate moist, and in a tightly corked bottle. A few spoonfuls taken soon after even a bad case of poisoning with Paris green or arsenic is a per-fect remedy. Persons who use Paris green to destroy potato-bugs should keep this always on hand, in a well-stoppered bottle.

Phosphorus. High pulse, onion taste, nausea, vomiting, purging, pain in stomach, convulsions. Children take it from eating some form of matches. Drink magnesia and water freely, or lime-water, then a milk emetic; keep up vomiting until symptons have abated.

Poison Dogwood or Poison Sumach (Rhus venenata) some-times has the effect of irritating the skin. It is known by its beautiful little red berry at the end of the twigs. Only a few persons are susceptible to poison from it. Keep the bowels free, and bathe the parts well with sweet oil several times a day. See Vegetable Poisons.—Poison Hemlock. See Hemlock.

Poison Ivy or Poison Oak (Rhus Toxicodendron). By touch-ing the hands or face in going through the woods, it poisons in a day or two after, by itching, then there is a red breaking out on the skin which soon shows little pellicles or blisters, with consid-erable swelling; the blisters deliver water and the skin peels off in about a week. Wash the parts well, four or five times a day, with lime-water. If the vesicles are broken apply sweet spir...

of nitre, and repeat next day. Take meanwhile a tablespoon or two of castor oil or other purgative, to give one free action of th: bowels once or twice a day, and live on coarse bread and fruit or berries, until the skin begins to peel off. See Vegetable Poisons.

Poison Sumach. See Poison Dogwood.

Poke, or Pokeberry Plant. See Hellebore.

Potash (or Potassa) leaves an acid taste; throat and stomach burn, clammy skin, colic, small pulse. Drink anything sour, and when relieved, take a dose of castor-oil.

Prussic (or Hydrocyanic) Acid. Instant weight and pain in the head, nausea, stupor, convulsions. Put hartshorn to the nose, apply mustard plaster to the whole chest, give some water; or if called at once, vomit with salt and mustard. Pour cold water on head and spine until the stupor and convulsions have disappeared.

Rhus Toxicodendron. See Poison Ivy.

Rhus venenata. See Poison Dogwood.

Rue, Oil of. See Oil of Rue.—Saltpetre. See Nitre.

Savin Oil. See Oil of Savin.

Silver, Nitrate of. See Nitrate of Silver.

Spanish Flies. See Cantharides.

Stramonium. See Thorn-Apple.

Strychnine, or Nux Vomica. Great bitterness in the mouth for an hour or more, violent convulsions, sometimes limbs are stiff and straight, jaws firmly closed as in lockjaw, drowsiness, hard breathing, fainting, and death. Give warm water or milk emetics; and when stomach is empty, take a glass of lemonade, or a tablespoon of vinegar in a cup of water, or drink largely of other acids.

Sugar (Acetate) of Lead. See White Lead.

Sulphate of Copper. See Blue Vitriol.

Sulphate of Zinc. See White Vitriol.

Sulphuric Acid. See Oil of Vitriol.

Sumach, Poison, or Swamp. See Poison Dogwood, and Vegetable Poisons.

Tansy Oil. See Oil of Tansy.—Tar Oil. See Oil of Tar.

Tartar Emetic (Tartrate of Antimony and Potassa). Burning and pain in throat and stomach and bowels, intense nausea, vomiting, cramps, colicky pains, hiccough, great purging, pulse small and hard and fast, dizziness, fainting. Stir five grains of quinine in a glass of warm water or milk, and drink it down; then drink a-cup of warm milk or water every five minutes, until a feather in the throat causes free vomiting; then drink a cup or two of strong tea, followed in half an hour by twenty drops of laudanum, or by flaxseed tea, or gum-arabic water.

Thorn-apple, Stramonium, or Jamestown Weed (Datura Stramonium). Excessive thirst, nausea, vomiting, sense of strangulation, anxiety, faintness, partial blindness, enlargement of the pupil of the eye, flushed and swollen face, cold and clammy sweat, weak pulse, dizziness, vertigo, delirium (furious or whimsical), tremor, stupor, convulsions, paralysis. Children often eat the seeds, which have a sweetish taste. Take salt and mustard and water, or other tepid emetic, at once; then 2 or 3 tablespoons of castor oil or salts to cleanse out the bowels · next 10 drops of laudanum every 3 hours for 3 times.

Tin. See Muriate of Tin.—Toad-stools. See Mushrooms.

Tobacco. Vomiting, headache, dizziness, convulsions, death. Vomit instantly with salt and mustard; give a dose of castor oil or salts, at least a tablespoonful of the latter and three or four of the former, followed with a tablespoonful of brandy in half an hour, repeated every hour until relieved.

Vegetable Poisons, such as opium, laudanum, morphia, hemlock, etc. Drink freely of vinegar or lemon-juice. If large quantities have been taken, by all means keep the patient walking about briskly, for sleep is death; if no other means avail, hold him still and pour cold water over head and shoulders as above stated, until he is fully awake and has no disposition to go to sleep again. Poison from ivy, dogwood, or swamp sumach is cured by bathing the parts, night and morning, with an ounce of copperas, that is, sulphate of iron, dissolved in a pint of water; be sure to keep the bowels free, and live on fruits and coarse bread.

Veratrum viride. See Hellebore.—Verdigris. See Blue Vitriol.

Vitriol. See Blue Vitriol, Oil of Vitriol, and White Vitriol.

White Lead (Carbonate of Lead), and Sugar (Acetate) of Lead. Mouth and throat dry, heat, pricking, thirst, distress at pit of stomach, nausea, vomiting, colic, skin cold, small pulse, perfect prostration, cramps, convulsions, and final insensibility. Take a tablespoonful of Epsom salts in sweet milk every hour until purging, and white of two eggs every half hour, for two or more hours;

or give the Epsom salts in a pint of warm water, drink freely of flaxseed or slippery-elm tea, or gum-arabic water; or give a salt and mustard and water emetic, an injection, next a brisk purgative of salts or castor oil, then a teaspoonful of magnesia in half a teacup of water every two hours four times.

White Vitriol (Sulphate of Zinc). Bitter taste, sense of choking, vomiting, colicky pains, purging, hard breathing, feet and hands cold, pulse rapid and feeble. Swallow at once the whites of half a dozen eggs in flour and milk, then cause vomiting by copious draughts of warm water; or swallow instantly white of eggs, or flour and water, or milk in large quantities; then, when relieved, drink a cup or two of strong green tea.

Wolf's-bane. See Monk's-hood.

Zinc, Sulphate of. See White Vitriol.

The general principles of action in reference to all poisons taken into the stomach are here repeated. Get the poison out as quick as possible, by drinking a teacupful of warm milk every two minutes, until the stomach is so full that vomiting is easily excited by a feather or finger; warm water is next best to warm milk; when free vomiting has been caused, then give an appropriate antidote, as learned from what has been already said; the most universally applicable is to swallow the whites of several eggs. If there is great burning in the throat and stomach and bowels, take an emetic as above of sweet oil and milk or water, or a teacupful of warm milk every three minutes, until the stomach is so full that the slightest feather or finger in the throat will cause vomiting; then take a tablespoonful of sweet oil. Great burning in the throat and stomach, and dry tongue, indicate that corrosive poison has been taken, such as acids, which eat off the mucous membrane; hence the milk, or better still, a tablespoonful of sweet oil in every cupful, stirred round and drunk quickly, is peculiarly applicable in all burning poisons. The first thing is to get them out of the stomach by warm water emetics or by tartar emetic, then give four or five tablespoons of castor oil at once, and a tablespoon every hour after until it begins to act; but as soon as the oil is taken, administer an enema; as soon as the oil begins to act on the bowels drink brandy and water, or any other stimulant, very freely, to keep up the strength; or use hartshorn or ether, or any kind of bitters that may be in the house.

45

MILK A MEDICINE.

IN the preceding the value of warm milk as an emetic and an emollient in giving relief from the effects of poisons is very apparent. Dr. B. Clark, an eminent English physician in the East Indies, says that sweet milk seldom fails to check and cure the most violent diarrhœa, stomach ache, and incipient cholera, if a pint is drank every four hours; it must not be boiled, but warmed enough to make it palatable. He says that it has never failed, in fifty times, to cure him of diarrhœa within six or eight hours. In one case of diarrhœa for eight months it acted like a charm; in two days the diarrhœa was gone, and in two or three weeks he became a hale, hearty man. In typhoid fever it promotes sleep, checks diarrhœa, cools the body, nourishes the system, wards off delirium, and prepares the way for cure. It will remain on the stomach sometimes when nothing else will. In scarlet fever give all the milk the patient will take; it keeps up the strength, and does good in other ways. It has been referred to in another page as a cure for diabetes; but when used in any of these cases, nothing else should be eaten or drank. Let the milk be the only food and beverage.

RHEUMATISM.

IF a hinge is dry or rusty or rough it moves heavily, harshly, and hard; every joint of the body is a hinge, and attached to each are certain little manufactories called

SYNOVIAL GLANDS,

whose office it is to prepare a lubricating fluid which answers to the joints the purpose of oil to a hinge; when this synovial fluid is dried up by fever, heat, inflammation, all which mean the same thing in this connection, the joints are dry, they do not move on one another easily, the slightest action gives pain; that is common rheumatism; this inflammation is the reaction of cold about the joints, rheumatism being the result of cold and wet to the joints or surrounding parts, and as it is caused by cold, its cure, in reality, is warmth ; but as it is deep-seated it requires a considerable time for the warmth to reach it, to exercise its sensitive influence, hence rheumatism is very tedious of cure. At the same time there are other causes of rheumatism besides cold and wet ; whatever can occasion heat about the joints and sheaths of the muscles can cause rheumatism ; hence there is :

1. Acute rheumatism, inflammatory rheumatism, or rheumati. fever.

2. Chronic rheumatism, affecting the joints and parts near them.

3. Syphilitic rheumatism of the long and flat bones, between the joints, not at them. The remedy for this, seldom failing, is ten, fifteen, or twenty grains of the iodide of potassium three times a day, until the symptoms have disappeared, and to be taken again should these symptoms return, and so often as they do return ; it is believed that this will cure where cure is possible ; it is a kind of inflammation of the live part of the bone, its outer covering, full of blood-vessels and nerves, called the

PERIOSTEUM.

This is always the result of venereal disease, from promiscuous sexual intercourse ; it sometimes fixes itself in the system for life, and perhaps from one single act, the work of almost an instant of time ! A merchant was on his way to Havanna in a steamer. Early one morning, as he was half dressed, a handsome Octoroon chambermaid, in the prime of young womanhood, was passing his stateroom door ; scarcely without a thought he threw out an arm about her, drew her in, and standing, there was an iniquitous consummation. Fourteen years later a physician was hastily called, he was laid in the middle of his own parlor, his wife and children about him, witnesses of his suffering and agony ; which he declared was unendurable—the result of that one act. For all these long years he had been a martyr to these tortures, at varying intervals. This is given more in detail, as an illustration of the infinite folly of any man trusting himself for one brief instant to any woman but his own lawful wife ; and also of the inconceivable weakness of intellect in any wife, who fails to afford those appeasements which nature calls for, and which, if not had in a rightful way, will be sought in a devious path, as above ; hence, any obstacles interposed, unless there be a positive physical necessity, endangering great injuries to the system or the constitution, tend to bring about domestic infelicities and infidelities, which but too often embitter the whole subsequent domestic life.

A WARNING TO YOUNG MEN.

Not long ago a young gentleman called for medical aid, a man of family, of high social position and of extensive business associations; he had been suffering from this form of rheumatism, which had located itself deep into the thigh bones; it was the daily bane of his life, the result of

ONE SINGLE ERROR,

long years ago. No hurry of business would keep those pains away; they were an incubus on every undertaking, sometimes disappearing for a time, and then without apparent cause suddenly returning; on 'change, at bank, at his counting-room; like an evil genius forever hovering around him; for many nights in succession sleep would be driven away for hours and hours together, until from sheer exhaustion he would forget himself in fitful slumbers as the morning dawned. He had sought medical advice in various directions; he had fled to the sea-shore, to the White Mountains, to the Pacific sea, to the Florida coast, and across the great waters to the opposite side of the globe; but there was that torturing pain which refused alike to be left in the burning sands of the south, the icebergs of the poles, on land or sea, and all for one transgression years ago. Let every unmarried man, every youth, take warning of this case, a representative one of millions of its kind, and never yield to the tempter, honorably reserving all for her, and her alone, who is or shall be the woman of his choice, his lawful married wife.

Arthritic rheumatism is a severer form of joint-affection attended with effusions, causing long-continued or permanent lameness.   Give the liver pill at ten days' interval, keeping the bowels acting freely and fully every day; between the pills follow rigidly the special fruit diet, and take thrice a day a tablespoon of the following mixture, into five ounces, or ten tablespoonfuls of peppermint water: one drachm of the wine of colchicum root, of the bicarbonate of potash and Rochelle salts, three drachms each.

MYALGIA,

or "muscle aching" literally, is the name given to that form of rheumatism which attacks the muscles of the body, as those of the chest, back, loins, and of the joints near these parts, and fibrous tissues generally.

LUMBAGO

is rheumatism of the loins, or joints of the small of the back.

SCIATICA

is rheumatism of the hip-joint.

PLEURODYNIA,

when the muscles of the chest are affected. Here again is an illustration of the "oneness of disease," and the oneness of the remedy. Various names are given, but the cause is one—inflammation, as a result of wet or cold applied to the part; the remedy is one—the liver pill and the special fruit diet; and notwithstanding the various names of the disease, as varied almost as the locality, the principles of treatment are the same—to relieve the "congestion" of the parts by means which act on the liver, which result in diminishing the quantity of the blood in the whole body, and, as a matter of course, the quantity in every part of it; this is done promptly, largely, and effectually, the liver pill not only acting on the liver, clearing out its channels, but the fruit diet cools the system and tends to clear out of it the contents of the bowels, thus largely also diminishing the total amount of blood. But in these varied rheumatic affections, whether acute or chronic, there are various aids to the medicine and diet; keep the parts warm every instant of time by soft woollen flannel bandages, or pads of cotton and wool, thick enough to keep up an abundant warmth.

Lemonade, half a gallon or more a day, between meals, pretty sour; next best is vinegar and water sweetened; all acids are cooling, but the vegetable acids are best.

In addition, if the bowels were made to act freely twice every day, a great point will be gained; do this, if it requires salts or castor oil or other laxative to be used every morning.

Rheumatic persons should stay in the house; time will be gained by it in the end, for slight dampness, slight cold drafts on a part bring back the pains; hence they will get well soonest of all these forms of rheumatism who most rigidly remain in the house, in a warm room, not under 65° in winter, taking care to keep it well ventilated when the joints or muscles are very painful.

HOT BATHS

are sometimes very grateful; they soothe the whole system; at other times relief is obtained by bathing the parts with tincture of arnica, or rubbing into the skin freely and well, twice a day, veratria ointment.

GONORRHŒAL RHEUMATISM.

Gonorrhœal rheumatism is caused by the absorption of gonor-rhœal matter into the blood; the speediest relief is attained by bleeding, but better to take a liver pill weekly and special fruit diet; take twice a day a dose of muriate of ammonia, and at night a quarter of a grain of sulphate of morphia in a teaspoonful of water on going to bed.

GONORRHŒA

itself is a disease from promiscuous intercourse; like syphilia, it never originates, it is always caught from another, like small-pox, hence those who live in lawful wedlock can never have either of them. Syphilia always affects the blood, and is never wholly ex-tricated from the system; the children born to such are always scrofulous, exhibiting itself in sore eyes, scabs on the scalp, and various forms of eruptions and ulcers, according to the constitu-tion of the patient and various attendant circumstances, occupa-tion and modes of life. Gonorrhœa is not such a disease. It comes on from one to ten days after exposure, and may last for weeks, sometimes leaving a chronic discharge which lasts indefinitely long, called a gleet. Gonorrhœa is always aggravated by walking or any form of exercise; it is cured certainly in a few days if the patient will go to bed, observe special fruit diet, and take Epsom salts night and morning, to keep the bowels acting freely twice every day without fail; if gonorrhœa is neglected, it is the more difficult to cure, and surgical assistance should be obtained. Gonorrhœa and syphilis are the only diseases resulting from impure intercourse; a single time is all-sufficient; simple introduction, without consummation, is all that is necessary; 'hence the infinite folly of voluntary exposure to such disgraceful and disgusting maladies. Both of them give out a yellowish matter, which is often left on the sheets in bed, and on privy seats, and handkerchiefs; if such matter should touch a sore part of another person, even the slightest scratch or abrasion, or the mucous surface of the eyes or nose or other part, the disease is as certainly imparted as small-pox would be if the same bed were occupied; hence the care which the intelligent and cultivated classes take while travelling never to sit on a privy seat so as to allow it to come in contact with the skin. Spread a paper over it by all means; if no paper, take a handkerchief, and then burn it; better walk a mile to the woods than run the risk, or manage in some way or other not to touch the seat with any part of the skin.

Hence also the keepers of all good hotels never put a guest in a bed on sheets which have been used by another; for this and other reasons good housekeepers in cities and large towns are very careful to have the sheets washed, even after a single night's use by a guest. In country places it is not thought necessary to have sheets washed oftener than once a month, and a dozen persons may sleep on them in succession; hence country hospitality does not cost much trouble.

Sometimes matter forms in the eyes, and a handkerchief is used; that handkerchief can impart the disease to the eyes of another, or to a chapped lip; sometimes the scalp is affected with ulcerous formations of the same kind; hence, never touch the handkerchief or comb or hairbrush of a stranger, any more than you would touch a carrion. These diseases have been adverted to, not so much with a view to give the treatment, as to impress upon the reader's mind the precautions just named, and also to fill it with utter detestation and abhorrence of impure sexual intercourse, and to give a hint to wives, that if husbands are driven by trifling excuses to obtain supplies elsewhere, these abominations may be brought home to them, and are brought home to them in multitudes of instances, to be infected themselves, and to have those infected with the degrading taint of blood who are born to them. Many a divorce originates in things like these, to be a living disgrace to father and mother and all the children for a whole life thereafter; for let it be remembered that in all cases of this sort, a cloud forever hangs around the character of divorced parties; however faultless and honorable and pure one party may be, the great public does not take pains to inform itself as to whether the grounds are just or not; it takes up the reproach greedily, rather likes it, often revels in it, especially when the parties are persons of position. The city physician has reason to believe that three divorces out of four can be traced to the fault of the wife; she pleads her husband's infidelity; the courts release her, for they look at the husband's dereliction, and are not authorized to go farther back and inquire what led him to infidelity to the marriage vow; if they did, they would find it in the conduct of a petted, spoiled, childish wife, taking her little revenges in interposing obstacles to accommodations, in spite sometimes, in mere waywardness often. In other cases where the husband is too honorable, too high-minded to commit a wrong himself because one has been committed by another, he may hold fast his integrity, but the charm is broken, the sun has gone behind a cloud, and happiness never dwells again in that household. These are suggestions not only for wives, but for mothers, to be made use of at a proper time, and thus enable their daughters to escape, and escape easily, the early stranding of the domestic ship.

There is, in connection with this subject, a

GONORRHŒAL OPHTHALMIA,

an inflammation of the eye caused by the matter of gonorrhœa coming in contact with the lid; it is the worst form of inflammation of the eyes; progressing very rapidly, and there is great danger of loss of sight. At first it seems merely a cold in the eye, but in a day or two matter begins to form at some spot in the eye; in colds the matter finds its way to the corners of the eyes, but in this form it is at one spot. Give at once a large dose of castor-oil, four tablespoons, and in a few hours, or at bedtime, a liver-pill, with a special fruit-diet, no meat, and keep the bowels acting twice every day with Epsom salts or castor-oil until the symptoms have entirely disappeared. After the oil has operated, apply a solution of nitrate of silver, five grains to an ounce of water, with a camel's-hair pencil. If gonorrhœa has been imparted to the mother before the birth of the child, it may take this form of eye-disease; if she suffers from leucorrhœa, the matter, in the passage of the infant, may come in contact with the eyelids, causing ··

PURULENT OPHTHALMIA.

In such case dissolve four grains of alum in two tablespoons of water, and with a little syringe wash the ailing part three or four times a day, keeping the bowels free, and giving nourishing food.

RHEUMATISM,

in the common acceptation of the term, is the result of a cold imparted to a particular portion of the body by a draught of air on it, or by damp clothing. If a person works hard, and perspires profusely, in a stooping position, especially if in the sun, the

"SMALL OF THE BACK,"

which embraces the loins, becomes very warm, the clothing next the skin is wet with perspiration; suppose it begins to rain, and the person has nearly completed the work in hand, there is an ambition to continue until it is done; but the rain is falling, and before he is aware the outer clothing is saturated with cold water, this chills the garment wet with perspiration, and the next morning the body is racked with

LUMBAGO.

Or suppose the same person, having completed the work, sits down to rest and the wind is blowing against his back, the clothing next the skin is cooled, there is a clammy dampness, more or less chilling the parts, causing lumbago, on the same general principles; if done a few times, either of these forms of exposure lays the foundation of

BRIGHT'S DISEASE,

so uniformly fatal. Hence rheumatism is a cold in the muscles or joints of the body, inducing inflammation; it is from a Greek word "rheuma," a flowing from, a defluxion, meaning thereby that rheumatism flows or shifts from one point to another, the essential idea of the word being motion, changing. Innumerable remedies have been advised for rheumatism; most of them give more or less of temporary relief, but the point is to eradicate it by removing the inflammation, which is a congestion of the arteries, as before explained.

For acute rheumatism the homœopathic remedies are aconite, when cheeks are red and there are shooting, tearing, racking pains, especially at night, preceded or followed by sulphur; belladonna, when there are burning pains; if pain is increased by every motion, give bryonia; if there is great restlessness, agitation, and tossing about, chamomilla is appropriate; give nux vomica when there is numbness, tightness, or partial paralysis; if there are burning, crampy, stitching pains in the muscles, give cimicifuga; if after getting better a relapse takes place, dulcamara is appropriate; if the pains are increased by the warmth of the bed, or towards morning, administer mercurius; lachesis, when there is pain, stiffness, or swelling in the part; if the pains are most in the wrists, finger-joints, and nape of the neck, take caulophyllum; if the stomach is deranged, or there is fever in the afternoon, followed with sweats, colchicum is serviceable, or veratrum viride; if the patient is scrofulous, give calcar. carb.

SPIRITS OF TURPENTINE,

rubbed freely and well into the skin over the rheumatic part, has been known to have an admirable and speedy effect in the removal of rheumatic pains. The skin should be covered with warm flannel.

Orris-root, carried in the pocket and chewed freely as tobacco is chewed, is said to have been efficacious. Permanganate of potash, in half-grain doses, although given in other ailments ten grains at a time, is said to be highly efficacious in acute rheumatism and where there are swellings in the joints. Take half a grain of the permanganate four times a day, in raspberry or other syrup, which makes it less nauseous. To be taken half an hour before meals, or two hours after, and once besides. Half an ounce of finely pulverized saltpetre, in half a pint of sweet oil, rubbed well into the skin, night and morning, gives welcome relief to pain. Flowers of sulphur, twenty grains, thrice a day in syrup, and good bandaging of the joint in fine old woollen flannel, do great good, says the London *Lancet.*

Oil of mustard, well rubbed into the skin of the part twice a day, is one of the most efficient remedies known.

As an internal remedy, take several lemons a day, or one every four hours, or drink freely of old or new cider. If either acts more than twice a day on the bowels, omit for awhile, but in all cases of rheumatism cause the bowels to act three times in two days, keep in a warm room of sixty-five degrees; do not go outside of the door until relieved, and live on the special fruit diet.

Rheumatism seems to be benefited at times by remedies which at others and in other persons are useless, and, as it is a very tedious and troublesome complaint, some of them are named; but no one need hope for any benefit from any source unless the patient keeps warmly dressed in a warm room, and avoids dampness in every form, whether in the air, or clothing, or skin. Keep the parts well rubbed with a mixture of hartshorn and sweet oil, half and half; rub it into the skin patiently and well, or a drachm of chloroform in two ounces of sweet oil. Either of these should be rubbed well into the skin, before the fire, on going to bed, and then wrap the part in soft, dry flannel, or keep oiled silk over it; at the same time, take in a little water thirty-five drops of the tincture of cohosh, with ten drops of elixir vitriol, twice a day.

On going to bed, bathe the parts well in very hot water, said to be more efficacious if potatoes have been boiled in the water; there would be one advantage in this course, the potatoes would be ready for breakfast next morning.

Acids seem to affect rheumatic pains favorably; as they have an influence on the action of the liver, it is worth the trial to take half a lemon four times a day, or drink largely of lemonade or buttermilk.   In very severe pains keep on a poultice of linseed meal and a strong decoction of valerian root.

————— ◦◦◦ —————

THE LUNGS.

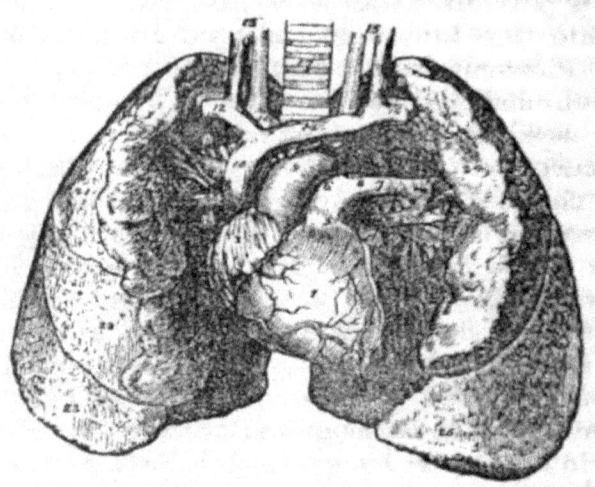

1. Is the heart's right ventricle or chamber.
7. The left pulmonary artery.
3. The right auricle.
4. Left auricle.
5. The pulmonary (lung) artery.
6. Right pulmonary artery.
8. Remains of the ductus arteriosus.
9. Aortic arch.
10. Superior vena cava.
11. Arteria innominata.
12. Right subclavian vein.
13. Right common carotid artery and vein.
14. Left vena innominata.
15. Left carotid artery and vein.
16. Left subclavian artery and vein.
17. Trachea or windpipe, the seat of croup and diphtheria.
18. Right bronchus, or branch of the windpipe.
19. Left bronchus.
20, 20. Pulmonary veins.
21. Upper lobe of right lung.
22. Its middle lobe.
23. Its inferior lobe.
24. Superior lobe of left lung.
25. Lower.

THE lungs are contained in a bag, called pleura; when it is inflamed, as by a bad cold, it is called

PLEURISY,

or more correctly, pleuritis, meaning inflammation of the pleura; if the lungs themselves are inflamed it is properly pneumonitis, or lung inflammation, generally denominated pneumonia, or lung fever. They are both dangerous diseases, especially pneumonia, usually fatal within a week, and even if the patient gets well, it is by painfully slow degrees, requiring weeks and months and even years. The treatment of both these diseases is essentially the same, both being congestion of the arteries, too full of blood ; formerly the old-school physicians emptied them speedily by bleeding the patient until he was about to faint ; no doubt in skilful and experienced hands it is still the quickest, safest, and best way, but there is such a prejudice against bleeding in these later years, that less decided means are almost universally relied on. Hydropaths use the wet sheet when called before there is much pain, but when the pain is decided, increased by cough, and there is difficult breathing, a wet compress or wrapper should be kept all over the chest, covered with a dry cloth ; it should be kept on without intermission, and in bad cases renewed every two or three hours. In addition, the tepid sitz-bath two or three times in twenty-four hours ; if the patient is weak, feet and hands cold, take the warm sitz-bath and warm foot-bath, even hot foot-bath rather than allow the feet to keep cold. Keep the bowels open twice a day with tepid enemas. If the expectoration is scant and sticky and hard to get up, drink warm water to the point of vomiting, and keep the body warm.

Homœopathy relies on aconite when there is arterial congestion, that is, inflammation. If intense pain in the side on the least motion, give cimicifuga racemosa ; if the phlegm is sticky and reddish and tough, take bryonia, and belladonna if the fever is rising. Phosphorus can be given to advantage in every stage of the disease, six globules in two tablespoons of water, one teaspoonful every three hours.

If there is great oppression, give antimonium ; and sulphur if there is any tendency to a relapse. Eat nothing whatever until the symptoms are certainly abating ; may drink toast water, whey, barley-water sweetened, and when the appetite begins to return eat very sparingly, and increase the amount very slowly.

The Allopathic treatment should be liver pill, acid drinks, live on fruits and coarse breads in very moderate quantities, keep quiet, warm, and composed. Pneumonia is a terrible disease to the feeble and the old. Thousands of clergymen die of it from going out of doors soon after speaking in a warm room, especially when they have to ride some distance immediately after service; it is pitiful to think how many useful and great men have been thus cut off in the flower of their age. For a man to ride on horseback, facing a raw, cold, damp wind, at any season of the year, soon after preaching, is almost as certain death within a week as standing before a rifle at the distance of fifty yards; and yet it is done, with greater or less aggravation, every year. Remaining in cold, damp rooms for a long time, or riding or walking in the cold, is a common cause of pneumonia. An old man walked against the wind on a very cold day, made a fire in his office and sat down to his law books, supposing that the room would soon get warm. He died of pneumonia in four days. The walk warmed him up, but before the fire kindled well he became chilled.

Sitting in damp clothing after having walked briskly, even in warm weather, is a sufficient cause for pneumonia. A great many old men die of it in the winter time, simply because they do not dress warm enough. Every man after forty years of age, north of thirty-five degrees, ought to put on his warmest clothing on the first day of November, and keep it on until the middle of June—that is, his inner clothing, the shirts which touch the skin of his body. This garment should be of thick, knitted yarn, thicker than any yarn stockings; on the first of December an article of the same kind should be worn as drawers. If this cannot be had, then two pair of woollen drawers, or at least one pair and a muslin pair over them; or, which may be still better, a common flannel shirt and over it a pervious doeskin shirt, or buckskin; it is soft and admirably adapted to keep the warmth of the body in, and to keep the cold wind from reaching it. In this climate, so changeable, damp, and raw from New Year's to the middle of April, a buckskin shirt should be worn over a woollen one by all women, by all sedentary persons, all students, and all men after fifty years of age. If any one man of intelligence can be induced to try it one winter fairly, and note the number of his days of indisposition, comparing them with any previous winter, there will be no difficulty in inducing him to repeat the experiment. To dress sufficiently warm, comfortably so, from the holidays to May, would prevent multitudes of bad colds, with their greater multitudes of ill results, and the suggestion is most earnestly pressed upon the attention of all concerned.

One of the reasons why a good covering for the body in winter is so highly beneficial is that the only point where the lungs are attached to the body is between the shoulder-blades behind, and that is the most important part of the chest to be protected; every observant person knows how soon he begins to take cold, even in warm weather, if the back is toward a door or window even if closed, because the little drafts of air coming through the cracks and crevices and joinings strike directly between the shoulders and chill the blood at the very fountain-head, the lungs. Hence, by all possible means, keep the space between the shoulder-blades behind well protected against the cold; a good expedient for gentlemen is to attach a padding of wool or cotton to the vest so as to cover the whole space; it will be found to be one of the greatest preventives of taking cold in winter-time ever tried, and costs but little of time or trouble or money.

No. 17 is the trachea or windpipe, the seat of that fearful disease

THE CROUP,

known to physicians as trachitis, or inflammation of the trachea. As stated elsewhere, croup is a congestion of blood in the arteries of the windpipe, congested to such an extent that the more watery portions of the blood exude and spread and thicken, until the windpipe is so nearly closed that breathing is difficult, and as the filling-up increases and the breathing becomes more labored, a kind of spasmodic contraction of the top of the windpipe takes place and the child is dead.

Croup is the result of cold, especially if connected with damp clothing or wet stockings. No mother should ever put her child, under seven years, to bed without feeling the feet, and if not warm, by all and every means warm them, as it may end in croup before the morning.

Being out of doors after sundown from November to May is a very frequent cause of croup in small children; in playing about their feet are very apt to get wet; or they get over-excited in their little play, are over-heated, and are very much inclined to stand in the wind, or at a corner on damp ground, or sit on a cold stone.

Croup usually comes on with a slight increase in the frequency of breathing about sundown or bedtime; the next morning it seems to be better and the mother is hopeful; but at night it is worse, and the third night or sooner it is regular croup; the child is restless, uneasy, it breathes hard and fast; the chest heaves, there is a kind of wheezing, barking, suppressed cough and dry; it does not seem to relieve any.

If mothers would apply remedies the first night, croup is as easily cured as a common cold, when taken in time.   The instant croupy threatenings are observed the child should be kept indoors, should eat very light food indeed, and not much of that, until the symptoms have abated.   Hydropathists invest the throat immediately in cloths, wet with water, very cold, as near ice-cold as possible, but so as not to dribble about; the wet cloth should be covered with a dry flannel one; these cloths should be renewed every two to ten minutes, according to the violence of the symptoms, to be continued by all means until the breathing is comfortably easy.

If there is not much fever, or if the skin is dry, put the child in a tepid bath of seventy-five degrees and then well wrapped up in a dry blanket until perspiration takes place.   But if there is much fever and hot skin, use the wet pack sheet, and renew until the fever abates; the bowels should be emptied at once with a warm-water enema; by all possible means keep the feet and hands warm.   If there is no expectoration and the child seems to be almost suffocating, give warm water copiously, until the use of a feather to tickle the throat induces vomiting; it is sometimes wonderful to see the good effects of this warm-water vomiting in cases of croup in children.

HOMŒOPATHIC TREATMENT.

As croup comes on with a short, difficult, or labored breathing, with a kind of whistling, squeaking sound, before the deep, hoarse-sounding cough is noticed, hepar sulphuris is given, with a warm bath; the temperature of the room to be not less than sixty-five; four globules in two tablespoonfuls of water, one teaspoonful every three hours until a decided change for the better; the moment the child comes out of the bath it should be warmly wrapped up in bed.

Use also a cold wet compress to the throat, covered with a piece of silk, overlapping the edges of the compress; if no silk, cover with a dry flannel; wet the rag as soon as it becomes hot and before it gets dry. When there is thirst, dry cough, and hurried breathing, take six globules of aconite in two tablespoonfuls of water, use one teaspoonful every half hour until there is a decided abatement of the symptoms. But if decided relief is not obtained in three or four hours, skin not getting moist, breathing no easier, but still difficult and wheezing, and the cough is dry, coarse, and hollow, then take spongia, six globules in two tablespoonfuls of water; a dose is one teaspoonful every half hour. Spongia is relied on of itself in many cases for the cure of croup when there is not very strong fever.

If the patient is cold, exhausted, and sinking, give three globules of arsenicum in a teaspoonful of water every ten minutes; if no prompt results, give, fifteen minutes after the third dose of arsenicum, three globules of antimonium tartaricum in a teaspoonful of water or in powder, put far back on the tongue every five minutes until decided improvement takes place. In general, continue to give hepar until all the diseased symptoms have passed away. It is of absolute importance in all practices to keep the patient abundantly warm throughout the attack, not less than sixty-five degrees; the slightest draught of air or chill should be carefully guarded against. The food should be warmed milk and water, half and half, during the sickness; increase the food very gradually at each meal, avoiding all stimulating drinks and irritating or hard food—fruits and bread and berries, with a little lean meat once a day.

ALLOPATHIC TREATMENT

goes on the principle that in no sickness is it of so much importance to do something in the earliest stages of the disease as in croup. Nauseating remedies are considered indispensable.

ALUM AND IPECAC.

Mix half a teaspoon each of powdered alum and ipecac in half a glass of tepid water, and give it as quickly as possible; if it does not vomit in ten minutes by the watch repeat the dose, with a teacup of warm water every five minutes until a feather or finger in the throat causes copious vomiting ; or, two grains of calomel every hour when the symptoms are not urgent ; but in the urgent cases, after vomiting, give two grains of calomel every three hours until the bowels are acted upon.

When there is a great deal of inflammation, indicated by high fever, the croupy cough and voice coming on very slowly and continuing steadily to increase, with the difficult breathing with a stridulous sound, then give ten grains of calomel mixed with one drachm of saltpetre, called nitrate of potash, divide into twelve powders, and give one every two hours.

The Greeks called croup the dog-choke, from its resemblance in the sound of the cough to the barking of a dog, as if something were drawn around his windpipe ; this choking sensation or result is owing, in part, to the filling up of the windpipe with unnatural secretions and exudations, as explained in the article on Congestion, which see ; this must be brought away, and vomiting is the remedy, and, however inconvenient and distressing to the child, the means should be persisted in until the most decided relief is obtained; sometimes half-teaspoon doses of powdered alum are sufficient, but it is better to be on the safe side and use the ipecac with it, or the child will die ; every moment adds to the chances of a fatal termination, and there should be no dallying or indecision. Croup is a disease which gets steadily worse every instant, but to wait, in hopes that it will pass away of itself, is trifling with life.

Some give with great success two drops of the tincture of veratrum viride. The great danger in croup is the hardening of the substance oozing out on the inside of the windpipe; it is known that lime antagonizes this hardening process, hence pour boiling water on unslaked lime, and cause the patient to breathe the steam of it ; but this is very difficult to do in cases of children. Perhaps the easiest plan would be to have the child in the mother's lap, envelop both with a blanket, and introduce the vessel so that its fumes rising up should come into the mouth of the child, which would be naturally kept open to get air under such circumstances. All these things are mentioned because croup is so common, is so urgently dangerous, the oozing out is so rapid, that it takes but a very short time to nearly fill up the child's windpipe, which is not more than a quarter of an inch in diameter at two years of age. To sum up all, in the Allopathic treatment of croup the best plan is, as soon as a child is seen to be restless at bedtime—for it is after night that the disease is most apt to manifest itself—and the breathing is labored and loud, the breast heaving a great deal more than natural, whether there be any cough or not, give two teaspoonfuls at once of Epsom salts in a cup of warm water, so as to unload the bowels as soon as possible, or use an enema; at the end of ten minutes give the alum and ipecac emetic as before-named; as soon as the vomiting has ceased, give every hour, until the bowels are acted upon, or at least until relief is most decided, one grain of calomel, five grains of nitrate of potash, with as much loaf sugar as would lie on a nickel cent; it can be given dry, put far back on the tongue, and washed down with water, or may be dissolved in two tablespoons or quarter of a teacup of water. If relief is not speedy put the child in a warm bath, its whole body, chin only above the water, having a cap on its head wet with cold water; in addition, dip flannels in boiling water, wring them out and apply to the throat, on the instant of applying, put a dry flannel over it to keep in the steam and renew every three minutes until decided relief has been obtained; ice-cold water, as advised by hydropathists, can be used in place of hot flannels, because a cold wet rag soon gets warm and conveys the heat away by evaporating rapidly. It may be known that the child is getting over the attack by the return to natural breathing, by coughing up the phlegm loosely, and becoming lively, instead of being restless and uneasy.

If the attack of croup is not very severe, if the cure is attempted at the beginning, the hydropathic method is simplest and best: ice-cold water to the throat, an enema, and warm water bath.

Or ice-water or hot flannel compresses to the throat will cure in most cases, without any medicine at all.

If a mother had once seen a case of child's croup treated, she would then know precisely what to do and how to do it; but to treat a case herself for the first time, and that, too, under the responsibility of its being her own child, it is scarcely possible to be too minute in the prescriptions, and to take it for granted that the young mother knows nothing.

Remember then, first, that the sooner you begin to treat a case of croup the more certain is the cure; that croup always comes on by restlessness, uneasiness, and a heaving of the breast in breathing; then the croupy, the barking, wheezing, imperfect cough; these may be all slight, and indeed no cough at all the first evening, and you may hope that it will pass off, that you may save yourself the trouble and the child the pain of treatment; and it may pass off, but to be more decided the next evening—for there is a tendency in most diseases to get worse at particular seasons, times, or hours—and the third evening it will come in all its violence; or the attack may have been so mild as not to have been observed;—the first thing then is an enema or laxative medicine, then the ice-cold compresses or boiling water flannel, to be renewed until the child is breathing easily, and is disposed to play or to be amused; if these encouraging symptoms do not soon appear, put the child in a warm bath, if you have no thermometer to measure seventy-five degrees put your hand in to see whether it is cold enough to shock, or hot enough to burn, let it be medium; put a cap on the head, wetted with cold water, not to dribble, put the feet in first, gradually sinking in the whole body in the course of a minute or two, then add hot water from time to time. The bath should be warmer when the child is taken out than when it was put in; keep it in until the breathing is easy, and the phlegm is loose; the instant of its coming from the bath, without taking time to wipe the body, envelop the child fully in a warm thick blanket, and in that blanket put it to bed.

In applying the hot or cold cloths to the throat, be careful that no water dribbles on the clothing, and keep the feet and hands warm; all the time held, if possible, in some one's hands.

Recapitulation.—The careful mother should keep an eye to children under seven in damp, raw, cold weather, to notice the very first appearing of croup, for then it is easily cured, being nothing more than a common cold which has not seated itself; one of the very first indications is carrying the hand towards the throat; then begin at once to apply the wet ice-cold bandages as elsewhere named, until the inflammation is entirely subdued, keeping the child in the same warm room with herself all the time, at least sixty-five degrees; be specially careful that there shall be no draught of air blowing on the child, and that the feet and hands are quite warm; do not ask the child to eat, but if hungry give some dry or toasted bread broken into hot tea, or gruel or sago, boiled rice, and the like, until all the symptoms have disappeared. It is singularly claimed that the worst cases are sometimes relieved by a stout, strong, healthy person drawing a full breath, and blowing it on the child's throat and chest, beginning under the chin ; repeat it breath after breath, and renew every ten minutes ; perhaps a bellows would do better on the principle of evaporation, and carrying off the heat. Onions cut into thin slices, each sprinkled over with loaf-sugar, soon yield a syrup ; a teaspoonful of this sometimes gives grateful relief, repeat every ten minutes.

SCROFULOUS SORES.

A FEW years ago a distinguished western millionnaire wrote of a favorite remedy for scrofulous ulcers : I have never heard of a case where it did not effect a speedy cure, and it can in no case do any injury. In several instances, where it has been applied to old sores, it has also speedily effected perfect cures. Put one ounce of aquafortis in a bowl or saucer ; drop in it two copper cents—it will effervesce—leave the cents in ; when the effervescence ceases, add two ounces of strong vinegar. The fluid will be a dark-green color. It should and will smart. If too severe, put in a little rain water. Apply it to the sore, morning and evening, by a soft brush or rag. Before applying it, wash the sore with water. Its first application known to me was a poor girl sent to our city from Memphis to have her leg cut off, as it was feared she might not live long enough to have it cut off in that hot climate. She was refused admittance to the poor-house, and was lying on the sidewalk, as she could not even stand up. From her knee to her foot one-third of the flesh gone and all the skin, except a strip about two inches wide. She was laid on a bed, and the remedy placed on a chair by it. She could rise up and apply it. In a few days her peace of mind returned, and she declared it was getting well. It was supposed it was a relief from the pain only, but when examined fresh flesh was found growing, and skin over it. She was soon running about and would work, which delayed the entire cure, leaving a small sore, which was in a few months entirely healed. A young girl, with scrofula in her neck, having a large open hole, and deemed incurable, came one month after, entirely cured, and recently married, with her husband, on their way to the East. I have never known a case where it did not effect a cure. This case is given to show how readily the organ of wonder is attached to what are called "simple" remedies. Everybody has seen a copper cent, every one knows or has heard of aquafortis. But pour some oil of vitriol, called sulphuric acid on some copper; let it evaporate, and bluestone will be the result; a teaspoonful of this, in a pint of water, and used as a wash, night and morning, will cure any common scrofulous sore; and it will kill, too, unless the bowels are kept freely acting every day, either with medicine or by the use a fruit and coarse bread diet, elsewhere described.

There is one general truth in reference to scrofula, which, if acted upon with a reasonable amount of intelligence, would save millions of money, millions of lives, and would prevent an incalculable amount of human suffering. In the first place, scrofula is utterly incurable by any human means. It is a blood impurity, a poison; and ever-watchful nature is constantly endeavoring to hustle it out of the system, as bees when an intruder is found in the hive. In throwing this humor out, it poisons the skin in its exit, giving a variety of appearances, according to the part of the skin on which it appears, and according also to a variety of other circumstances of condition, habit, constitution, about which little is as yet certainly known as in tetter, ringworm, sore eyes, itchings, pimples, splotches, and dozens of other things. Everything done to "cure" any kind of breaking-out on the body, or to dry it up, or drive it in, is an absurdity; it is a fighting against nature, and will always meet with a disastrous defeat. There are only two things to be done: 1st. Improve the general health. 2d. Keep the bowels acting, averaging three times in two days. In addition, never touch these things with anything stronger than pure water or glycerine.

ALLOPATHIC PRESCRIPTIONS.

It is believed that the following "recipes" of the most eminent medical men who have lived within the last third of century are not equalled in numbers and value in any book yet published, for they are the result of the life-long experience and observation of members of the profession, who, by their ability, have earned the respect and confidence of the most distinguished living physicians; and these are placed in the hands of the young practitioner, giving him at once advantages which others had at the close of life only.

The names of the authors of these prescriptions are seldom given, in order to prevent too implicit reliance on them; that if in any given case the desired results were not promptly observed, other means might be used without loss of time. The list has been brought down to the present year, so as to have the fullest advantage of the very latest discoveries and improvements, making this alone worth many times the money value of the entire volume to beginners in medicine and to all country practitioners, for the recipes are mainly from the books and private memoranda of city physicians at home and abroad, who have had large and varied and wide fields of observation; and in this respect the author hopes to have not only private families his debtors, but the whole medical profession, making it at once the interest of the people and of physicians of all schools to have the work in their libraries. Special attention should be given to what follows, as in many cases life and death hang on the proper understanding of a prescription. Various prescriptions are given for the same disease; first, because all of the ingredients of one may not be had; second, sometimes one medicine may be poisonous to one person or inert in another, according to some peculiarity of the constitution or condition of the patient, just as some persons "cannot bear" one kind of healthful food, as onions, while many are passionately fond of them; third, a medicine often has a good effect for a short time, and then becomes useless; in such cases it is of great importance to know some other remedy which is closely allied to it; in protracted cases it is often necessary to change several times.

Although the following prescriptions are in plain English, and figures are not used for fear of mistakes, an alphabetical table or dictionary of the signs and terms used by medical men is given, that medical prescriptions may be safely interpreted when not otherwise clearly explained. Bear in mind that sixty drops make one teaspoonful; four teaspoonfuls make one tablespoon; two tablespoons make one ounce; four tablespoons make one wineglass; two wineglasses make one gill; four gills make one pint. To save space, drachm, meaning one teaspoonful of liquid or sixty grains in weight, is spelled dram; and when there is the measure of a fluid ounce, the word fluid is left out, and oz. is a contraction for ounce.

ABBREVIATIONS OF MEDICAL FORMS.

It will be noticed that almost all the terms are Latin. Where water is used to mix up medicines, it is to be understood that rain or snow water is best, or distilled water, or water which has been boiled. Spring or well or river waters have various ingredients, and some of them antagonize some medicines. But nine times out of ten the water used for drinking purposes is good enough.

MEDICAL ABBREVIATIONS.

B. *Recipe*, take.
A. ββ, *ana utriusque*, of each.
℔. *Libra*, a pound.
℥. *Uncia*, an ounce.
f℥. A fluid ounce.
℈. *Drachma*, a dram.
f℈. A fluid dram.
℈. *Scrupulum*, a scruple.
℔. *Minimum*, a minim.
ss. *Semissis*, half; jss., one and a half.
j. One; ij., two; iij., three.
Abs. Febr., in absence of fever.
Ad., add.
Ad lib. *Ad libitum*, at pleasure.
Altern. hor., every other hour.
Aq. *Aqua*, water.
Aq. comm. *Aqua com.*, common water.
Aq. bull., boiling water.
Aq. ferv. *Aqua fervens*, hot water.
Aq. font. *Aqua fontis*, spring water.
Bib. *Bibe*, drink.
Bis. ind. *Bis indies*, twice daily.
Bol. *Bolus*, a large pill.
Bull. *Bulliat*, let it boil.
Cap. *Capiat*, let him take.
Chart. *Chartula*, a small paper.
Cochl. *Cochleare*, a spoonful.
Cochl. ampl. *Cochleare amp.* a tablespoonful.
Cochl. mod., a dessertspoonful.
Cochl. parv., a teaspoonful.
Col. *Cola*, strain.
Collyr. *Collyrium*, an eye-water.
Comp. *Compositus*, compound.
Conf. *Confectio*, confection.
Cons. *Conserva*, conserve.
Cont. *Continuetur*, be continued.
C. or cong. *Congius*, a gallon.
Coq. *Coque*, boil.
Cort. *Cortex*, bark.
C. M. *Cras mane*, to-morrow morning.
C. N. *Cras nocte*, to-morrow night.
Crast. *Crastinus*, for to-morrow.
Cuj. *Cujus*, of which.
Cujusl. *Cujuslibet*, of any.
Cyath. *Cyathus*, a glassful.
Cyath. theæ, a cup of tea.

D. *Dosis*, a dose.
D. *Detur*, let it be given.
Decub. *Decubitus*, lying down.
Dec. *Decanta*, pour off.
De D. in D., from day to day.
Dep. *Depuritus*, purified.
Dieb. altern., every other day.
Dieb. tert. *Diebus ter.*, every third day.
Dig. *Digeratur*, let it be digested.
Dil. *Dilutus*, dilute.
Dim. *Dimidius*, one-half.
Dist. *Distilla*, distil.
Div. *Divide*, divide.
Ejusd. *Ejusdem*, of the same.
Enem. *Enema*, a clyster.
F. *Fiat*, let it be made.
F. pil. *Fiat pil.*, make into a pill.
Feb. dur., fever continuing.
Fl. *Fluidus* and *Flores*, fluid and flowers.
Gr. *Granum*, a grain.
Gtt. *Guttæ*, drops; Gt., *Gutta*, a drop.
Guttat. *Guttatim*, by drops.
Hor. decub. *Horâ decubitûs*, at bedtime.
Hor. interm., at intermediate hours.
H. S. *Horâ somni*, at bed-time.
Inf. *Infunde*, infuse.
Ind. *Indies*, daily.
Liq., liquor.
Lb. or lib. *Libra*, a pound weight.
M. *Misce*, mix.
Mac. *Macera*, macerate.
Man. *Manipulus*, a handful.
Man. prim. *Mane primo*, early in the morning.
Mic. pan. *Mica panis*, crumb of bread.
Min. *Minimum*, the sixtieth part of a dram.
Mitt. *Mitte*, send.
Mist. *Mistura*, a mixture.
Muc. *Mucilago*, mucilage.
O. *Octarius*, a pint.
Ol. *Oleum*, oil.
Omn. bih. *Omni bihorio*, every two hours.
Omn. hor. *Omni horâ*, every hour.

Omn. man. *Omni mane*, every morning.
Omni nocte, every night.
Oz. *Uncia*, an ounce.
P. Æ. *Partes æquales*, equal parts.
Pil. *Pilula*, a pill.
P. R. N. *Pro re natâ*, as occasion may be.
Pulv. *Pulvis*, a powder.
Q. S. *Quantum sufficit*, as much as wanted.
Rad. *Radix*, a root.
Rep. *Repetatur*, let it be repeated.
Rec. *Rectificatus*, rectified.
S. A. *Secundum artem*, according to art.
Sem. *Semen*, seed.

S. *Sumat*, let him take.
Solv. *Solve*. Dissolve. SS. *Semi*, one-half.
Semi-H. *Semi horâ*, half an hour.
Sesquih. *Sesquihora*, an hour and a half.
Si op. sit. *Si opus sit*, if there be need.
St. *Stet*, let it stand.
S. V. *Spiritus vini*, spirit of wine (alcohol).
S. V. R., spiritus vini rectificatus.
Syr. *Syrupus*, syrup.
Tr. and tinct., tinctura, tincture.
Trit. *Tritura*, triturate.
V. O. *Vitellum ovi*, yolk of egg.

ANÆMIA AND DEBILITY.—Extract of hemlock, one dram; sesquioxide of iron, two drams; tincture of colomba, two oz.; syrup of tolu, half an oz.; oil of partridge-berry, ten drops; water, two oz. Take one teaspoonful night and morning.

Sesquioxide of iron, four drams; extract dandelion, six drams; sherry wine, five oz.; tincture of partridge-berry or gaultheria, three fluid drams; water, four oz. One tablespoonful twice a day.

Citrate of iron, two and a half drams; syrup of orange-peel, two and a half oz.; peppermint water, two oz.; water, four oz. One teaspoonful four times a day.

Phosphate of iron, sixty grains; sulphate of quinine, twelve grains. Mix and divide in twelve powders. Take one three times a day.

Liquor of the iodide of iron, half an oz. Take fifteen drops in water, thrice daily.

Tincture of chloride of iron, half an oz.; take twenty drops thrice daily.

Citrate of iron, two drams; water, five oz. and a half; simple syrup, half an oz. Take from a teaspoonful to a tablespoonful thrice daily, before or after meals, for children.

AMENORRHŒA.—Powder of aloes, one to two scruples; oil of cloves, five drops. Mix, and divide into twenty pills. Take one twice or thrice daily.

Aloes, twenty grains; Quevenne's metallic iron (per hydrogen), half a dram; oil of cloves, four drops. Mix, and divide into twenty pills. Take one thrice daily.

Compound decoction of aloes, three oz.; borax, one dram; compound tincture of aloes, four drams; tincture of castor, half an oz.; water, two oz. Take a tablespoonful three times a day.

Proto-iodide of mercury, three grains; iodide of potassium, two drams; tincture of gentian, three oz.; water, two oz.; simple syrup, one and a half oz. Take a teaspoonful three times a day.

Powdered guaiac, four ounces; carbonate of soda and carbonate of potassa, each fifty grains; powdered allspice, one dram; alcohol, one pint. Macerate four days, and add five fluid drams of spirits of ammonia. Take a teaspoonful three times a day in a glass of sweetened milk.

Sulphate of iron, one and a half drams; iodide of potassium, two drams; tincture of cardamom, one oz.; simple syrup, one and a half oz.; water, one oz. Mix, and take a teaspoonful three times a day.

Carbonate of iron, three drams; tincture of colomba, two fluid drams; syrup of ginger, two fluid drams. One teaspoonful night and morning.

Powdered alum, twenty grains; sulphate of iron, sixteen grains; calomel, five grains. Make sixteen pills. Take one thrice daily.

Iodide of potassium, two drams; wine of colchicum, one and a half fluid drams; syrup of sarsaparilla, three oz.; water, one oz. One teaspoonful three times a day.

Powdered aloes, two drams; sulphate of iron, forty grains; powdered myrrh, two drams. Divide into forty pills. Take two twice a day; bowels need moving.

Wine of colchicum seed, one oz.; tincture of stramonium, four drams; tincture of black snakeroot, or cimicifuga, one and a half oz. Take a teaspoonful three times a day, for painful menstruation.

Citrate of iron, two drams; syrup of orange peel, two and a half oz.; peppermint water, two oz.; water, three oz. One teaspoonful three times a day.

ANGINA PECTORIS, RETROCEDENT GOUT.—Chloroform and aromatic spirit of ammonia, each two fluid drams; Hoffman's anodyne and paregoric, each half an oz.; mucilage of gum-arabic, one oz. Mix. Take a teaspoonful at once.

ANGINA PECTORIS, OR GOUT OF THE STOMACH.—Bicarbonate of soda, four scruples; aromatic spirit of ammonia, one fluid dram; compound spirit of ether, one oz.; compound tincture of cardamom, three fluid drams; water and mucilage of gum-arabic, each an oz. and a quarter. Mix. Take a dessert-spoonful or tablespoonful at once.

ASTHMA.—Tincture of lobelia and wine of ipecacuanha, each an oz. Take one-half teaspoonful every half hour until expectoration or nausea occurs.

Tincture of lobelia, one oz. Give two teaspoonfuls every half hour until vomiting.

Blood-root, seventy grains; hot water, half a pint. One tablespoonful every ten minutes until vomiting.

Solution of strychnine, two drams; tincture of lobelia, two drams; syrup of tolu, two oz. Take teaspoonful four times a day.

Iodide of potassium, two drams; decoction of seneka, five oz.; tincture of lobelia, one oz.; paregoric, one oz. Take teaspoonful three times a day.

BRONCHITIS.—Nitrate of potassa, two drams; oxymel of squills, one oz.; tincture of digitalis, a fluid dram; vinegar, a tablespoonful; sugar and gum-arabic, each two drams; water, enough to make in all six oz. Mix. Take a tablespoonful every three hours.

BRONCHITIS WITH DRY COUGH.—Tartar-emetic, one grain; syrup of squills, three oz. Take a teaspoonful every four hours.

Hydrocyanic acid, sixty drops; sulphate of morphia, three grains; tincture of blood-root, one fluid oz.; wine of ipecac, three drams; almond emulsion, four fluid oz. Take a teaspoonful three times a day.

Hydrocyanic acid, thirty drops; wine of antimony, half an oz.; syrup of tolu, three drams; mucilage of gum-arabic, two oz. One teaspoonful four times a day.

Hydrocyanic acid, one dram; liquor potassa, half an oz.; infusion of colomba, two oz.; almond emulsion, three and a half oz. Take a teaspoonful three times a day.

Syrup of squills, four oz.; paregoric, one oz. Take a teaspoonful three times daily, and two at night.

Muriate of ammonia, four drams; mucilage of gum-arabic, four oz. Mix. Take a tablespoonful four times daily.

Balsam of copaiba, four fluid drams; compound spirit of lavender, two fluid drams; white sugar and gum-arabic, each two drams; water, enough to make six oz. Mix. Take a tablespoonful thrice daily.

Decoction of seneka, four oz.; iodide of potassium, two and a half drams; wine of antimony, four drams; syrup of tolu, two oz. Mix, and take a teaspoonful three times a day.

Decoction of seneka, five oz.; syrup of tolu, two fluid drams; paregoric, two and a half fluid drams; tincture of squills, two fluid drams; carbonate of ammonia, twenty grains. Mix, and take a teaspoonful three times a day.

Ammoniac mixture, six oz.; syrup of squills, one and a half oz.; paregoric, half a fluid dram; tincture of hyoscyamus, one fluid dram; wine of ipecac, three fluid drams. Mix, and take a tablespoonful as required.

Decoction of seneka, three oz.; honey of squills, two drams; wine of ipecac, two drams; wine of antimony, four drams. Give twenty drops every fifteen minutes until vomiting occurs, afterwards five drops every two hours.

Decoction of seneka, five oz.; iodide of potassium, three drams; paregoric, one and a half oz.; syrup of tolu, one and a half oz. Take a teaspoonful twice a day.

Iodine, six grains; iodide of potassium, one and a half drams; tincture of cardamom, one and a half oz.; compound syrup of sarsaparilla, three oz. Take a tablespoonful twice a day, for scrofulous cases.

Syrup of the iodide of iron, seven drams; iodide of potassium, twelve grains; pure glycerine, one and a half oz.; syrup of lemons, one oz.; water, three and a half oz. One tablespoon thrice daily.

Dover's powder, or compound powder of ipecac, sixty grains; tartar emetic, three grains; calomel, twelve grains; mucilage of gum-arabic, a sufficient quantity to form a pilular mass. Divide in twelve pills. Take two morning and night.

Powdered ipecac, sixty grains; infusion of Virginia snake-root, six and a half oz.; paregoric, two and a half drams. Take a teaspoonful every hour.

Tartar emetic, two drams; powdered camphor, seventy grains; fresh lard, one oz. Mix and form ointment. Wet the skin on front of the chest with strong vinegar, and then rub on thoroughly the ointment to produce pustular eruption.

BILIOUSNESS.—Take a powder of rhubarb root, magnesia, and prepared charcoal powder, each a teaspoonful; powdered ginger, one teaspoonful. Mix, and divide into three parts. Take one every morning.

Tartar emetic, four grains; powdered ipecac, twenty grains; water, four oz.; one tablespoonful every twelve minutes, until vomiting.

Extract of gentian and powder of rhubarb, each half a dram; blue mass, four grains; oil of cloves, four drops. Mix, and divide into twenty pills. Take one three or four times daily for a few days, for bilious colic.

Aromatic spirit of ammonia, and spirit of camphor, each a fluid dram; tincture of ginger, two fluid drams; bicarbonate of soda, four scruples; peppermint water, enough to make four oz. Dose, a tablespoonful.

BALDNESS, PREMATURE.—Aromatic spirit of ammonia, spirit of rosemary and glycerin, each an oz.; tincture of cantharides, three fluid drams; water, enough to make six oz.; mix and rub into the scalp daily.

BALDNESS.—Balsam of tolu, two drams; oil of rosemary, thirty minims; tincture of cantharides, two fluid drams; castor oil, four fluid drams; lard, an oz. Rub it into the head daily.

BLADDER, IRRITATED.—Dissolve one oz. of borax and three oz. of glycerin in two oz. of water. Of this, for use, add two or three teaspoonfuls to four oz. of warm water. Inject into the bladder through a catheter.

Benzoic acid, two drams; water, six oz. Dissolve. Take a tablespoonful thrice daily.

BRAIN CONGESTION: AS A CATHARTIC.—Resin of jalap, half a dram to a dram; squills, fifteen grains to a scruple. Mix, and divide into twelve powders. Take one twice a day.

Carbonate of manganese, one dram; carbonate of iron, one and a half dram; powdered white sugar, one and a half dram. Mix, and divide into fifteen powders. Take one thrice daily.

Carbonate of manganese, two drams; carbonate of iron, two and a half drams.

CHLOROSIS.—Tincture of colomba, three oz.; syrup sarsaparilla, four oz. One tablespoonful twice daily.

Sixteen grains each of aloes and sulphate of iron; make sixteen pills. Take one or two thrice daily.

Syrup of iodide of iron. Take twenty-five drops thrice a day.

CHOREA, OR ST. VITUS' DANCE.—Extract of hyoscyamus, one dram; valerianate of iron, two drachms. Mix, and divide in sixty pills. Take one three times a day; or purge, and then take—

Black snake-root, one ounce; boiling water, one pint. Two tablespoonfuls three times a day.

Extract of hyoscyamus, forty grains; valerianate of zinc, forty grains; subnitrate of bismuth, sixty grains. Mix, and divide in forty pills. Take one three times a day.

CONSUMPTION.—Cod-liver oil, thirty drams; alcohol, twelve drams; essence of peppermint, twenty-four grains. Mix. Take a dessert-spoonful thrice daily.

Iodide of potassium, three drams; syrup of ipecac, two oz.; water, four oz. One teaspoonful thrice a day.

Iodide of potassium, two drams; hydrocyanic acid, forty drops; sarsaparilla syrup, three oz.; water, one oz. Take one teaspoonful night and morning.

Muriate of ammonia, thirty grains; powdered opium, ten grains; powdered digitalis, twenty grains; powdered squills, twenty-five grains. Make thirty pills. Take one every six hours, to promote expectoration in early stages.

Phosphate of manganese, two drams ; tincture of Peruvian bark, three oz. ; syrup of sarsaparilla, four oz. ; mucilage of gum-arabic, one and a half oz. ; oil of partridge-berry, twenty drops. Take two teaspoonfuls three times a day ; shake before taking.

Phosphate of manganese, two drams ; phosphate of iron, three drams ; tincture of colomba, two and a half oz. ; syrup of tolu, three and a half oz. ; essence of partridge-berry, one dram. Shake and take two teaspoonfuls three times a day.

Malate of manganese, two drams ; tincture of Peruvian bark, two oz. ; simple syrup, four oz. ; essence of lemon, one and a half drams. Take a teaspoonful night and morning.

Iodide of potassium, two drams ; tartar-emetic, two grains ; syrup of ginger, two and a half oz. ; water, three oz. Take a teaspoonful twice a day.

Iodide of potassium, two and a half drams ; syrup of ipecac, two oz. ; water, four and a half oz. Take a teaspoonful three times a day.

Syrup of the iodide of iron, six drams ; iodide of potassium, twelve grains ; pure glycerine, one oz. ; syrup of lemons, one and a half oz. ; water, three and a half oz. Mix, and take a tablespoonful three times a day, before meals.

Tincture of blood-root or sanguinaria, a fluid dram ; acetate of morphia, three grains ; antimonial wine, or wine of tartar-emetic, three fluid drams ; wine of ipecac, three fluid drams ; syrup of wild cherry bark, three oz. Mix, and take a teaspoonful three times a day.

The above is said to be the original formula for "Ayer's Cherry Pectoral."

Tincture of blood-root or sanguinaria Canadensis, one oz. ; tincture of opium or laudanum, two fluid drams ; wine of ipecac, six fluid drams ; syrup of tolu, two and a half oz. Mix, and take sixty drops four times a day.

Tincture of blood-root, one oz. ; sulphate of morphia, one and a half grains ; tincture of foxglove or digitalis, three drams ; wine of tartar-emetic, one-half oz. ; oil of partridge-berry, fifteen drops. Take thirty drops three times a day.

Glycerine, three oz. ; syrup of iodide of iron, four drams ; sulphate of morphia, two grains. Take a teaspoonful four times a day.

Glycerine, three oz. ; hypophosphite of soda, one oz. ; sulphate of morphia, three grains. Take a teaspoonful four times a day.

Iodide of potassium, one dram ; proto-iodide of mercury, ten grains ; ointment of rose-water, one oz. Mix and form ointment. Rubbed on night and morning over the diseased lung, the above forms an excellent counter-irritant.

COLIC.—Chloroform, a fluid oz. ; camphor water, water, and mucilage of gum-arabic, each a fluid oz. Mix. Dose, from a teaspoonful to a tablespoonful, *repeated cautiously.*

Bicarbonate of soda, half a drachm ; aromatic spirit of ammonia, half a fluid dram ; solution of morphia, half a fluid dram ; syrup of ginger, half an oz. ; water, enough to make two oz. Mix. Dose, a teaspoonful, repeated if necessary.

Carbonate of magnesia, sixty grains ; tincture of assafetida, half a fluid dram ; tincture of opium, forty drops ; white sugar, two drams ;

water, two oz. Mix, and give thirty drops as often as required; especially useful in flatulent colic, sour stomach, and diarrhœa of young children. Or : prepared chalk, sixty grains ; white sugar, sixty grains; powdered gum-arabic, two drams ; cinnamon water, four oz. Mix, and give a teaspoonful three times a day.

Spiced syrup of rhubarb, compound tincture of cardamom, paregoric, and water, each an oz. Mix. Dose, from a dessertspoonful to a tablespoonful.

CANCER.—Dissolve in absolute alcohol as much pure tannin as it will dissolve in two days. Then add enough washed ether to make the thick tincture quite fluid. Saturate this with xyloidin or gun-cotton. Lastly, add twenty drops of tincture of benzoin.

Dissolve one dram of pure tannin in as little absolute alcohol as will dissolve it, and then add it to one oz. of collodion. Use externally.

Fowler's solution of arsenic, two oz. ; compound liquor of the iodide of potassium, four drams. Take five drops in a little water three times a day, and use the following ointment externally :

Iodide of lead, two drams ; lard, two oz. Mix thoroughly, and rub the cancerous or other indolent tumor with it twice a day.

CHOLERA.—Chloroform, laudanum, spirit of camphor, and aromatic spirit of ammonia, each a fluid dram and a half ; creasote, four drops ; oil of cinnamon, eight drops ; alcohol, two fluid drams. Twelve drops in some water is a dose.

2. Chloroform, two fluid drams ; spirit of camphor, a fluid dram ; alcohol, three drams. Mix. Dose, fifteen drops in water.

COMMON SUMMER CHOLERA MORBUS.—Magnesia, a dram ; aromatic spirit of ammonia, a dram ; water, four oz. Mix. To be shaken before administration. Take a teaspoonful every half hour.

Chloroform, half a troy oz. ; camphor, one dram ; the yolk of one egg ; water, six oz. Rub the yolk in a mortar, first by itself, then with the camphor, previously dissolved in the chloroform, and lastly with the water, gradually added. This is the "Mixture of Chloroform," of the United States Pharmacopœia. Dose, two teaspoonfuls.

INCIPIENT CHOLERA INFANTUM.—Calomel, three grains ; bicarbonate of soda, one scruple ; powder of ginger, twelve grains. Mix, and divide in twelve powders. Give one three or four times daily.

EARLY STAGE OF CHOLERA INFANTUM.—Mercury with chalk, and powder of cinnamon, each fifteen grains. Mix, and divide into twelve powders. Give one thrice daily.

CHOLERA INFANTUM. — Aromatic spirit of ammonia, twenty drops; paregoric, half a fluid dram to a fluid dram ; spiced syrup of rhubarb, an oz. ; peppermint water, enough to make two oz. Mix. Give a teaspoonful every three hours.

To check the DIARRHŒA OF CHOLERA INFANTUM.—Tincture of krameria and paregoric, each a fluid dram ; sugar and gum arabic, each half a dram ; water enough to make two oz. Give a teaspoonful every three hours.

CONSTIPATION.—Rhubarb root and Castile soap, each forty grains ; oil of anise, four drops. Mix, and divide into twenty pills. Take one or two as required.

Rhubarb, Castile soap, and compound extract of colocynth, each thirty-five grains. Mix, and divide into twenty pills. Take one or two as required.

Rhubarb, two scruples; aloes, one scruple; extract of nux vomica, five grains. Divide into twenty pills. Take one at a time.

Bicarbonate of soda, one dram; compound tincture of cardamom, one oz.; spirit of camphor, one fluid dram; syrup of rhubarb, half an oz.; water, enough to make four oz. Take a teaspoonful at once.

Resin of podophyllum, two grains; fluid extract of rhubarb and fluid extract of senna, each an oz.; oil of cloves, five drops; syrup of ginger, half an oz.; mucilage of gum-arabic, enough to make four oz. Dose for an adult, a tablespoonful.

To ACT UPON THE BOWELS.—Cut a piece of good yellow soap to the shape, and rather less than the size, of the last joint of the little finger. Dip it in lard, and introduce it within the rectum.

FOR TORPOR OF THE BOWELS.—Compound extract of colocynth and white soap, each forty grains; extract of nux vomica, five grains. Mix, and divide into twenty pills. Take one night and morning.

HABITUAL CONSTIPATION.—Rhubarb and aloes, each half a dram; extract of belladonna, four grains; oil of cloves, three drops. Mix, and divide into twenty pills. Take one twice daily.

CONSTIPATION IN INFANTS.—Resin of podophyllum, one grain; simple syrup of rhubarb, an oz.; oil of fennel, one drop. Mix. Dose, half a teaspoonful.

Calomel, sixty grains; ten drams white sugar, into five-grain powders, one at bedtime, put far back on the tongue, and rinse mouth well.

Extract of podophyllum, one dram; aloes, three drams. Make sixty pills; one to four at bedtime.

Extract of podophyllum, two drams; calomel, one dram; oil of cajeput, six drops. Make into sixty pills. Dose, two to five.

Podophyllin, fifteen grains; powdered ginger, thirty grains; extract of gentian, forty grains. Make thirty pills. Take one to three, at bedtime.

Podophyllin, sixty grains; white sugar, two oz. Mix thoroughly. Dose, six grains of the powder. An excellent substitute for calomel.

Saturated tincture of blood-root or sanguinaria, two oz.; compound tincture of aloes, two oz. Take sixty drops, twice a day.

Powdered blood-root, and powdered rhubarb, each one dram; Castile soap, fifty grains. Mix and divide in thirty-two pills. Take one night and morning.

COUGH.—Musk, two scruples; syrup of orange-peel, 2oz.; mucilage of gum-arabic, three oz. Mix. Take a tablespoonful every two or three hours.

VIOLENT, TROUBLESOME COUGH.—Dilute hydrocyanic acid, twenty drops; syrup of wild cherry and camphor-water, each one oz. Mix. Dose, a teaspoonful every two or three hours.

Syrup of wild cherry and syrup of lactucarium, each two oz. Mix. Take a tablespoonful at night, or one or two teaspoonfuls during the day.

Syrup of squills, two oz.; Hoffman's anodyne (compound spirit of ether) and solution of morphia (one grain in the oz.), each an oz.; camphor-water and mucilage of gum-arabic, of each an oz. and a quarter. Mix. Dose, from a teaspoonful to a tablespoonful.

Decoction of seneka, four oz.; syrup of tolu, half an oz.; sulphate of morphia, one grain; extract of wild cherry bark, four drams. Take a tablespoonful as required.

Canadian balsam, one oz.; liquor potassa, one oz.; wine of ipecac, four drams; syrup of tolu, one and a half oz.; water, two oz. Take a teaspoonful three times a day.

Canadian balsam, six drams; cyanide of potassium, one and half grains; tincture of aconite, one dram; liquor potassa, one dram; syrup of tolu, five drams; water, three oz. Mix, and take a teaspoonful when required.

CATARRH.—Saturated tincture of blood-root, or sanguinaria, two oz.; wine of ipecac, two oz. Take fifty drops every four hours. An excellent febrifuge.

Tincture of blood-root, one oz.; laudanum, two drams; wine of ipecac, six drams; syrup of tolu, two and a half oz. Take sixty drops four times a day.

Decoction of seneka, four oz.; iodide of potassium, 2 drams; wine of antimony, four drams; syrup of tolu, two oz. Mix, and take a teaspoonful four times a day.

Powdered seneka, two drams; powdered ipecac, one dram; honey, two oz.; hot water, six oz. Take a teaspoonful, repeating as circumstances require.

Balsam copaiba, four drams; paregoric, one oz.; wine of ipecac, half an oz.; syrup of gum-arabic, two and half oz.; oil of partridge-berry, twenty drops. Take a teaspoonful three times a day.

Acetate of morphia, four grains; cyanide of potassium, three grains; wine of antimony, and wine of ipecac, each two drams; tincture of blood-root, five drams; syrup of tolu, three oz. Mix, and take a teaspoonful four times a day.

CROUP.—Powder of ipecacuanha and powder of alum, each a teaspoonful. Mix with water. Repeat in ten minutes until vomiting.

INFLAMMATORY.—Calomel, fifteen grains; nitrate of potassa, one dram; sugar, one scruple. Mix, and divide into twelve powders. Take one every three hours.

MEMBRANOUS.—Nitrate of silver, ten grains; water, half an oz. Dissolve. Apply with a camel's-hair pencil to the throat.

Tartar-emetic, one grain; powdered ipecac, ten grains; warm water, four oz. Give a teaspoonful every fifteen minutes until the child vomits.

Sulphate of zinc, ten grains; powdered ipecac, twenty grains; warm water, four oz. Give a teaspoonful every ten or fifteen minutes until vomiting.

Turpeth mineral, or yellow sulphate of mercury, ten grains; simple syrup, five drams. Mix, and give a teaspoonful every twelve minutes until vomiting.

Blood-root, sixty grains; hot water, half a pint. Mix and macerate for an hour, and give teaspoonful every fifteen minutes until the child vomits.

Wine of ipecac, three drams; syrup of tolu, four drams; mucilage of gum-arabic, one oz. Mix, and give a teaspoonful every two hours.

Powdered ipecac, sixty grains; infusion of Virginia snakeroot, or serpentaria, six oz.; paregoric, two drams. Mix, and give a teaspoonful every hour or every half hour.

CATHARTIC.—Resin of jalap, thirty grains. Divide into three parts. Give one every four hours till they operate.

CATHARTIC AND CHOLAGOGUE.—Resin of podophyllum, three grains; Turkey rhubarb, eight grains; oil of anise, two drops. Divide into eight pills. Take one or two at once.

AS A POWERFUL CATHARTIC, IN RARE CASES.—Croton oil, five drops; crumb of bread or conserve of roses, a sufficient quantity to make four pills. Mix, and divide. Take one every four hours, until they operate.

PROMPT CATHARTIC.—Mix a tablespoonful each, of castor oil and molasses, with a pint of warm water, in which a little Castile soap has been dissolved. Inject into the rectum with a syringe.

FOR FLATULENT PAIN IN THE BOWELS.—Oil of cajeput, half a dram; compound spirit of lavender, an oz.; syrup of ginger, two fluid drams; mucilage of gum-arabic, enough to make two oz. Take a dessert-spoonful at once.

DYSPEPSIA.—Hydrocyanic acid, sixty drops; extract belladonna, ten grains; tincture colomba, one oz.; simple syrup, one and a half oz.; water, one and a half oz. Mix, and take a teaspoonful four times a day.

Extract nux vomica, thirty-two grains; tincture cardamom, one and a half oz.; syrup of ginger, one oz.; water, one and a half oz. Take twenty-five drops three times a day.

Extract nux vomica, four grains; extract opium, six grains. Divide into sixteen pills. Take one night and morning.

Nux vomica, forty grains; oxide of silver, sixteen grains; extract gentian, one and a half drams. Mix, and divide in sixty pills. Take one three times a day.

Subnitrate of bismuth, one dram; powdered colomba root, three drams; powdered gum-arabic, two drams. Mix, and divide into twenty pills. Take one three times a day.

Strychnine, twelve grains; acetic acid, sixty drops; alcohol, one and a half oz.; water, ten oz. Mix, and take ten drops, slowly increasing to thirty, three times a day.

Solution strychnine, half an oz.; tincture cardamom compound, three oz. Mix, and take a teaspoonful three times a day.

Bichloride of mercury, or corrosive sublimate, four grains; tincture of nux vomica, half an oz.; compound tincture of rhubarb, two oz.; Syrup of orange-peel, one and a half oz. Mix, and take a teaspoonful three times a day.

Pill of carbonate of iron (Vallet's mass), two scruples; or, Quevenne's metallic iron, per hydrogen, thirty grains; sulphate of quinia, one scruple; alcoholic extract of nux vomica, five grains. Mix, and divide into twenty pills. Take one thrice daily.

Compound tincture of gentian, and tincture of rhubarb, each three oz. Mix. Take two teaspoonfuls before each meal.

Extract of gentian, and powder of rhubarb root, each half a dram. Mix, and divide into sixteen pills. Take two thrice daily.

DROPSY.—Extract hemlock, or conium, one dram; powdered cantharides, forty grains; calomel, thirty grains; powdered ipecac, twenty grains. Mix, and divide into forty pills. Take one three times a day.

Tincture of black snake-root, or cimicifuga, one oz.; tincture of

47

myrrh, six fluid drams; tincture of opium, one dram; tincture of Cayenne pepper, one and one-half drams. Take forty drops four times a day.

Compound powder of ipecac, sixty grains; tartar-emetic, three grains; calomel, twelve grains. Make twelve pills. Take two night and morning.

Infusion of juniper, six oz.; spirits of nitric ether, one oz.; compound tincture Peruvian bark, one oz.; tincture of cardamom, four drams. Mix, and take a tablespoonful every four hours.

Infusion of digitalis, or foxglove, six oz.; corrosive sublimate, or bichloride of mercury, two grains; tincture of Spanish flies, or cantharides, two drams; peppermint water, two ounces. Take a tablespoonful three times a day.

Camphor mixture, seven ounces; spirits of nitric ether, one and one-half oz.; tincture of digitalis, or foxglove, four drams; tincture of opium, two drams; tincture of colomba, one oz. Take a tablespoonful twice a day.

Tincture of colchicum, one-half oz.; infusion of juniper, six oz.; compound tincture of orange-peel, one oz.; carbonate of potassa, two drams; nitrate of potassa, or saltpetre, one dram. Take two tablespoonfuls four times a day.

Wine of colchicum, two drams; tincture of digitalis, six drams; iodide of potassium, two and one-half drams; compound syrup of sarsaparilla, two oz.; pure water, three oz. Mix, and take a teaspoonful four times a day; or,

Elaterium, or wild cucumber, five grains; powdered digitalis, or foxglove, fifteen grains; extract of gentian, forty grains. Make twenty pills. Take one morning and night.

Sweet fennel water, six oz.; tincture of Spanish flies, or cantharides, two drams; spirits of nitric ether, one oz.; syrup of orange-peel, one oz. Mix, and take a tablespoonful twice a day.

Compound tincture of Peruvian bark, three oz.; compound tincture of cardamom, two and one-half ounces; tincture of Spanish flies, three drams; syrup of gum-arabic, one oz. Take two teaspoonfuls three times a day.

Juniper berries, two oz.; saltpetre, or nitrate of potassa, four drams; white wine, two pints. Take two tablespoonfuls three times a day.

DROPSICAL EFFUSION.—Bruised juniper berries, one oz.; infuse for three hours in a pint of hot water; pour off, and add a tablespoonful of bitartrate of potassa. Stir and drink it through the day.

Citrate of potassa, two hundred grains; tincture of squills, two fluid drams; wine of colchicum root, two fluid drams; liquor of acetate of ammonia, two fluid drams; infusion of digitalis, two oz.; peppermint water, enough to make eight oz. Mix. Take half a wineglassful thrice daily.

Take of bitartrate of potassa, an ounce; extract of taraxacum, half a dram; decoction of taraxacum, six oz. Mix. Take half a wineglassful two or three times a day.

Bruised juniper berries, mustard seed, and ginger, each half an oz.; bruised horseradish and parsley root, each an ounce; sound old cider, a quart. A wineglassful thrice a day.

DIARRHŒA.—Compound spirits of lavender, an oz.; spirit of camphor, a fluid dram; laudanum, half a fluid dram; sugar and gum-arabic, each a dram; cinnamon water, enough to make six oz. Mix. Dose, a tablespoonful once in three hours.

Obstinate.—Acetate of lead, fifteen grains; acetate of morphia, one grain; gum-arabic, two drams; cinnamon water, enough to make eight oz. Mix. Take a teaspoonful every three or four hours.

Slight Diarrhœa.—Spiced syrup of rhubarb, half an oz.; magnesia, twenty grains; cinnamon-water and camphor-water, each two fluid drams. Mix. Take in two doses, three hours apart.

Prepared chalk, two drams; white sugar and gum-arabic, each a dram and a half; tincture of kino, two fluid drams and a half; laudanum, thirty drops; peppermint water, enough to make six oz. Mix. Dose, a tablespoonful.

Extract nux vomica, four grains; extract of opium, six grains. Make into sixteen pills. Take one night and morning.

Powdered ipecac, fifteen grains; peppermint water, four oz. Take tablespoonful every ten minutes until vomiting supervenes.

Tincture of catechu and paregoric, each half a fluid oz. Mix. Take a teaspoonful every three hours.

To Check Diarrhœa.—Tannic acid, thirty-six grains; powder of opium, three grains. Divide into ten pills. Take one every three hours.

INCIPIENT DYSENTERY.—Blue mass, twelve grains; powder of ipecacuanha, six to twelve grains. Mix, and divide into ten pills. Take one every three hours.

INCIPIENT ACUTE DYSENTERY.—Mix one tablespoonful of castor-oil thoroughly with three tablespoonfuls of spiced syrup of rhubarb, and administer it immediately after mixture. To the above prescription add ten, or twenty, or thirty drops of laudanum. Useful in incipient acute dysentery.

Opium, ten grains; camphor, three grains; white soap, twenty grains; nitrate of silver, eight grains. Make thirty pills. One thrice daily.

Tincture of catechu, one and a half fluid drams; cinnamon water, five drams; tincture of opium, two drams; simple syrup, one and a half oz. Mix, and take a tablespoonful after every evacuation.

Oil of turpentine, two drams; tincture of opium, two drams; powdered gum-arabic and white sugar, each three and a half drams; water, two and a half ounces. Mix, and give a teaspoonful every twenty minutes.

EARLY STAGE OF DYSENTERY.—Blue mass, ten grains; ipecacuanha, six grains; camphor, twelve grains. Mix, and divide into twelve pills. Take one every three hours.

DYSENTERY.—Camphor, eighteen grains; ipecacuanha, six grains; opium, five grains. Mix, and divide into twelve pills. Take one every three or four hours.

Acetate of lead, twenty-five grains; opium, three to twelve grains. Mix, and divide into fifteen pills. Take one every four hours.

Nitrate of silver, eight grains; powdered opium, twenty grains. Make twenty pills. One every two hours until relieved.

Cascarilla, one oz.; cinnamon, four drams; gentian, two drams; nux vomica, two drams; water, eight oz. Mix, and form infusion, and add four oz. of white sugar. Dose, from two to four tablespoonfuls, repeated according to circumstances.

Prepare half an ounce of starch, thin enough to be drawn into a syringe; add sixty or more drops of laudanum, according to the case, mix, and inject into the bowel.

OBSTINATE CHRONIC DYSENTERY.—To four fluid oz. of flaxseed tea, made without boiling, add fifty drops of laudanum, and from four to ten grains of sulphate of zinc. Mix, and inject into the rectum.

ASTHENIC, MALARIOUS DYSENTERY.—Quinine, thirty grains; camphor, two scruples; ipecacuanha, five grains; opium, ten grains. Mix, and divide into twenty powders (or pills). Take one every three or four hours.

Tincture of camphor, one and a half oz.; tincture of Cayenne pepper, half an oz.; compound spirits of lavender, one and a half oz.; tincture of opium, one oz. Mix, and take sixty drops every hour.

Chalk mixture, six oz.; spirit of cinnamon, one and a half oz.; aqua ammonia, one and a half dram; tincture of opium, fifty drops. Take two tablespoonfuls, as circumstances require.

DYSMENORRHŒA.—Spirits of camphor, one fluid dram; paregoric, three fluid drams; tincture of ginger, half a fluid dram; compound spirit of lavender, half an oz.; water, enough to make three oz. Mix. Take a dessertspoonful every hour or two.

Extract of belladonna, eight grains; powdered camphor, one dram; sulphate of quinine, forty grains. Make thirty pills. Take one every two hours until pain is relieved.

Extract of belladonna, eight grains; powdered ipecac, ten grains; sulphate of zinc, thirty grains. Make thirty pills. Take one every four hours until pain is relieved.

DIPHTHERIA.—One part of muriatic acid, and three parts of honey; apply to the throat in diphtheria with a soft sponge, fastened to a piece of whalebone.

Chlorate of potassa, three drams; peppermint water, five oz. Dissolve. Take a tablespoonful every three hours.

Chlorate of potassa, two drams; tincture of chloride of iron, one dram; simple syrup and water, each two fluid oz. Mix. Take a tablespoonful every three hours.

Carbolic acid, twenty-five minims; acetic acid, half a dram; honey, two drams; tincture of myrrh, two drachms; water, enough to make six oz. Mix together the acids first, and then, gradually, the honey and water.

DELIRIUM TREMENS.—Solution of sulphate of morphia, and fluid extract of valerian, each two oz. Take two teaspoonfuls at a time until quietude is secured.

EPILEPSY.—Take of iodide of potassium, one dram; bromide of potassium, one ounce; bromide of ammonium, two drams; bicarbonate of potassa, two scruples; infusion of colomba, six oz. Dissolve. Dose, a teaspoonful before each meal, and one tablespoonful at bedtime. Brown-Séquard.

Mix together eight grains of crystallized carbolic acid and two oz. each of water and mucilage of gum-arabic. Dose, a tablespoonful every three or four hours.

Dissolve half an oz. of hydrate of chloral and twenty-five drops of essence of peppermint in four oz. of pure glycerine. Dose, a dessert-spoonful (two teaspoonfuls) *with water.*

EMACIATION.—Fusel oil, thirty drops; syrup, four oz. One teaspoonful for a child of six months, thrice a day.

ECZEMA.—Powder of krameria, half an oz.; prepared chalk, 3 drams; dry starch, an oz. and two drams. Mix. To be dusted on the skin.

Carbonate of potassa, two drams; glycerine, two drams; lard, two oz. Mix.

ERYTHEMA.—Acetate of zinc, two grains dissolved in one fluid dram of rose-water. Mix with one oz. of cold cream. Apply externally.

Carbonate of lead, five grains; glycerine, two teaspoonfuls; simple cerate, one oz. Mix.

Sulphate of copper, six grains; water, two oz. Dissolve. Use as lotion.

ERUPTIONS ON THE FACE.—Oxide of zinc, three drams; lard, one oz. Mix. Apply locally.

EARACHE.—Glycerine and warm water, each one teaspoonful. Mix. Pour into the ear from a teaspoon night and morning.

Mix half a teaspoonful of warm olive oil with three drops of laudanum. Pour it into the ear.

EMOLLIENT.—Mix together two drams of starch and three oz. of Price's glycerine, cold; heat gradually to 230° Fahr., stirring all the time; then let it cool.

EYELIDS.—To an oz. of water add one drop of Goulard's extract of subacetate of lead. Apply this with a camel's-hair pencil to the outside of the lids twice a day.

EYE-WATER.—Three grains of alum; water, one oz. Dissolve. Drop into the eye from a quill or a hair-pencil once or twice daily.

Nitrate of silver, five grains; distilled water, one oz. Dissolve. Apply to the inside of the lids with a hair-pencil, or drop between the lids.

Carbonate of lead, two drams; simple cerate, one oz.

OPHTHALMIA.—Carbonate of lead, seventy grains; glycerine, four oz. Mix. As a local application for ophthalmia (to the outside of the lids with a hair-pencil).

Sulphate of atropia, two grains; water, one oz. Dissolve. Drop into the eye once or twice daily, to dilate the pupils.

FEVER.—Epsom salts, one oz.; tartar-emetic, one-half grain; syrup, one oz.; pure water, six oz. Mix, and take a tablespoonful every hour.

Liquor of the acetate of ammonia, two oz.; spirits of nitrous ether, four drams; wine of antimony, four drams; syrup of gum-arabic, one oz. Take a teaspoonful every hour.

Tartar-emetic, two and a half grains; cinnamon water, two oz.; syrup, four drams; water, four oz. One teaspoonful hourly.

Dissolve fifty grains of carbonate of ammonia in four oz. of water, and add pure vinegar slowly, until it ceases to effervesce. This will substitute the "liquor ammoniæ acetatis," or spiritus Mindereri.

Dose, two tablespoonfuls with as much of water, every two hours, as a diaphoretic.

Bicarbonate of potassa, twenty grains; paregoric, two drams; water, eight oz. Mix, and take a tablespoonful every half hour.

Carbonate of soda, forty grains; spirits of nitric ether, one oz.; syrup of ginger, one oz.; water, one and a half oz. Take two tablespoonfuls every two hours.

Nitrate of potassa, three drams; tartar-emetic, one grain; water, six oz. Mix, and take two teaspoonfuls every two hours.

INTERMITTENT FEVER.—Sulphate of cinchona, fifty grains; aromatic sulphuric acid (elixir of vitriol), a fluid dram and a half; compound tincture of cardamom, half an oz.; water, enough to make four oz. Take a teaspoonful or two as required.

IN THE CHILL OF PERNICIOUS FEVER.—Powdered capsicum, a dram. Divide into twelve pills. Take one every hour.

Sulphate of quinine, forty grains; aromatic sulphuric acid (elixir of vitriol), a fluid dram and a half; oil of cloves, four drops; mucilage of gum-arabic, an oz.; peppermint water, enough to make in all four oz. Mix. Take a teaspoonful or two every three or four hours in asthenic pneumonia; but larger doses, or the same at shorter intervals, for intermittent fever.

Divide twenty grains of sulphate of quinine into ten pills. Take one every two hours.

PERNICIOUS FEVER, No. 4.—Calomel, quinine, and camphor, each eight grains; opium, two grains. Divide into six pills. Take one every hour or two.

LOW FEVER.—Nitro-muriatic acid, half a fluid dram; sweet spirits of nitre, half an oz.; camphor-water, five and a half oz. Dissolve. Take a tablespoonful every two hours.

TYPHUS FEVER.—Nitric acid, forty drops; water, six oz. Dissolve. Take one or two tablespoonfuls every three hours.

FEVER.—Citrate of potassa, two drams; lemon syrup, half an oz.; water, three oz. Mix. Dose, a tablespoonful every two hours, with one of water. The lemon syrup may be omitted without disadvantage.

TYPHOID FEVER.—Liquor of acetate of ammonia, three and a half oz.; sweet spirits of nitre, half an oz. Mix. Take a tablespoonful every two hours.

FAVUS, where two hairs grow in a yellow crust.—Bichloride of mercury, four grains; alcohol and distilled water, each an oz. Dissolve.

GASTRALGIA—STOMACH-ACHE.—Extract belladonna, twelve grains; sulphate quinine, thirty grains. Make thirty pills. Take one three times a day.

Laudanum, three drams; tincture Cayenne pepper, two and a half drams; sulphuric ether, three and a half drams; tincture camphor, three drams; chloroform, one dram. Take a tablespoonful when needed.

Extract hyoscyamus, one dram; nitrate silver, ten grains; subnitrate muth, two drams. Make forty pills. Take one night and

ot lupulin, one dram; nitrate of silver, twenty grains; subnitrate of bismuth, two drams; sulphate of quinine, forty grains. Make forty pills. Take one three times a day.

Extract conium, one drachm; nitrate silver, ten grains; powdered Cayenne pepper, forty grains; sulphate quinine, forty grains. Make forty pills. Take one three times a day.

GRAVEL.—Bicarbonate of soda, three drams; sweet spirits of nitre, five fluid drams; peppermint water, enough to make six oz. Dissolve. Take a tablespoonful three or four times daily.

Bicarbonate of soda, two drams; phosphate of soda, half an oz.; benzoic acid and gum-arabic, each three drams; sweet spirits of nitre, half an oz.; peppermint water, enough to make six oz. Mix. Take from a teaspoonful to a tablespoonful occasionally.

GOUT.—Carbonate of potassa and nitrate of potassa, each two and a half drams; water, seven oz. Dissolve. Take a tablespoonful thrice daily.

GOUT AND GOUTY RHEUMATISM.—Wine of colchicum root, one fluid dram; Husband's magnesia, one drachm; water, four oz. Mix. Take a tablespoonful thrice daily.

Wine of colchicum root, one fluid dram; bicarbonate of potassa and Rochelle salts, each two and a half drams; water, four oz. Mix. Take a tablespoonful thrice daily.

Tincture of rhubarb and senna, one and a half oz.; syrup of ginger, four drams; laudanum, one fluid dram. Mix. Take a teaspoonful at once in hot water.

GONORRHŒA, No. 2.—Copaiba, half an oz.; compound spirit of lavender, two fluid drams; sugar and gum-arabic, each two drams; water, enough to make six oz. Take a tablespoonful thrice daily.

Oil of cubebs, two drams; sweet spirit of nitre, half an oz.; sugar and gum-arabic, each two drams; water, enough to make six oz. Mix. Take a tablespoonful thrice daily.

INJECTION FOR GONORRHŒA, No. 1.—Sulphate of zinc, four grains; water, two oz. Dissolve. Use once daily.

No. 2.—Solution of subacetate of lead (Goulard's), one dram; water, five oz. Use once daily.

No. 3.—Chloride of zinc, two grains; glycerine and water, each an oz. Dissolve. Use once daily.

GARGLE.—Dissolve seven drops of creasote in two oz. of glycerine, diluted with an equal bulk of water; one pint of water, two heaping tablespoons of common salt, a heaping teaspoonful of powdered alum, and a level tablespoonful of ground red-pepper; or, a pint of red-pepper tea, and a level tablespoonful of salt and alum.

HEMORRHAGES.—Gallic acid, two drams; syrup of cinnamon, four oz. Mix. Take a dessert-spoonful every two, three, or four hours.

Oil of turpentine, three drams; compound spirits of lavender, half an oz.; laudanum, twenty minims; sugar and gum-arabic, each two drams; water, enough to make six oz. Mix. Take a tablespoonful at once.

Ammonio-ferric alum, two scruples; water, four oz. Dissolve. Take a tablespoonful every two or three hours, in hemorrhages.

ASTRINGENT IN HÆMATEMESIS.—Creasote, twenty drops; conserve of roses (or extract of gentian), one dram. Mix, and divide into sixteen pills. Take one every two, three, or four hours.

HOOPING-COUGH.—Hydrocyanic acid, twenty-five drops; wine of ipecac, two drams; syrup of tolu, one and a half oz.; water, three oz. Take a teaspoonful every four hours.

Blood-root, one dram; hot water, half a pint. Give from a teaspoonful to a tablespoonful, according to age, every fifteen minutes, until vomiting.

Tincture of lobelia, one oz.; syrup of squills, one oz. Twenty-five drops three times a day.

Iodide of potassium, one and a half drams; bitter almond water, three drams; paregoric, two drams; tincture of musk, two drams; alcohol, two drams; water, four oz. Take a teaspoonful as often as needed.

Syrup of ipecac, two fluid drams and a half; syrup of squills, one tablespoonful; mixture of assafœtida, enough to make two oz. Mix. Give one or two teaspoonfuls thrice daily.

SEVERE HOOPING-COUGH. — Extract of belladonna, one grain; mucilage of gum-arabic, three oz. Mix. Give two teaspoonfuls thrice daily.

Fluid extract of hyoscyamus, half a fluid dram; orange-flower water, or camphor water, three oz. Mix. Give two teaspoonfuls every three hours.

HYPERTROPHY OF THE HEART.—Acetate of lead, half a dram; opium, four grains; crumb of bread, a sufficient quantity. Mix, and divide into twenty pills. Take one thrice daily.

Norwood's tincture of veratrum viride, half an oz. Take four drops every four hours. If nausea or prostration follow, withdraw or diminish the dose.

OVER-RAPID ACTION OF THE HEART.—Powder of digitalis, one grain, thrice daily.

Tincture of digitalis, half an oz. Take ten drops thrice daily, in water.

Iodide of potassium, two and a half drams; tincture of hyoscyamus, four drams; tincture of digitalis or foxglove, half an oz.; compound syrup of sarsaparilla, six oz. Take a teaspoonful night and morning, for heart enlargement.

For irregular action of the heart, Dr. Austin Flint, who is high authority, relies on digitalis to increase the power of ventricular contractions. For difficult breathing he recommends ethers, dry cuppings, and revulsive applications. For general dropsy, elaterium comes first as a cathartic of water, as it can be given for a long time without depression. For anæmia, as a result of heart-affection, he commends a nutritive diet, chalybeate tonics; to cease nursing, or whatever else may debilitate.

HEADACHE.—A cup of strong tea is sometimes a temporary remedy; but for sick headache take two teaspoonfuls of pulverized charcoal in half a glass of water.

Headache from Sour Stomach, or Sick Headache.—Aromatic spirit of ammonia, six drams; bicarbonate of soda, one and a half drams; infusion of cascarilla, eight oz. Take two tablespoonfuls twice a day.

Carbonate of magnesia, thirty grains; sulphate of magnesia, or Epsom salts, two and a half drams; aromatic spirit of ammonia, one dram; tincture of rhubarb, half an oz.; tincture of hyoscyamus, four drams; water, half a pint. Take one tablespoonful thrice a day.

Twenty or thirty drops of turpentine, every hour or two, not only removes headache, but has a delightfully soothing influence in frontal headache resulting from protracted physical exertion or mental effort, as also that severe headache to which nervous and hysterical women are subject.

For periodical headaches.—First, what is proper to be done during the attack; second, what is proper in the interval. In such cases there is always constipation of the bowels, consequently if he begins treatment during the interval, he gives one or two of the following pills: Blue mass, extract of colocynth, Socotrine aloes, each twelve grains; ipecac, six grains. Make twelve pills. To be followed by one (1) dram of sulphate of magnesia. Then he begins with three drops of liquor potassæ arsenitis, to be taken in a dram of water after each meal.

If the patient is delicate and complains of the coldness of the extremities during the attacks, and frequent chilliness during the intervals, he substitutes the following:

Liq. arsenicalis hydrochloric............half a dram.
Quiniæ disulphat.....................twelve grains.
Liq. ferri perchloridi..................two drams.
Aquæ...............................six drams.

One tablespoonful in a wineglassful of water, twice a day after meals.

Whichever one of these is given, it is to be interrupted once in three weeks, and the first prescription given.

When the attack begins he places the patient in a chair, with the head elevated, the feet in a hot mustard bath, the hands in warm water, and a bag of ice on the head, if it can be borne, and gives the following prescription:

Potassii bromid........................six drams.
Ammon. bromid.......................two drams.
Potassii iodid ....six grains.
Infus. calumbæ ....three oz.

One dessert-spoonful in an ounce of water.

This treatment persevered in three or six months, will cure nearly every case.

HYSTERIA, says the eminent professor, Dr. Austin Flint, "is a term used to denote an abnormal condition of the nervous system and the mind, which as a morbid element enters largely into a great variety of affections. Hysteria involves a morbid susceptibility to emotions, and a defective power of the will to restrain their manifestations, whether in male or female, weeping or laughing irrepressibly on inadequate occasions, making it very incongruous with abrupt transitions." The phases of the disease are various, hence a number of prescriptions are given.

HYSTERIA.—Bromide of ammonium, two drams; water, three oz.; aromatic spirit of ammonia, one fluid dram. Dissolve. Take a dessert-spoonful thrice daily.

Compound tincture of lavender, one and a half oz.; spirits of caraway, two oz.; tincture of opium, one dram; sulphuric ether, four drams; water, four and a half oz. Mix, and take a tablespoonful every hour.

Valerianate of zinc, twelve grains; tincture of valerian, four drams; simple syrup, one oz.; spring water, four oz. Take one tablespoonful.

Extract hyoscyamus, forty grains; valerianate of zinc, forty grains; subnitrate of bismuth, thirty-five grains. Make forty pills. Take one three times a day.

Valerianate of ammonia, one dram; syrup of tolu, one oz. Mix, and take a teaspoonful every four hours.

Musk, sixty grains; sulphuric ether, one and a half drams; tincture of opium, one and a half drams; cinnamon water, three oz.; simple syrup, one oz. Take a tablespoonful three times a day.

Tincture of castor, one and a half oz.; tincture of assafetida, one and a half oz.; camphor-water, one oz.; aromatic spirit of ammonia, four drams; syrup of gum-arabic, one and a half oz. Take a tablespoonful as circumstances require.

Tincture of castor, one and a half oz.; sulphate of morphia, four grains; tincture of valerian, one and a half oz.; syrup of gum-arabic, one oz. Take a dessert-spoonful every two hours.

Tincture of valerian, one oz.; carbonate of magnesia, two drams; tincture of opium, one dram; peppermint water, three and a half oz.; oil of anise, forty drops. Take a teaspoonful every hour.

Assafetida, one dram. Divide into eighteen pills. Take one every two hours.

Twenty or thirty drops of spirits of turpentine every hour or two has a charming, good effect in some cases of this sort.

Assafetida, one and a half drams; sulphate of morphia, five grains; castile soap, forty grains. Make forty pills. Take one or two at a time.

Assafetida, sixty grains; sulphate of morphia, three grains; powdered camphor, forty grains. Make thirty pills. Take one three times a day.

Musk, sixty grains; assafetida, one and a half drams; powdered camphor, thirty grains; extract of gentian, a sufficient quantity. Make thirty pills. Take one three times a day.

HEMORRHAGES.—From the nose. Lie down, and place cloths dipped in ice-water, or vinegar and water, over the forehead and sides of the nose.

Powdered ipecac, twenty grains; penny-royal water, four oz. Take a tablespoonful every fifteen minutes, until vomiting.

Blow into the nostrils, through a quill, some powdered gum-arabic, or the dust of tea from a canister; or,

Ice-water to the genitals; or stand up and raise the arm above the head, on the side of the bleeding, until the blood ceases to flow.

Gallic acid, sixty grains; mucilage of gum-arabic, two oz.; syrup of orange-peel, two and a half oz.; water, three and a half oz. Take one tablespoon four times daily.

Internal bleedings of all kinds are frequently relieved by taking two or more grains of ipecac every ten minutes until nausea is excited. Spitting blood has been relieved at once by taking ten grains of ipecac, in the form of pills.

Powdered opium, ten grains; powdered camphor, three grains; white soap, twenty grains; acetate of lead, one dram; powdered ipecac, fifteen grains. Make thirty pills. Take one for a dose, and repeat according to circumstances.

Sugar of lead, thirty grains; digitalis, or foxglove, twenty grains; powdered opium, five grains; conserve of roses, forty grains. Make twenty pills. Take one four times a day.

Sugar of lead, sixty grains; tincture of opium, two drams; vinegar, five drams; water, three oz. Take a teaspoonful, repeating as required, every two hours, or oftener.

Acetate of lead, sixty grains; tincture of opium, one and a half drams; cinnamon, two oz.; water, four oz. Take a teaspoonful four times a day.

Tannic acid, sixty grains; extract of gentian, forty grains. Make twenty pills. Take one every three hours.

Tannic acid, sixty grains; extract opium, ten grains; conserve of roses, thirty-five grains. Make thirty pills. Take one four times a day for uterine hemorrhage.

In extreme cases give the following:

Two grains of sugar of lead, three tablespoons of water; vinegar, half a dram; five drops of black-drop; one teaspoonful of syrup. Take all this at once, and repeat three or four times in twenty-four hours.

Gallic acid, two drams; powdered gum-arabic, two drams; syrup of tolu, two ounces; water, two and a half ounces. Take a tablespoon thrice daily.

Nose-bleed in advanced life indicates apoplexy; best prevented by a seton in the neck, or fruit diet, and have the bowels act very freely every day.

Decoction of bearberry, four ounces; tannic acid, sixty grains; tincture of opium, two drams; syrup of gum-arabic, two and a half oz. Take a teaspoonful four times a day.

INTERMITTENT FEVER.—Any case can be cured with a pound of Epsom salts, then a liver pill, next when it begins to act, take two grains of quinine in two tablespoons of water every two hours except during the six hours including midnight; stubborn cases may require larger doses of both medicines; the liver pill not to be taken oftener than twice a week.

Quinine, thirty grains; powdered pepsin, twenty grains; one grain of strychnine. Make ten pills, and take one thrice a day.

Quinine half a dram; one oz. of muriated tincture of iron; two drams of a solution of strychnine, and two of water. One teaspoon every three hours during the absence of fever.

A teaspoonful of liquid hartshorn in water, just before a chill, sometimes arrests it; good also in delirium tremens and to promote sleep.

IMPOTENCE.—One-twelfth of a grain of strychnine taken in the form of a pill three times a day, the bowels being kept free, the body clean with a cold hip-bath twice a day.

ITCH.—Iodide of potassium, one oz.; glycerine, three oz. Is a good wash in itch; or, twenty grains of cyanide of potash in seven oz. of water.

Iodide of potassium, half an ounce; iodide of sulphur, a dram; glycerine and water, each two fluid oz.; oil of bitter almonds, four drops.

Petroleum and alcohol, each one oz.; balsam of Peru, one dram; oil of rosemary and oil of lavender, each twenty drops. Use as a wash.

Aromatic, or even common vinegar rubbed in with a sponge twice a day, with a daily warm bath, or smear the parts with equal parts of liquid storax and sweet oil.

ARMY ITCH.—Iodide of sulphur, twenty-five grains; lard, one oz.

ITCHING OF THE SKIN IN PRURIGO SENILIS.—Oil of juniper and alcohol, each an oz.; water, four oz. Use as a wash.

OBSTINATE ITCHING.—Muriatic acid, twenty drops; water, five oz. Employ as a lotion.

Sulphur, one hundred grains; carbonate of potassa, one dram; lard, one oz. Use as an ointment; or, rub common soap into the skin until it tingles severely, then wash off with warm water every other day. The most troublesome itchings of the private parts are relieved at once by dissolving twenty-five grains of the cyanide of potash in half a pint of water, or two grains of corrosive sublimate in six ounces of water, with regular bowels, and "special fruit diet," either to be used as a wash twice a day.

Prof. Gunning S. Bedford, in cases of final cessation of menses, advised a vegetable and fruit diet; to have the bowels act every day; used as a wash twice a day a teaspoonful of powdered alum in half a pint of water, or a powder of twenty grains of camphor, and two drams of starch, and powder the parts well twice a day. At other times wash the parts with twenty grains of the nitrate of silver and two oz. of water; the author recommends in addition a cold hip-bath, night and morning, and a strict fruit diet. This itching is sometimes fearful, causing the patient to scratch the parts to bleeding; sometimes she is compelled to step into an alley way and scratch; free bowels, fruit diet, and hip-baths, or cold-water vaginal injections will cure.

INFLUENZA, or the "La Grippe" of the French, is best treated by being kept warm; use active purging with salts or oil in vigorous patients; in the old or feeble it is better to "take sweats."

Liquor of the acetate of ammonia, two oz.; wine of antimony, four drams; paregoric, four and a half drams; syrup of tolu, one oz. Take a teaspoonful thrice daily.

Liquor of the acetate of ammonia, two oz.; camphor mixture, four oz.; wine of ipecac, four drams; syrup of tolu, two oz. Take one teaspoonful every three hours.

A specific for influenza, if taken early, a powder made of six grains of quinine and ten grains of compound powder of opium and ipecac; that is, Dover's powders. Take all at once.

LICE.—Bichloride of mercury, a scruple; water, five oz. Use as a wash; or,

Seeds of cocculus indicus, eighty grains; prepared lard, an oz. Bruise the seeds well in a mortar, and mix with the lard.

TO DESTROY LICE, OR RELIEVE PRURITUS.—Carbolic acid, one or two drams; glycerine, an oz.; water, enough to make eight oz. Mix. Use as a lotion; or,

Bruise one oz. of seed of cocculus indicus, add a pint of alcohol, and wash the head well; it will kill every louse and nit in a minute.

LEUCORRHŒA, OR WHITES.—Alum, two drams; water, eight oz. Dissolve. Inject into the vagina twice daily, first washing out the parts well with cold water.

This is often such an unmanageable disease that a number of prescriptions are given; premising, however, that the feet must be kept warm, the bowels regular, and live on special fruit diet until cured, with plentiful syringing with cold water three times a day; such a course will often cure without any medicine whatever.

Extract hyoscyamus, one dram; nitrate of silver, ten grains; powdered cantharides, fifteen grains; sulphate quinine, forty grains. Make forty pills. Take one twice a day.

Sulphate of zinc, forty grains; extract of opium, ten grains; aromatic confection, thirty grains. Make forty pills. Take one three times a day.

Leucorrhœa is a discharge from the womb or the vagina alone; if from the womb it is thick, gelatinous, adheres to the fingers; if from the vagina it is white, creamy and opaque, except during the menstrual flow.

Sulphate of copper, ten grains; extract of opium, ten grains; confection of roses, thirty-five grains. Make thirty pills. Take one four times a day.

Decoction of oak-bark, seven oz.; alum, thirty grains; wine of galls, one oz. Use as an injection twice a day.

Compound liquor of alum, half a pint; water, half a pint. Mix, and use as an injection twice a day.

LINIMENTS.—Sweet oil, one ounce; hartshorn, one oz. Mix. To be rubbed on with a piece of flannel.

Lime-water, two oz.; flax-seed oil, two oz. Mix. Apply in cases of burns.

Spirits of turpentine, one oz.; linseed oil, one oz.; lime-water, one oz. Mix. Useful in cases of burns.

Sulphuric acid, one dram; spirits of turpentine, one dram; olive oil, three drams. Mix the oil and turpentine first, then gradually add the acid. A valuable liniment for chilblains. Rub two or three times daily.

Oil of marjoram, four drams; tincture of camphor, half an oz.; Granville's lotion, three drams; chloroform, three and a half drams; tincture of aconite, half an oz.; tincture of Cayenne pepper, half an oz.; oil of sassafras, thirty drops; compound soap liniment, one oz. Good in neuralgic affections.

Spirits of hartshorn, oil origanum, gum camphor, laudanum, spirits of turpentine, one part each; and soft soap, three parts. This may be relied on.

The best known for sprains, bruises, flesh wounds, etc., for man or beast:—One pint of alcohol; one oz. of origanum oil; one oz. wormwood oil; one oz. hemlock oil; one oz. camphor gum; four oz. aqua ammonia. Add, if you have it, the liquid of one beef's gall. Mix, and it is immediately ready for use.

Tincture of arnica, one oz.; aqua ammonia, one oz.; spirits of camphor, four drams; tincture of opium, four drams; olive oil, one oz. Make a liniment. Excellent in the commencement of sore throat, rubbed on well with the hand, or a flannel cloth.

Tincture of aconite, tincture of opium, tincture of camphor, and chloroform, each one ounce.

Dr. Stokes, of Dublin, thought highly of the following: three oz.

spirits of turpentine, two oz. rose-water; one oz. yolk of egg (yellow); half an oz. acetic acid; one dram lemon oil. Or,

Three oz. of soap liniment, and one oz. chloroform. Or,

Camphor, five drams; chloroform, four drams; oil of turpentine, four drams; tincture of opium, one oz.; oil of olives, one oz.

Take fifteen grains of iodine and seven oz. of water. Dissolve and add one dram each of the oils of rosemary and lavender, two drams of camphor, and one oz. of the water of ammonia.

Croton oil, one dram; compound soap liniment, one oz. Make a liniment. Or,

Croton oil, thirty drops; sulphuric ether, one oz. Mix, and apply externally. Apply so as to make an eruption.

Liniment cured a fourteen years' rheumatism: one quart alcohol, one quarter gill beef's gall, one oz. of oil of origanum, one oz. gum camphor. All well shaken, rub in well with the hand twice or more a day; parts rubbed not to be wetted with water while using this. Or,

Take the whites of two eggs, beaten to a froth; a wineglass of spirits of turpentine, and a wineglass of alcohol, beating it all the time. This liniment must be put together in the order mentioned above, or it will not be thoroughly incorporated. We find this very superior in all cases of sprains, bruises, etc. This is the famous St. John Long's liniment; was to be applied with a sponge; its good effects are proportioned to the vigor of the rubbing and the length of time it is followed up. It will often bring about marvellous good results.

LOOSE BOWELS.—Tinct. of catechu, half an oz.; laudanum, two drams; spirits of camphor, two drams; tinct. of myrrh, two drams; tinct. of Cayenne, two drams. Mix. Dose, from half to a teaspoonful. Or,

Syrup of orange-peel, one oz.; acetate of morphia, two grains; tinct. of cinnamon, six drams; tinct. of cardamom, two drams. Mix. Dose, a teaspoonful. A valuable remedy in diarrhœa.

Bind woollen flannel tight around the abdomen, so as to be double in front; this supports the bowels, keeps them warm, draws the fluid to the surface, and so confines the intestines in a narrow space that their vermicular or natural motion is arrested, as it is the excess of this motion which is the immediate cause of the disturbance. Or,

Keep quiet in bed, because in loose bowels every step taken increases the disturbance, and nature points to rest, by taking away the disposition to move about, while to sit or recline is delightful.

Rest and the flannel bandage, eating nothing but boiled rice with boiled milk, every six hours; better still if the rice is first parched brown like coffee; this alone will cure any ordinary case, without any medicine whatever.

Half an oz. of elixir vitriol in eight oz. of water. Dose, one oz. every two hours as long as necessary.

Five years old, fifteen drops elixir vitriol every hour with syrup.

MOUTH CANKER.—Keep the bowels acting daily, eat thrice a day of nourishing food, nothing whatever between meals, and use a wash of half an oz. of the liquor of chlorate of soda in five ounces of water, and take at the same time four grains of the chlorate of potash in a little syrup, four times a day. Cases of several years' standing may be cured in a short time thus.

Keep the skin clear. Avoid all salt food and stimulants, including tea and coffee, live mainly on fruits, berries, coarse breads, cracked wheat, sago, tapioca, boiled rice, and the like.

Chlorate of potassa, half an oz.; water, half a pint. Take a tablespoonful every three hours.

Labarraque's solution of chlorinated soda, one dram; good glycerine, and water, each two oz.

MOUTH WASH.—Creasote, three drops; good glycerine, and water, each half an oz.

Alum one dram, dissolve in six oz. of water, add two oz. of brandy, for salivated sore mouth.

NEURALGIAS are almost without number. If one remedy fails, use another; but to cure any of them permanently the bowels must be made to act every day, the feet must be kept warm, the special fruit diet kept up, and three hours spent in out-door activities every day; these alone will cure in many cases; when they fail, use some one of the following:

Extract of hyoscyamus, half a dram; sulphate of morphia, three grains; strychnine, two grains; powdered Cayenne pepper, thirty-five grains; sulphate of zinc, fifteen grains. Make thirty pills. Take one every five hours.

Valerianate of ammonia, one teaspoonful twice a day, increased to three, in water.

Extract hyoscyamus, half a dram; valerianate of iron, one dram. Make thirty pills. Take one three times a day.

Extract hyoscyamus, half a dram; valerianate of zinc, one scruple. Make thirty pills. Take one three times a day. Or,

Half a dram of sal ammoniac in an oz. of camphor water, to be taken a teaspoonful at a dose, and the dose repeated several times, at intervals of five minutes if the pain be not relieved at once. An admirable California remedy.

Extract of aconite, ten grains; arsenic, one grain; sulphate of quinine, thirty grains. Make twenty pills. Take one every four hours.

Extract of belladonna, ten grains; powdered iron, thirty grains; quinine, twenty grains. Make twenty pills. Take four or five every day.

Subcarbonate of soda, one and a half drams; water, one pint; dilute sulphuric acid, one dram; aromatic confection, four drams; peppermint water, half an oz. Mix. Two tablespoonfuls twice a day.

Chloroform and olive oil, four oz. each, prevented from evaporating by oiled silk, acts as a strong rubefacient, burning like mustard.

Veratria, ten to twenty grains; pure lard, one oz. Mix. Applied to the part.

Lime-water, eight oz.; calcined magnesia, thirty grains; aromatic spirit of ammonia, three drams; compound tincture of cardamom, one oz. Take two tablespoonfuls twice a day, or oftener.

Veratrum, five grains; lard, one dram. Make into ointment.

Veratrum, twenty grains; ointment of rose-water, one oz. Mix and form ointment. Rub a small portion behind the ear night and morning, in nervous deafness.

Saturated tincture of aconite root rubbed gently into the skin.

Neuralgias of the severest kind in the head or other parts of the body are often delightfully relieved by a mixture of equal parts of tincture of aconite root and chloroform; dip into it a piece of woollen cloth, spread it over the spot, and then cover with a larger cloth.

Prof. Gross, of Philadelphia, uses forty grains of quinine, one grain of morphia, one grain each of strychnine and arsenious acid, with ten grains of extract of aconite, made into twenty-one pills. Take one four times a day.

Extract hyoscyamus, fifteen grains; extract stramonium, four grains; extract hops, one and a half drams; sulphate morphia, one and a half grains. Make thirty pills. Take one every half-hour until pain is relieved.

Sulphate quinine, forty grains; sulphate morphia, ten grains. Make twenty pills. Take one when needed.

Strychnine, twelve grains; acetic acid, sixty drops; alcohol, one and a half oz.; water, ten oz. Take ten drops, slowly increasing to thirty, three times a day.

Solution of strychnine, three oz.; Magendie's solution of morphia, one and a half drams; tincture of gentian, two oz.; syrup of gum-arabic, two oz. Take a teaspoonful three times a day; or,

Bicarbonate of potassa, one dram; hydrocyanic acid, twenty-four drops; solution of sulphate of morphia, twenty-four drops; camphor water, four oz. Take two teaspoonfuls, as circumstances require.

Valerianate of ammonia, one dram; syrup of tolu, one oz. Take a teaspoonful every four hours.

OZÆNA.—Tannic acid, one oz.; glycerine, four oz. Mix, and dissolve by a gentle heat. Inject or snuffle up twice a day to remove ill-smelling discharges from the nose; or,

One oz. of carbolic acid (melted); nine oz. of Boner's or Price's glycerine. Mix over a water-bath at 120° Fahr., stirring until incorporated. Use as injection, in ozæna, etc., diluted with ten or twenty times its bulk of water; but to cure this disagreeable affection the general health must be built up, which article see.

OTORRHŒA, or offensive discharges from the ear, are corrected and cured by letting fall into it daily, or carefully injecting into it, a mixture of one dram of carbolic acid, once oz. of glycerine, and five oz. of water, well mixed.

OINTMENTS.—Iodide of potassium, one dram; proto-iodide of mercury, twelve grains; ointment of rose-water, one oz. A counter-irritant in consumption, rubbed in night and morning over the chest.

Iodine, twelve grains; iodide of potassium, one dram; fresh or prepared lard, one oz. Mix, and form ointment.

Oil of tobacco, six drops; white precipitate of mercury, twenty grains; simple cerate, one oz. Mix, and form ointment.

Extract of henbane, or hyoscyamus, one oz.; extract of belladonna, one oz.; extract of hemlock, or conium, one oz.; iodide of potassium. Good for all indurations.

Tartar-emetic, two drams; powdered camphor, thirty grains; fresh lard, or prepared lard, one oz. Make an ointment.

In chronic bronchitis, or other deep-seated inflammations in the chest, first wet the skin with strong vinegar.

Tartar-emetic, one and a half drams; powdered ipecac, fifty grains;

simple cerate, or lard, one oz. Make an ointment; or for children use,

Tartar-emetic, thirty grains; Croton oil, twenty drops; powdered ipecac, sixty grains; rose ointment, one oz.; red oxide of mercury, five grains; simple cerate, one-half oz. Mix and form ointment, for sore eyes.

Ointment or salve for wens and other tumors: equal parts of soot, spirits of camphor, turpentine, and soft-soap, to be well rubbed in thrice a day, and a plaster of it kept on the parts in the mean while.

PNEUMONIA, called by various names, as lung-fever, inflammation of the lungs, and pneumonitis, is always a dangerous disease, and should be attacked most promptly.

Wine of antimony, four drams; nitrate of potassa, or "saltpetre," two drams; liquor of the acetate of ammonia, three oz.; syrup of tolu, one oz.; water, three and a half oz. Take a dessert-spoonful every three hours.

Powdered ipecac, sixty grains; infusion of Virginia snakeroot, or serpentaria, six oz.; paregoric, two drams. One teaspoonful every hour; or,

Two oz. of saturated solution of tartar-emetic; sixty grains of iodide of potash, with half an oz. of oil of turpentine; or use the sat. sol. of tar.-em. alone, so as to cause an eruption; or,

Tartrate of antimony and potassa, two grains; water, five oz. Take two teaspoonfuls every three hours.

Sulphate of quinine, half a dram; elixir of vitriol, one dram and a half; oil of cloves, five drops; mucilage of gum-arabic, an oz.; water, to make in all four oz. Take a teaspoonful every three hours.

Nitrate of potassa, two drams; powder of gum-arabic, or white sugar, two drams. Divide into ten papers. Take one every two hours.

Calomel, and ipecacuanha powder, each eight grains; nitrate of potassa, half a dram, or a dram. Mix, and divide into twelve powders. Take one powder every three hours.

Acetate of potassa, five drams and a half; sweet spirits of nitre, two fluid drams; water, enough to make eight oz. Dissolve. Take a tablespoonful every three hours, in debilitated cases.

PLEURITIC EFFUSION.—Acetate of potassa, six drams; sweet spirits of nitre, two fluid drams; water, enough to make half a pint. Take a tablespoonful every three hours, as a diuretic; or,

Powder of squills, half a dram; powder of digitalis, fifteen grains. Mix, and divide into sixteen pills. Take one thrice daily.

Compound spirit of juniper, two ounces. Take one or two teaspoonfuls thrice daily, in water.

Calomel, six grains; opium, three to six grains; tartar-emetic, a grain and a half. Mix, and divide into twelve powders. Take one every three or four hours, in water, for an acute attack of pleurisy.

PNEUMONIA.—From five to ten drops of the tincture of arnica will so control the action of the heart in pneumonia as to lead to a cure if continued every three hours for two days, bringing the pulse down to forty in a minute, where it sometimes remains for several days after its administration has ceased, as is the case with veratrum viride.

PERITONITIS.—Calomel and opium, each six grains. Mix and divide into twelve pills. Take one every two, three, or four hours.

48

PARALYSIS in some forms is greatly benefited by taking carefully, and making out of half a grain of strychnine sixteen pills. Take one at a time thrice a day, until relieved.

PILES.—If bleeding, take an injection, twice a day, of thirty grains of tannic acid dissolved in a third of a pint of ice-water; powder of galls, two drams; opium, twelve grains; lard, one oz., as ointment.

Ointment of spermaceti, glyceryl, one oz. each; opium, twelve grains. Use as ointment.

PAINFUL PILES.—Extract of belladonna, seventy grains; spermaceti ointment, an oz. Mix. Use as ointment.

Stramonium ointment, one oz.; carbonate of lead, one dram; powdered opium, one and a half drams. Make an ointment, and use twice a day.

Ointment of stramonium, one oz.; powdered galls, one dram; powdered camphor, three drams. Make an ointment, and use it twice a day.

Opium, one or two grains; soap, a sufficient quantity. Mix, and introduce it solid into the rectum; or,

Extract of belladonna, five grains; soap, a sufficient quantity. Mix, and introduce into the bowel.

One dram of powdered galls; two drams of opium; two drams of the liquor of the acetate of lead. Make into an ointment with hog's lard.

PSORIASIS.—Reddish, scaly eruptions in patches over the skin, has been treated with great success by the administration of large doses of balsam copaiba, given with a little liquor potassæ, mucilage, and water. The physician will be able to discharge his patients sooner under this treatment than by any other.

RICKETS.—Take of concentrated lactic acid, one oz.; magma of freshly precipitated phosphate of lime, a sufficiency; orange-flower water, one and a half oz.; white sugar, eleven oz. Mix the lactic acid with two fluid ounces of pure water, and saturate it with the magma; put the liquid upon a filter, and add enough water to make eight oz. of filtrate; pour this upon the sugar in a bottle; shake until dissolved, and strain. Dose, for a child, one or two drams; for an adult, a tablespoonful thrice daily.

RHEUMATISM.—Free bowels, plenty of flannel, time, and sulphur will cure most cases.

Take a teaspoonful of the tincture of guaiacum thrice daily, with free bowels; mix two oz. of lime and eight oz. of sugar in a mortar, and pour over them a pint of boiling water. Take teaspoonful three times daily in milk; or,

Take the juice of one lemon every four hours; removes the most acute pains in two to five days.

Oil of turpentine, spirit of camphor, water of ammonia, and olive oil, each two tablespoonfuls. Externally applied; or,

Nitrate of potassa, two oz.; sulphur, an oz.; guaiacum, half an oz.; add two nutmegs, and a half pint of molasses. Take two teaspoonfuls at night.

Oil of marjoram, half an oz.; oil of turpentine, half an oz.; tincture of opium, one oz.; aqua ammonia, one oz.; olive or sweet oil, one oz.

Make a liniment to be rubbed on externally in rheumatism, or rheumatic pains about the chest and back.

Oil of marjoram, aqua ammonia, tincture of opium, and olive or sweet oil, each two oz. Mix. A liniment; rub on thoroughly with the hand, and wet a flannel, lay it over the affected joint, and cover it with oiled silk. Once a celebrated patent remedy for rheumatism.

Iodide of potassium, one to two drams; cinnamon or peppermint water, six oz. Take one tablespoon thrice a day for syphilitic rheumatism.

Two drams of saltpetre; powdered opium, twelve grains; ipecac, twenty grains. Divide into twelve powders. Take one every night.

Sulphate of quinine, forty grains; sulphate of morphia, ten grains. Make twenty pills. Take one according as circumstances require.

Corrosive sublimate or bichloride of mercury, four grains; extract of opium, ten grains; extract of gentian, four grains. Make forty pills. Take one three times a day.

Dissolve two grains corrosive sublimate in a few drops of water, enough to moisten a sufficient quantity of crumbs of bread and white sugar to make forty pills. Take two night and morning.

The London *Lancet* contains the history of a series of cases of this disease treated successfully by Dr. O'Conner, one of the physicians of the Royal Free Hospital, by the use of sulphur and flannel bandaging.

Corrosive sublimate, four grains; tincture of gentian and common syrup, each three oz. Take one tablespoonful thrice a day.

Citrate of potash, two oz.; Rochelle salts, two drams; wine of colchicum, fifteen drops; laudanum, ten drops. Take it at a draught three or four times a day.

The celebrated Dr. Arbuthnot says that a diet of whey and bread is a cure for rheumatism. A physician in the Philadelphia *Medical Journal* says: "I have been using cider in acute rheumatism with much satisfaction. I think more of it than of lemon-juice. I allow my patients to drink freely of it; either new or old cider answers equally well. From this fact I am convinced that lemon-juice operates in rheumatism more from a peculiar vegetable principle than from its acid properties, which principle resides in the apple as well as in many other fruits. It sometimes purges; if so, I lessen the quantity."

Iodide of potassium, three drams; liquor potassa, two and a half drams; tincture of colchicum, two drams; tincture of cardamom, two and a half oz.; syrup of sarsaparilla, three and a half oz. Take a tablespoon thrice daily; or,

Thirty grs. each of antimonial powder and calomel, with ten grs. of opium. Make twenty pills, and take one four times a day.

A mixture of half an oz. of pulverized saltpetre and half a pint of sweet oil is a certain cure for the inflammatory rheumatism. The mixture must be applied externally to the part affected, and a gentleman who has witnessed its application in a number of instances says it will infallibly effect a cure, and that right speedily.

Or one oz. of tincture of black snakeroot; two drams of iodide of potash; syrup of ipecac, one oz.; and two oz. of water. One tablespoon thrice daily.

Oil of mustard is a rubefacient, being first diluted in its own weight of alcohol at forty degrees. Some patients may object to its pungent odor; but that is temporary, while the remedy in some cases proves a permanent cure. Make the application at least twice a day, and protect the part with a soft flannel. Mustard mills are in operation in the cities generally, at which the oil may be procured, it being an article not much in demand in the arts. Were it not for detecting it by a pungent odor, this oil would have become a secret remedy for rheumatic pains years ago.

Two oz. each of tincture of squills and veratrum viride. Take six drops every three hours in water. It rapidly reduces the pulse in all fevers and inflammation. Two drops for children under three years.

SCROFULOUS SORES.—Iodine, ten grs.; iodide of potash, one dram; dissolve in syrup of rhubarb and water, each two oz. Take one tea-spoonful thrice daily. Or,

Twelve grains of iodine; sixty grains of iodide of potash; liquor of potash, one oz.; syrup of sarsaparilla, four oz. Take one teaspoonful thrice a day.

Make an ointment of twelve grains of the proto-iodide of mercury; one dram of the iodide of potash; one oz. of simple cerate. Rub into the skin thoroughly twice a day, where these are hardening.

Oxide of zinc, half a dram; glycerine, five oz. Apply as an emollient. Shake before using it. Or,

Six drams of iodine; of potash iodide, one and a half oz.; water one pint. Take five drops in water thrice a day.

SLEEPLESSNESS.—Epsom salts, two drams; elixir of vitriol, or aromatic sulphuric acid, two drams; tincture of opium, two drams; water, two oz. Take a teaspoonful as required. An excellent remedy to procure rest or allay pain when opium alone disagrees.

Powdered opium, one dram; powdered camphor, fifteen grains; white soap, two drams. Make sixty pills. Take one as required.

Take eight grains of sulphate of morphia; add six tablespoons of water, and two tablespoons of alcohol or other spirits. Take one tea-spoonful about ten minutes before going to bed; as four teaspoonfuls make a tablespoonful, there is one quarter of a grain of morphia to each dose. It should not be taken oftener than once in twenty-four hours; the above quantity will last a month, if a dose is taken every night.

Assafœtida, sixty grains; sulphate of morphia, four grains. Make sixteen pills; take one at bedtime.

Bromide of potassium, half an oz.; peppermint or cinnamon water, or pure water, six oz. Dose, a dessert-spoonful.

STYPTIC.—M. Pagliare, an Italian pharmacien, is the discoverer of a liquid possessing so extraordinary a power of coagulating blood, that if to a large basin containing this fluid one drop of the styptic be added, complete solidification ensues, so that the basin may be inverted without causing any blood to be lost. The practical advantages of this styptic are consequently very great, inasmuch as, by its timely application, the bleeding from large and dangerous wounds may be immediately stanched. In addition to the other valuable qualities of this liquid it is totally devoid of poisonous agency, and easily prepared as follows:

take eight ounces of gum benzoin, one pound of alum, and ten pints of water; boil all together for the space of eight hours in an earthenware glazed vessel, frequently stirring the mass, and adding water sufficiently to make up the original quantity of that lost by ebullition, adding the water gradually, so that boiling may not be suspended. The liquid portion of the compound is then strained off and preserved in well-corked bottles.

Spider's web sometimes stops bleeding wounds promptly; also the dust from a tea box, or a steady pour of spring or ice water.

SWELLINGS OF JOINTS.—Oil of sassafras, two fluid drams; water of ammonia, a tablespoonful; camphorated soap liniment, four oz. Rub in thoroughly night and morning.

SICK HEADACHE.—Bathing the head in cold water every morning, and frequently through the day in warm weather, is a preventive; also the free use of salt.

An emetic of ipecac in an infusion of boneset often gives relief by its revulsive action upon the nervous system, even though there may be nothing of moment in the stomach.

SYPHILIS.—Powder of opium and powder of ipecacuanha, each six grains. Mix, and divide into twelve pills. Take one every three hours. Or five drams of liquor of the iodide of mercury and arsenic in half a pint of the compound syrup of sarsaparilla. Take one teaspoonful thrice daily.

For eruptions take three grains of iodide of arsenic; twenty-five grains of extract of hemlock; make thirty-two pills. Take one thrice a day, for lepra.

Four drams of the compound liquor of the iodide of potash, in two and a half ounces of Fowler's solution. Four drops in water thrice daily.

Green iodide (protiodide) of mercury, ten grains; conserve of roses, a scruple. Divide into twenty pills. Take one twice daily.

Secondary Syphilis.—Liquor of the iodide of mercury and arsenic, half a fluid oz. Take four drops thrice daily. Or,

Four oz. of syrup of the iodide of manganese. Take twenty drops thrice daily in water, for constitutional syphilis. Or,

Extract of gentian, fifty grains; powdered silver, twenty-five grains; podophyllin, sixteen grains. Make sixteen pills. Take one nightly.

Corrosive sublimate or bichloride of mercury, three grains; dissolve in half an oz. of alcohol, and add decoction of Peruvian bark, eight oz.; tincture of myrrh, four ounces; honey of roses, one and a half oz. Gargle frequently in ulcerated sore throat of syphilis.

Chloride of lime, seventy grains; powdered opium, two drams; water, eight oz.; use as lotion to sores or chancres after being cauterized. Apply frequently on lint. Keep it wet.

For nodes and pains in the bones, syrup of sarsaparilla, seven oz.; syrup of poppy, one oz.; iodide of potash, sixty grains. Take one tablespoonful thrice daily.

Protiodide of mercury, three grains; iodide of potassium, two drams; tincture of rhubarb, one and a half oz.; compound syrup of sarsaparilla, two and a half oz. Take a teaspoonful thrice daily.

Iodide of potassium, two drams; protiodide of mercury, two and a half grains; tincture of gentian, two oz.; compound syrup of sarsaparilla, two and a half oz. Take a teaspoonful three times a day.

Extract of hemlock or conium, one and a half drams; protiodide of mercury, four grains; iodide of potassium, three drams; tincture cardamom, one and a half oz.; compound syrup of sarsaparilla, five oz. Good for all eruptions from bad blood. Take a teaspoonful thrice daily.

SKIN-DISEASES.—Creasote, eight drops; tincture of krameria, two fluid drams; hydrocyanic acid, ten drops; water four oz. As a wash twice daily.

PUSTULAR DISEASES OF THE SKIN.—Wine of colchicum root, and wine of ipecac, each two fluid drams. Mix. Take twenty drops in water thrice daily.

CHRONIC DISEASES OF THE SKIN.—Sulphite of soda, two oz.; glycerine, four oz.; water, enough to make a pint. Mix. Use as lotion.

OBSTINATE SKIN-DISEASES.—Oil of juniper, soft soap, and alcohol, each an oz. Use as an ointment.

STOMACH.—For irritated condition of stomach and bowels, take from 10 to 20 grains of subnitrate of bismuth in rice, at the beginning of each meal, or six grains of nitrate of silver, and 3 grains of opium; make twenty pills. Take one at each meal.

Two drams of bicarbonate of potash in a gill of water. A tablespoonful of this to a tablespoon each of water and lemon-juice in water, thrice daily.

Nitro-muriatic acid, half an oz.; muriatic acid, three drams. Dose, three drops, thrice daily in a teacup of water; or, if there is general debility, carbonate of ammonia, one dram; mucilage of gum-arabic, five fluid oz.; water, two oz.; one tablespoon hourly.

SCARLET FEVER.—Carbonate of ammonia, sixty grains; paregoric, two oz.; wine of ipecac, forty drops; water, six oz. Give one tablespoon in some lemonade, or vinegar and honey every three hours.

VOMITING.—Equal parts of clear lime-water and milk. Take a tablespoonful at a time.

For nausea and vomiting. Bicarbonate of potassa, one dram; compound tincture of cardamom, an oz.; syrup of ginger, two fluid drams; water, enough to make four oz. Take a dessert-spoonful.

Powdered cloves, ginger, and cinnamon, each two teaspoonfuls; wheat flour, a tablespoonful; brandy, enough to make a paste to spread upon flannel, and apply to the abdomen.

Bicarbonate of soda, four scruples; aromatic spirit of ammonia, one dram; solution of morphia, two drams; water, enough to make four oz. Take two teaspoonfuls.

Creasote, ten drops; bicarbonate of soda, one dram; solution of morphia, a dram and a half; peppermint water, enough to make four oz. Take two teaspoonfuls at a time.

Vomiting is caused instantly by swallowing one dram of carbonate of hartshorn in half a pint of warm water.

Calomel, two grains; half a teaspoon of white sugar, divide into eight powders. Take one every two hours; or a calomel pill of five grains at once.

TONICS.—Take thrice daily in water, at meals, six grains of phosphate of iron; or,

Take one hour's walk after each meal, for a week, and live on coarse bread, lean meats, and fruits and berries; or,

Three grains of quinine in half a glass of water at each meal, when fever and ague is present; or,

Thirty grains of quinine, sixty grains of carbonate of iron, into sixteen pills. Take one thrice daily; or,

One dram of elixir vitriol; compound tincture of Peruvian bark, three oz.; syrup of juniper, two oz. One teaspoonful thrice a day for protracted fever and ague.

Seventy grains of quinine; two grains of arnica; conserve of roses, forty grains. Make thirty-two pills. Take one night and morning.

Syrup of the iodide of iron, one oz.; tincture of black snakeroot, half an oz.; tincture of aconite root, three drams. Take twenty-five drops three times a day.

Sulphate of iron, two drams; iodide of potassium, one and a half drams; tincture of colomba, one and a half oz.; syrup of ginger, three oz. Take a teaspoonful thrice daily.

Fowler's solution of arsenic, one and a half drams; tincture of Peruvian bark, half an oz.; syrup of orange-peel, one oz. Take a teaspoonful three times a day for obstinate agues.

Iodide of manganese, two drams; tincture of cardamom, one oz.; syrup of sarsaparilla, six oz. Mix, and take a teaspoonful three times a day. Specially useful in glandular enlargements.

Carbonate of manganese, one dram; carbonate of iron, two drams; iodide of potassium, two drams; compound tincture of gentian, two and a half oz.; compound syrup of sarsaparilla, three and a half oz. A teaspoonful thrice daily.

ULCERS OR SORES.—Chloride of lime, one dram; powdered opium, one and a half drams; water, six oz. Use as lotion applied on lint, keeping the lint moist with the lotion. Useful in old and indolent ulcers of the leg and other parts of the body; also applied in same way to chancres after being cauterized.

Sixteen grains of blue vitriol in a pint of water is the best application known for all ulcers, or old sores, whether scrofulous or otherwise, and will cure all curable cases, making two applications daily as a wash; but two things must be done at the same time, the bowels must be made to act once in every twenty-four hours, and the patient must eat plain nourishing food three times a day, and nothing between meals, nor any fluid at any meal. In stubborn cases the amount of blue vitriol may be doubled; in all cases it should be made strong enough to cause considerable smarting when applied. It is very efficient in healing up ulcerations from salivation. The author makes this known from personal observation of its efficiency in the past thirty years.

WASHES.—Chlorate of potash, a quarter of an oz.; muriatic acid, forty drops; water, one-half pint to one pint. Mix. An excellent wash for chronic fetid ulcers, soon converting a foul ulcer to a healthy-looking one. A good gargle.

Powdered golden seal, one dram; powdered cranesbill, one dram; powdered witch-hazel bark, one dram. Mix and pour upon these a pint of boiling water. Let it stand till cold. Used to swab an ulcerated sore throat in scarlet fever, and for other purposes.

Another : Pulv. Cayenne, one dram ; salt, one dram ; boiling water, one gill. Mix and let stand fifteen minutes. Then add one gill of vinegar. Let it stand one hour, and strain. Put a teaspoonful in a child's mouth once an hour in malignant scarlet fever.

Creasote, twenty-four drops ; tincture of myrrh, four drams ; compound tincture of lavender, four drams ; simple syrup, one and a half oz. ; water, three and a half oz. Mix, and use frequently as a gargle for inflammatory sore throat ; or,

Creasote, twenty drops ; tincture of Cayenne pepper, two drams ; tincture of myrrh, half an oz. ; compound tincture of lavender, four drams ; simple syrup and water, one oz. each ; or,

Lunar caustic, or nitrate of silver, forty grains ; rose-water, four oz. Mix, and dissolve the caustic in the rose water, and use as a gargle as often as it seems to do good ; or,

Nitrate of potassa, two drams ; honey of roses, one oz. ; water, five oz. ; or,

Decoction of white-oak bark, seven oz. ; alum, thirty grains ; wine of galls, one oz.

Tincture of Cayenne pepper, one dram ; alum, one dram ; honey, one oz. ; water, four oz.

For the eye : One grain of corrosive sublimate ; two drams of wine of opium ; and water, half a pint. Bathe the closed lids with this several times a day. Or,

A teaspoonful of vinegar and half a pint of water. Make several folds of muslin ; dip in this, and let them lie on the closed eyes loosely, and if sore, let fall three drops into each eye, night and morning.

Laryngitis : Gargle often with a dram of guaiacum in a pint of tepid water, and take twenty grains internally thrice a day.

A good gargle is made of two parts water and six of glycerine.

If there are ulcers in the mouth, apply a powder of equal parts of chalk and gum-arabic ; or,

Twenty grains of sulphate of zinc in an oz. of water, in severe cases ; do not swallow any of the mixture.

Biborate of soda, two drams ; powdered myrrh, one dram ; water, six oz. Use as a mouth-wash.

Wine of ipecacuanha, half an oz. Take thirty drops every two or three hours, in a tablespoonful of water, for inflamed tonsils.

Tannin, thirty grains ; water, an oz. Applied with a hair-pencil to swollen tonsils.

One of the best gargles for common sore throat, and to loosen phlegm, is, one dram of tincture of capsicum to a pint of water, adding a level tablespoon each of salt and alum.

For ulcerated sore throat, as a gargle, half an oz. of liquor of chloride of lime in six oz. of water ; or,

Six oz. of decoction of pearl-barley ; as much tincture of myrrh ; tincture of opium, two drams ; honey of roses, one oz. Gargle. Or,

Six oz. of tincture of myrrh and one oz. of honey.

SYPHILITIC GARGLE.— Corrosive sublimate, three grains ; dissolve in half an oz. of alcohol, and add decoction of Peruvian bark, six oz. ; tincture of myrrh, four oz. ; honey of roses, one oz.

Chloroform liniment, tincture of camphor, and laudanum and sweet oil, each half an oz. Excellent for all pains.

Breaking out on the skin, with intolerable itching, is cured by wrapping the parts with cloths dipped in a solution of one dram of carbonate of potash in a pint of water; keep the cloths wet with it.

TAPE-WORMS result from eating meats, especially pork not well cooked. A full-grown worm has over one thousand joints; the most certain cure is to take mashed pumpkin-seeds before breakfast, not eating anything for six hours after; or,

Five drams of pink-root in a pint of hot water. Take one tablespoonful every three hours, having preceded it with a liver pill the night before, followed next morning with an oz. of castor-oil every hour until the bowels act, then take the pumpkin-seed; or,

Four drams each of pink-root and senna; sixty grains of anise in a pint of hot water. Take two tablespoonfuls every three hours, beginning on rising, and not eating anything sooner than noon.

Three grains of santonine twice a day, with a tablespoonful of castor oil night and morning, or twelve drops of worm-seed oil in an oz. of molasses. Take one teaspoonful on rising, on retiring, and at noon.

Powdered male fern is considered a superior remedy; two oz. in two oz. of molasses. Take one teaspoonful night and morning on an empty stomach.

Kousso is also an excellent remedy, taken on an empty stomach; take half an oz. in half a pint of water. Take half of this on rising in the morning; the other half in an hour; two hours after take two oz. castor-oil; an hour later take the first meal of the day.

Pin-worms, or ascarides, are sometimes insufferably troublesome; for children, an injection of three oz. of castor-oil every few days is efficient; or an injection of half a grain of iodide of potash and 1 grain of biniodide of mercury in two pints water; repeat this daily for four days; omit two weeks and begin again; one-quarter for children.

Take night and morning, on an empty stomach, three teaspoonfuls of the fluid extract of spigelia and senna, or two drams of quassia in a pint of boiling water; cool and inject.

Santonine, fifteen grains; cocoa butter, a sufficient quantity to make four suppositories. Mix and divide. Introduce one into the bowel at bedtime. Infallible for pin-worms.

Santonine, half a dram; divide into twelve pills. Take one thrice daily; half for a child.

Leaves of senna, and root of spigelia, each half an ounce; boiling water, a pint and a quarter; infuse, covered for two hours. Take a wineglassful morning and night.

WASTING DISEASES.—Cod-liver oil, syrup of ginger, and mucilage of gum-arabic, each two oz.; oil of cloves, eight drops. Mix. Take a tablespoonful thrice daily; or,

Cod-liver oil and glycerine, each two oz.; gum-arabic, two drams; oil of bitter almonds, three drops; oil of cloves, ten drops. Take a tablespoonful thrice daily.

Take of citrate of ammonia, iron, and quinine, ten grains; cod-liver oil and glycerine, each two oz. Mix. Dose, a tablespoonful.

Some of these six hundred formulæ are original, others have been taken from the private and published memoranda of the most eminent medical men of the century. Abernethy, Hunter, Marshall Hall, Liston, Parrish, Jackson, Warren, Dunglison, Hartshorne, Professors B. W. Dudley, John Eaten Cook, Barker, Flint, Post, Draper, Clark, Carnochan, and others; some of the most valuable are from the Essentials of the Principles and Practice of Medicine, by Henry Hartshorne, A.M., M.D., Professor of Hygiene in the University of Pennsylvania, (some of them original with himself), Henry C. Lea, Philadelphia, publisher, a volume which ought to be in the library of every intelligent practitioner in the country.

ALIMENTS FOR THE SICK.

EXTRACT OF BEEF.—Take one pound of rumpsteak, mince it like sausage meat, and mix it with one pint of cold water. Place it in a pot at the side of the fire to heat very slowly. It is well to let it stand two or three hours before it is allowed to simmer, and then let it boil very gently for fifteen minutes. Skim and serve; a tablespoonful of fresh sweet cream to a teacupful of this beef-tea renders it more nourishing, or thicken with a little flour.

Children, and even adults, will frequently take the raw meat simply minced when they are suffering from great debility. One teaspoonful of such meat should be given every four hours. If disagreeable, mix two parts of pounded white sugar and one part of meat.

ESSENCE OF BEEF.—Take one pound of beef free from skin and fat, chop it up as fine as mince meat, pound it in a mortar with three tablespoonfuls of soft water, and let it soak for two hours. Then put it in a covered earthen jar with a little salt, cementing the edges of the cover with pudding paste, and tying a piece of cloth over the top. Place the jar in a pot half full of boiling water, and keep the pot on the fire four hours; give two teaspoonfuls frequently. Useful in great debility, diphtheria, typhus, exhaustion from hemorrhage, etc.

BEEF ESSENCE—ANOTHER MODE.—Take a pound of good beef, free from fat, cut into small bits, and put into a porter bottle, loosely corked. Place the bottle in a kettle or pan of water, and keep it there until the water has been boiling at least an hour. As the boiling goes on the cork may be made a little more secure to prevent the contents of the bottle from escaping. The juices of the beef are thus forced from the fibre and are collected in the bottle, constituting the essence; season to suit. It was a favorite diet with the late Dr. Parrish.

BEEF-TEA is less nutritious than essence of beef. Boil a pound of lean beef with a quart of water for an hour; the resulting juice can be taken in much larger quantities, and with grated crackers or toasted bread makes a pleasant soup.

PANADA.—Take white bread, one ounce; ground cinnamon, one teaspoonful; water, one pint. Boil until well mixed; add a little sugar and nutmeg. Wine or butter may also be added if desirable. Or cut two slices of stale bread half an inch in thickness; toast them to a nice brown; break them up, place them in a bowl, sprinkle a little salt over them, add some sugar, and pour on a pint of boiling water; grate a little nutmeg.

CALVES'-FEET JELLY.—Boil two calf's feet in one gallon of water to a quart; strain, and when cold skim off the fat and take up the clear jelly. Put the jelly into a saucepan with a pint of wine, half a pound of loaf sugar, the juice of four lemons, the white of six eggs beaten to a froth. Mix well. Set the saucepan upon a clear fire and stir the jelly till it boils. When boiled ten minutes pour it through a flannel bag till it runs clear.

TOAST-WATER.—A slice of bread half an inch thick, toast it brown without scorching, pour over it a pint of boiling water; when cool strain and drink.

RICE-WATER.—Boil two ounces of rice for one hour in two quarts of water, add salt or sugar, and nutmeg. A good drink in diarrhœa.

OATMEAL GRUEL.—Pour a pint of boiling water on two tablespoonfuls of oatmeal, add half a pint of milk, and a little salt; simmer in a saucepan for half an hour, may add a few raisins; strain and drink, seasoned with nutmeg.

VEGETABLE SOUP.—Put three potatoes, one onion, and a piece of bread into a quart of water; boil it down to a pint. Then throw in a little chopped parsley and salt. Cover, remove from the fire, and allow it to cool.

BREAD-AND-BUTTER BROTH.—Spread a slice of bread with butter; sprinkle with salt and black pepper. Pour on a pint of boiling water; cover, and let it cool.

LIME-WATER AND MILK.—Take of clear saturated lime-water and fresh milk, each a wine-glassful. Mix. Take tablespoonful or less. This will sometimes remain upon an irritable stomach which will retain nothing else.

CHICKEN BROTH.—Clean half a chicken and remove the skin; pour on a quart of cold water, and salt to taste; add a tablespoonful of rice, and boil slowly for three hours; skim well, and add a little salt.

COMPLIN'S BRAN-LOAF FOR DIABETES.—Take two or three quarts of wheat bran, boil it in two successive waters for ten minutes, each time straining it through a sieve; then wash it well with cold water (on the sieve), until the water runs off perfectly clear; squeeze the bran in a cloth as dry as you can, then spread it thinly on a dish, and place it in a slow oven. If put in at night, let it remain until the morning, when, if perfectly dry and crisp, it will be fit for grinding. The bran thus prepared must be ground in a fine mill, and sifted through a wire sieve of sufficient fineness to require the use of a brush to pass it through: that which does not pass at first ought to be ground and sifted again, until the whole is soft and fine.

Take of this bran-powder three troy ounces; three fresh eggs; an ounce and a half of butter, and rather less than half a pint of milk. Mix the eggs with part of the milk, and warm the butter with the other portion; then stir the whole well together, adding a little nutmeg and ginger, or other spice. Just before putting into the oven, stir in, first, thirty-five grains of bicarbonate of soda, and then three drams of dilute hydrochloric acid. Bake the loaf in a basin, well buttered, for an hour and a quarter.

EXTRACT OF RAW BEEF.—Cut lean beef *very fine*, put in cold water (half a pint to a pound) in a bottle. Soak it for twelve hours, shaking it half a dozen times during that time; strain it off with pressure through a cloth. Mutton or chicken may be used in the same way.

LIEBIG'S BROTH.—Chop half a pound of beef, mix it well with one dram of table salt, four drops (ten would be better) of muriatic acid, and eighteen ounces of distilled water. Macerate for an hour, and strain through a fine hair sieve. Dose, a teacupful. This contains the *soluble* constituents of the meat, but not all its nutritive elements.

LIEBIG'S FOOD FOR INFANTS.—Mix together half an ounce of wheat flour, the same of malt flour, seven and a quarter grains of bicarbonate of potassa, and an ounce of water. Add five ounces of fresh milk, and put the whole upon a gentle fire. When it begins to thicken, take it from the fire, stir it for five minutes, heat and stir again until it becomes quite fluid; finally boil it for a short time. Filter through a sieve to separate the bran; it is then ready for use.

PANADA.—Take two slices of stale bread, without crust; toast them brown, cut them into squares of two inches, sprinkle with salt and a little nutmeg. Pour on a pint of boiling water, and cool.

ARROW-ROOT.—Mix a tablespoonful with cold water, to make a paste. Boil a pint of water, stir in the arrow-root, and boil it a few minutes. Sweeten with white sugar. Wine may be added if necessary. A little orange-peel added before boiling will improve the flavor.

TAPIOCA.—Cover three tablespoonfuls of tapioca with a teacupful or more of cold water, and soak for two or three hours, or over night. Put it into a pint of boiling water, and boil it until it is clear and of the desired consistence. Sugar, nutmeg, or wine, etc., may be added as required.

SAGO JELLY.—Mix four tablespoonfuls of sago, the juice and rind of one lemon, and a quart of water. Sweeten, and boil it, stirring constantly until clear; add four tablespoonfuls of wine.

APPLE WATER.—Slice two large apples, put them in a jar, pour over them a pint of boiling water, cover close for an hour, pour off the fluid and sweeten if needed.

APPLE TEA.—Roast eight fine apples, put them in a jar with two teaspoonfuls of sugar; pour on a quart of boiling water, let it stand near the fire for an hour, and take it as desired.

MUTTON BROTH.—Put a pound of lean mutton in a saucepan with two pints of water and a little salt, let it simmer for two hours, strain it through a sieve, and when cold, remove all the fat, and thicken with arrow-root, boiled rice, or bread crumbs; for weak stomachs, or for persons recovering from severe illness, this is excellent.

WINE WHEY.—Boil half a pint of milk, add a wineglass of Madeira or sherry wine. Separate the curd by straining through muslin or a sieve. Sweeten the whey to taste, and grate upon it a little nutmeg.

EGG AND WINE, OR BRANDY.—Beat up a raw egg, and stir in two tablespoonfuls of wine. Sweeten according to taste.

CAUDLE.—Beat a raw egg with a wineglassful of sherry, and add to it half a pint of hot gruel. Flavor with orange-peel and sugar.

MILK PUNCH.—Into a tumblerful of milk put two tablespoonfuls of brandy, whiskey, or Jamaica rum. Sweeten, and grate in nutmeg.

FERRUGINOUS CHOCOLATE.—Mix sixteen ounces of chocolate with half an ounce of carbonate of iron. Divide the mass into sixteen cakes. One may be dissolved in half a pint of hot milk, to be taken night and morning.

ANNOTATIONS.

THERE are many practical things in relation to health and disease which may be stated in a few words or sentences, without the necessity of separate chapters ; a number of these are presented here.

At least half the diseases and deaths of children under two years could be prevented by the attention of mothers to the following points :—

1. Regular feeding, not an atom between times.
2. Clean skin.
3. Good ventilation, especially while asleep.
4. Loose dressing, yet sufficiently warm.

A man had an ulcer twenty years and which obstinately refused to heal. Three pea-sized pieces of skin were taken from his arm and stuck on in patches upon the granulated sore ; in seven days they began to enlarge, and the entire ulcer was eventually covered with a healthy skin ; a bald head can be made to have hair grow on it in the same way as a tooth from one man's mouth will grow in the socket from which another was taken.

Tonics not only fail to do good in many cases, but cause injurious effects by not being preceded with medicines which remove engorgements of the liver and spleen. Hence never take a tonic unless preceded twenty-four hours by a liver pill.

Quinine fails to remove fever and ague permanently in many cases because it was not preceded by a dose of calomel.

The reader should remember that all that is new is not true necessarily, for example, the quibble that calomel does not act on the liver ; but that it some way brings bile from the system cannot be denied, that is all that is wanted ; and as the bile is made in the liver, the result is the same.

Bromide of iron has been successfully used in chronic diarrhœa, in doses of fifteen grains twice a day ; while bromide of potash is available in rheumatism, ten grains thrice daily.

The tincture of aconite is very valuable as an external application to the skin in bruises, hurts, and pains ; this is best done by protecting the skin of the finger with silk or rubber cloth, or tie a bit of sponge or soft rag to the end of a stick.

CASTOR OIL.—Is one of the mildest, safest, and surest remedies known for moving the bowels, but it is so disagreeable to take that many have to forego its benefits. It may be made almost tasteless thus :—one dessert-spoonful of castor oil ; magnesia, one dessert-spoonful ; oil of peppermint, one drop. Rub together into a paste. Children will take it generally without opposition.

To a pint of oil add a teaspoonful of oil of wintergreen and the same quantity of oil of origanum. Mix thoroughly.

Mix one tablespoonful of castor oil thoroughly with two tablespoonfuls of spiced syrup of rhubarb, and give it immediately after mixture. Child's dose, one teaspoonful.

BURNING FLUIDS.—Rock oil was first given as the name of what is now called petroleum, as it first comes from the well, or coal oil.

Coal oil is artificially made from cannel coal.

Camphene is distilled turpentine.

Burning fluid is made of two parts of turpentine and ninety-eight parts of alcohol.

Phosgene is made from alcohol and turpentine, and is really impure or diluted alcohol, or ten parts of alcohol and one of camphene.

Kerosene is the lightest product of coal oil.

THE WONDERS OF CHEMISTRY.—Aquafortis and the air we breathe are made of the same materials. Linen and sugar and spirits of wine are so much alike in their chemical composition, that an old shirt can be converted into its weight in sugar, and the sugar into spirits of wine. Wine is made of two substances, one of which is the cause of almost all combination of burning, and the other will burn with more rapidity than anything in nature. The famous Peruvian bark, so much used to strengthen the stomach, and the poisonous principle of opium, are found to be of the same materials.

DANDRUFF is cleaned from the scalp by rubbing into the roots of the hair, every morning, with the balls of the fingers, the following mixture: Stir one ounce of flowers of sulphur into a quart of water which has been boiled and cooled; next day strain off the water and use it.

USES OF SWEET OR OLIVE OIL.—Compresses wet with warm oil and applied, speedily remove pain and swelling of wasp and hornet stings, etc. Sweet oil is also used to destroy or dislodge insects in the auditory (ear) passages when swelling prevents other methods being used to remove them.

A gill of sweet oil drank every quarter of an hour until a pint and a half was taken, expelled a tape-worm from a gentleman within twenty-four hours.

Olive oil in large doses administered internally, and the warm oil used by friction upon the affected limbs, has repeatedly proved successful in cases of bites of venomous reptiles.

FRECKLES REMOVED.—Powdered alum, one ounce; lemon-juice, one ounce; rose-water, one pint. Shake and dissolve. Apply two or three times a day.

The following is one of the most elegant and efficacious washes for chapped hands, face, etc.: Pulverized borax, ten grains; glycerine, one dram; rose water, one oz. Mix.

EFFLORESCENCE OF THE FACE, so very annoying to young persons, females especially, has been treated with a solution of borax with happy results: Pulverized borax, two drams; orange-water and rose-water, each two oz. Wash the face five or six times a day with the mixture. Sometimes its powers are increased by adding two to four grains of corrosive sublimate. A proper regimen and healthy condition of the stomach, liver, and alimentary canal are essentials to be observed.

DR. RINEHART employed the following with great success in scaly tetter of the hand: Powdered borax, one-half dram; water, one oz. Employed twice a day.

ALUM curd is readily formed by agitating a lump of alum (say the size of a nutmeg) in the whites of two eggs. The curdled albumen, placed between pieces of fine gauze, and applied to the eye laboring under inflammation, affords much relief and is extremely grateful to the patient.

CHAFINGS OF CHILDREN.—Dust the parts with flowers of zinc, and give internally small doses of rhubarb and the best magnesia to correct the secretions.

ELIXIR VITRIOL in doses of ten drops, with or without half the quantity of laudanum, is very useful in *cholerine and profuse* diarrhœas.

COUGH OR EXPECTORANT REMEDY USED MUCH IN ENGLAND.—Take of wine of ipecac, two drams; syrup of tolu, four drams; gum-arabic, pulv., two drams; water, sufficient to make six oz. Dose.—For a child, one, for a grown person, two teaspoonfuls every four hours.

ANTI-BILIOUS PHYSIC TEA.—Take pulverized senna, one oz.; pulverized jalap, one-half oz.; pulv. ginger, one-fourth oz. Mix. A heaping teaspoonful of this powder steeped in half a cup of boiling water and sweetened with a teaspoonful of sugar, forms an excellent purgative draught; should be taken at bed-time or early in the morning. It is mild, yet active, equaled by few and surpassed by none as a general purge.

If the pulse suddenly decreases largely in any disease, it is going to the brain.

Asthma is often greatly relieved by rubbing chloroform liniment well into the skin over the chest, night and morning. Prompt relief has been given thus: Three ounces of the tincture of assafœtida, with one oz. of tincture of lobelia; forty drops at a time in water.

MEASLES.—Do not cause sweating to "bring out" the measles, but drink freely of cold water when thirsty; it is a great comfort.

GONORRHŒA AND GLEET.—Permanganate of potash in one ounce of water as an injection, or two grains of sulphate of zinc in an ounce of water; inject six times a day, and keep it up for a week after the discharge ceases, causing the bowels to act twice daily.

INGROWING TOE-NAIL.—Scrape the centre of the nail longitudinally to the quick, keep it well scraped in a line the eighth of an inch broad, then cover some yarn with mercurial ointment and press it under the edge of the toe-nail as far as you can, and keep it there ; or cut a triangular portion of the centre of the nail, having a wide base at the free edge of the nail, and a fine point at or near the matrix. This will cause the nail to contract from the edge towards the centre, and if kept up for six months will quite alter the shape of the nail, making it filbert-shaped and prominent in the centre. The edges of the nail should be raised and separated from the soft parts into which they intrude with a piece of worsted coated with mercurial ointment, or Monsel's solution of iron.

When very sensitive granulations exist, some extract of belladonna and resin ointment rubbed together form a good application.

Pulverized blood-root, sprinkled on old sores, often removes "proud flesh" and promotes healing.

PHYSICAL PROPERTIES.—Garlic, as kept by druggists, is a compound spherical bulb, flattened at the bottom and drawn towards a point at the summit ; covered with a white, dry, membranous envelope of several laminæ, with which the small *bulbs*, five or six in number, are arranged around the stem, each having a separate coat. They have a disagreeable pungent odor, so peculiar as to be termed *alliaceous.*

The active properties reside in a volatile oil, easily separated by heat. So penetrating is this oil and odor of garlic, that if a poultice even be applied to the soles of the feet, or taken internally, the odor will be exhaled from the lungs and the taste will be perceptible. The flesh of fowls, their eggs, as well as milk and butter, are liable to be impregnated by it.

MEDICAL PROPERTIES AND USES.—The use of garlic, both as a medicine and condiment, can be traced up to the highest antiquity. Moderately employed as a condiment it is beneficial in enfeebled digestion and flatulence.

A syrup of garlic is used with decided benefit in chronic catarrh and other pectoral affections, especially of children, as well as in the nervous and spasmodic coughs to which they are liable. A few drops of the juice has been used to check nervous vomiting, and to relieve earache, applied warm.

The expressed juice is an ancient remedy for *deafness*. Garlic, rubbed to a pulp with as much sugar as can be incorporated with it, is readily taken by young children, and is frequently efficacious as a vermifuge. Dioscorides advised garlic as a remedy for *tape-worm*, *venomous* bites, coughs, etc. ; and Celsus employed it to prevent the paroxysms of *ague*. One of the oldest uses was to apply it to the spine of young children affected with *whooping-cough*. The external use of garlic is more extensive, and perhaps more important than its internal. Bruised and applied to the feet, it relieves, by revulsive action, disorders of the head ; and in febrile disorders of children it quiets restlessness and promotes sleep.

WIVES are many times worked to death literally, brought to such a state of exhaustion from excessive family care and household labor, that there is no capability of resisting the onsets of disease, and being attacked, there is no power of recuperation, and death follows. But a great deal of hard work may be avoided by a little thought and planning sometimes. In the manner of washing clothing, for example, better than the old plan of half a century ago, better than any washing-machine of the present day, is the simple device of dissolving two pounds of soap in three gallons of water as hot as the hands can bear, to this add one tablespoon of turpentine and three of aqua ammonia, the mixture to be well stirred. Linens are steeped in this preparation two or three hours, care being taken to keep the boiler covered as closely as possible. The cloths are afterwards simply washed out and rinsed in the usual way. The preparation may be used the second time by the addition of half as much turpentine and ammonia. The process saves a great amount of time, labor, and fuel. The fabrics do not suffer, there is no necessity for rubbing on the washboard, while the cleanliness and color are perfect. Ammonia and turpentine possess strong detersive qualities, without injurious effect. The former evaporates at once after removal, and the smell of the latter, if too much has not been used, disappears during the process of drying. If the clothes are then submitted to a wringer, not only are the injurious effects of soda and potash avoided, but three-fourths of the hard work is avoided.

Dr. Boyd cures inflammatory rheumatism in from three to seven days, by producing free vomiting with tartar-emetic, then give five drops each of landanum and tincture of colchicum every three hours. In addition take every hour a teaspoonful of a mixture of four ounces of potash dissolved in half a pint of water, eating nothing whatever until all pain ceases, then take two tablespoons of milk or an oyster thrice a day, gradually increasing the amount daily.

Incontinence of urine is sometimes a troublesome symptom in old people. Take two drops of tincture of iodine thrice a day; a girl of twelve was cured of a two years' habit in two days, thus: Fifteen grains of hydrate of chloral every night, and to eat or drink nothing from 6 P.M. to 7 A.M.; the first night she did not get up at all, when before she had to get up four or five times; after the third day diminish two grains every night to nothing.

Croup, hoarseness, and loss of voice are promptly relieved sometimes by inhaling pure glycerine, fifteen minutes at a time, at every half hour's interval; it increases the secretion, that is, unloads the congestion of the parts. Inhale through an atomizer.

Fever and ague are cured in the Australian Hospital for Soldiers thus: Half an oz. of aloes; camphor, four scruples; orange-peel and elecampane root, each eight oz.; bruise, and let it stand in ten pints of alcohol or whiskey for eight days; then press it out, adding twelve oz. of dilute sulphuric acid; six oz. of sulphate of quinine; tincture of opium, one and a half oz. Give two drams three hours before the expected chill, eating but little. On the seventh, fourteenth, and eighteenth day after the last attack the same dose is given, and seldom fails. It is better to begin with an injection or a castor-oil purgative.

The only safe cans for preserving fruits, berries, or vegetables are glass jars; all others are liable to fatal poison.

POSITION OF HEAD IN SLEEPING.—The pillow should be only thick enough to allow the head to be on a line with the shoulder when lying on the side, that is, to be a very little above a horizontal line, for then it is easier for the heart to throw the blood to the head through the arteries, while there would be a little incline to favor the descent through the veins.

There is no advantage in sleeping in a room where water freezes, because the deadly carbonic acid settles towards the floor, and is so breathed by the sleeper. The chamber should not be lower than forty, and the fire-place should be open all the time. The sunniest room in the house should be the sleeping-room; the sun should shine in every family-room all day.

A room should not be repapered until the old paper has been removed.

To keep milk sweet several days put a teaspoonful of fine salt or horse-radish in a gallon pan; or it may be kept fresh for a year thus:—Procure bottles which must be perfectly clean, sweet, and dry; draw the milk from the cow into the bottles, and as they are filled, immediately cork them well, and fasten the cork with pack-thread or wire. Then spread a little straw in the bottom of a boiler, on which place the bottles with straw between them, until the boiler contains a sufficient quantity. Fill it up with cold water, and as soon as it begins to boil draw the fire and let the whole gradually cool. When quite cold, take out the bottles and pack them in sawdust in hampers, and stow them away in the coolest part of the house.

The best beverage in the world is cold water, but sometimes a different kind is needed, and is made thus:—Take of dilute sulphuric acid, concentrated infusion of orange-peel, each twelve drams; syrup of orange-peel, five fluid oz. This quantity is added to two imperial gallons of water. A large wineglassful is taken for a draught, mixed with more or less water, according to taste. All may drink this with pleasure. It is being consumed in large quantities daily, and I am convinced it will be the means of warding off a great deal of sickness.

A cooling wash for hands and face in fever is made thus:—One tablespoonful each of cologne, vinegar, and water; apply with a linen rag.

CROUP is sometimes instantly relieved by giving a teaspoonful of powdered alum in a little syrup, molasses, or oil; it vomits speedily.

Sore throat is often relieved by gargling every two hours with a teaspoonful of chlorate of potash dissolved in a glass of water.

Freckles are constitutional, always present, for which there is no remedy; or they are accidental, appearing only in summer in persons who have a very delicate skin. Into half a pint of milk squeeze the juice of a lemon, add a tablespoonful of brandy, boil, skim, add a tablespoonful of alum ; apply to the face night and morning.

Or, into a half pint of sour milk, scrape half as much horse-radish, next day strain, and apply morning, noon, and night.

Or, put a teaspoonful each of powdered borax and sugar into the juice of one lemon ; put it into a glass bottle and apply twice a day.

Pimples on the Face. To four tablespoonfuls of water add two grains of corrosive sublimate and apply night and morning.

Boxing the ears of children is a dangerous and inhuman punishment ; the drum of the ear, of paper-like thinness, is often ruptured by a single slap on the side of the face, causing an incurable and life-long deafness. All strokes on the head of children with an angry hand are brutal and criminal. A school-teacher once made a motion to hit a young child on the head with a closed penknife ; the blade flew out, and striking the skull at one of its joinings, the brain was penetrated, resulting in instant death. A generous, humane, and wise parent should allow a night to intervene between the commission of a fault on the part of a child and any decided punishment. The veriest thief is allowed time lest the law should be vindictive and wrathful. And shall a man or woman punish an unresisting child with angry inconsideration, with unreasoning wrath in the heart ? It is monstrous.

Thermometers are now coming into use for determining the grade of fevers, instead of the more uncertain pulse. In health there is a heat in the armpits of ninety-eight degrees Fahrenheit, winter and summer, day and night. In fevers it goes up to a hundred and six or eight, or more.

Softening of the brain is becoming a more common disease than formerly ; as it is utterly incurable, attention should be given to its causes. This softening is caused by an inflammatory condition or a gradual degeneration of the substance of the brain, arising from intense mental excitement, as a result of study, of the use of spirituous liquors, or allowing the mind to dwell on one subject unpleasantly, especially when there is no real cause, as in fancied slights, conjectured injuries, or injustices and the like, moping over them, cherishing thoughts of them. This lamentable malady comes on at one time with a sudden head or ear ache, at another with difficulty of speech, or numbness, or convulsions, or paralysis, or actual insensibility ; at other times there is simply a decline of the power of the senses, sight, hearing, speech, and the mental powers generally. The same disease is caused by the want of something to do, when there is no compulsion to mental effort or muscular exertion. To ameliorate a malady arising from causes so diametrically opposite, antipodal means should be employed, less work to the overworked, more work for those who have nothing to do.

Clergyman's sore throat is almost always found to have its origin in the stomach, thus : The voice-organs are always heated and wearied by public speaking ; then going out into a cold air too soon, they are too soon cooled off, are chilled, then comes the reaction of fever and inflammation, which relieves itself by an extra secretion of a viscid phlegm ; this adheres to the delicate vocal cords, preventing them from vibrating freely, as glue on a fiddlestring ; nature seems to know the cause, and there is an instinctive effort to hawk or hem or clear it away, and if successful, the voice is clear enough for awhile until a re-accumulation of phlegm takes place, to be hemmed away as before. These coolings off being frequently repeated, a habit of hemming is set up, to the very great annoyance of both speaker and hearers. But the real cause is far back of this. If there had been sufficient vigor of circulation of general health the parts would not have been so easily cooled and chilled ; this want of vigor in the circulation arose from the want of a vigorous, a healthy digestion, resulting in poor, bad blood. This want of a vigorous digestion comes from two causes—eating too much. exercising too little ; hence a European trip generally cures clergymen's sore throat, because there is a great deal of exercise and either a very little to eat, or the food is prepared in such a way that much cannot be eaten. Any ordinary case of clergyman's sore throat, called chronic laryngitis, can be cured by adhering to the suggestions under the heading of "General Health."

Catarrh is an extra discharge from the nose, coming down from the head, and is of two kinds—it has no odor, or it has an offensive one ; if it has no odor, three things will cure every case : avoid colds, keep the bowels acting every day, and

49

maintain the general health ; it can scarcely be called a disease, it is simply an effort of nature to relieve herself of a cold in the head by an extra discharge. As long as it remains in the head, it is a protection of the lungs against disease settling on them. It can only be made a serious disease by snuffing things up the nose to cure it. There never was a case of ordinary catarrh that either did not get well of itself, or that could not be cured perfectly and permanently in a reasonable time in the way named at the beginning of the article. This is said in the full knowledge of the fact that the newspapers have abounded in advertisements stating that it was a dangerous disease, and that it could be always cured for one, two, or ten hundred dollars. The other form of catarrh is where the odor is so offensive that it is perceived almost the moment the patient enters the room ; this is a catarrh connected with a scrofulous constitution, and never has been cured by any drug known ; the best plan is to let it alone, except to keep up the general health and free bowels ; if the offensiveness of the discharge continues, a weak solution of the chloride of potash, snuffed up the nose, night and morning, simply removes the odor, and that is all that ought to be done in any case to the nose directly. The representations made in the newspapers and in the pamphlets of irresponsible persons about the dangerous nature of any form of catarrh, and the ruinous results from neglect of paying a thousand dollars to get it cured, are utterly absurd. The real nature and meaning of what is designated by catarrh is a cold in the head, and that is the very safest place in which a cold can settle ; and if treated at all, it should be treated as any other cold. If the reader has any extra discharge from the nose, all that he has to do is to keep the bowels freely acting every day, live temperately, avoid colds, and exercise or work in the open air a great part of every day.

Paralysis is loss of motion in the body, in whole or in part ; sometimes half of the whole body, as in paraplegia ; sometimes of a single limb or muscle ; in some cases there is partial motion, but the mind cannot control it ; the limb moves, but not under the direction of the will ; this is because the nerves of motion are not nourished—are not strengthened enough to perform their proper service ; it is the blood which conveys the requisite nourishment, but it does not flow ; it stagnates—becomes congested ; muscular motion promotes the flow of the blood, but the patient has not the power to exercise ; in such cases artificial motion must be resorted to, either by the hand of another or by machinery ; this is the very essence of " THE MOVEMENT CURE," to which public attention has been directed of late years, it having been first reduced to a system in Sweden. It is applicable in that great variety of cases where exercise is needed and yet the patient is too weak to engage in it, or cannot take enough to answer any effective purpose. The author considers it a humanity to direct the attention of any of his paralytic readers to the subject, since it is a malady over which medicine has but little if any control.

NEURALGIA is literally "nerve ache," hence all pains are neuralgic, yet there are various kinds of pain. Rheumatism (see page 704) is pain in the joints, called arthritic rheumatism ; there is also a rheumatism of the muscles—that is, of the fibres which compose the muscles ; the blood-vessels which supply the nerves are too full of blood—are distended more than is natural, and press against the nerve pulp, causing pain ; that is, the blood-vessels which supply the nerves with nutriment, or are in immediate proximity to them, are congested ; if the congestion is in the arteries, it is a sharp, acute, racking, or throbbing pain ; if the veins are congested, the pain is dull or heavy or grumbling. If the latter, a mustard plaster will relieve it at once ; if the former, the direct abstraction of blood by leeches or the lancet is the most immediate remedy. If the pain is in the face or teeth, twenty grains of the hydrate of chloral, or one grain of iodoform sometimes gives speedy and permanent relief.

CROUP and diphtheria are characterized by a membrane forming around the inside of the windpipe ; it must be removed or dissolved, or death is certain. Sometimes the steam of hot water will do this ; at others, it is admirably done by mixing one grain each of bromine and bromide of potash in two tablespoons of rain or snow or distilled water ; dip a sponge in this, place it in a funnel or funnel-shaped pasteboard or paper, hold it to the mouth and nose of the child for five minutes every half hour ; infants breathe these fumes very well.

PURIFICATION OF HOUSES.—All cellars should have a fire-place in them, in the same stack with the kitchen-fire ; and in all houses where there are water-closets, there should be a pipe inserted just below the water-trap, as also below that of the kitchen-sink, the other end to terminate in the flue of the kitchen chimney, where there is always a draft upwards which would carry off all gaseous impurities in a constant stream.

COLDS ON THE CHEST.—All stuffings up and oppressions there, may be removed by applying a large cold-water compress over the whole chest and another over the throat ; if there is hoarseness for two or three hours in the morning soon after rising, see the article on compresses and their management.

DRINKING WATER may be carried to excess, and is often done under an impression that it washes out the system, cleans it of its impurities. The more fluid of any kind a person drinks, the more labor must be performed by the system in carrying it out of the body, and the more it is fatigued by such an operation ; hence persons may very easily drink too much of cold water, however pure it may be. The less water we drink the better ; in fevers, we may drink all we want, or swallow all the ice we desire ; but it is not healthy to drink much of any kind of liquid, as a general rule, except when thirsty.

BATHING.—Cold baths are always dangerous in the after-part of the day, in proportion as the person is tired or warm ; under such circumstances, the warm bath is very reviving and refreshing if not more than ten or fifteen minutes are spent in it, as the warm water dissolves the impurities which obstruct the pores of the skin, and also draws the blood to the surface, thus removing the congestions of the internal organs which are oppressed by them ; but after a warm bath in the evening it is best to go to bed, to avoid taking cold ; in this way a delicious sleep is often promoted.

"RAIN OR SHINE" should be the motto of all sedentary persons in reference to daily exercise, because a certain amount of it is needed to digest the food and work the accumulated wastes and impurities out of the system ; the fact of its raining does not prevent these accumulations. If exercise cannot be taken on any particular day, then but half the usual amount should be eaten, on the same principle, that, as on Sundays we exercise but very little in proportion to other days, but little should be eaten, and that should be of plain, untempting food, thus escaping sleepiness at church and the disagreeable unrest and discomfort so common in the after-part of Sundays.

BRIGHT'S DISEASE is simply a congestion of the blood-vessels of the kidneys, always brought on by intemperance or sudden changes from heat to cold, as by checking perspiration, injudicious changes in clothing, or the application of dampness to the small of the back. It is comparatively rare in latitudes where the weather is steadily cold or warm ; if promptly attended to it is easily cured, but, like consumption, it is incurable if neglected too long. More than one-half the cases in New York hospitals are among intemperate persons, hence are preventable ; most of the other cases are preventable because they result from colds, dampness, or chills ; an extra strip of flannel, or of buckskin outside the flannel, should be worn along the spine, covering the space between the shoulders, widening out, until at the bottom it should cover the whole of the small of the back, by all who are liable to any affection of the kidneys or in that region. It is of more importance to keep the spine well protected than the chest, because the latter is protected by a bony covering ; all observant persons know how soon a draught on the back will give a cold. It is said that one death in fifty in New York is from Bright's disease, one in ninety in London, one in two hundred and fifty in Paris, one in twenty-eight hundred in Bombay. It is our liquor-drinking, our hurry-scurry break-neck life, and the neglect of wearing the heaviest knitted woollen flannel next the skin from the first day of November to the first day of June, which cause the amazing disparities just stated. Such a garment, thus worn by all classes, especially the sedentary, the frail, and all above fifty, would diminish full one-half, in New York City, the diseases and deaths from coughs, colds, pleurisies, and especially inflammation of the lungs, that terrible scourge of our city. There is scarcely a family connection of any extent in which there is not made a gap every year by this sudden and rapidly fatal disease.

FEVER AND AGUE, of many weeks' continuance, may be promptly eradicated thus :—Put into a glass bottle sixty grains of sulphate of quinine, then add one hundred and twenty drops, that is, two teapoonsfuls or two drams, of elixir vitriol; to this add a pint of water or sixty tablespoonfuls; this gives about one grain of quinine in one tablespoon of water. Two tablespoonfuls or two grains make a dose. The vitriol is added to dissolve the quinine more effectually, and thus make it more efficient. Take one dose six hours before the expected chill, and repeat every hour until there is a decided singing, ringing, roaring, or rumbling in the ears. This will prevent the chill from coming on. Then take from five to ten grains of calomel or one or two liver-pills, according to the aggravation of the case; if they do not act on the bowels within twelve hours, take salts or castor-oil, or an injection. Repeat this process six hours before the time for the next chill; keep this up three or four days; it is not often necessary to repeat it oftener than once. This is the most certain and speedy cure for fever and ague ever put in print hitherto.

INGROWING TOE-NAIL is a fearfully painful ailment. The safest and best cure up to this time is to find the edge of the toe-nail with a probe, remove with a knife all the granulations and overgrowth, or proud flesh, on both sides, and nothing more whatever is needed except a bread-and-milk poultice, or any other, to remove the inflammation, securing a very free action of the bowels; or apply freely a few drops of perchloride of iron, night and morning, to the tender flesh, which it benumbs and hardens in a few days, so that it can be cut off or can be softened in water and removed with the finger-nail.

BILIOUS COLIC of the most painful and dangerous character may be promptly cured by putting a dram of chewing tobacco in a pint of boiling water; use half of it as an injection, keep it in awhile, and, within half an hour, all pain will be gone, and then free evacuations will take place. If the symptoms return within a few days, repeat the injection, using a light diet meanwhile. It is an admirable remedy for all forms of obstructed bowels, from its relaxing effects, and might be efficient in cases of intussusception—one part of the bowel running into another, as is seen in the finger of a glove sometimes—in drawing it off. Applicable, also, in lockjaw and strangulated hernia. These suggestions are very important, as the ailments named are often fatal in a few hours. When there is very great pain in the bowels without much fever, add to half a teacupful of warm water, twenty grains of hydrate of chloral, twenty drops of laudanum, and twenty pennyweights of tincture of belladonna, use it as an injection, and retain it a few minutes.

Summer complaint of infants and young children is often cured by giving from three to fifteen grains of pepsin, after having removed all undigested food from the bowels; sometimes half a grain or more of subnitrate of bismuth may be added to each dose.

NEURALGIA in any part may be removed promptly by the *continuous* application of galvanism for about two minutes, not removing the magnet or sponge from the skin, but moving them about on the skin.

CATARRH just commencing is thus treated by Hagner, of Berlin:— Mix five parts each of carbolic acid and spirits of hartshorn with fifteen parts of alcohol and ten parts water, kept in a dark glass bottle with ground-glass stopper. When the catarrh is commencing, lay a few drops on three layers of blotting or other soft paper, place this at the nose, shut the eyes and mouth, and draw up the breath forcibly and deep, as long as any smell is perceptible---repeat every two hours, until cured. It seems to cut short the disease at once.

SWEATING FEET, excessive. Dip them in cold water for a minute every morning, and sprinkle pulverized tannin freely in the bottom of the shoes every other day, wash the feet in warm water at night, afterwards dipping them in cold water for an instant.

ST. VITUS' DANCE, OR CHOREA, is an irregular twitching contraction of some of the muscles of the body, limbs, face or fingers, but not during sleep; in many cases it is an excess of nervous energy, and more or less dependent on an ill condition of the bowels or stomach before fourteen years of age. Laughing at children, or scolding them, only aggravates the malady, often fixing it for life. The best remedy is regular eating, to be doing something out-of-doors all day, and to keep the bowels acting once and sometimes twice every day, by the following mixture:—One dram of the citrate of iron, one dram of tincture of belladonna, two drams of the tincture of nux vomica, one fluid oz. of tincture of aloes and twelve ounces of lemon syrup; give one teaspoonful, more or less, night and morning, so as to secure one full, free evacuation of the bowels every day. Continue all these until a cure is effected.

PILES, or hæmorrhoids, is a very painful and troublesome affection about the end of the bowels, or intestinal canal; it is literally a blood flow, and is very common, generally affecting persons who sit a great deal, especially on soft, warm seats or cushions; resulting often from costiveness, then aggravated by looseness, straining too much at stool, or remaining too long at stool, or pregnancy, or whatever else may cause congestion, or too much blood flowing into the small blood-vessels on the inner side of the lower end of the rectum, causing the sides of these little blood-vessels to distend or bulge out, as the blood is more and more crowded or wedged in, making little knobs, sometimes inside, sometimes outside, called internal and external piles; when these little knobs burst, they are called bleeding piles; if they do not, "blind piles;" these are the most painful, for the bleeding ones relieve themselves. After stooling, the finger ends or balls should be placed on the parts, and pushed upwards as the patient rises, so as not to have the pile caught on the outside of the purse-string-like apparatus of the parts, for then it will get larger and more painful as more blood accumulates in it, while none can return in consequence of the constriction. Persons subject to piles must guard against costiveness in all ways possible, and night and morning and after each stool should place themselves over a basin of cold water, and flap it up against the parts until they fairly ache with cold; this tends gradually to invigorate the blood-vessels and give them power to pass the blood onwards as fast as it arrives, and thus prevent congestion. If, after a fair trial, these remedies do not avail, and the blood escaping from the piles, under the mucous membrane, forms tumors from time to time, which break and discharge blood freely, then take an injection of cold water, three times a day, retaining it until warmed a little, the object being to cool the parts; after each injection, or otherwise, grease the parts well with sulphur or any other ointment or pain-killer, the object being to soothe and cool the parts. Twice a day sit over a close vessel, containing hops, on which boiling water has been poured; or the leaves or seed of the stramonium, that is, thorn-apple, known by some as the "Jimson," or Jamestown weed. Very many "pile ointments" are sold; none of them have any virtue beyond a little sweet oil, or glycerine, or hog's lard, or a level teaspoonful of powdered sulphur, mixed well with two ounces of hog's lard. A quicker way in many cases is to apply to a surgeon, who will tie the foot of the pile with floss silk, tightening it every day or two, when the pile comes off. Some physicians prefer to cut them off at once, and be done with it. Regular bowels, hard seats, and cold water flappings and injections will prevent and cure most cases, if the diet is light and cooling, and rest on a bed is observed until relief is obtained. An ointment made of equal parts of lard, powdered galls and opium or laudanum, is very soothing. If the bowels are very costive, take sulphur or castor-oil in small and frequent doses.

SICK HEADACHE is a result of too much blood, congestion in the veins of the brain, and too little arterial blood in the arteries; the congestion gives disturbed vision and cold feet and nausea; the lack of blood in the arteries causes debility, faintness, and similar symptoms; hence lay the patient flat without a pillow, with the arms extended above the head; these aid the heart in sending more blood to the brain; then bathe the feet in hot water, may add mustard, or encase them in hot ashes or hot salt; this draws the excess of venous blood from the head to the feet, or equalizes the circulation, which may be still further energized by any diffusible stimulant, strong red pepper or ginger-tea, or a few drops of hartshorn or camphor in a little water. If much pain in the head, keep a cloth wrung out of hot water on it all the time, and drink freely of very warm water until vomiting is induced, and if the bowels are costive, take an injection. The hot cloths to the head disperse the congested blood of the veins and invite the arterial flow.

HEARTBURN, OR ACIDITY.—Aitkin, of Edinburgh, gives as his favorite remedy a powder thrice a day of fifteen grains of bicarbonate of soda and three grains of nitrate of potash; carbonate of ammonia, one grain; extract of gentian, two grains; in form of pill, thrice a day for a weak digestion; but in either case a liver pill should be taken at bed-time, not to be repeated within a month, aided by a strict fruit diet and plentiful out-door exercise.

COSTIVENESS.—Dr. Aitkin induces one gentle motion of the bowels daily by giving early in the morning a pill made of four grains of the compound extract of colocynth with half a grain each of sulphate of iron and extract of nux vomica.

MINERAL ACID.—Drs. Aitkin and Bence Jones think that, as a general rule, sulphuric acid is astringent, hydrochloric acid promotes digestion, while nitric acid, or aquafortis, largely diluted, aids the secretions.

INDIGESTION, from want of the proper amount of gastric juice, is aided by Da Costa's remedy: one dram of nitro-muriatic acid in two oz. of wine of pepsin. After each meal take one teaspoonful, keeping the bowels free, using meats mainly, and avoiding sweets and starches.

CHLOROFORM should never be taken in surgical or dental operations except under three conditions: 1, the person should not be brought under its influence in a shorter time than twenty minutes; 2, the force or volume of the pulse should not be perceptibly diminished; 3, nor should the skin be darkened. With these three conditions chloroform, as an anæsthetic, it may be considered safe.

HYDRATE OF CHLORAL, to promote sleep, should not be taken in doses exceeding thirty grains; should not be taken when there is fever, or dysentery, or chronic diarrhœa, or rheumatism, or typhus, or heart affections, or hysteria; it should never be taken except dissolved in some liquid in proportion of twenty parts to a hundred; it is best taken in beef-tea, or syrup of orange-peel, or as an enema in gruel.

ANTIBILIOUS PILLS have been used for thirty years by a Georgian physician; if any one wants to make them purely vegetable antibilious pills, use soap instead of the calomel.

Sixty grains each of calomel, aloes, and rhubarb, mixed with twelve grains each of capsicum, gamboge, podophyllin, and extract of hyoscyamus, make it into a mass with water or syrup and divide into twenty-two pills; dose from two to four at bed-time; if they do not act on the bowels in twelve hours take a tablespoonful of castor-oil or Epsom salts every two hours until the bowels move.

BURNS.—To one hundred parts of glycerine add three parts of freshly precipitated hydrate of lime and three parts of chlorinated chlorohydric ether; this makes a clear, transparent liquid, using more or less of the glycerine. This is a favorite application of De Bruyne, of Brussels. Wet several folds of fine linen thoroughly with this preparation and lay it on the part, covering it with oiled silk, india-rubber cloth, or even flannel, to prevent evaporation; it is also an excellent preparation for ill-conditioned and noisome wounds, sores, and ulcers, and in dry, scaly, and itching conditions of the skin.

LINIMENT for small-pox, erysipelas, rheumatism, sprains, gout, and carbuncle, soothing and cooling, also raging inflammations; it is sometimes almost wonderful in its effect; it also disinfects as well as cools: Gasoline, one pint; gum camphor, one ounce; pulverized sulphite of soda, one dram; pure carbolic acid, thirty drops. Sponge the whole body with this mixture every two hours in small-pox, or other more limited diseased parts, taking ten drops in sweetened water every three hours during daylight. It also checks all forms of ulceration; its main virtue lies in its great power of evaporation; a bottle of it with ground stopper may be well kept in every family.

WORM MEDICINES should be given in their most concentrated forms, hence early in the morning when there is no food or fluid on the stomach to dilute them, and for the same reason do not eat or drink anything for two or three hours, and then before eating take a dose of castor-oil to carry off the worm medicine and the worms with it. Worms thrive on the diseased mucous membrane of the intestines; worms cannot exist in a healthy condition of the alimentary canal and digestive functions. Hence, after having got rid of any kind of worms, means should be taken to improve the general health or they may return. What kills one kind of a worm may not hurt another. The most efficient worm medicines are the areca nut, filix mas, kamela, kousso, mucuna, pomegranate root bark, pumpkin seed, santonine, scammony, Tin powdered, turpentine spirits. Santonine is almost a specific for thread worms; two or three grains in a teaspoonful or two of castor-oil every morning for three or four mornings. Mixed with castor-oil and albumen as an injection, santonine kills thread worms in ten minutes.

LUMBAGO of a virulent form is reported by Homœopaths to have been permanently cured by giving one drop of the spirit of Venice turpentine on a lump of loaf sugar, thrice a day.

BEST BEEF TEA.—Lay a thin steak on a board, scrape it with a knife until nothing but the fibrous tissue is left; mix what is scraped off with three times as much cold water, stir it most thoroughly, put it over a moderate fire and let it come slowly to a boil, stirring it well all the time to keep it thoroughly mixed and to prevent the burning or caking of the pulp; as soon as it comes to a boil, remove, let it cool, and season it to the taste; take from two to six tablespoonfuls at a time; this is the best concentrated meat fibre, the most nutritious beef-tea that can be made.

PSORIASIS is a scaly eruption of the skin. Wash and rub off the scales with warm water and soap, then paint the skin with acetic acid or strong vinegar; it smarts considerably, so operate on two or three square inches at one time; scales form, and in two or three days fall off, then renew the application; but apply it three times a day, until the skin whitens and puffs up; a cure is effected within a month if the bowels are made to act daily and the food consists only of coarse breads and fruits.

HEMORRHAGES, or bleedings and aneurisms of *every* description,—lungs, nose, menorrhagia, etc., etc.,—seem to have been controlled by five drops of Norwood's tincture of veratrum viride hourly for five or six hours. In aneurisms, increase one drop every hour, until the sedative effects are seen.

BLISTERS on the inner side of the thighs have been exceedingly efficient in swelled testicle, chronic gonorrhœa, and labial abscess.

COUGHING PAROXYSMS, sore throat, and hoarseness are often wonderfully relieved by carrying in the pocket a piece of rich pine, and when needed, cut off a few shavings with a pen-knife; hold them in the mouth, which is to be kept closed; the air coming in at the nostrils and reaching the throat and lungs, after it has passed through the shavings, more or less carries their odorous particles along with it; it seemed to cure in one case of twenty years' standing.

PIN-WORMS IN HORSES are cured by mixing with their food every other day a gill of wood-ashes, because there is acidity causing a diseased condition of the inner covering, the mucous membrane of the bowels; in this worms thrive; the ashes form an alkali with the fluids of the stomach and correct the acidity; hence a little saleratus or half a dozen drops of hartshorn or any other alkali, in a little water at each meal, is sufficient sometimes to dislodge pin-worms. Or from half to a whole teaspoonful of the iron scales around the anvil, powdered in syrup, every morning, and a teaspoonful of flowers of sulphur at bed-time for ten or fifteen days; omit a week, then repeat, if the worms have not disappeared. Dr. Butler, of the Philadelphia *Medical and Surgical Journal*, says he has cured epilepsy in the same way repeatedly, and other nervous affections from similar causes.

TOOTHACHE is modified on the principle of derivation in many cases, by partly filling a large-mouthed vial with the bisulphuret of carbon and placing it against the cheek, near the tooth, with the stopper out for a minute or two by the watch; re-apply if the pain returns; it is a temporary but a very welcome relief; if the pain arises from ulceration or decay, the teeth must be removed. In about a minute a slight burning is felt on the cheek, from the fumes of the article coming in contact with the skin.

FROSTED FEET cause intolerable itching, because of contact with the oxygen of the air; if there is no swelling, dissolve gum shellac in alcohol and spread it over the part thickly; it dries without sticking to the stocking, and thoroughly excludes the air. If there is swelling and pain, cover with any good sticking-plaster or salve; if there is great inflammation and pain, keep it covered from the air with any moist poultice.

DYSMENORRHŒA.—Begin two days before the time and take night and morning, in water, from ten to twenty drops of the following mixture; dissolve one ounce each of gum guaiac and Canada balsam in four ounces of alcohol, let it stand three days, then pour off the clear liquid, to which add four ounces of alcohol in which has been dissolved one scruple of corrosive sublimate. When the flow is established, omit until next time, keeping the bowels active daily and using a fruit diet.

STOMACH IRRITABLE OR CHOLERA MORBUS, not from organic cause, has been successfully treated for ten years thus : one drop of creosote in one ounce of lime-water ; give five drops every ten minutes, or one drop every three minutes.

STOMACH IRRITATION, OR "MORNING SICKNESS" OF PREGNANT WOMEN, if nothing is eaten after a noonday dinner, but a cracker or some bread-crust broken into a cup of tea for supper, is cured thus: take twelve grains each of lactate of iron, citrate of iron and strychnine, and sulphate of quinine ; make into twelve powders, and take one every four hours during the day-time.

CHAPPED NIPPLES.—M. Van Holsbeck recommends the following formula as of great service :—Oil of cade (empyreumatic oil of juniper) 3½, oil of almonds 2, glycerine 3. When the chaps are very large and deep the proportion of oil of cade must be increased. It is to be applied every time the child has sucked by means of a badger's-hair brush. The child exhibits no repugnance to it. For a short time the application causes a little heat ; but in a few days the sores are healed.

PILES, external, have often been cured by the use of rectified oil of amber as a wash, or made into an ointment with sweet oil, lard, or glycerine, and rubbed well into the parts night and morning with the finger. It smarts at first only.

DIPHTHERIA.—Dr. Bailhache of Springfield, Illinois, says : " The local applica-tion of a solution of persulphate of iron (Liquor ferri persulphatis), in cases of diphtheria and ulcerated sore throat, acts almost as a specific in arresting the ul-cerative inflammation of these two alarming diseases. It should be applied un-diluted by means of a probang (or a rag securely fastened upon one end of a bent stick) immediately to the ulcerated patches or sloughs. Two or three such appli-cations, together with the usual tonic treatment, will restore the parts to a healthy condition in twenty-four hours."

DYSENTERY.—Creosotum, 10 drops ; acetic acid, 20 drops ; sulphate of mor-phine, 2 grains—all mixed in an ounce of distilled water. A teaspoonful of this is given every three or four hours to adults ; smaller doses are given to children, in gum-arabic mucilage. Drs. McMath and Weilder consider it nearly, if not entire-ly, a specific in dysentery.

CHOLERA PRESCRIPTION.—The Board of Health of New York city recom-mends the following prescription in severe cases of diarrhœa, when the services of a physician cannot be immediately obtained.

Tincture of opium, tincture of camphor, tincture of capsicum, of each 1 drachm ; chloroform, half a drachm ; mix and take half a teaspoonful after every evacua-tion. This will in most instances cure a diarrhœa, but it does not follow that it will cure cholera. The typhoid symptoms which the disease leaves behind it in the system must have other treatment ; but much has been gained when these characteristics have been overcome. By the use of the above remedy until a pa-tient can be seen by a physician, a recovery may occur which would be hopeless if the disease were permitted to go unchecked into a full or even partial col-lapse.

CROUP, and the forming stages of diphtheria, have been cured during a practice of seventeen years thus : Have four or five folds of muslin or linen, large enough to cover the whole throat from ear to ear and the upper part of the breast nearly down to the nipples ; dip this cloth into ice water or even fresh spring or well water, wring it out just enough to prevent dripping ; cover this with several thicknesses of dry woollen flannel, then secure all with a silk handkerchief ; as soon as the first cloth has become warm, have another ready to apply in its place, and continue until perfect relief, which takes place as soon as the skin over the throat comes down to its natural warmth. The water must not dribble on the clothing.

ASTHMA.—All that a man has will he give for relief in the dreadful paroxysms of asthma. A remedy is sometimes efficient to-day and useless to-morrow, and may be as good as ever next week; hence several are here named. The smoke of the dried leaves of stramonium, that is the thorn-apple or "Jimson" weed. Burn the leaves in a funnel turned upside down, conducting the smoke into a wide-mouthed bottle turned upside down, hold the nose, take the bottle-mouth in the mouth, draw in the fullest breath, close the mouth, hold it as long as you can, then let the air out of the lungs, and then inhale again ; continue until relieved. The fumes of burning coarse paper which has been soaked in saltpetre-water and dried can be inhaled in the same way. Chloric ether breathed sometimes relieves; at others, ten grains of common alum in fine powder, plastered far back on the tongue, is often beneficial, if allowed to dissolve, and then swallowed. The fumes of burning tobacco, inhaled like the stramonium, sometimes give grateful relief. Strong Mocha coffee, a swallow or two at a time, is good. If the attack is from mental causes, an injection of two grains of the sulphate of morphine with a drachm of the tincture of assafœtida in a little water, so as to be retained, has given almost instantaneous relief when all other things have failed. Any person subject to attacks of this most agonizing malady, should have all these remedies on hand, in the house, all the time, and, if he goes on a journey, should take them with him.

SKIN DISEASE FROM SYPHILIS is often removed thus: Two grains of corrosive sublimate and two grains of the iodide of potash, dissolved in eight ounces of water; take near one tablespoonful thrice a day.

LINIMENT, of extraordinary value in all forms of skin-heat, fever, and inflammation. Sponge the parts every two or three hours, until relieved, and give five or ten drops in sweetened water every three hours in carbuncle, erysipelas, gout, rheumatism, spasms; in small-pox, reducing its heat, neutralizing its odor, preventing exhalation and pitting, and soothing the whole body. One pint of gasoline, one ounce of gum camphor, one drachm of pulverized sulphite of soda, and thirty drops of pure carbolic acid. Every family owes it to itself to keep a bottle of this invaluable liniment on hand, all the time, marked " Poison," in large letters, as a drink of it would be fatal; but its external application has amazing value, in reducing the fiery rage of inflammation in very many cases.

MILK CURE.—Fresh, sweet, warmed, not too hot to be drank, nor boiled, has great curative powers, if judiciously used; its safety and efficiency in all poisons has already been noticed, and the reader's special attention is solicited to what follows. The London *Milk Journal*, on the authority of Dr. Benjamin Clark, states that in the East Indies warm milk is regarded by many as a specific, which means an almost certain cure, for diarrhœa; it is used in the United States, in the form of ice-cream, for the cure of loose bowels in children. One pint of warm, fresh sweet milk every four hours, will often check the most violent diarrhœa, stomach-ache, dysentery and cholera. A gentleman states he has tried it as often perhaps as fifty times in his own case, with unvarying success in from six to twelve hours. One man seemed to be dying from diarrhœa of eight months' standing; in three weeks he was a hale, hearty man. The *Medical Times and Gazette* states that in 26 cases of typhoid fever, it did not fail to be of great value; it checks the diarrhœa and nourishes and cools the body. Every man ought to remember that nourishment is as imperatively needed in disease as well as in health, especially in nervous diseases, and warm sweet milk will remain on the stomach, in many cases, when nothing else will, not even cold water, and not only nourishes but soothes and cools, promotes sleep, and averts delirium. In scarlet fever, give the patient as much warm milk as can be taken; it nourishes, sustains, and in many cases is a blessed remedy, as above applied.

SMALL-POX is almost infallibly modified, as well as scarlet fever, thus: Sulphate of zinc, one grain; fox glove (digitalis), one grain; half a teaspoonful of water. Mix most thoroughly, then add four ounces of water or eight tablespoonfuls, take one to four teaspoonfuls every hour.

CONSTITUENTS OF FOOD.—Scientific investigation has determined the following as being the proportion of constituents, in the ordinary articles of food which are utilized in the nourishment of the human body, and may be studied by all with interest and profit. The table is to be read thus: One hundred pounds of artichokes contain two pounds or two per cent. of nitrates, that is of that quality or ingredient of the food which helps to make muscle or flesh; nineteen per cent. of carbon or that which warms the body. Fats, oils and sugars are nearly all carbon, can be burnt, leaving nothing; so also table-butter, lard and suet; so the carbonates warm. The nitrates give strength of body, the phosphates feed the brain and bones, and strengthen both, of which there is only two per cent. in the artichoke, while seventy-six per cent. is water and one part waste, that is, cannot be used in any way and is voided from the body. It will be seen that the largest portion of ordinary food is water; thus persons in common life and in good health really need very little fluid of any kind, unless they exercise a great deal or are overheated. The general use to be made of the table is in four directions:—

1. If costive, use the food which has the most waste; this accumulates in the lower bowel, distends it, like an injection.

2. If the bowels are too loose use the most concentrated food, having little waste or water, as rice.

3. If the body is chilly in cold weather, the oils, the food which has the most carbon, is appropriate, if it can be digested. The Greenlanders luxuriate in oil and fats.

4. If the system is feverish, use the fruits, for they are nearly all water, having little nutriment and no waste, hence do not oppress the system, but cool it off, keep it open and free; a blank means an inappreciable quantity.

ARTICLES.	Nitrine.	Carbonates.	Phosphates.	Water.	Waste.
Artichoke	2	19	2	76	1
Asparagus	1	5	1	93	
Bacon	8	63	1	28	
Barley	32	15	4	14	17
Beans	24	40	3	15	18
Beef	19	14	2	68	
Buckwheat	9	53	2	14	23
Butter		100			
Cabbage	1	6	1	91	1
Carp	18	1	3	78	
Carrots	1	12	1	83	3
Cauliflower	4	5	1	89	1
Corn, Southern	12	68	1	14	5
Corn, Northern	35	39	4	14	8
Cheese	31	28	5	36	
Cherries	1	21	1	76	1
Chicken	21	2	3	74	
Chocolate	9	88	2		1
Clams	12	1	3	74	
Codfish	16	1	2	80	
Cream	4	5		91	
Cucumbers	1	2	1	95	1
Currants	1	7		81	11
Dates, Fresh		74		24	2
Eels	17	4	4	75	
Eggs, White of	13		8	86	
Eggs, Yolk of	17	30	2	51	
Figs	5	58	3	20	14
Flounders	15	3	4	78	
Green Gages	1	26	26	45	2
Haddock	14	1	8	83	
Halibut	18	3	4	75	
Ham	35	32	4	29	
Herrings	18	3	4	75	
Horse-radish		5	1	76	16
Kidney	21	1	1	76	
Lamb	20	14	2	64	
Lard		100			
Lentils	26	39	2	14	20
Liver	26	4	1	69	
Lobster	14	1	5	79	
Milk, Cow	5	8	1	86	

ARTICLES.	Nitrates.	Carbonates.	Phosphates.	Water.	Waste.
Milk, Human	8	7	1	89	
Oats	17	51	3	14	15
Onions	1	5	1	93	
Oyster	13			87	
Parsnips	2	14	1	79	3
Pearl Barley	5	78	2	9	8
Pears		10		86	4
Peas	23	41	3	14	19
Pigeon	23	2	3	72	
Potatoes	2	16	1	73	8
Potatoes, Sweet	2	22	3	67	6
Pork	17	17	2	66	
Prunes	4	79	5	12	
Radishes	1	7	1	89	1
Rice	5	82	5	10	3
Rye	7	75	1	13	4
Salmon	20	1	6	73	
Smelt	17	2	6	75	
Sole	17	1	2	80	
Suet		100			
Trout	17	1	4	78	
Turbot	14	1	5	80	
Turnips	1	4	1	90	4
Veal	18	14	2	66	
Venison	20	8	3	66	
Vermicelli	47	88	1	14	
Wheat	15	66	2	13	4
Whey		5	1	94	
Whiting	15	6		79	

URINATION.

Very many persons keep themselves in a constant state of disquietude by inspecting the urine, and drawing adverse conclusions from its quantity, frequency, and color, when in reality the conditions are the natural results of the varying circumstances of human life ; only an experienced physician is competent to decide what indicates disease and what health. If the weather is cold or becomes so suddenly, the pores of the skin are closed and the fluids are driven inwards, and what would have been gotten rid of by perspiration, must be carried out of the system through the kidneys and the bladder, then the urine is of a lighter or amber color and in much larger quantities.   If a person perspires a great deal, works hard in warm weather, then most of the water passes from the body by perspiration ; and thereby, so wonderful are the economics of nature in her operations, this very useless matter, useless because it has subserved its purposes, is made a means of cooling the body by its evaporation, as it escapes from it, carrying away in steam the extra heat of the system, as witness the dry condition of the skin in fever, how it burns up the body and soon wastes away the life unless subdued.

When persons perspire profusely, the more fluid portions of the waste water escape by the skin ; the more solid parts are conveyed away through the interior channels ; hence, in warm weather, the urine is scant, is of a high color, and deposits more or less sediment, usually reddish ; these more solid particles frequently cause irritation or burning in their passage, and the discharges are frequent and scant.   Articles of food and drink greatly influence the color and quantity of the urine ; buttermilk, lemonade, flaxseed tea, watermelons, &c., largely increase the amount of water.   Although free urination is a sign of health, as a general rule, it must not be concluded that the freeer it is, the more healthful we must be, and therefore that it "is healthy" to drink large quantities of cold water because it "washes out the system."   Drinking cold water has ruined the health of thousands, it has brought on chills at the dinner table, in feeble persons, resulting in death in a few days, in a few hours sometimes.   Multitudes have brought on life-long dyspepsias, simply by getting into the habit of drinking a glass or two or more of ice water at meals ;   this ice water is at forty degrees ;   it must be warmed up to ninety-eight degrees before the stomach can go on with the work of digestion ;   this abstracts, absorbs so much of the heat of the system as sometimes to cause a feeling of chilliness at the dinner table, even on a summer's day—quite a common thing in feeble constitutions—and every chill must be followed by a fever and this is a cold, hence drinking a glass of ice water may give a person a cold, may abstract heat from the system so rapidly as to chill it, and the chill falling on the lungs may induce Pneumonia in a few hours.   A French general of artillery, in the Crimean war, having exerted himself in bringing some cannon to an eminence, found himself tired, thirsty, and perspiring ;   he drank in his haste, a glass or two of snow water, a chill followed ; inflammation of the lungs set in, and he died in a few days, very generally regretted, for he was a good officer and a brave man ; it was not that it was snow water, it was the coldness of it which killed him. A glass of spring or ice water may be taken at a repast with impunity, for a time at least, by robust persons, but it is an injurious habit for all that, in all cases. If persons must drink something at meal time, the liquid should be hot ; persons who are not robust, all old persons, require a single cup of hot drink, and the best thing is a cup of tea ; that kind of China tea, which of the very many different kinds, seems to agree with the person using it ; but in all cases where any discomfort whatever follows drinking a cup of tea or drinking anything else, that thing should be let alone : common sense teaches that. If a person is chilly or very tired on sitting down to a meal, a cup of hot tea is very comforting, very refreshing, and very healthful, an unmistakable good, physiologically speaking, without any possible ill ; a single cup ; for if any fluid is largely drunk, even cold water, it should be remembered that every drop of it must be worked out of the system at the expense of a certain amount of nervous power ; hence, to over-drink without being thirsty, to force fluids down into the stomach, requiring, absolutely, an effort to swallow them, whether simple cold water or medicinal water, as at the various springs of the country, is a physiological absurdity, a delusion and a snare, always does an injury, never does an unmixed good, whatever may be the general prejudice to the contrary. No beast drinks without feeling like it ; and why should man guzzle down whole quarts of villainous compounds, sulphurous and fiery, when his whole nature rises in repugnance against it ? If the instincts crave these things or cold water between meals, then they are grateful and will do good. Small wonder is it that fanatical water people, persons who swallow whole tumblerfuls before breakfast every morning, to "wash out the system," and continue at it until the habit is forced on the body,—and it is called for just as liquor is called for when it becomes a habit to indulge in it—small wonder is it that the strength of the system is wasted away and body and brain all become watery together, simply because so much of the nervous energy is used up in working these immense amounts of liquid out of the body, there is not enough left to carry on the machinery of the mind. These things certainly merit the consideration of all intelligent minds, because they are of practical occurrence every day. Now and then a glass of ice water at dinner is admissible, if only three or four swallows are taken at a time ; it is the regular habit which is opposed. The general truth is, it is better to take but little liquid at meals, and what is taken will do more good in almost all cases if it is something less than scalding hot ; by the warming up the stomach it kindles a fire in the center of the system at once, the heat alone rousing up the circulation and imparting new life, especially if in the form of tea, but to use strong hot China tea largely at almost every meal, will undermine the health and shorten the life of all who practice it. Returning to the subject of urination, it is important to remember a few practical every-day facts. A gentleman of forty called, complaining that the water dribbled away all the time, attributing his misfortune to the fact that while he was a young clerk he was so anxious to please his employers that he made every effort possible to avoid leaving his desk, and to that end got into the habit of retaining his urine from morning until night ; this set up a slow inflammation resulting as above.

Medical works record cases where persons have died in a few days from inflammation of the bladder caused by resisting the call of nature for an evacuation, from a false sense of modesty or apparent necessity, as sitting in stage coaches, being kept in crowded assemblies. Children should be early taught to urinate before going on a visit, or going to church, or any public gathering, for when the bladder is distended to a certain point it loses its power of contracting upon its contents, inflammation follows and death ensues within a week unless surgical means are applied.

As persons grow old the desire for urination increases in frequency, making it necessary after fifty, to get up several times in the night, not however that there is any disease. Many persons are greatly annoyed from misapprehension as to this point. Urination should never be attempted unless the parts are very flaccid ; otherwise rupture of the canal and stricture follow, involving expensive surgical appliances or life-long discomfort.

PARALYSIS OR PALSY FROM THE BRAIN,

causes a cessation of growth of the nails on the palsied side ;

when the nails begin to grow again, it indicates that the person is recovering, but they grow slowly, requiring four or five months for an entire new nail; the nail may be stained with nitrate of silver just where it joins the skin, this indicates the rapidity of growth.

ECZEMA

is a "boiling out," an eruption of vesicles close together without fever or inflammation at the base; keep the bowels free, live on berries, fruit, and coarse bread, and wash the parts thrice a day with the following solution: two drams of Hydrate of Chloral to a pint of water.

"WETTING THE BED"

at night by children; give one drop of Creosote combined with two grains of Asafœtida, thrice a day.

HEMORRHAGE AND ANEURISMS

are often arrested permanently by giving 5 drops tinct. Veratrum viride, increasing it one drop at each dose, at three hours' interval until the full sedative effect, cessation of bleeding, &c., occurs, requiring sometimes two weeks' perseverance.

ULCERS

of the legs are sometimes cured by uniform pressure with strappings and bandages, uncovering only once or twice a week, plain food, fresh air, and free bowels.

DROPSY OF THE LIVER

has been cured by giving Hydrochlorate of Ammonia, in thirty drop doses, every five hours, diluted with water to the extent of making it agreeable; valuable in other affections of the liver.

NERVOUS PERSONS,

whose hands shake when stretched out, who are easily agitated, or annoyed, may find great relief by eating stalks of blanched celery, in moderation, two or three times a day.

SOUP

to be nourishing, should have potatoes or bread or other solid substance in it, as there is some, but very little nutriment left, if the fat is skimmed off and the meat or flesh is removed; still if taken hot, it has a stimulating, appetizing effect on the system.

HAY FEVER

In all its forms, is promptly averted, arrested and cured, at least for the time being, by a residence in the island of Mackinaw; the same has been said of the White Mountains and some other localities; but few persons comparatively, who suffer from the annual visitation, have the means to enable them to make a yearly pilgrimage to this delightful spot. See page 208.

NEURALGIA OF THE FACE

and other parts is sometimes almost instantaneously removed thus: one dram or tea-spoonful of white of egg, 4 oz. of Riga Balsam, and one ounce each of Collodion and Chloroform; shake it well and often during twenty-four hours, when it becomes jelly-like and retains this form for months, but it is ready for use after the first shaking; to be applied with a brush or mop, along the direction of the nerve and rubbed into the skin briskly with the fingers.

INGROWING TOE NAIL

is cured by Dr. Finch, who says: " Neither of the cutting operations is at all necessary for the complete and rapid cure of ingrowing toe-nail. If a small, thin, flat piece of silver plate be bent at one edge into a slight, deep groove, and, after the toe has been poulticed twenty-four hours, slipped beneath the edge of the nail, so as to protect the flesh from its pressure, and the rest of the plate bent round the side and front of the toe, being kept in position with a small portion of resin plaster passed round the toe, a speedy and almost painless cure will take place; and the patient, after the first day, has the additional advantage of being able to walk. I have followed this method in numerous cases with uniform success."

SICK HEADACHE

Is so common and so distressing, that a multiplicity of remedies are given, so that some of them may be had in almost any locality (see pages 670, 755, and 771); whether induced by mental emotion, or a disordered stomach, empty the bowels promptly by an enema, or Seidlitz powder, or castor oil, or salts, then take a heaping tea-spoonful of pulverized charcoal in half a glass of water; this at once absorbs the gases and relieves the distended stomach which caused the headache, by pressing against the nerves which extend from the stomach to the head. Relief is at other times obtained by taking two or three table-spoons of liquid magnesia, followed with ten or fifteen grains of chloral hydrate, combined with five grains of chloride of potash. More than one-half the cases of sick headache are believed to arise from the too free use of tea, such are generally cured by total abstinence from the use of tea. At the same time persons having sick headache, who do not use tea, are relieved by drinking a weak infusion. Sick headache arising from nervous irritation is sometimes permanently relieved by sitting ten or fifteen minutes in hot water in which has been dissolved a table-spoonful or two of carbonate of soda.

ITCHING OR PRURITUS OF WOMEN.

In one ounce of distilled water dissolve thirty grains of the sulpho-carbonate of zinc. Bathe the parts thoroughly in tepid water, then wash with the preparation twice a day, allowing it to dry in; keep on week after week, until entirely relieved; have a daily action of the bowels. Itching of the fundament arises from the presence of worms, or from a scrofulous irritation; if from the former, see page 270; if from the latter, keep the bowels acting daily and flap up cold water against the parts three minutes, night and morning, but never touch them in any way to relieve the itching, as it causes soreness and troublesome abrasions.

ASTHMA SPASMODIC,

often follows the use of flax seed poultices, and so does the handling of powdered ipecac, which also causes symptoms of Catarrh. Marked relief is often given in Asthma by taking, every hour or two, until relieved, a tea-spoonful of the following mixture: One and a half ounces of sulphuric ether, tincture of lobelia one ounce, tincture of stramonium or thorn apple four drams, and tincture of opium or laudanum four drams.

50

HEMORRHAGIC BOWELS, TYPHOID.

Give from twenty to sixty drops of oil of turpentine, hourly, until relieved.

SMALL POX.

Take twelve grains of sulphate of soda every three hours for a week ; to materially shorten the duration of the disease, and prevent pitting, add a few drops of water to carbolic acid, to make it of syrup consistency ; apply one drop of this to each pustule with a camel's-hair pencil from the 7th to the 12th day ; if it has become confluent, then wash the whole skin in the same way ; the pustules should turn black and fall off the third day, leaving no mark whatever.

ERYSIPELAS

is prevented from spreading in the commencement of the disease, by painting the healthy skin outside of the diseased part for the space of two or three inches, with collodion ; fill the cracks, if any appear by painting them over with the preparation.

PROSTRATION

of a very distressing kind sometimes follows a long sickness, or severe labor of body or mind ; it is a result, also, of various typhoid ailments and other low fevers ; a good remedy is one dram of carbonate of ammonia, three ounces of gum arabic mucilage, and four ounces of water ; take one table-spoonful every hour or two as occasion may require.

PNEUMONIA

is an inflammation of the substance of the lungs, coming on with a chill, then fever ; the skin is hot and dry, the pulse a hundred or over, pains about the chest increased by lying on the side ; there is a constant dry, short cough ; in addition to these, there is oppression at the top of the breast bone, a reddish expectoration, like brick dust, although this may not appear until the second or third day ; the phlegm is so tenacious, that if it were to fall on the bottom of a vessel it would not fall out if it were turned upside down.   When these symptoms appear and a thermometer in the armpit rises towards a hundred and five degrees or over, the case should be regarded as a dangerous attack of Pneumonia or Lung Fever, which will, in all probability, prove fatal within a week if not promptly met with appropriate remedies; not a moment's time should be lost in using expectorants, in steaming, or other mere experiments. The first best remedy, in most cases, is to place the patient in a sitting position in bed and cause blood to flow from the arm until fainting is almost induced; but there is such a general prejudice against blood letting and such a little appreciation of the dangerous character of the disease, that few are willing to adopt the remedy.

The next best treatment is to put a large blister plaster, eight inches by four, along the space between the shoulder blades behind; if the case is not very urgent, this also may be omitted; small blisters are ineffectual and irritate. Next to a beginning with bleeding or blister plasters, the most efficient treatment is to unload the bowels by an enema, or by taking two or three table-spoonfuls of castor oil or salts, and repeat every two hours until there is an operation, but without waiting for that, take within an hour, one or two liver pills and wrap up warm in bed. Within two hours there will be more or less relief, which becomes more decided as time passes. As soon as the bowels begin to act freely by the pills, the feeling of relief will be regarded with surprise and gratification. During all this time, nothing must be taken but warm toast-water or barley-water, or whey may be drank. The after treatment in all cases must be the same. The room should be kept at a temperature not lower than sixty-five degrees, and as much higher as will enable the patient to feel comfortably warm; a feeling of chilliness should not be allowed for an instant, and by no means leave the room until the appetite is fully restored and then go cautiously out of doors in such a way as to avoid fatigue and the slightest chilliness. Fatal relapses often take place from going out of doors too soon.

When the cough is tight, take the tincture of Ipecac or the compound syrup of squills to the extent of loosening the phlegm, but not to vomit, nor within an hour of eating.

The diet should consist of light food, soups, and teas with bread broken in, taken at five hours' interval. Grapes may be freely eaten in the forenoon and afternoon, and as the appetite and strength increase, lean meat may be gradually added.

If the pulse continues over eighty, bring it down to sixty and not let it rise above seventy by taking, every three hours, from five to ten drops of the tincture of aconite or the tincture of veratrum viride or poke root, in half a table-spoonful of water; or take one-sixth of a grain of tartar emetic in a table-spoonful of water, every two hours; such a treatment promptly given will seldom fail of a speedy cure of this dangerous malady, sometimes called Lung Fever, so dangerous, that with the best treatment, the patient recovers very slowly, in the course of months, and for a long time after, is very liable to attack, from very slight causes.

Pneumonia is a disease which lays the most robust in the grave within a week, and which has numbered among its victims some of the greatest and best and most eminent men of modern times, especially public men, generals, senators, and clergymen; hence, its symptoms, its nature, its dangerous character, and its speedy and efficacious treatment, ought to be thoroughly understood by the people generally. Promptitude is vital, and in nine cases out of ten, makes all the difference between a speedy convalescence and months of sickness, or between recovery and the grave within a week. The great fatality of the disease, arises from the fact of its slow development, in many cases; the very best physicians hope and hesitate, and while they are waiting for convincing proof that it is a true case of inflammation of the lungs, the critical time has passed for saving life. The clear, sharp rule should be, if a person, from a bad cold, or from any other cause, has a sense of oppression at the top of the breast bone, with a frequent hacking or short cough, and more or less of pain any where, especially if the pulse beats over ninety times in a minute, and a thermometer in the arm pits rises from its natural state of ninety-eight degrees Fahrenheit, to a hundred and five or six or more, it should be set down as a case of inflammation of the lungs. It will simply amaze and delight an intelligent observer to contemplate the speedy, general, and complete relief which will uniformly follow a prompt unloading of the lower bowels by an injection of a pint or more of water warm or tepid, or instead, by giving two table-spoons of castor oil or common salts, and within an hour or two administering one or two of the liver pills, according to the violence of the symptoms; let the patient keep warm in bed and promote perspiration by hot drinks; keep the arms under the bed clothes, which should come up to the chin, and include the shoulders. By such a treatment the patient will be cured within eighteen hours, and all that will be required after that is good nursing; by which is meant taking the food and drink already named, and remaining in a warm room for a week afterwards, until the appetite becomes vigorous, then gradually accustom the patient to out-door air and exercise, avoiding with the greatest possible care two things, chilliness and fatigue. In Pneumonia there is a constant fever which rapidly wastes the strength of the system, endangering the complication of typhoid-pneumonia, to prevent which, the pulse should be kept down to sixty beats in a minute by giving from five to ten drops of the tincture of aconite every three hours at any stage of the disease. The general reader may think that too much space has been given to Pneumonia, but if he ever has the disease, or sees any one dear to him suffering from it, he will have a different opinion.

A BAD COLD

is simply a mild form of Pneumonia, for it is an inflammation of the breathing organs, from the tip of the nose up through the head, down along the windpipe to the little hollow at the bottom of the neck, extending to the branches of the windpipe, &c., to the very bottom of the lungs; all these parts are too hot; have too much blood in them, more than is natural, hence the lungs are preoccupied and air enough cannot get in to supply the wants of the system, causing the patient to complain of oppression, of a want of breath, expressing himself as being all "stuffed up," he feels dull and stupid and restless.

In such cases the body is too full, and nature seeks to relieve herself by diminishing the amount of the fluids of the system, the eyes water, there is an increased discharge from the nose and a direct attempt to relieve the lungs themselves by exciting a cough, or hawking and expectoration of a heavy yellowish substance with which all are familiar.

What is about to be said, in conjunction with the statements made relative to Pneumonia, will be worth ten times the value of this book, to every family, to every individual, old or young, even if the money had to be earned by working for ten cents a day, "board and lodging included," because

COLDS ARE TAKEN

during the whole course of life, and in a great many cases they are the agencies which kindle into fatal activity a variety of forms

of disease. All invalids have noticed, and will notice to the end
of time, that a cold makes them worse, always aggravates the
malady under which the body already labors. If a person suffering from a cold feels stuffed up, oppressed, too full, and nature, in
the ways above described, endeavors to unload the body of its
surplus, common sense dictates the propriety of helping nature to
get rid of the oppressing and depressing surplus. Yet, with incomprehensible perversity, the people begin, forthwith, to work
against nature by more "stuffing"; by eating, even when instinct
takes away the appetite, under the delusive plea, that if they do
not eat they will get weak, and will soon be confined to the bed.
But as it is a very uncomfortable operation to eat without an appetite, some resort to tonics and bitters and brandy to

GET UP AN APPETITE.

But not content with this outrage against nature, another form
of warring against her is, as soon as there is a cough, which is
her method of helping us to get rid of the matters which are in
the lungs, and so fill them up that breath enough cannot get in,
medicines are resorted to which are said to be

GOOD FOR A COUGH,

meaning thereby that they cure the cough, cause it to cease and
disappear; and that medicine works with a charm which is the
greater in proportion to the promptitude with which it acts in the
direction of causing the cough to disappear, as far as the lungs are
concerned in young children, to take refuge in the head, causing
convulsions and water on the brain; in older persons, the cough
ceases, the lungs become more oppressed, and pneumonia or heart
disease, or other more critical malady takes the place of the
cough.

In every decided cold, three things are always to be considered.

First.—Nature takes away the appetite; then eat nothing, not
an atom; drink nothing, not a drop. You are too full already,
and nature is using all her efforts to unload the system as a means
of relief, and every atom, every drop requires that much more
strength to convey it out of the body, thus imposing more work,
thus hindering instead of aiding.

Second.—In all colds there is a chilliness; instinct prompts to get warm ; we almost get into the fire ; while we are warming one side, the other gets chilly. Chilliness is the stagnation of the blood ; there is no animation, no activity, no cheeriness. But all know that warmth promotes the circulation ; instinct urges us to procure that necessary warming ; hence a person suffering with a cold should occupy a room comfortably warm to him, even if it requires a heat of over a hundred degrees. Ordinarily, in fire-time of year, it is warm enough if the thermometer marks seventy degrees, five feet from the floor, near the window. But the patient must not decide from figures ; he must be guided by principle, not by numbers, or by the experience of others ; the room must be comfortably warm to him ; and in that warm room he must remain, and never go outside of the door, until he becomes hungry, feels strong, with a pulse not over seventy-five a minute ; then he may resume his ordinary occupation by degrees, guarding most of all against chilliness and over-fatigue or over-work as in Pneumonia.

Third.——As nature, in all cases, attempts to cure the system of a cold by unloading it of the surplus which oppresses it, we can greatly aid her in this operation by first taking an injection, which will remove a pound or two from the body in a few moments ; or by swallowing one or two table-spoonfuls of castor oil, or Epsom salts, dissolved in a glass of warm water ; there will be a more efficient action than from an injection, requiring, however, a longer time, an hour or two or more. All that is now necessary to be done is to keep comfortably warm in bed in a warm room, with a pure air ; if perspiration is induced by drinking hot water or hot teas of any kind, the cure will be hastened and will be more complete. Follow the instructions for convalescence which were recommended in getting well of Pneumonia, in reference to warmth, eating, drinking, and exercise. All observant persons know how easy it is to renew a cold ; so easy sometimes, that it is almost impossible not to think that it comes of itself. In all cases, the renewal is owing to a slight chilliness attacking some part of the body in going out into the cold air, before the gloves are drawn over the hands ; very many persons wait until they get out of the door before they begin to draw on their gloves, hence the fingers become cold before it is accomplished ; at other times you stand on the door stone in thin slippers, or without a hat ; or talk a moment to a parting visitor with the door partly open ; or you undress or rise in a cold room; or you fail to get into bed without a slight chilliness running over you; or the feet may get a little damp or cold; in short, any chilly or cold sensation to any small portion of the body, is capable of renewing a cold, when there is one already present; hence, the necessity has been insisted on, of every person who has a cold, keeping himself comfortably warm for every instant of time until his cold is cured. A young gentleman came home the other evening with a very severe cold; some one advised him to steam himself by breathing the vapor of hot water; he did so, went to bed, and arose next morning feeling almost entirely well; he was perfectly delighted, and so were his friends, at the good effects of so simple a remedy. He went down town to his business after breakfast, returning in the evening, feeling that he had increased his cold; he became very ill during the night, has been very low, and for days together life has been despaired of by all the attending physicians; the lesson is, do not be in a hurry to get out of doors when you have a cold. An idea is repeated here with great emphasis, in the belief that it is of incalculable importance to every reader. If a cold is attacked as above within twenty-four or thirty-six hours after it has been taken, it will be cut short and perfectly cured in a day; but if it is neglected for several days, nothing will cure it; it will hang on and run its course of two or three weeks, as measles will run its course, and wear itself out.

If nothing is done for a cold for several days after it has been taken, resort should be had to one or two of the liver pills, instead of salts or oil. No one should ever forget to notice what gives a cold; then carefully avoid it. Different persons are susceptible to cold from different causes, and each one should observe for himself what gives him a cold, and act accordingly, for it is impossible for a cold to occur without a cause, and it is as unreasonable to expect the finger should not be burned by putting it in the fire, as for a person to escape a cold if he exposes himself to those causes which give him a cold. A miracle will never be worked; the operations of nature will never be suspended to save even an angel from the infraction of a law of nature; and yet many have some indistinct impression that they will escape or be protected in some way, especially if in the performance of some good work. The great and good John Howard, of immortal memory, lost his life by an unauthorized exposure in visiting a young lady who was suffering from the plague and of which she died. Our wisdom lies in noticing what causes disease and then scrupulously guard against such causes ever after. It is better to store the memory with items of knowledge which will preserve the health, than to be satisfied with possessing a remedy which will cure disease. There are persons who are careless of getting sick, because they think they have at hand an infallible remedy, hence do not take the same pains to use means for the preservation of their health, which they would otherwise do. Attention to this point as a matter of principle, in reference to the avoidance of colds, will prevent an incalculable amount of sickness and suffering. Many persons have noticed if while laboring under a cold, there is an attack of diarrhœa or loose bowels there is an immediate abatement of all the symptoms of the cold, and the diarrhœa is said to "carry off" the cold; this fact having been noticed by the common people, they very naturally concluded that if the spontaneous intervention of a diarrhœa cured a cold, the artificial production of diarrhœa will also cure a cold, hence resort is had to castor oil, salts, and other purgatives. A gentlemen took some pills the other day with this end in view, they acted well and all the symptoms of the cold were abating, and wishing to expedite matters, he kept taking the pills every day, not observing that he was getting weaker with the result, that the increasing debility arising from continued purgation allowed the system to fall into a typhoid condition and he died, showing that while one or two free actions of the bowels are beneficial in colds, continued looseness day after day is injurious, and even dangerous.

Some persons are constantly taking little colds but are not aware of it, because they think that if they had a cold, there would be more or less of cough; that would be the case if the cold fell on the lungs, but it does not always do so, only when the lungs are the weak point of the system; but if they are healthy and strong and the person is suffering from any ailment in another part of the system, that part is the weaker point, the cold settles there, aggravates the trouble, while the lungs are not affected by it at all. Thus a person may keep up a malady, for an indefinite time by a constant succession of little colds, without the patient knowing anything about it, hence the importance of guarding against taking fresh colds in all forms of sickness, by studiously avoiding all the causes of cold, and the best way is to use all the means possible and necessary to keep the body continuously warm.

Let it be remembered that most colds can be cured by warmth and abstinence from all food for a day or two, without any medicine whatever; it is only in the severer forms that enemas and medicines are necessary. Whenever a person is suffering from any disease and any symptom gets worse, he may conclude he has renewed his cold or the bowels have become costive.

If anything is needed to impress on the reader's mind the importance of remaining in doors, while suffering from a cold, especially the old and frail and feeble, it is the fact, that the immediate cause of the death of one of the most distinguished men in the nation's history, William H. Seward, was the renewal of a cold by taking a two hours' drive. The weather was not cold, but he was feeble and returned home thoroughly chilled, and died in a few days.

MORAL CHARACTER TRANSMITTED.

Hereditary influence on page 622 finds confirmation in the following narrations of the Rev. William Fulton:

"Some years ago, a young man in the town of N———, in Prussia, indulged in mocking the little singing birds of the forests, and wherever he succeeded in catching one, he cut out its tongue! By and by he got married, and in the course of time had seven children born to him, all of whom came into this world without tongues to speak! This can be certified by a person from the town of N———, now living in my own family."

"Among the people with whom I worshiped in earlier years, there was a gay young man, the most prominent trait in whose character was that of scoffing; he married, and his wife it seems caught the moral contagion. In their eyes every body was slighted; every child was defective; every beggar was taunted; every lady was gibed, and every gentleman jeered at. This pair of scoffers had nine or ten children born to them; but every child was deformed— some of them so much so as to demand surgical operations!"

The physical constitution of the child is to a certain extent molded by the mother's habits during gestation. The first teetotal temperance preacher was an Angel, who enjoined upon a woman, that until the child was born there should be an entire abstinence from all that could intoxicate, and also that she should not eat any "unclean" (unhealthy) food. The woman was faithful to the injunction, a son was born to her three thousand years ago, Samson, one of the judges of Israel. Manoah's wife had never had a child; the father wanted to know what was the nature of the work which the child would be expected to perform; and in answer to the question, how the child should be ordered, what should be done, which would be best calculated to fit him for his life's work, the reply was as above stated, showing, at that early time in the world's history, that there was an adaptation of means to an end; that the avoidance of injurious drinks and eating healthful food, would be the means of securing the birth of a strong, healthy child. The principle cannot be less true now, than in the earlier ages of the world. In connection with the habits during gestation, there is a practical question which comes before all intelligent married persons; ought there to be marital indulgence during gestation and nursing? There ought to be, to the fullest extent required by maternal instincts; because the parts connected with reproduction are in a state of extraordinary excitement, and if not appeased, precisely as in hunger, the mind is physically compelled to dwell on the sensation until it is satisfied; and if any other appetite calls for appeasement, the result is the same. If the mind is dwelling upon the subject and instinct remorselessly calls for appeasement, the being to be born will have these same yearnings, with just as much uniformity as the child born to a drunken parent will inherit the propensity for drink. As it has been asserted with extraordinary positiveness that indulgence during the time thus referred to is a fruitful cause of scrofula, without any even plausible proof, readers must decide for themselves, as there is not space for argument here; this may be done in the light of a single question, "Is it not better to gratify the tastes, appetites, and inclinations of the mother that is to be, than to oppose them, when they are known to be natural, not artificial?" There must be health and happiness in the temperate gratification of the natural appetites, as there is health and happiness in the temperate use of all the good things of this life which the Almighty One has given us "richly to enjoy."

In 1840 the very eminent Dr. Combe published a work on "Infancy" in which he gives many cases proving that mental and physical impressions were made on the unborn child as the result of the mental states of the mother during gestation. William Hunter, the greatest medical philosopher of his age and nation, advocates the same doctrine; hence the physician should frankly inform the pregnant woman that the physical constitution of the child, and to a great extent its moral character, very much depend on herself, and that it is her highest duty to act accordingly during the whole time of gestation. Dr. Hunter believed that from the first hour of conception to the consummation of the birth, the states of mind and body and heart of the woman were constantly molding those of the child; such being the case, we ought as true benefactors of the race to do what in us lies, to make that mold as near perfection as possible and thus give a happy direction to the tastes, habits, feelings, and inclination, that the bent of them may be in the right direction from the first, then it will prove emphatically true that "as the twig is bent, the tree's inclined." Thoughts like these will excite peculiar interest during the whole of gestation and make the term of it a period of absorbing consideration. Dr. Williamson of Cincinnati thus writes in a Medical Journal for February, 1870:

"Mrs. B——, of Virginia, an excellent lady, of fine cultivation, the wife of a tradesman, became *enceinte;* this so enraged the husband that, during her entire term of pregnancy, he treated her with great brutality, forced her to take emmenagogues with the view of destroying the embryo, but all to no purpose, and in due season she gave birth to a fine male child. When the boy was old enough to distinguish one person from another, he became afraid of his father, and nothing could appease his fear. As he grew older his fear turned to hatred. The once brutal husband was now a devoted father, and loved his promising son with great affection, but he was at last compelled to send him from home to school, from which he never returned during the lifetime of his father. For fifteen long years they never saw each other. About three years ago the father died, while the son, a noble young man, now stands high as a jurist in his native state. He deplored his unnatural feeling, and often declared, with tears, that he could not tell why it was so."

The growing and burning affection of the mother may stamp the image of the idol of her heart upon the fœtus in utero.

"Mr. W——, my uncle, once employed a Miss Hoffman as teacher in his family. Her powers of mind, virtues of heart, and charms of person could not be excelled. Her right inferior extremity, however, was some three or four inches shorter than her left. She had a lustrous brown, and a laughing blue eye. Mrs. W——, who is one of the kindest and most affectionate of women, formed an attachment for Miss H——, which was, perhaps, as holy as that which bound Damon and Pythias together. Becoming *enceinte*, she gave birth to a female child, whose right leg, like that of Miss H——, was three or four inches shorter than her left, and one eye is brown while the other is blue. The girl is now grown, and could hardly be distinguished from Miss H——, were they both of the same age."

"The mother's mind, through sympathy, pleasure, or hatred, may bear with such power upon the nerves of sensibility, as to entirely transform the perfect human form of the embryo into that of the lower order of animals, and instead of a perfect child being born to gladden the mother's heart, she becomes the wretched parent of a human monster. These facts should not be overlooked by the mother, as the observance of them is a duty which she owes alike to herself as well as to the well-being of her children."

THE FAMILY MEDICINE CHEST.

In every household there should be a family medicine chest, for in every household there will be more or less midnight sickness, sudden attacks of illness, of accident, and death, and to be able to do something promptly, although a physician may be within ten minutes' call, sometimes makes all the difference between a life saved and a life lost; but especially is it needful for every family in the country and at the farm house, where a physician may not be had for hours, to have some few remedies at hand which may meet ordinary emergencies. Under the head of the articles named, will be found the uses which may be made of them, and the manner of their employment.

1. Half pound of ground mustard in an unopened box.
2. A self-injecting apparatus.
3. One dozen liver pills.
4. Two dozen dinner pills.
5. Half a pint each of castor oil, tincture of arnica, tincture of veratrum viride, tincture of camphor, tincture of hartshorn, and chloroform liniment.
6. Two ounces each of the tincture of opium and ipecac.
7. One box of pain extractor.

There is scarcely any form of suffering arising from disease which may not be relieved, modified, or cured by the judicious use of one or more of the remedies named ; the main object however is to abate bodily pain, and to soothe and quiet the mind until the doctor comes.

The reader is requested to bear in mind two things in reference to all statements made in this book which is here brought to a close :

First.——There are exceptional cases to the statements made, whether of principle or fact, of theory or practice ; it was intended to say what was generally true.

Second.——Numerous remedies are given for some of the more common ailments,because in different and distant localities one or more of them cannot be had ; then again a person cannot tolerate some particular medicine, but can readily take another ; besides most remedies lose their power in time, then another must be employed which is similar, then after a while the first can be returned to with advantage.

Third.——In all cases of sickness procure the services of a practicing physician if you can, for it will take a load of responsibility from your own mind, and will save that painful groping in the dark which is inseparable from the administration of medicine on your own judgment. The strictly medical part of the work is for the emergencies of sickness and accident which may occur at midnight, or in most inclement weather, or in remote places where there is neither drug nor doctor ; meanwhile, in all forms of sickness whether moderate or severe,

Keep quiet. Keep warm. Keep clean.

Keep up a free exposure to a pure atmosphere and the life-giving sunshine.

RINGING OR BUZZING IN THE EARS,

called Tinnitus Aurium, arises from congestion, a too great amount of blood about the organs of hearing; in some cases it is one of the attendants of increasing age, then there is no cure. Persons in good health sometimes have it without any appreciable cause, in which cases it passes away without treatment; sometimes it is the temporary result of a cold, and will disappear with it. If large amounts of Quinine are taken, a troublesome ringing in the ears is a result, but disappears in time. Sometimes this ringing is caused by diseased humors working their way out of the system at the ear; for this there is no cure except in the direction of improving the general health by purifying the blood. See page 273. It is a result also of nervous debility, and can only be cured by getting rid of that malady. Sometimes it attends a diseased condition of the brain, and there is no relief except in the removal of that condition. All these causes produce one effect, " congestion," the only remedy is the removal of the cause; hence, for the cure of Tinnitus Aurium, we will look in vain for relief to applications to the ear itself, and yet that is the very course pursued almost in every case, not only losing valuable time, but endangering the hearing still more. If the ringing is caused by fever or inflammation, these must be removed by general principles. If inflammation tends to the ear, it sometimes gives ear-ache instead of ringing, then relief is given by warm poultices of any kind to the ear, or rubbing back of the ear with warm lard or warm hartshorn and water. But if the inflammation or congestion goes to one side of the head or face instead of the ear, it is called " Face Ache," or Neuralgia, giving short or sharp darting pains; if in the muscles of the parts, causing stiffness in moving the head from side to side, it is Rheumatism of the Head. Pain on the top of the head indicates Uterine Disease. When a pain in the head is constant, or comes at intervals, but always at the same spot, there are tumors or serious functional brain disorders. When there is a throbbing headache, there is fever or poisoning.

Sometimes the ear aches because insects have crawled into it; lay the head on the side, drop in a little sweet oil; this will kill the insect or cause it to come out. If a solid substance falls into the ear, make a loop of fine wire, carefully introduce it down to the drum of the ear, twist it around until it catches the substance, then draw it out.

In all cases of running at the ear keep it scrupulously clean by gentle syringing with tepid water several times a day.

SKIN DISEASES

cannot be foretold. They must make their appearance on the surface before it can be told what they are. They have a multitude of premonitory symptoms which are common to all of them, and it would only cumber the book to no purpose to enumerate them, besides confusing the reader. But when they make their appearance the exact nature of the malady is known at once; hence, in small pox, measles, and the like, extended descriptions are omitted. To save space, sometimes half a dozen different pages are referred to in the index as treating of one disease, because the symptom is connected with as many different and distinct diseases, and when a man has a symptom he naturally wants to know the different ailments in which it is present. This makes the book much more satisfactory, as showing the various connections in which the particular symptom or disease is manifested.

FEVER BLISTERS

are troublesome little sores which often appear on the lips, outside and in; they show that the system has been feverish, and that nature is pushing it out, and is relieving herself, and is a " good sign," as boils are a " good sign." Their immediate cause is bad blood, a cold biliousness, or constipation. Take promptly a liver pill, or live exclusively on cracked wheat and fruits for a few days; keep the bowels free, the skin clean, and be out of doors in the open air several hours daily; in less than twenty-four hours the symptoms would begin to abate, and a cure would be certain.

W. W. HALL, M. D.

New York, March 15, 1873.

FEVER BLISTER.

This ailment is a form of skin disease, of which there are perhaps a hundred different manifestations or varieties. It would require a good sized volume to describe these with sufficient minuteness to enable any one not a physician, to distinguish one from another with even reasonable certainty; hence it is better to understand the nature and the cure of these diseases in general; that they are diseases of the blood, what medical men call " constitutional diseases;" they are functional, belonging merely to the working of the human machine—it is clogged up—no wheel or cog is missing; it simply needs cleaning, and all that the patient needs is pretty well expressed in the common phrase, " a good cleaning out," which means that the general health should be improved, whereby two things are accomplished, the body is relieved of its excess of blood, and the blood itself becomes pure. This is, in truth, the only safe method of treating affections of the skin, and is applicable alike to every ordinary form of skin disease between a hive or fever blister up to measles and small pox. Hydropathists treat all these maladies without medicine of any kind; careful and experienced Allopaths give little or no medicine, and if any, it is of a mild character, even in small pox. Hydropaths use warm baths, cooling and simple food, such as coarse bread and fruits and berries and melons, being careful to secure one full, free action of the bowels every twenty-four hours, and sedulously avoiding everything in the least calculated to cause a chilly or cold sensation to any part of the body. The only special difference in the treatment between the Hydropathist and Allopath is that the latter uses medicine when needed to keep the bowels free. The treatment of both is constitutional, intended to purify the blood, and thus secure a more equable and healthy circulation.

These views have been strikingly confirmed, since the first edition of this book was printed, by Dr. Fox, physician to the skin department of University College Hospital, London, who says, in reference to skin diseases: " The general treatment of them is everything, the local treatment is of little value, comparatively, as they are the direct consequence of disturbances of general nutrition," meaning thereby that they arise from bad blood, and

51

yet, the very first thought, in almost every case, the moment any-thing seems to be the matter with the skin, is to put something on it, as if driving it out of sight was to cure ; and yet a single hive on the skin of an infant, driven in, has induced convulsions with-in an hour ; anything cold, a damp cloth, or a raw wind, may drive in any eruption, and death often follows, or the patient does not get over it in a lifetime, as the commonest observers have noticed in the " striking in " of measles ; hence the safest and best method of treating superficial maladies is to avoid applica-tions to the skin itself, and seek to improve the general health by cleanliness, regularity in using cooling and loosening food and drinks, and occupying well ventilated rooms ; but the benefits of all these will be greatly increased by a plentiful exposure to the out-door air in moderate activity, and the careful avoid-ance of everything calculated to give a cold, or induce a chilly feeling.

SHINGLES

is a species of Herpes or Tetter, a skin disease with different names, according to locality ; if on the lips it is called a

FEVER BLISTER ;

If in half circles on the skin, it is called by the familiar name of

RINGWORM,

which on the skin is called *Tinea Circinnatus,* if on the scalp it is *Tinea Decalvans,* or

" SCALD HEAD."

Both forms require perfect cleanliness ; wash the parts twice a day, gently and well, with soft soap and warm water, and when dry, rub the parts with a linen rag dipped in hartshorn made from gas tar, or mild preparations of carbolic acid or creosote ; but keep the bowels free and live lightly. When Herpes attacks the waist and runs half around the body, physicians call it *Herpes Zoster,* the common people "Shingles." The blisters have a red, inflamed surface, sometimes with severe pains, generally affecting the right side, lasting a week or two in vigorous persons; in the frail and feeble there is a strong tendency to tedious and dangerous ulcera-tions. The patient should be confined to the bed. Use any fa-miliar anodyne if the pains are severe.

At least one free action of the bowels should be secured every day, with a diet of fruit, brown bread, wheaten grits, oat meal porridge and the like. Belladonna ointment affords great relief in some cases. When on the lips it may be repressed by the frequent application of Cologne water. Keep it well covered with pulverized magnesia. Carefully avoid picking the sore ; it protracts the cure, and may become cancerous. Before the blister breaks it is cooled and moistened by frequent applications of glycerine ; still, the best treatment of a fever blister, in all cases, is to secure a speedy action of the bowels, and let the diet be as above named until the sore is healed ; make no application to it whatever, and it will get well in a few days.

The fever blisters on the body, or Shingles, are sometimes an inch or more across, are flat and oval shaped, called *Bullae-Rupia* if small, and *Pemphigus* if large. These, as well as the various forms of

ECZEMA,

whether simple red, infantile, or " Water Blisters," are all, in reality, of the same general nature, and are uniformly cured by the same general treatment as recommended for shingles, endeavoring in all cases to build up the general health. It is certainly safer to avoid all external applications to the Shingles, except before the blisters break glycerine may be applied, and when they break cover them with powdered magnesia. A warm bath does good if taken every day or two. The water-cure treatment of Shingles is the use of fruit and coarse bread diet ; drinking cold water freely, frequent hip baths, at least twice a day, and wet cloths worn around the body all the time. If the parts itch a great deal, or are tender, they are soothed by the use of warm or tepid water.

If Eczema in any form is troublesome, take five drops of Fowler's Solution of Arsenic twice a day, increasing one drop every dose until it amounts to twelve or fifteen drops at a time.

If there is any syphilitic taint, give three drops of Donovan's solution twice a day, increasing one drop daily. This is a mixture of arsenic and mercury, to be had at any good drug store. Feeble children and scrofulous persons are benefited by cod liver oil, unless it deranges the stomach or bowels. It is worth special remembrance that there is one mode of treatment alike applicable to all forms of skin diseases.   Their names, number and appearances are multitudinous, and instead of burdening the reader with whole pages of nicely drawn distinctions, in the effort to enable him to distinguish one from the other in their endless variety, it will be safer and better to have before the mind certain general principles of treatment.

The *London Lancet* is considered high authority the world over, in all that pertains to medical progress. In its latest issue, since the publication of the third edition of this book, there is the most gratifying confirmation, from the latest investigations and discoveries in medicine, of some of the most important and wide-reaching principles stated in the previous pages. Among these are that

BRIGHT'S DISEASE

has for its immediate cause a "congested" condition of the kidneys, preceded by a "congestion" of the liver, which, says Dr. Hood, "If more carefully studied by the Profession, would be found to guide us toward the prevention of maladies otherwise impossible of cure."

LIGHTNING RODS.

For protecting ordinary buildings, there are eleven specifications :

First.—The rod should be of round iron not less than one inch in diameter.

Second.—This rod should be continuous along its whole length if possible ; if pieced, welding is best ; next to that, screw the parts together by a coupling ferule.

Third.—Keep off rusting by having them well covered with black paint.

Fourth.—The top should terminate in a single point, covered with a sheathing of platinum one-twentieth of an inch in thickness.

Fifth.—Carry the rod to the earth as direct and straight as possible.

Sixth.—Fasten the rod to the building with iron eyes.

Seventh.—The rod should terminate in water or very wet earth, and for that reason it should reach down a yard or more ; whenever possible let the rod end in a well, or stream, or spring of water, or in gas mains or water pipes in cities.

Eighth.—The west side of the house is best in United States latitudes, and still better if attached to a chimney where a current of heated air is ascending.

Ninth.—When roofs are covered with metal there should be a good metallic connection between the two ; solder strips of copper to the roof and gutters and leaders.

Tenth.—The top of the rod should be ten feet above the building if protection is desired for twenty feet in all directions ; the rule being at least one-half as high as the diameter of the protection.

Eleventh.—If there are large masses of metal in a building the rods should be connected with it.

DYSPEPSIA

can only be radically cured by eating the right kind of food, using the right kind of drink, being out of doors as much as possible, and avoiling great fatigue of body or brain.

COOK'S PILLS.

The author has heard Dr. Cook many times in lectures delivered in the course of two years, describe his own method of making his very famous and very efficient pills. His confidence in them increased with increasing years ; he eventually seemed to think if his pills did not cure, nothing else would, and he seldom prescribed anything else as a means of relieving and curing ordinary diseases, his theory being that all disease is a congestion in some part of the body, that is, excess of blood, and the remedy was to get rid of that excess, and that was done by diminishing the whole amount of the fluids of the system, and that diminished the amount proportionably in the part affected, and that his pills would diminish largely the whole amount of the fluids of the body in half a day, could be proven in any case by giving a single dose, which was ordinarily two or three at a time. If they did not operate within twelve hours, his imperative direction was to give double the dose ; for, said he, " If you want to knock a man down you must strike with a certain force ; if you fail, you need not expect to do so by striking him the second time with the force of the first; so, not to lose valuable time, and to be sure of the desired results, you had better knock twice as hard as you did at first." He always seemed to think that this illustration was equal to a demonstration.

In those days a pill machine was never heard of, and physicians made their own pills; and to be able to divide them nearly equal, he directed to mix together well, sixty-four grains each of calomel, aloes, and rhubarb; mix with water only, so as to make of it a mass which could be rolled into a convenient length, then divide it in the middle, and keep on dividing each piece in the middle until 32 were made; thus thirty-two pills would be made of about equal size, and containing two grains each of calomel, aloes, and rhubarb. Nothing but pure water was to be used in mixing up the ingredients, because if anything thicker was employed the pills would be too large. The author believes that this real Cook Pill is the best combination of medicines ever devised for efficiently reaching a large class of human ailments.

APERIENT REMEDIES,

which act gently, and which, by being taken continuously, do not poison the system as mineral medicines and others would certainly do, are exceedingly useful in a great variety of circumstances where it is not important to act on the liver, but simply to unload the bowels in a gentle manner, without griping, debilitating, or other special discomfort. Among these is the Dinner Pill, which became famous over a hundred years ago in Paris, as named on page 499.

The great Marshall Hall's "Dinner Pill" is made thus: Equal parts of powdered aloes, extract of liquorice powder and soap, each pill weighing four grains.

Abernethy was one of the most eminent and successful physicians of his century. His favorite aperient pill was thus made: Powdered aloes forty-eight grains, extract of henbane forty-eight grains, twenty-four grains of blue mass, and twenty grains of ipecac, all mixed with water, and divided into twenty-four pills—good to act on liver and bowels—one or more at bed-time.

Mandrake Pills: Take thirty grains of compound extract of colocynth, and three grains of resin of podophylum; (May apple) make into twelve pills ; dose, two at bed-time. A good substitute for Abernethy's when it is not designed to take mercury, and still have the liver acted upon.

Dr. Parrish made a similar pill of twenty-four grains of aloes, twenty grains of resin of podophylum, and four drops of oleo-resin of ginger ; make into twenty-four pills—one for a laxative, two or more for a purgative.

Indian Vegetable Pills : Aloes one pound, powdered gamboge six ounces, three ounces each of compound extract of colocynth, Castile soap and scammony, two ounces of extract of butternut, Cayenne pepper half an ounce, oil of cloves one dram ; mix well, and make into four-grain pills.

Make an impalpable powder of six drams each of senna leaves and liquorice root, three drams each of fennel seed and sulphur, with eighteen drams of refined sugar ; take a level teaspoonful or more of this in water at bed-time. It neither sickens nor purges : it makes a pleasant drink, and children like it. It is, perhaps, the mildest and most agreeable aperient known.

When it is taken into account what multitudes of persons there are who are more or less troubled with costiveness, which always, in all cases, and inevitably undermines the constitution, and renders life miserable, there can be no reasonable objection to the number of remedies given, especially as one may act very well for a short time and then seem to lose its effect, when another should be employed, and thus may the round of the whole of them be made repeatedly and with advantage. At the same time, let the reader be advised, that taking drugs all the time simply to secure a daily action of the bowels, is injurious and unnatural. A diet of coarse bread and fruits and berries and grains, will seldom fail to accomplish the same results, if patiently persevered in, and accompanied with a reasonable amount of daily out-door activities.

Lee's Antibilious Pills had a wide reputation, and were valuable : Half an ounce each of pulverized aloes, jalap and rhubarb, calomel three drams, pulverized gamboge one dram ; made into a mass with syrup, four grains of each in a pill—take one, two, or more at bed-time.

PERISTALTIC PERSUADERS,

from the alliterative designation, attracted considerable attention. The idea is that the pills have an effect to gently increase the natural action or motion of the intestines, that motion being designated by physicians Peristaltic, literally, placing around, referring to that vermicular, worm-like motion of the intestines, by which the contents are worked downwards and outwards. If that motion is tardy we are costive; if it ceases we die. The Peristetic Persuader is the gentlest of the remedies which create a freer motion of the intestines: Two drams of powdered Turkey rhubarb, ten drops of caraway oil, simple syrup one dram by weight; mix well and divide into forty pills; dose, two to four on rising in the morning, or at bed-time, acting on the bowels usually within twelve hours.

PURGATIVE PILLS,

referred to in pages 28 and 30, are very efficient in their action, and may be used instead of the milder Liver Pills where there is greater urgency. Each one contains five grains of calomel, one grain each of rhubarb, aloes and gamboge, with one-fifth of a grain of tartar emetic.

FELON,

or Whitlow, is, properly speaking, a boil on the bone, under the tendon, fascia or " Whitleather," a term used to designate that part of the muscle which is attached to the bone; it is as impervious as leather, and quite as tough. When a Boil forms on any part of the body, it becomes painful in proportion as it swells, until the skin breaks, then there is the most agreeable relief in a minute; and it may well be imagined what agony must be endured when the yellow matter cannot escape, confined as it is, not by a thin piece of skin, but by a thick material, tougher than leather. The general treatment of a boil is to endure it until it breaks, taking care to keep upon it a bread and milk poultice, or anything else which will keep the skin soft and moist, as a means of cooling it; a flax-seed poultice is very soothing: beyond this poulticing, it is better not to interfere with an ordinary boil, but let it run its course, keeping the bowels free, and live on fruits and coarse bread, grits, cracked wheat, and the like. But no poultice can reach a felon with any efficiency, for it cannot be touched; the whit-leather is between the poultice and the boil on the bone. There is only one speedy, efficient remedy for Felon; take a lancet and thrust it down through the skin and flesh and tendon, to the very bone; and to make sure of it, scrape it on the bone, first cutting one way and then another in the form of a cross; the re lief is instantaneous, as the yellow matter comes out as it does from a boil which " breaks." Care should be taken to adopt the same diet as in boils, and to keep the bowels very freely acting at least once every twenty-four hours. Felons are caused almost always by bruises, which, in their influences, reach the bone, seeming to be confined mostly to the forefinger, which ever after remains stiff unless the lancet is used in a timely manner. On the other hand, boils are the result of bad blood, and their appearance is proof that nature is endeavoring to throw the poison out of the system, that she has strength to make the effort, thus giving proof of vitality, hence the appearance of boils is in that connection encouraging, and the effort should be made at once to improve the general health, and thus get rid of the bad blood. A salve is sometimes made for felons thus: Take the yellow part of an egg, burn a teaspoonful of copperas, powder it and mix well, then apply, after soaking the part in warm water for ten minutes; do this night and morning. When the felon is under the fascia there may be no soreness or swelling on the surface or in the skin, but sometimes the felon is above the fascia, nearer the surface, and makes a change in the skin; it is rather a bastard felon. Make a " fly plaster" as large as the thumb nail, keep it on the spot six or eight hours, then the " core " may be seen and pricked out with a needle. An onion poultice, applied fresh, thrice a day is good; or thrust the finger in a lemon for twenty-four hours, or until easier; or use an ointment made of equal parts of opium, soap and gum camphor, with spirits of turpentine enough to make a salve. These and various remedies are proposed with great confidence; they are beneficial in superficial ailments, bearing some resemblance to felons, but for the real felon, the " Bone Felon," so-called because it is located on the bone, any other than the lancet treatment is loss of time, involving intense suffering. It has been advised to starve the felon by tying a string around the finger, thus preventing a supply of blood on which it is supposed to " feed," but the torture is unendurable.

NETTLE-RASH OR URTICARIA,

little pimples, oval or round, red or white in patches, sometimes
go and come in an hour, over arms, body and legs, burning, stinging, itching, most at night in bed, lasting for weeks sometimes,
arising from disordered stomach or biliousness. Diet for a few
days on fruits, berries, melons, and brown bread or wheaten grits,
keeping up a full free action of the bowels every twenty-four
hours; if it is stubborn, take a liver pill, use the same diet, be
out in the open air, and take plenty of exercise. Cold applications are dangerous, tending to drive in the rash and induce dangerous internal disorders. If anything is applied externally, it
should be starch powder, or milk and water, vinegar and water,
or glycerine with rosewater. The same treatment is applicable
to most skin eruptions, it being always safe, mild and effective.

LONGINGS.

Many believe that a great desire for any special article of food
during pregnancy, will have the effect, if not procured, of making
a mark on the child. The best plan is to have all reasonable desires gratified as soon as possible. It is the duty of the husband
to do all that is in his power to meet his wife's wishes; to make
her as comfortable as possible. If this requires sacrifices of time
and means, let them be made promptly and cheerfully; made, too,
in love and affection, and in generous sympathy.

Any shock, mental or physical, experienced by the expectant
mother, may leave an impression—physical, mental, or moral—
on the unborn babe; hence reasonable precautions should be taken
to prevent them, to avoid places and times and circumstances
which might be calculated to occasion them, and instead, secure
surroundings which are in every way encouraging, pleasurable,
elevating, and delightful.

DYSMENORRHŒA,

or painful monthlies, has been successfully treated thus: Give the
following pill thrice a day for five days, beginning three days before the time, and continue two days after it comes on. Begin
the same treatment the next time. Usually a regular, painless
monthly flow is established in five or six months: One-third
of a grain of the extract of datura stramonium seeds, that is, the

thornapple or·"Jimson weed," two grains of the sulphate of quinine, one-third of a grain of opium, and two grains of gum camphor, with two grains of powdered ipecac. The bowels should be made to act every day; the feet should be kept comfortably warm, with as much out-door exercise in the sunshine as practicable, all the time eating plain, nourishing food at regular intervals. It will greatly add to the good effects if the mind is fully employed in something animating and pleasurable. As the malady is one which sometimes lasts for many years, and occasions a great deal of suffering, it is well worth while to make a steady and persistent effort for its removal.

For the immediate relief of pain, take a warm hip-bath, then wring out a flannel dipped in hot water, sprinkle it with spirits of turpentine and apply it to the "small of the back." It is really a neuralgic affection, and great comfort will be derived from the warm hip-bath as a means of immediate relief from suffering.

GONORRHŒA

is claimed in the *London Lancet* as late as June, 1873, to be cured in from two to six days, by injecting a solution of the permanganate of potassa, ten grains or more to an ounce of water, four times a day, made more certain by remaining at rest in a room all the time; better still if lying down fifteen hours of the twenty-four.

PHAGEDENIC CHANCRE

is now treated at St. George's Hospital, London, by taking every four hours twenty drops of laudanum with half a dram of compound spirits of hartshorn.

CIRCUMCISION.

In performing this operation excessive bleeding sometimes takes place. If all other remedies fail, let a piece of iron be heated to whiteness, and apply it to the bleeding surface. Other dangerous bleedings may be arrested in the same way if they are the result of wounds.

TEDIOUS LABOR

has been managed successfully in 731 cases out of 732 by Professor Hamilton, thus:

1st.—Never interfere with the first half of labor, however prolonged ; thus allowing the mouth of the womb to be dilated naturally by the bag of membranes.

2d.—The second stage of labor should never be allowed to go on more than two hours without the application of forceps, greased with India rubber paste. He avoids ergot, and thinks the child's life is often lost by delaying the use of instruments longer than two hours.

DEFICIENCY OF MOTHER'S MILK

is often remedied if the mother has a great relish for good fresh milk, and can drink it freely, without any discomfort, in addition to three regular meals a day ; if not relieved, it does more harm than good.

Vomiting in pregnancy is often relieved by taking three times a day the following mixture: Two ounces of sweet tincture of rhubarb and one ounce of compound tincture of gentian—one teaspoonful at a time : or, one dram of the carbonate of magnesia, half ounce tincture of colombo, five ounces of peppermint water ; take one tablespoon three times a day.

SORE NIPPLES.

The agony endured by some mothers from this affection is greatly mitigated and soon cured thus : First arrest the bleeding by smearing the parts with benzoin tincture, then take a soft handkerchief, carefully dry the parts, then cover all the sore parts with a solution of gutta percha ; when dry, repeat the coating several times, so as to completely exclude the external air and prevent abrasions. While nursing the child the nipple should be protected by some of the shields made for that purpose. In a very few days the cure will be complete. The solution above is made by putting a dram of gutta percha in a bottle, then add three drams of chloroform and shake it well. As soon as the coating wears off apply another. This is a most admirable remedy.

GENERAL INDEX,

ALPHABETICAL, ANALYTICAL, AND EXPLANATORY.

In this index, "a." stands for "article;" "H." or "h." for "homœopathic;" a figure in parenthesis after the page, denotes occurrence so many times on that page; words in italics are Latin, French, &c.

52

INDEX. **837**

Suffocation, 229-1, 259, 469-9; see Drowning.
Sugar [= *Saccharum*], Composition of, 763, 775.
In water, 812. Use for food or drink, 123, 186
(little). 233. 279 (2; good, bad), 249 (2; good,
little or none), 291, 332, 843, 369, 414 (avoid),
529, 582 (omit), 558, 659, 680 (brown) 687
(little), 688, 760 (4; white, loaf, &c.), 761, 762
(4; white, &c.): for medicine, usually refined,
loaf or white, 132, 393, 401. 433, 479, 675
(brown), 674, 675 (3), 681, 699, 721, 723, 728, 729,
730, 731, 782 (2), 733 (2), 731, 737 (3), 738, 741
(3) 751, 752 2), 753, 755, 784, 785, 787 (external
use), 773, 805; of smoke of, 167 (brown), 396
(brown), 479; see Sweetening.—Sugar (= acetate) of lead, poison and antidote, 701, 702-3
(q.); see under Lead.
Suicide and cause. 585-7, 579, 623.
Sulphur [= Brimstone in a dr. 824. Use of, 211,
479 (on coals), 745, 751 (2), 758, 771, 805.
Flowers of, or Sublimed 281, 713, 764, 773. H.
use of, 214, 399, 453, 433, 431, 655 2, 645, 712,
715; tincture and wash, 423. Iodide of, 745,
745. Ointment, use and recipe, 771.—Sulphate
of copper, iron, soda, &c.; see Copper, Iron,
Soda, &c.—Sulphureted hydrogen, 430.—Sulphuric acid [= *acidum sulphuricum*, or oil of
vitriol], astringent, 772; corrosive, 257; in
wheat, 657; poison and antidote, 699 (a.), 701.
External use of, 170, 724, 747. Internal use of,
115; diluted, 749, 765 (2). H. use of (Acid
sulph.), 214. Aromatic sulphuric acid [made
of sulphuric acid, ginger, cinnamon, and alcohol, = Elixir of vitriol, which see.—Sulphuric
ether, made of sulphuric acid, alcohol, potassa,
and distilled water, is commonly called simply
Ether, which see.
Sumach, Poison from Poison or Swamp [= *Rhus
venenata*], with antidote, 700 (a.). 701, 702.
Summer-complaint [= *cholera infantum*; also
diarrhœa, dysentery], 290, 398-9 (a.); origin,
5x6, 604; difficulty, 609; remedies, 782, 770;
see Diarrhœa, Dysentery. Summer-excursions,
291-3 (a.), 441-50.
Sunrise and Sunset, 131, 172, 202, 550-1.—Sunshine, Use of, 9, 51-2, 148, 419, 585, 550, 790.—
Sun-stroke, 86, 397-7 a.
Suppers, Hearty, 311-5 (a.); and late, 210-11,
615. Light and early, 87, 88, 197, 224, 290,
649. Omit, 195, 211. See Eating, Food, Fruit
diet, General health, Temperate living, &c.
Suppository [= a solid medicine introduced by the
anus], Use of, 752, 759, &c.
Suppression; see Lochia, Menstruation, Nocturnal, Sore, Urination.
Supra renal; see Capsules.
Suretyship, 246, 345.
Surgical roller = a bandage rolled up, in order
to be applied to a wounded limb, &c., by being
unrolled and evenly fitted, Use of, 89, 90, 92-3
(8), 94.
Swallow, The, 187 (cut), 233; see Throat, &c.—
Swallowing prevented, or difficult, or painful,
97, 255, 370, 674, 691; see Injection, Œopha-
gus, &c.
Swamp fever, see Fever; sumach, Poison from,
with antidote, 700 (a.), 701, 702.
Sweat, Cold or clammy, 696, 702.—Sweats in
rheumatism, II. remedy, 712; see Night-sweats,
Mode of taking, 66-7, 75-6, 186, 197, 203, 3-9,
403-4, 674, 685, 691. Use of, 21. 433, 746, 784
(no), 788, 789.—Sweat-glands, 877 (cut). See
Diaphoretic, Perspiration, Pores.
Sweet-bread (see Pancreas) as food, 406; cake
(see Pastry), 332-8; oil = Olive oil, which see;
potato [= *Convolvulus Batatas*, or *Batatas
edulis*, Carolina potato], 105, 777 (constituents):
see Apples, Milk.—Sweetening used in food and
drink, 290 (little), 832, 529, 544, 605 (2), 715,
762 (6); in medicine, 727, 772, 775. Avoid, 772.

Consequence of excess, 293. See Molasses,
Sugar.
Swelling beneficial, 108, 110, 304-5; from poison,
700; of lymphatics, 140. Abdominal, 696, 698.
Treatment of, 5-6, 78, 95 (2), 96 2), 151, 157-8,
161, 294-6, 485, 612, 673. 674 755 (joints), 764;
see Bronchocele, Bruises, Burns, Erysipelas,
Fractures, Inflammation, White swelling.—Swollen limbs, remedy, 5-6.
Sympathy, Want of, 488-9; see Benevolence.
Symptoms of disease, 708, &c.; see Principles,
and the various diseases. Symptoms of poison,
643-703.—Symptomatic asthma, 207-11.
Synovial fluid and glands, 704; membrane injured, 187.
Syphilis, = the venereal disease, the pox], 287, 292,
708-9; prescriptions, 755-6.—Syphilitic gargles,
prescriptions, 753; rheumatism, 705, 753 (prescriptions); skin disease, prescriptions, 775,
801.
Syringe [= squirt], Use of, 583 (2), 711, 735, 747,
798; see Injection.
Syrup common or simple syrup = refined sugar
dissolved in heated water to saturation: medi-
cated syrups have sugar incorporated with
vegetable infusions, decoctions, expressed juices,
fermented liquors, or aqueous solutions], Use of,
102, 241, 529, 659, 675, 688 (2), 692, 699, 713 (2)
727 (2), 728, 731, 734, 735, 737, 738, 739 (3), 744
(2), 745, 754 (2), 753, 758 (2), 769, 772, 778, 805,
806; see Ipecac, Lemons, Orange-peel, Rhubarb,
Sarsaparilla, Senna, Soothing, Squills, &c.
System, Lack of, 10

Tag-locks, Use of smoke from, 169.
Tallow, Use of, 470; see Mutton-tallow, Suet.
Tannic acid or Tannin, Use of, 183, 373, 803, 599
(2), 732 (2), 737, 745 (3), 750. 752, 758, 770.
Tansy oil, poison and antidote, 699 (a.), 701.
Tape-worm [= *Tænia solium*, *Tænia medioca-
nellata*, &c.], 194, 269-71 (a.); remedies, 5, 271,
420-2 (a.), 759, 764, 765.
Tapioca [= the fecula or starchy matter from
the root of *Janipha* (or *Jatropha*) *Manihot*, the
cassava plant], Use of, 188, 292, 375, 808-9, 406,
428, 483, 527, 528, 632, 681, 682, 689, 749;
recipe, 762; see Starch.
Tar, 168; burned or smoked, 371, 479; plaster,
674; see Gas.—Tar oil, poison and antidote,
699 (a.), 701.
Taraxacum = Dandelion, which see.
Tartar, Cream of; see Potassa (Bitartrate of).
—Tartaric acid, Use of, 471.—Tartar-emetic
[= tartrate of antimony and potassa], poison
and antidote, 701-2 (a.); use, 11, 30, 31, 34-6,
83. 114, 119. 203 (2), 310 (2), 403, 695, 708, 728,
729 (3), 731, 734, 735, 739 (2), 740, 750 (2), 761
(3), 766, 768, 8 6; saturated solution, 761 (2).
Wine of [= wine of antimony, or solution of
tartar-emetic], 731 (2). See under Antimony.
Taste, Bad; see Biliousness, Castor Oil, Metallic,
Mouth, Onion.
Tea [= usually a decoction or infusion in boiling
water of the dried leaves of *Thea Bohea*, or
Thea viridis (black or green tea), but applicable
to any infusion or decoction of dried leaves,
&c.], after medicine, 35, 36; constringes, 626;
see Astringent. Avoid excess in, 196, 197, 788.
Avoid strong, 162, 730. Take strong, 700, 702,
703 (green), 742. Use of hot, 9, 29, 47, 66, 107,
111, 114, 120, 121. 142, 161. 184, 195 (2), 224,
233 (2), 287, 249, 266, 276, 281 (2). 289, 403, 406
(black), 412, 427, 429, 452, 513, 581, 664 (2), 674,
687. 722, 749 (no), 774. 779-80, 783 (use; no
use), 785, 789. See Antibilious, Beef, Bran, Catnip. Cundurango, Flax seed, Gourd-seed, Pumpkin seed, Saffron, Sassafras, Slippery elm,
Water-melon, &c.—Tea-berry, 11; see Winter-
green.—Tea-dust, Use of, 232, 744, 755.—Tea-

117386

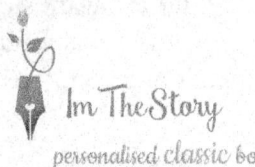
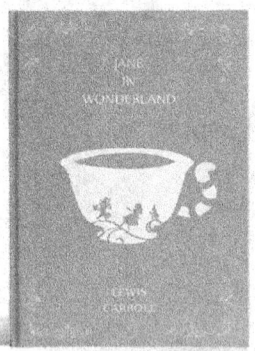

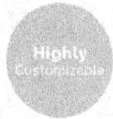

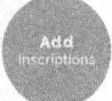

CPSIA information can be obtained
at www.ICGtesting.com
Printed in the USA
BVHW060553280819
556854BV00001B/49/P